Local Drug Delivery for Coronary Artery Disease

EDOARDO CAMENZIND MD
Division of Cardiology
University Hospital of Geneva
Geneva, Switzerland

IVAN K DE SCHEERDER
Katholieke Universiteit Leuven
Campus Gasthuisberg
Leuven, Belgium

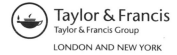
Taylor & Francis
Taylor & Francis Group

LONDON AND NEW YORK

© 2005 Martin Dunitz, an imprint of the Taylor & Francis Group plc

First published in the United Kingdom in 2005
by Martin Dunitz, an imprint of the Taylor & Francis Group plc, 2 Park Square, Milton Park, Abingdon, Oxfordshire OX14 4RN

Tel.:   +44 (0) 20 7017 6000
Fax.:   +44 (0) 20 7017 6699
E-mail: info.medicine@tandf.co.uk
Website: www.tandf.co.uk/medicine

Although every effort has been made to ensure that all owners of copyright material have been acknowledged in this publication, we would be glad to acknowledge in subsequent reprints or editions any omissions brought to our attention.

A CIP record for this book is available from the British Library.

ISBN 1-84184-045-9

Distributed in the USA by
Fulfilment Center
Taylor & Francis
10650 Toebben Drive
Independence, KY 41051, USA
Toll Free Tel.: +1 800 634 7064
E-mail: taylorandfrancis@thomsonlearning.com

Distributed in Canada by
Taylor & Francis
74 Rolark Drive
Scarborough, Ontario M1R 4G2, Canada
Toll Free Tel.: +1 877 226 2237
E-mail: tal_fran@istar.ca

Distributed in the rest of the world by
Thomson Publishing Services
Cheriton House
North Way
Andover, Hampshire SP10 5BE, UK
Tel.: +44 (0)1264 332424
E-mail: salesorder.tandf@thomsonpublishingservices.co.uk

Composition by EXPO Holdings, Malaysia

Printed and bound in Great Britain by CPI Bath

Contents

VII Clinical studies

Catheter-based intravascular delivery

Inert coatings and stent-based intravascular delivery

VIII Alternative methods for local vascular drug delivery

IX Local drug delivery: a critical perspective

List of contributors

Alexandre S Abizaid
Institute Dante Pazzanese of Cardiology
Av. Dr. Dante Pazzanese 500
Setor Angioplastia
Sao Paulo - SP- 04012-180
Brazil

Mariano Albertal
Department of Interventional Cardiology
Instituto Cardiovascular de Buenos Aires
Blanco Encalada 1543
Codigo Postal 1428
Buenos Aires, Argentina

Juan Jose Badimon
Director, Cardiovascular Biology Research
Laboratory
Mount Sinai School of Medicine
One Gustave L Levy Place
PO Box 1030
New York NY 10029
USA

Peter Barath
Previously at: Loyola University Medical
Center
2196 South First Avenue,
Maywood, IL 60153, USA

Frederick J Barry
Parkway Cardiology Association
80 Vermont Avenue
Oak Ridge TN 37830
USA

Antonio L Bartorelli
Director, Catheterization Laboratories
Centro Cardiologico Fandazione 'Monzino'
IRCCS
University of Milan
Via Parea. 4
20138 Milan
ITALY

Andreas Baumbach
Bristol Heart Institute
Bristol Royal Infirmary
Bristol
BS2 8HW
UK

Johan M Bosmans
Division of Cardiology
Faculty of Medicine
University of Antwerp (CDE)
Universiteitsplein 1
B-2610 Wilrijk
Belgium

Lutz Buellesfeld
Heart Center Siegburg
Cardiology/Angiology
Ringstrasse 49
53721 Siegburg
Germany

Hidde Bult
Division of Pharmacology
Faculty of Medicine
University of Antwerp (CDE)
Universiteitsplein 1
B-2610 Wilrijk
Belgium

Edoardo Camenzind
Cardiac Catheterization Laboratory
Division of Cardiology
University Hospital of Geneva
Rue Micheli-du-Crest 24
1211 Geneva
Switzerland

Bernard Chevalier
Centre Cardiologique du Nord
Département de Cardiologie Interventionelle
32/36 rue des Moulins Gémeaux
93207 Saint-Denis Cedex
France

Anthony Collias
Biocompatibles Ltd.
Farnham
Surrey, GU9 8QL, UK

Antonio Colombo
Director, Cardiac Catheterization Laboratory
EMO Centro Cuore Columbus Srl
Via M Buonarroti 48
20145 Milano
Italy

Ivan K De Scheerder
Consultant Stent R&D
Global Medical Services
Keeromstraat, 5A
B-3020 Herent
Belgium

Andrew Farb
Department of Cardiovascular Pathology
Armed Forces Institute of Pathology
Room 2005
Building 54
14th Street and Alaska Avenue NW
Washington DC 20306
USA

Aloke V Finn
Department of Cardiovascular Pathology
Armed Forces Institute of Pathology
Washington, DC 20306
and
Massachusetts General Hospital
Boston, MA
USA

Roger Foo
Department of Cardiology
Glenfleld Hospital
Leicester LE3 9QP
UK

Richard Gallo
Montréal Heart Institute
5000, Bélanger Street
Montréal (Québec) H1T 1C8
CANADA

Anthony H Gershlick
Consultant Cardiologist
Department of Cardiology
Glenfleld Hospital
Groby Road
Leicester LE3 9QP
UK

Herman K Gold
Massachusetts General Hospital
Boston, MA 02114
USA

Juan Granada
Section of Cardiology
Baylor College of Medicine
Baylor One Plaza
Houston, TX 77030
USA

Steve Grantz
Atrium Medical Corporation
5 Wentworth Drive
Hudson, NH 03051
USA

Eberhard Grube
Chief, Department of Cardiology / Angiology
Heart Center Siegburg
Ringstrasse 49
53721 Siegburg
Germany

Julian Gunn
Consultant Interventional Cardiologist &
Senior Lecturer in Cardiology
University of Sheffleld
Northern General Hospital
Herries Road
Sheffleld S5 7AU
UK

Christoph Hehrlein
Department of Cardiology
University of Freiburg
Hugstetterstraβe 55
79106 Freiburg
Germany

Alan W Heldman
Johns Hopkins University School of Medicine
Baltimore
Maryland
USA

Christian Herdeg
Bristol Heart Institute
Bristol Royal Inflrmary
Bristol
BS2 8HWUK

Bernd Heublein†
Leibniz Research Laboratories for
Biotechnology and Artiflcial Organs
Hannover Medical School
Podbielskistr. 380
D-30569 Hannover
Germany

Richard Heuser
Phoenix Heart Center
Phoenix St Luke's medical Center
525 North 18th Street, Suite 504
Phoenix AZ 85006
USA

Berthold Höfling
Medical Clinic 1, Grosshadern Clinic
Ludwig Maximilan University
Munich
Germany

Sjoerd H Hofma
Department of Interventional Cardiology
Erasmus University
Thoraxcenter
3015 GD, Rotterdam
The Netherlands

Dongming Hou
Indiana Center for Vascular Biology & Biology
Krannert Institute of Cardiology
975W. Walnut Street, IB441
Indianapolis, IN 46202, USA

Yanming Huang
Department of Cardiovascular Medicine
The Cleveland Clinic Foundation
9500 Euclid Avenue
Cleveland, OH 44195, USA

Tanya Y Huehns
The Wellcome Trust
215 Euston Road
London NW1 2BE, UK

Patrick Iversen
Senior Vice President, Research and
Development
AVI-BioPharma,
One SW Columbia
Suite 1105
Portland, OR, 97258, USA

Stefan Janssens
Department of Cardiology
Katholieke Universistiet Leuven
Campus Gasthuisberg
Herestraat 49
BE-3000 Leuven
Belgium

Aaron V Kaplan
Associate Professor of Medicine
Director, Device Department Development
Laboratory
Dartmouth-Hitchcock Medical Center
Section of Cardiology
One Medical CenterDrive
Lebanon, NH 03756, USA

Karl R Karsch
Department of Cardiology
Bristol Royal Inflrmary
Bristol
BS2 8HW
UK

R Stefan Kiesz
Southeast Endovascular and Heart Institute
Port Arthur, TX
USA

Nicholas Kipshidze
Lenox Hill Heart and Vascular Institute
130 East 77th St
New York NY 10021
USA

Bruce D Klugherz MD
Abington Medical Specialists
1235 Old York Road
Ste. 222, Levy Medical Plaza
Abington, PA 19104, USA

Frank D Kolodgie
Department of Cardiovascular Pathology
Armed Forces Institute of Pathology
Washington, DC 20306
USA

Michael Kuehler
B. Braun Melsungen AG – Vascular Systems
Sieversufer 8
12359 Berlin
Germany

Michael JB Kutryk
Department of Cardiology
7081 Queen's Wing
St Michael's Hospital
30 Bond St
Toronto, Ontario
M5B 2W8
Canada

Guy LeClerc
Laboratory of Molecular Cardiology
CHUM, Hôpital Notre-Dame
1560, Sherbrooke East
Montreal, Quebec
Canada, H2L4 M1

Martin B Leon
Chairman, Cardiovascular Research Foundation
Associate Director, Center for Interventional
Cardiovascular Research, and Professor of
Medicine, New York Presbyterian
Hospital/Columbia University Medical Center
New York, NY, USA

Maddalena Lettino
CCU - Department of Cardiology
San Matteo Hospital,
Piazza Golgi 2
27100 Pavia, Italy

Robert J Levy
William J Rashkind Professor of Pediatrics
Cardiology Department
Children's Hospital of Philadelphia
34th Civic Center Boulevard
Philadelphia PA 19104
USA

Andrew Lewis
Research and Technology Director
Biocompatibles UK Ltd.
Farnham Business Park
Weydon Lane
Farnham
Surrey GU9 8QL, UK

Shengqiao Li
Katholieke Universiteit Leuven
Campus Gasthuisberg
Herestraat 49
BE-3000 Leuven
Belgium

A Michael Lincoff
Cleveland Clinic Foundation
Department of Cardiology, F25
9500 Euclid Avenue
Cleveland OH 44195
USA

Keith L March
Indiana Center for Vascular Biology & Biology
Krannert Institute of Cardiology
975W. Walnut Street, IB441
Indianapolis, IN 46202, USA

Paul Martakos
Atrium Medical Corporation
5 Wentworth Drive
Hudson, NH 03051
USA

Jack L Martin
Jefferson Health System – Main Line
Department of Cardiology
Radnor, PA
USA

Gabor Matos
Loyola University Medical Center
2196 South First Avenue,
Maywood, IL 60153, USA

Guido RY De Meyer
Division of Pharmacology
Faculty of Pharmaceutical, Vetinary and
Biomedical Sciences
University of Antwerp (CDE)
Universiteitsplein 1
B-2160 Wilrijk
Belgium

Geoffrey Moodie
Atrium Medical Corporation
5 Wentworth Drive
Hudson, NH 03051
USA

Jeffrey W Moses
Department of Interventional Cardiology
Lenox Hill Hospital
100 East 77th Street
New York, NY 10021
USA

Gishel New
Director of Cardiology
Centre for Heart and Chest Research
Monash University Department of Medicine
Clayton
Melbourne
VIC 3168, Australia

Sigrid Nikol
Molekulare Kardiologie/Angiologie
Medizinische Klinik C, Universitätsklinikum
Albert-Schweitzer-Strasse 33
48129 Münster
Germany

Martin Oberhoff
Bristol Heart Institute
Bristol Royal Inflrmary
Bristol
BS2 8HW UK

Gerard Pasterkamp
Department of Cardiology
University Medical Center
Utrecht
The Netherlands

Klaus Pels
Charite – Universitätsmedizin Berlin
Campus Benjamin Franklin
Medizinische Klink II;
Vaskulaerbiologisches Labor
Hindenburgdam 30
12200 Berlin
Germany

Alexander Popov
Cedars-Sinai Medical Center
8700 Beverly Blvd
Los Angeles, CA 90048
USA

Herbert Radisch
InterVentional Technologies Inc.
3574 Ruffln Rd., San Diego
CA 92123, USA

Nicolaus Reifart
Kardiologisches Institute
Kronberger Strasse 36
65812 Bad Soden
Germany

Bernhard Reimers
Centro Cuore Columbus
via Buonarroti 48
20145 Milan
Italy

Jörg Rodermann MD
University Hospital Essen
West German Heart Centre
Department of Cardiology
Huferland str. 55
45122 Essen
Germany

M Marius Rozek
Department of Medicine
Clinical Epidemiology and Cardiology
University of Texas Health Science Center
Mail Code 7873
7703 Floyd Curl Drive
San Antonio, TX 78229
USA

Koen J Salu
Division of Cardiology
Faculty of Medicine
University of Antwerp (CDE)
Universiteitsplein 1
B-2610 Wilrijk
Belgium

Amit Segev
Heart Institute
Chaim Sheba Medical Center
Tel-Hashomer 52621
Israel

Patrick W Serruys
Thoraxcenter, Bd 416
University Hospital - Dijkzigt
DR Molewaterplein 40
3015 GD Rotterdam
The Netherlands

Marion J Sierevogel
Department of Cardiology
University Medical Center
3584 CX Utrecht
The Netherlands

Peter Sinnaeve
Department of Cardiology
University Hospitals Gasthuisberg
Herestraat, 49
B-3000 Leuven
Belgium

J Eduardo Sousa
Institute Dante Pazzanese of Cardiology
Av. Dr. Dante Pazzanese 500
Setor Angioplastia
Sao Paulo - SP- 04012-180
Brazil

James Spratt
Dept of Internal Medicine
University Hospital of Geneva
Rue Micheli-du-Crest 24
1211 Geneva
Switzerland

Cezar Staniloae
Cardiology Research Fellow
Montreal Heart Institute
5000, Bélanger Street
Montréal (Québec) H1T 1C8
CANADA

Bradley H Strauss
Roy and Ann Foss Interventional Cardiology
Research Program
Terrence Donnelly Heart Center
St Michael's Hospital
University of Toronto
Toronto, Ontario
Canada

Neil Swanson
Cardiology Clinical Sciences
Glenfleld Hospital
Leicester LE3 9QP, UK

Vincenzo Toschi
Chief, Department of Hematology and Blood
Transfusion - Thrombosis Center
Ospedale San Carlo Borromeo
Via Pio II, 3
20153 Milano, Italy

Daniela Trabattoni
Centro Cardiologico 'Monzino' IRCCS
Institute of Cardiology
University of Milan
Italy

Willem J Van der Giessen
Department of Cardiology
Thoraxcenter, BD412
Academic Hospital Dijkzigt
Dr Molewaterplein 40
3015 GD Rotterdam
Netherlands

Eric Verbeken
Department of Pathology
University Hospitals Gasthuisberg
Herestraat, 49,
B-3000 Leuven
Belgium

Renu Virmani
Department of Cardiovascular Pathology
Armed Forces Institute of Pathology
Room 2005
Building 54
14th Street and Alaska Avenue NW
Washington DC 20306
USA

Chris J Vrints
Head of Cardiology
Faculty of Medicine
University of Antwerp (CDE)
Universiteitsplein 1
B-2610 Wilrijk
Belgium

Kai Wang
Department of Cardiovascular Medicine
The Cleveland Clinic Foundation
9500 Euclid Avenue
Cleveland, OH 44195, USA

Lan Wang
Department of Pathology
University Hospital Gasthuisberg
University of Leuven
Belgium

Robert Wilensky
Associate Professor of Medicine
Director of Experimental Intervantional
Cardiology
University of Pennsylvania
Philadelphia PA 19104
USA

Xianshun Liu
Katholieke Universiteit Leuven
Campus Gasthuisberg
Herestraat 49
BE-3000 Leuven
Belgium

Zhongmin Zhou
Department of Cardiovascular Medicine
The Cleveland Clinic Foundation
9500 Euclid Avenue
Cleveland, OH 44195, USA

Preface

The purpose of this book is to give the reader (both physicians and students) a comprehensive and up-to-date overview on site-specific therapy for the treatment of arterial disease.

The first section of the book deals with both the purpose of site specific treatment, reaching from arterial-wall passivation to restenosis prevention, and also the physico-chemical challenge linked to this treatment modality. A summary of the performed experimental and clinical work using the different catheter- and stent-platforms as well as the different molecular approaches is provided in the syllabus section. In the third section each chapter represents an in-depth description and elaboration of the different issues summarized in the syllabus. Lastly a critical overview of the drug eluting stents is given to allow the reader to develop a critical and knowledgeable opinion on the impressive clinical results obtained with these new technologies.

Edoardo Camenzind, MD
Ivan K De Scheerder, MD

1

The purpose of site-specific therapy

Cezar Staniloae, Richard Gallo, and Juan J Badimon

Introduction • Treatment of local thrombus • Modification of the disease process
• Addressing or inhibiting restenosis • Conclusions

INTRODUCTION

The acute coronary syndromes are ultimately the clinical manifestations of a disease process that begins and perpetuates at a localized segment of the coronary artery. The disruption of an atherosclerotic plaque in a coronary artery is fundamental for the development of arterial thrombosis and myocardial ischemia. Thrombosis is central to the pathogenesis of the acute coronary syndromes. Platelet activation and aggregation not only causes blood flow obstruction, but also their phospholipid-rich surface acts as a catalyst for fibrin deposition and thrombus extension. In addition, platelets adhered to the site of injury interact continuously with the arterial wall and other circulating factors.

There are presently three strategies to improve outcome in patients with acute coronary syndrome:[1] (1) restoration and maintenance of coronary flow at the site of a culprit lesion; (2) prevention of reperfusion injury and reduction of the infarct size; and (3) stabilization (passivation) of the coronary arterial wall and its interaction with the bloodstream. These strategies are achieved by either mechanical or pharmacologic means but they are limited either by insufficient local concentration of the pharmacologic agent or by late coronary restenosis. Despite extensive investigation into

a variety of adjunctive therapies and mechanical techniques, it can be anticipated that approximately 30–40% of patients with successfully treated coronary lesions will develop restenosis.[2]

Local drug delivery offers a unique opportunity to provide site-specific drug therapy, achieving high local concentrations without systemic elution or side effects.[3] The goals of the site-specific passivation of the arterial wall include:[4] (1) treatment of local thrombus; (2) modification of the atherosclerotic disease process; and (3) addressing or inhibiting restenosis.

TREATMENT OF LOCAL THROMBUS

Thrombolytic therapy has been used as an adjunct to balloon angioplasty to treat intracoronary thrombus before intervention or during the course of the procedure. Nevertheless, this practice has been limited by systemic complications. Local delivery of agents at the site of thrombus formation has therefore many potential advantages. It may allow the simultaneous use of antithrombotics and thrombolytics in adequate local concentrations without exposing patients to an increased risk of bleeding.

Platelets are rich reservoirs of growth factors and their activation can stimulate smooth muscle growth therefore contributing to restenosis.

Local deposition of an antithrombotic agent may attenuate this process and decrease the rate of restenosis. Prolonged systemic infusion of r-hirudin has been shown to reduce intimal hyperplasia in a porcine model of balloon angioplasty.[5] Using a double balloon perfusion catheter, Meyer and colleagues have demonstrated that the specific antithrombin r-hirudin can be successfully delivered in high concentrations to the intima of porcine coronary vessel after balloon angioplasty negating the potentially dangerous side effects of prolonged systemic infusion.[6]

As a result of injury to the vascular endothelium, local vasoconstriction and platelet–vessel wall interactions continuously occur.[7–9] The interaction between the de-endothelialized surface and the activated circulating platelets activates intimal smooth muscle cells and causes synthesis of extracellular matrix and both platelet-mediated and thrombin-dependent vasoconstriction. The arterial wall is 'activated' and perpetuates a cascade of events that can lead to further thrombus formation.

Antithrombotic and antiplatelet agents have become the mainstay in the treatment of the acute coronary syndromes. Newer and more powerful antithrombins, such as the specific thrombin inhibitors, hirudin and hirulog, have been widely investigated with varying results.[10,11] Studies to date have shown that systemic infusions of low doses of these agents show only a marginal benefit, while higher doses are limited by excess bleeding complications,[12,13] illustrating the limitations of systemic administration and the promise of site-specific delivery. Glycoprotein IIb/IIIa receptor antagonists are of proven benefit in preventing adverse cardiac events, such as death, myocardial infarction, and reocclusion, after coronary angioplasty or acute coronary syndromes.[14] They may also lead to greater coronary artery patency rates when used as adjuncts to thrombolysis in the setting of acute myocardial infarction.[15–17] Bleeding complications remain of major concern when using combinations of antithrombotic agents systemically.

Some early trials suggested that abciximab, a glycoprotein IIb/IIIa receptor antagonist, could have some antirestenosis properties by its non-specific inhibition of the $\alpha_v\beta_3$ receptor.[18] This receptor has been identified as a potential target for site-specific therapy. Other potential therapeutic targets for site-specific therapy include glycoprotein 1b/IX, tenase complex, tissue factor VII, amplification of endogenous anticoagulants, such as heparin cofactor 2, and recombinant activated protein C.[19] Local delivery may make these agents more attractive by permitting higher local concentrations and eliminating their negative systemic side effects.

MODIFICATION OF THE DISEASE PROCESS

Long-term passivation of the arterial wall may represent the main future purpose of local drug delivery. By counteracting the progressive and accelerated coronary arteriopathy characterized by vascular inflammation, endothelial dysfunction, and coagulopathy, or by limiting the arterial wall response after mechanical injury, further ischemic events could be prevented.

Agents, such as lipid-lowering drugs, anti-inflammatory drugs, antibiotics, antioxidants, antiproliferative or numerous others hold promise in altering the natural evolution of atherosclerosis. Agents that interfere with platelet–vessel wall interaction, inflammation, proliferation, and matrix production have shown positive results in vitro. As an example, when fibrous caps of human atherosclerotic plaques were incubated with human monocyte-derived macrophage in cell culture, there was biochemical evidence of increased collagen degradation, which was inhibited in the presence of a matrix metalloproteinase (MMP) inhibitor.[20] Inhibition of pathogenic processes at the local level may become possible means for achieving plaque stabilization.

ADDRESSING OR INHIBITING RESTENOSIS

Systemic pharmacological therapy for restenosis has generally been unsuccessful, or impractical. While numerous animal studies have identified agents that can reduce intimal hyperplasia associated with balloon angioplasty, clinical results have been less than enthusiastic. One possible reason for the repeated failure of clinical drug studies has been that agents given systemically do not attain sufficient therapeutic levels in the injured artery wall to significantly impact the restenotic process, without producing serious systemic side effects. Site-specific delivery of therapeutic agents could achieve these higher local tissue concentrations than systemic administration.

Local delivery of heparin has been tested for the prevention of restenosis.[21] Continuous release of heparin from a periadvential system has been shown to inhibit neointimal proliferation and local thrombus formation without significant systemic anticoagulation.[22] Other agents delivered locally, such as doxorubicin, colchicine, methtrexate, angiopeptin,[23–26] failed to inhibit the development of intimal hyperplasia. These various results could be explained by differences in the delivery vehicle, physiochemical properties of the drug, and timing of administration in relation to cell cycle properties.

Newer agents that have been shown to diminish smooth muscle cell proliferation in several animal models when delivered both systemically and locally are sirolimus and paclitaxel. Sirolimus is a cytotactic agent (arrests cell replication) that inhibits the smooth muscle cell cycle. In a porcine model, systemic administration of sirolimus has been shown to reduce neointimal hyperplasia after balloon injury to coronary arteries. However, because of its immunosuppressive effects, undesired systemic effects were observed.[27] Animal studies have shown that high local concentrations of this agent can be administered by specially formulated coated stents. Clinical trials are now evaluating this concept by using intracoronary stents as a platform for local drug delivery of agents, such as sirolimus and paclitaxel.

Parallel to local delivery of pharmacological agents, much attention has focused on the concept of site-specific gene therapy.[28] Although intravenous delivery of recombinant DNA is feasible, local delivery of DNA would be expected to increase the efficacy and reduce the risk of peripheral contamination. The resulting gene products can be selected to modulate biologic processes in the vascular wall, such as cell proliferation or matrix production. Local intravascular gene therapy may also prove useful for secretion of angiogenic growth factors intended to facilitate regional revascularization of ischemic myocardium,[28] or for overexpression of protein products, such as recombinant urokinase, designed to prevent thrombosis.[29] Ongoing studies are presently testing the effect of a variety of antisense oligonucleotides administered locally to inhibit arterial narrowing.

The local delivery of radiation to the arterial wall validates the concept of directed therapy and the evolution of this procedure will serve as a model for further development of local drug delivery. Radioactive stents have also been evaluated and they have shown the ability to diminish neointimal proliferation.[30,31]

CONCLUSIONS

In an attempt to passivate an injured arterial wall, local drug delivery holds the promise of reducing thrombus formation and growth, as well as reducing the local inflammatory process that is present before and after a percutaneous coronary intervention. Further studies to evaluate the safety and efficacy of various devices, drugs and delivery techniques will optimize the use of therapeutic agents at the site they are most required.

REFERENCES

1. Schwartz GG. Exploring new strategies for the management of acute coronary syndromes. Am J Cardiol 2000; 86(suppl):44J–50J.
2. Dangas G, Fuster V. Management of restenosis after coronary intervention. Am Heart J 1996; 132:428–36.
3. Riessen R, Isner JM. Prospects of site-specific delivery of pharmacologic and molecular therapies. J Am Coll Cardiol 1994; 23:1234–44.
4. Bailey SR. Local drug delivery: current applications. Prog Cardiovasc Dis 1997; 40:183–204.
5. Gallo R, Padurean A, Toschi V, et al. Prolonged thrombin inhibition reduces restenosis after angioplasty in porcine coronary arteries. Circulation 1998; 97:581–8.

6. Meyer BJ, Fernandez-Ortiz A, Mailhac A, et al. Local delivery of r-hirudin by a double-balloon perfusion catheter prevents mural thrombosis and minimizes platelet deposition after angioplasty. Circulation 1994; 90:2474–80.

7. Bogaty P, Hackett D, Davies G, Maseri A. Vasoreactivity of the culprit lesion in unstable angina. Circulation 1994; 90:5–9.

8. Willerson JT, Golino P, Edit J, et al. Specific platelet mediators and unstable coronary artery lesions: experimental evidence and potential clinical implications. Circulation 1989; 80:198–202.

9. Kinlay S, Selwyn AP, Libby P, Ganz P. Inflammation, the endothelium, and the acute coronary syndromes. J Cardiovasc Pharmacol 1998; 32(suppl 3):S62–S66.

10. Organization to Assess Strategies for Ischemic Syndromes (OASIS) Investigators. Comparison of the effects of two doses of recombinant hirudin compared with heparin in patients with acute myocardial ischemia without ST elevation: A pilot study. Circulation 1997; 96:769–73.

11. White HD, Aylward PE, Frey MJ, et al. Randomized, double-blind comparison of hirulog versus heparin in patients receiving streptokinase and aspirin for acute myocardial infarction (HERO). Circulation 1997; 96:2155–9.

12. The Global Use of Strategies to Open Occluded Arteries (GUSTO) IIb Investigators. A comparison of recombinant hirudin with heparin for the treatment of acute coronary syndromes. N Engl J Med 1996; 335:775–80.

13. The Global Use of Strategies to Open Occluded Arteries (GUSTO) IIa Investigators. Randomized trial of intravenous heparin versus recombinant hirudin for acute coronary syndromes. Circulation 1994; 90:1631–5.

14. The CAPTURE Investigators. Randomized placebo-controlled trial of abciximab before and during coronary intervention in refractory unstable angina: The CAPTURE Study. Lancet 1997; 349:1429–33.

15. Coller BS. Inhibitors of the glycoprotein IIb/IIIa receptor as conjunctive therapy for coronary artery thrombolysis. Coron Artery Dis 1992; 3:1016–21.

16. Gold HK, Coller BS, Yasuda T, et al. Rapid and sustained coronary artery recanalization with combined bolus injection of recombinant tissue-type plasminogen activator and monoclonal antiplatelet GP IIb/IIIa antibody in a canine preparation. Circulation 1988; 77:670–5.

17. Shebuski RJ, Stabilito IJ, Sitko GR, Polokoff MH. Acceleration of recombinant tissue-type plasminogen activator-induced thrombolysis and prevention of reocclusion by the combination of heparin and the Arg-Gly-Asp-containing peptide bitistatin in a canine model of coronary thrombosis. Circulation 1990; 82:169–74.

18. Topol EJ, Califf RM, Weisman HF, et al. Randomized trial of coronary intervention with antibody against platelet IIb/IIIa integrin for reduction of clinical restenosis: Results at 6 months. Lancet 1994; 343:881–6.

19. Theroux P, Fuster V. Acute coronary syndromes: Unstable angina and non-Q-wave myocardial infarction. Circulation 1998; 97:1195–200.

20. Shah PK, Falk E, Badimon JJ, et al. Human monocyte-derived macrophages induce collagen breakdown in fibrous caps of atherosclerotic plaques. Potential role of matrix-degrading metaloproteinases and implications for plaque rupture. Circulation 1995; 92:1565–9.

21. Guyton JR, Rosenburg RD, Clowes AW, et al. Inhibition of rat arterial smooth muscle cell proliferation by heparin: in vivo studies with anticoagulant and nonanticoagulant heparin. Circ Res 1980; 46:625–34.

22. Edelman ER, Adams DH, Kamovsky MJ. Effect of controlled adventitial heparin delivery on smooth muscle proliferation following endothelial injury. Proc Natl Acad Sci USA 1990; 87:3773–7.

23. Nabel EG, Plautz G, Nabel GJ. Site-specific gene expression in vivo by direct gene transfer into the arterial wall. Science 1990; 249:1285–8.

24. Cumberland DC, Gunn J, Tsikaderis D, et al. Initial clinical experience of local drug delivery using a porous balloon during percutaneous coronary angioplasty. J Am Coll Cardiol 1994; 23:19A (abstract).

25. Hong MK, Farb A, Linger EF, et al. A new PTCA balloon catheter with intramural channels for local delivery of drugs at low pressure. Circulation 1992; 86:I–380 (abstract).

26. Franklin SM, Kalan JM, Cunier JW, et al. Effects of local delivery of doxorubicin or saline on restenosis following angioplasty in atherosclerotic rabbits. Circulation 1992; 86:1–52 (abstract).

27. Gallo R, Padurean A, Jayaraman T, et al. Inhibition of intimal thickening after balloon angioplasty in porcine coronary arteries by targeting regulators of the cell cycle. Circulation 1999; 99:2164–70.

28. Takeshita S, Zheng LP, Asahara T, et al. In vivo evidence of enhanced angiogenesis following direct arterial gene transfer of the plasmid encoding vascular endothelial growth factor. Circulation 1993; 88(Suppl I):I–476 (abstract).

29. Dichek DA. Gene transfer in the treatment of thrombosis. Thromb Haemost 1993; 70:198–201.

30. Hehrlein C, Zimmermann M, Metz J, et al. Radioactive stent implantation inhibits neointimal proliferation in nonatherosclerotic rabbits. Circulation 1993; 88:I–65 (abstract).

31. Laird JR, Carter AJ, Kufs WM, et al. Inhibition of neointimal proliferation with a beta particle emitting stent. Circulation 1996; 93:529–36.

2

Local drug delivery: impact of pressure, substance characteristics, and stenting on drug transfer into the arterial wall

Martin Oberhoff, Andreas Baumbach, and Karl R Karsch

Introduction • Pressure • Substance characteristics • Stenting

INTRODUCTION

Apart from the properties of the delivery device and the underlying principle of delivery, the variables of application pressure, substance characteristics, and stenting may have a strong influence on transfer efficiency. Due to the complexity of these variables a prediction of transfer efficiency is almost impossible.

PRESSURE

Several studies using different delivery devices were performed to evaluate the effect of application pressure on transfer efficiency. A linear relationship between the applied pressure and penetration of horseradish peroxidase has been described. Full penetration of the media was achieved by application of 300 mmHg pressure for 45 sec with a porous balloon catheter.[1]

The adverse effects of high-pressure delivery were demonstrated in porcine coronary arteries using the porous balloon catheter – 3 ml of normal saline were delivered with either 2, 5 or 10 atm. Infusion with 2 atm showed adequate adventitial penetration with minor focal medial edema and disorganization. However, at delivery pressures of 5 or 10 atm significantly more injuries and intimal hyperplasia were observed.[2]

Using a channelled balloon, the transfer efficiency of [³H]-heparin with a pressure of 2 and 4 atm were compared. The mean efficiency was comparable in both groups with 48% of expected counts in the 2 atm group and 24% in the 4 atm group.[3] Another channelled balloon catheter (Transport™) was used to deliver normal saline or indocyanine green to rabbit iliac arteries with different infusion pressures (0–12 atm). A deep vessel penetration showed a different extent of vascular injury. Therefore, infusion pressure seems to be a key determinant of vascular injury during local delivery, with lower pressure causing the least neointimal response.[4]

One group could demonstrate the importance of the support pressure of the underlying balloon catheter using the InfusaSleeve™ catheter. A 6-fold greater mean transfer efficacy using 6 atm instead of 1 atm support pressure was documented.[5]

Tritiated preparations of hydrophilic low molecular weight heparin and lipophilic paclitaxel were used to investigate the influence of different delivery pressures using the InfusaSleeve II™ catheter. Using a support pressure of 6 atm, different injection pressures (40–100 psi) did not result in a significant difference of delivery efficiency for both drugs. In addition, a comparable transfer efficiency could be achieved with the low pressure double balloon catheter.[6] It is noteworthy that from these data and from the comparison with the double balloon catheter, there is no apparent advantage of active injection systems over so-called passive devices.

The transfer efficacy of high pressure versus low pressure local heparin delivery was compared using technetium-99-labeled heparin in patients. With the low pressure device Dispatch™ catheter, 18 ml NaCl 0.9% with 1800 IU of heparin and an application pressure of 127 ± 47 mmHg were delivered. In comparison, the InfusaSleeve™, Transport™, and Multichannel™ catheter were used as high pressure devices and 6 ml NaCl 0.9% with 1800 IU of heparin were delivered with 5 ± 1 atm. Scintigraphic evaluation was performed and revealed a comparable transfer efficiency of $3 \pm 3\%$ of the total infused dose in the low pressure group and $2 \pm 1\%$ in the high pressure group.[7]

SUBSTANCE CHARACTERISTICS

Only a few studies performed a direct comparison between two substances in regard to transfer efficiency, mainly hydrophilic and lipophilic drugs. As already mentioned, a study compared the transfer efficacy of the hydrophilic low molecular weight heparin and the lipophilic paclitaxel with two different catheter systems. The percentage activity delivered to the vessel wall was substantially greater in the paclitaxel group as compared to reviparin delivery. The mean concentration of reviparin in the artery was 20 to 33 times higher than in the myocardium. For paclitaxel the factors were 110 to 243.[6] Another in vitro study compared the average arterial deposition of paclitaxel and

heparin. It was found that the average deposition for paclitaxel when compared with heparin is 19.4-fold higher after endovascular and 25.6-fold higher after perivascular application. The difference between both compounds was explained by the ability of paclitaxel to bind to many more non-specific sites in the arterial wall than heparin. This binding allowed the tissue concentration of hydrophobic paclitaxel to exceed the applied concentration.[8]

Another study could demonstrate that agents with increased binding to cellular or extracellular components can exhibit prolonged intramural retention. Iodine-125-labeled fibroblast growth factor-αβ (FGF-αβ) and platelet-derived growth factor (PDGF) with increased binding properties were compared with albumin. The radioactivity was measured up to 5 days after delivery with the microporous balloon. The intramural retention of PDGF after 3 days was 10-fold higher compared to FGF-αβ and 1000-fold higher compared to albumin.[9]

STENTING

The influence of stenting on transfer efficiency was investigated in an in vitro and a clinical study. Using the explanted porcine heart model the efficacy of radiolabeled drug transfer to the arterial wall before and after stenting was investigated. In porcine coronary arteries the local delivery of low molecular weight heparin and paclitaxel before and after stenting showed no significant difference in regard to delivery efficiency.[6] Comparable results were achieved clinically when the local delivery of heparin with the Channel™ balloon was compared pre- and poststenting. Site-specific administration of technetium-99-labeled heparin prestenting in six patients and poststenting in two cases was performed. The Channel™ balloon was inflated with 3 atm and 6.8 ml NaCl 0.9% containing 300 IU/ml of labeled heparin were delivered. The local activity was measured using scintigraphic acquisition. The authors found $3.4 \pm 2.4\%$ of the infused total dose in the prestenting cases and $3.3 \pm 1.1\%$ in the poststenting cases and concluded that delivery efficiency is not affected by stenting. However, they found a difference in half-life with 1.08 ± 1.18 hours in the prestent group and 2.51 ± 0.18 hours in the poststent group, which might be due to the compressed tissue after stent implantation.[10]

REFERENCES

1. Goldman B, Blanke H, Wolinsky H. Influence of pressure on permeability of normal and diseased muscular arteries to horseradish peroxidase. A new catheter approach. Atherosclerosis 1987; 65(3):215–25.

2. Santoian EC, Gravanis MB, Schneider JE, et al. Use of the porous balloon in porcine coronary arteries: rationale for low pressure and volume delivery. Catheter Cardiovasc Diagn 1993; 30(4):348–54.

3. Hong MK, Wong SC, Farb A, et al. Feasibility and drug delivery efficiency of a new balloon angioplasty catheter capable of performing simultaneous local drug delivery. Coron Artery Dis 1993; 4(11):1023–7.

4. Kimura T, Miyauchi K, Yamagami S, et al. Local delivery infusion pressure is a key determinant of vascular damage and intimal thickening. Jpn Circ J 1998; 62(4):299–304.

5. Gottsauner-Wolf M, Jang Y, Penn MS, et al. Quantitative evaluation of local drug delivery using the InfusaSleeve catheter. Catheter Cardiovasc Diagn 1997; 42(1):102–8.

6. Baumbach A, Herdeg C, Kluge M, et al. Local drug delivery: impact of pressure, substance characteristics, and stenting on drug transfer into the arterial wall. Catheter Cardiovasc Interv 1999; 47(1):102–6.

7. Camenzind E, Reijs A, Bakker W, et al. Scintigraphic evaluation of efficacy of high pressure versus low pressure local heparin delivery in man after balloon angioplasty. Circulation 1995; 92(suppl I).

8. Creel CJ, Lovich MA, Edelman ER. Arterial paclitaxel distribution and deposition. Circ Res 2000; 86(8):879–84.

9. Wilensky R, Medhi K, Baek SH, March K. Molecules with increased cellular and extracellular matrix binding exhibit prolonged intramural retention following local drug delivery. Circulation 1996; 94(suppl I).

10. Camenzind E, Reijs A, Bakker W, et al. Evaluation of efficiency of local intracoronary drug delivery pre-stenting versus post-stenting using a new drug delivery device (channel balloon) in human. Circulation 1996; 94(suppl I).

3

Catheter-based and stent-based treatment for coronary artery disease

James Spratt and Edoardo Camenzind

Catheters • **Inert stents** • **Stents with immobilized heparin** • **Drug-eluting stents**
• **Preclinical studies: catheter-based delivery** • **Preclinical studies: inert stents**
• **Preclinical studies: stent with immobilized heparin** • **Preclinical studies: drug-eluting stents**
• **Clinical studies: catheter-based delivery** • **Clinical studies: inert stents**
• **Clinical studies: stent with immobilized heparin** • **Clinical studies: eluting stents**

CATHETERS

The use of catheter platforms was originally explored in the 1980s with the 'double balloon' catheter in dog brachial arteries. Although this demonstrated the feasibility of local drug delivery by this diffusion-based method, the double balloon catheter was not suitable for arterial segments with side branches and due to the necessity of prolonged arterial occlusion. Future developments have therefore focused on shorter administration modalities as either convection-based method or direct intramural injections. Local drug delivery (LDD) using catheter platforms has been most explored in the coronary circulation for drug delivery – gene therapy and cell therapy.

Catheter platforms offer a considerable degree of flexibility in LDD in the context of percutaneous coronary intervention. In cases of balloon angioplasty without stent implantation, catheter platforms still allow LDD, and are flexible enough to permit LDD also when stents are used. This allows tailored LDD for prevention of thrombosis and restenosis. The limiting factor of catheter-based LDD has been poor drug kinetics and, in the case of gene delivery, poor transvection efficiency. Table 3.1 lists different catheter platforms used for transmural, intracoronary LDD.

INERT STENTS

Stainless steel stents, although efficacious for the treatment of elastic recoil and early vessel closure, have inherent problems of thrombogenicity and restenosis.

Although the transition to more aggressive antiplatelet treatment has significantly reduced the incidence of acute in-stent thrombosis, bleeding complications and cost issues remain of significance. A stent coating to reduce stent thrombogenicity, thereby allowing lower doses of antiplatelet medication would have considerable advantages.

In addition, there is evidence that in-stent thrombosis can be precipitated by allergic

Table 3.1 Catheters used for local drug delivery

Catheter (Company)	Trade name	Delivery modality	Type of catheter	Perfusion (Y/N)	Source
Double balloon catheter (USCI-Bard/Medtronic)	NA	Pressure-mediated diffusion	Over-the-wire	No	Atherosclerosis 1987; **65**:215–25 Semin Interv Cardiol 1996; **1**:27–9
Coil balloon catheter (Boston Scientific)	Dispatch catheter	Pressure-mediated diffusion	Fast exchange	Yes	Circulation 1995; **91**:785–93 Semin Interv Cardiol 1996; **1**:39–40
Hydrogel-coated balloon catheter (Boston Scientific)	NA	Pressure-mediated diffusion	Fast exchange	No	J Am Coll Cardiol 1994; **23**:1570–7 Semin Interv Cardiol 1996; **1**:45–6
Iontophoretic drug delivery system (Cortrak)	NA	Iontophoretic-mediated diffusion	Over-the-wire	No	Circulation 1994; **89**:1518–22 Semin Interv Cardiol 1996; **1**:40–2
Porous balloon catheter (Boston Scientific)	Wolinsky balloon	Convection	Over-the-wire	No	J Am Coll Cardiol 1990; **15**:475–81 Semin Interv Cardiol 1996; **1**:28–9
Microporous balloon catheter (Cordis/J&J)	NA	Convection	Fast exchange	No	Coronary Art Dis 1993; **4**:469–75 Semin Interv Cardiol 1996; **1**:30–1
Dual balloon catheter (Boston Scientific)	Transport catheter	Convection	Fast exchange	No	J Am Coll Cardiol 1994; **23**:186A Semin Interv Cardiol 1996; **1**:31–3
Multichannel balloon catheter (Boston Scientific)	Remedy	Convection	Fast exchange	No	Coronary Art Dis 1993; **4**:1023–7 Semin Interv Cardiol 1996; **1**:34–5
Infusion sleeve catheter (LocalMed)	InfusaSleeve	Convection	Over-the-balloon	No	Circulation 1995; **92**:2299–305 Semin Interv Cardiol 1996; **1**:36–8

Table 3.1 Continued

Catheter (Company)	Trade name	Delivery modality	Type of catheter	Perfusion (Y/N)	Source
Nipple balloon catheter (Boston Scientific)	Infiltrator catheter	Active injection/ Infiltrator nipples penetrate the tunica media	Over-the-wire	No	Semin Interv Cardiol 1996; **1**:41 J Vasc Interv Radiol 1999; **10**:817–24 Cath Cardio Diagn 1997; **41**:333–41
Needle injection catheter (Bavaria Medical)	NA	Active injection	Over-the-wire	No	Coron Art Dis 1995; **6**:329–34 Semin Interv Cardiol 1996; **1**:42
Intracoronary microsyringe (Endobionics)	Hornet	Single intramural injection	Over-the-wire	No	Am J Cardiol 2002; **90**:117H

NA, not available.

reactions to trace metals found in stainless steel stents, suggesting a role for inert stents in patients with established metal allergies. In this patient subgroup an inert metal stent would be expected to show lower levels of inflammation and therefore restenosis. Table 3.2 lists stainless steel stents with a specific surface treatment, with the aim of greater vasculo-compatibility.

STENTS WITH IMMOBILIZED HEPARIN

Heparin is covalently bound to the polymer coating of the stent, thereby preventing elution. The main development aim for these stents has been the prevention of acute stent thrombosis by local heparin coating, thereby obviating the need for systemic anticoagulation and the associated complications (Table 3.3).

DRUG-ELUTING STENTS

The main thrust in this modality is the prevention of restenosis by reducing neointimal formation. This mode of local drug delivery is stent-based with the most efficacious mode of delivery still open to question. These stents have mainly used a proprietary matrix as a delivery vehicle, yet this may cause increased restenosis. The alternative is matrix-free delivery, which can lead to poor control of delivery kinetics (Table 3.5).

Table 3.2 Stainless steel stents with specific surface treatment

Stent name (Company)	Coating	Coating: Method of application	Source
NIR royal (Medinol/Boston Scientific)	Gold (7 µm)	Heating via 2-stage procedure	J Am Coll Cardiol 1998; **31**:413A Circulation 2001; **103**:429–34
Inflow (Inflow dynamics)	Gold (5 µm)	Galvanic chemical layer process	Thromb Haemost 1997; **105**:426
Tenax or Lekton (Biotronik)	Silicon carbide	Plasma-assisted physical vapor deposition (PVD)	Tex Heart Inst J 1996; **23**:162–6
Carbostent (Sorin)	Turbostratic carbon (0.3–0.5 µm)	Plasma-assisted physical vapor deposition in high vacuum (PVD)	Int J Artif Organs 1986; **9**:115–18
Arthos Inert (AMG)	Carbon	Ion implantation	Z Kardiolol 2000; **89**:(suppl 6)
Diamond flex (Phytis)	Diamond-like carbon (DLC)	Plasma-assisted physical vapor deposition technique (PVD)	Infus Ther Transfus Med **27**:200–6
Yukon (Translumina)	Diamond-like carbon (DLC) (0.1 µm)	Plasma-assisted physical vapor deposition technique (PVD)	Thromb Res 2000; **99**:577–85
Helistent Titan (Hexacath)	Titanium nitride oxide	Physical vapor deposition in high vacuum (PVD)	Biomol Eng 2002; **19**:97–101
BiodivYsio (Abbott/Biocompatibles)	Phosphorylcholine (PC)	Attached to methacrylate polymers	Catheter Cardiovasc Interv 2001; **53**:182–7 Biomaterials 2002; **23**:1697–706

Table 3.3 Stents with immobilized heparin

Stent name (Company)	Dose/Surface area	Coating/ Abbreviation	Coating: Method of application	Source
Flexmaster Hepacoat (JoMed)	0.5–1 μg/cm^2	Inert polyamine layer	Covalent coupling of unctionalized surface with mid or end point attachment ('Corline' surface coating)	Biomaterials 2001; **22**:349–55
Bx Velocity Hepacoat (Cordis/J&J)	1–4 IU depending on size of stent	Polyethylene-imine & Dextran sulfate	Covalent bonding of underlying polymer layer ('Carmeda process')	J Long Term Eff Med Implants 2000; **10**:19–45
Wiktor/HepaMed (Medtronic)	0.6–10 μg/mm^2	Poly(vinylsiloxane)/ copolymer/ Polyethyleneimine	Patented covalent bonding	Blood Coagul Fibrinolysis 1998; **9**:435–40

Table 3.4 Drug-eluting stents

Stent name (company)	Drug (dose/mm² or mm stent length)	Coating	Source
Dexamet (Abbott)	Dexamethasone (0.5 µg/mm²)	Phosphorylcholine (PC)	Circulation 2001; **104**:1188–93
Cypher/Bx Velocity (Cordis/J & J)	Sirolimus = rapamycine (1.4 µg/mm²)	Poly(ethyl methacrylate)	Coron Art Dis 2002; **13**:183–8
BiodivYsio (Abbott)	ABT-578 (rapamycine analog) (10 µg/mm stent length)	Phosphorylcholine (PC)	J Am Coll Cardiol 2000; **35**:13A
Driver (Medtronic)	ABT-578 (10 µg/mm stent length)	Phosphorylcholine (PC) on cobalt-based alloy	ENDEAVOR I/II study in progress, no published data
Challenge (Guidant)	Everolimus (no data)	Bioerodable polymer	Am J Cardiol 2002; **90**:72H
JoMed Flex (JoMed)	Tacrolimus (0.7 µg/mm²; 1.4 µg/mm²)	Nanoporous ceramic (AL_2O_3) coating	Proceedings 8th LDDR; 2002
Supra G stent V-Flex plus (Cook)	Paclitaxel (up to 3.1 µg/mm²)	No polymer	N Engl J Med 2003; **348**:1537–45
NIR (Medinol/Boston Scientific)	Paclitaxel (1 µg/mm²; total dose for 15 mm stent = 85 µg)	Hydrocarbon-based polymer	J Am Coll Cardiol 2000; **36**:2325–32
Express (Boston Scientific)			

Table 3.5 Preclinical studies: catheter-based delivery

Catheter name	Drug	Amount/ Concentration	Vol (ml)	Animal model	Follow-up (days)	Histomorphometry: Area (mm²) Diameter (mm)	Comment	Source
Double balloon catheter	Heparin/ hirudin	100 IU/kg / 0.3 mg/kg/ 0.7 mg/kg	NA	Porcine carotid arteries	1 h	NA	Dose-dependent reduction in platelet deposition and thrombus formation vs systemic delivery	Circulation 1994; **90**:2474–80
Porous balloon catheter	Clivarin	1500 IU	4	Canine	14	NA	Reduction in thrombus; medial and perivascular haemorrhage following PTCA	Eur Heart J 1996; **17**:1538–45
Infusasleeve	Reviparin	375 IU/ml	5	Porcine	28	NIA: 2.48 ± 0.9 (LDD)/ 2.36 ± 1.1 (control)	No reduction in NIF; increase in media area	Basic Res Cardiol 2000; **95**:173–8
Porous balloon catheter	Reviparin	1500 anti-Xa-units	4	Rabbit atherosclerotic model	56	Endothelial cells (n): 207 ± 13 (LDD)/ 160 ± 25 (control)	Increased re-endothelialization seen	Cardiovasc Res 1998; **38**:751–62
Transport catheter	Anti-thrombin III	250 IU	2.5	Porcine	28	Media area: 1.06 ± 0.2 (LDD) 0.89 ± 0.1 (control)	No effect on NIF or area of stenosis	Coron Artery Dis 2001; **12**:31–6
InfusaSleeve	17-β-estradiol	~30 µg/kg	5	Porcine	28	NIA: 0.4 ± 0.1 (LDD) 0.8 ± 0.2 (PTCA) 1.1 ± 0.3 (vehicle)	Reduction in NIF	J Am Coll Cardiol 2000; **36**(6)

Table 3.5 *Continued*

Catheter name	Drug	Amount/ Concentration	Vol (ml)	Animal model	Follow-up (days)	Histomorphometry: Area (mm^2) Diameter (mm)	Comment	Source
Porous balloon catheter	Methotrexate vs saline	25 mg	4	Porcine carotid artery	30	Mean thickness (μm): 59 ± 30 (LDD) 56 ± 25 (vehicle)	No significant reduction in NIF	J Am Coll Cardiol 1992; **20**:460–6
Porous balloon catheter	Doxorubicin	0.3 mg	2	Rabbit iliac arteries	28	Angioluminal diameter (mm): 1.0 ± 0.3 (LDD) 0.6 ± 0.4 (control)	NSD in NIF Increased restenosis with PBC	Circulation 1992; **86**:I-52
Double balloon catheter	Paclitaxel	10 μmol/L	10	Porcine	28	NIA: 1.0 ± 0.4 (LDD) 0.7 ± 0.3 (control)	No reduction in NIF	Cath Cardiovasc Interv 2001; **53**:562–8
Double balloon catheter	Paclitaxel	10 μmol/L	10	Rabbit atherosclerotic model	56	Mean luminal area: 0.75 ± 0.2 (LDD) 0.42 ± 0.2 (control)	Increase in mean luminal size and reduction in NIF	J Am Coll Cardiol 2000; **35**:1969–76
Porous balloon catheter	Paclitaxel	10 μmol/L	4	Rabbit atherosclerotic model	56	NIA (%): 2.4 ± 2.4 (LDD) 8.4 ± 4.9 (control)	Significant reduction in stenosis after 8 weeks, trend to reduction in NIF	Basic Res Cardiol 2001; **96**:275–82
Microporous balloon	Paclitaxel	10 μmol/L	4	Rabbit atherosclerotic model	28	Mean intimal wall area: 0.21 ± 0.1 (LDD) 0.36 ± 0.3 (control)	Reduction in NIF	Circulation 1997; 15:**96**: 636–45

Table 3.5 *Continued*

Catheter name	Drug	Amount/Concentration	Vol (ml)	Animal model	Follow-up (days)	Histomorphometry: Area (mm^2) Diameter (mm)	Comment	Source
Hydrogel-coated balloon catheter	Naked plasmid DNA encoding vascular endothelial growth factor (VEGF$_{165}$)	10 µg/L	NA	Rabbit iliac arteries	28	Maximal intimal area: 0.61 ± 0.09 (LDD) 1.44 ± 0.13 (control)	Accelerated re-endothelialization and reduced NIF	J Am Coll Cardiol 1997; **29**:1371–9
Porous balloon catheter	*c-myc* antisense oligomers	1 mg/vessel	2	Porcine	28	NIA: 0.24 ± 0.06 (LDD) 0.80 ± 0.17 (control)	Reduction in NIF	Circulation 1994; **90**:944–51
Porous balloon catheter: Dispatch Catheter	S-dC28 (cytidine homopolymer)	NA	NA	Porcine	49	NIA: 1.00 ± 0.7 (LDD) 0.77 ± 0.6 (control)	No reduction in NIF	Antisense Nucl Acid Drug Dev 1999; **9**:549–53

PTCA, percutaneous transluminal coronary angioplasty; LDD, local drug delivery; NIA, neointimal area; NIF, neointimal formation; NA, not available.

Table 3.6 Preclinical studies: inert stents

Stent name (Company)	Coating	Animal model	Follow-up (days)	Histomorphometry: Area (mm²) Thickness (mm)	Angiography: Late loss (mm)	Comment	Source
NIR royal (Medinol/Boston Scientific)	Gold (7 μm layer)	Porcine	28	NI thickness: 0.21 ± 0.05 (gold coating) 0.15 ± 0.02 (heat-treated) 0.14 ± 0.02 (control)	NA	Increased NIF with gold coating which was normalized by heat processing	Circulation 2001; **103**:429–34
Freedom (Global Therapeutics/Cook)	Hydrogenated diamond-like carbon films (DLC, a-C:H)	Porcine	42	Lumen area: 2.31 ± 0.89 (DLC) 1.71 ± 0.66 (control)	Area stenosis (%): 41 ± 17 (DLC) 54 ± 15 (control)	Trend to reduction in NIF was observed, reduced area of stenosis	J Invasive Cardiol 2000; **12**:389–94
Carbostent (Sorin)	Turbostratic carbon	Porcine	60	NI thickness: 0.22 ± 0.05	NA	No placebo comparison made; low level of platelet deposition and NIF seen	Am J Cardiol 1998; 65S
BeStent (non-proprietary)	TINOX-1 (ceramic) TINOX-2 (titanium nitride oxide)	Porcine	42	NIA: 1.47 ± 0.8 (TIN-OX-1)/ 1.39 ± 0.9 (TIN-OX-2)/ 2.61 ± 1.1 (control)	NA	Reduced platelet adhesion with TINOX-1 & 2 (1 < 2). Reduced NIF with TINOX-1 & 2	Circulation 2001; **104**:928–33
Palmaz-Schatz (Cordis/J&J)	Poly(ethylmeth-acrylate)	Porcine	21–28	NIA: 1.97 ± 0.9 (coated) 2.27 ± 1.3 (control)	NA	Reduced NIF in coated stents	J Biomed Mater Res 2000; **52**:193–8

Table 3.6 Continued

Stent name (Company)	Coating	Animal model	Follow-up (days)	Histomorphometry: Area (mm²) Thickness (mm)	Angiography: Late loss (mm)	Comment	Source
Palmaz-Schatz (Cordis/J&J)	Phosphoryl-choline (PC)	Porcine/ Rabbit	28	Porcine: NIA: 1.51 ± 0.97 (PC) 1.34 ± 0.55 (control) Rabbit: NIA: 0.59 ± 0.2 (PC) 0.58 ± 0.3 (control)	Porcine: 0.5 (PC) 0.5 (control) Rabbit: 0.17 (PC) 0.17 (control)	nsd in either NIF or angiographic late loss	Scand Cardiovasc J 1998; **32**:261–8
BiodivYsio (Abbott)	PC	Porcine	28	NIA: 2.43 ± 0.19 (PC) 2.58 ± 0.34 (control)	0.3 ± 0.1 (PC) 0.2 ± 0.1 (control)	nsd in either NIF or angiographic late loss	J Invasive Cardiol 2001; **13**:193–201

NI, neointimal; NIF, neointimal formation; NIA, neointimal area; NA, not available; nsd, non-significant difference.

Table 3.7 Preclinical studies: stent with immobilized heparin

Stent name (Company)	Animal model	Follow-up (wks)	Histomorphometry: Area (mm^2) Thickness (mm or μm)	Angiography: Mean luminal diam. Late loss (mm)	Comment	Source
Palmaz-Schatz/ Hepacoat (Cordis/J&J)	Porcine	12	NI thickness (μm): 152 ± 61 (heparin) 198 ± 49 (control)	Mean luminal diameter: (mm) 3.2 ± 0.4 (heparin) 2.8 ± 0.2 (control)	Eliminated subacute thrombosis vs control stent. nsd in NIF	Circulation 1996; **93**:423–30
Non-proprietary stent/Duraflo II Heparin coating technic	Porcine	6	NIA: 1.21 ± 0.6 (heparin) 1.01 ± 0.8 (control)	Late loss: 0.13 ± 0.25 (heparin) 0.13 ± 0.01 (control)	Reduced thrombogenicity; no change in NIF or luminal area	Circulation 1997; **95**:1549–53
Wiktor/ HepaMed (Medtronic)	Porcine	4	NIA: 2.58 ± 1.07 (heparin) 4.58 ± 1.41 (control)	Late loss: 0.5 (heparin) 0.8 (control)	Reduced NIF and angiographic stenosis	Catheter Cardiovasc Interv 1999; **48**:324–30
Multi-link/ Ionically bound heparin/120 μg per stent (Guidant)	Porcine	4	NIA: 2.94 ± 0.4 (heparin) 4.41 ± 0.4 (control)	Mean luminal diameter: (mm) 2.32 ± 0.14 (heparin) 1.81 ± 0.17 (control)	Reduced NIF	J Cardiovasc Pharm 2002; **39**:513–22

NIF, neointimal formation; NIA, neointimal area; nsd, no significant difference.

Table 3.8 Preclinical studies: drug-eluting stents

Stent name (Company)	Coating	Drug	Animal model	Follow-up (days)	Histomorphometry: Area (mm²) Thickness (mm or μm)	Angiography: Late loss (mm)	Comment	Source
Palmaz-Schatz (Cordis/J&J)	Polylactic polymer (biodegradable)	Hirudin/ Iloprost	Sheep/ Porcine	28	Sheep: NIA: 1.92 (LDD) 2.50 (control) Pig: NIA: 3.11 (LDD)/ 4.13 (control)	NA	Reduced NIF	Circulation 2000; **101**:1453–8
Multi-Link Tristar (Guidant)	Duraflo coating	Heparin	Porcine	28	NIA: 2.12 (LDD) 3.92 (control)	Diameter: 2.32 (LDD) 1.81 (control)	Reduced NIF and in-stent restenosis	J Cardio Pharm 2002; **39**:513–22
Gianturco-Roubin (Cook)	Cellulose polymer coated	Monoclonal anti-rabbit platelet glycoprotein (GP) IIb/IIIa antagonist	Rabbit iliac arteries	28	NI thickness: 0.12 ± 0.04 (LDD) 0.09 ± 0.03 (control)	NA	No effect seen on NIF, reduced platelet deposition and improved arterial patency	Circulation 1996; **94**:3311–17
Wiktor tantalum wire stent	Poly-L-lactic acid (PLLA, 0.4 mg)	Dexa-methasone (0.8 mg)	Porcine	28	NA	NA	nsd in NIF	J Am Coll Cardiol 1997; **29**:808–16
Strecker stent	Biodegradable membrane	Dexa-methasone	Canine femoral arteries	168	NI thickness: 0.18 ± 0.03 (LDD) 0.26 ± 0.06 (control)	Angiographic restenosis (%): 22 ± 5.4 (LDD) 31 ± 11.7 (control)	Reduced NIF; increased level of stent thrombosis	Cardiovasc Intervent Radiol 1998; **21**:487–96

Table 3.8 *Continued*

Stent name (Company)	Coating	Drug	Animal model	Follow-up (days)	Histomorphometry: Area (mm²) Thickness (mm or µm)	Angiography: Late loss (mm)	Comment	Source
Bx Velocity (Cordis/J&J)	Poly(ethyl methacrylate)	Dexa-methasone (DEX) Sirolimus (S)	Porcine/ Canine	28	NIA: 2.47 (S) 2.42 (S+DEX) 4.31 (DEX) 5.06 (control)	NA	Reduced inflammation and NIF No additional effect seen with DEX	Circulation 2001; **104**:1188–93
Bx Velocity (Cordis/J&J)	Non-erodable polymer	4 groups: Sirolimus (S) high dose 196 µg (SHD)/low dose 64 µg (SLD)/ Polymer (P)/ Bare stent (BS)	Rabbit	28	NIA: 0.66 (SHD) 0.92 (SLD) 1.26 (polymer) 1.2 (control)	NA	Dose-dependent reduction in NIF	Coron Artery Dis 2002; **13**:183–8
Stainless steel	Bioerodable polymer	Everolimus: low dose (ELD)/high dose (EHD) Sirolimus: low dose (SLD)/high dose (SHD) polymer only (P)/bare stent (BS)	Porcine	30	% area stenosis: 39 (ELD) 38 (EHD) 43 (SLD) 51 (SHD) 70 (P) 62 (BS)	Late loss: 0.27 (ELD) 0.23 (EHD) 0.32 (SLD) 0.29 (SHD) 0.56 (P) 0.44 (BS)	Everolimus & sirolimus significantly reduce NIF	Am J Cardiol 2002; **90**:72H
Stainless steel	Phosphoryl-choline (PC)	ABT-578 (rapamycin analog)	Porcine	28	NIA: 2.81 (LDD) 1.61 (control)	NA	Reduced NIF and diameter stenosis	J Am Coll Cardiol 2000; **35**:13A

Table 3.8 *Continued*

Stent name (Company)	Coating	Drug	Animal model	Follow-up (days)	Histomorphometry: Area (mm²) Thickness (mm or µm)	Angiography: Late loss (mm)	Comment	Source
BiodivYsio (Abbott)	Phosphoryl-choline (PC)	Angiopeptin	Porcine	28	NIA: 2.78 (LDD) 2.73 (control)	NA	NSD in NIF	J Invasive Cardiol 2002; **14**:230–8
NIR (Boston Scientific)	Poly(lactide-co-σ-caprolactone) copolymer	Paclitaxel (200 µg/stent)	Rabbit	180	NIA: 0.40 (LDD) 0.98 (control) (28 days)	NA	Prolonged reduction in NIF	J Am Coll Cardiol 2000; **36**:2325–32
ACS Multi-Link (Guidant)	Gelatin-chondroitin sulfate coacervate (GSC)	Paclitaxel 42.0 µg, n = 6/ 20.2 µg, n = 7/ 8.6 µg, n = 5/ 1.5 µg, n = 6/ Control GSC coating alone, n = 24	Rabbit	28/90	NI thickness: 0.34 (42 µg) 0.43 (20.2 µg) 0.61 (8.6 µg) 0.62 (1.5 µg) 0.7 (control)	NA	Dose-dependent reduction in NIF at 28 days; not maintained at 90 days	Circulation 2001; **104**:473–9
Palmaz-Schatz (non-proprietary)	None – dip-coating	Paclitaxel (187 µg/stent)	Porcine	28	NIA: 2 (LDD) 1.4 (control)	0.05 (LDD) 0.35 (control)	Dose-dependent reduction in NIF and increase in luminal diameter	Circulation 2001; **103**:2289–95
Gianturco-Roubin II (Cook)	Linear chain of aromatic hydrocarbons	Paclitaxel (175–200 µg/stent)	Porcine	28	NI thickness (µm): 403 (LDD) 669 (control)	Diameter stenosis (%): 27 ± 27 (LDD) 51 ± 27 (control)	Reduced NIF and diameter stenosis	Coron Artery Dis 2001; **12**:513–15

NIA, neointimal area; NIF, neointimal formation; NA, not available; nsd, no significant difference; LDD, local drug delivery

Table 3.9 Clinical studies: catheter-based delivery

Catheter name	Drug	Trial: Name or Acronym	Type of study/ number	Type of lesion: B2–C (%)	DM (%)	MACE (% at 6 mths)	Angiography: Binary restenosis rate (%)	Angiography: Late loss (mm)	Comment	Source
Dispatch catheter	Heparin	Camenzind et al.	Registry/ 22	A–B2	NA	20	7	0.27 ± 0.51 (stent) 0.18 ± 0.43 (POBA)	No MACE observed	Circulation 1995; **92**:2463–72
Infusion sleeve	Heparin: 1000 IU/ ml in 2–4 ml	Bartorelli et al.	Registry/ 35	A–B2 (18% B2)	20	9	12	0.94 ± 0.78	Low level of restenosis was seen	Catheter Cardiovasc Diagn 1997; **42**:313–20
Porous balloon catheter	Reviparin: 1500 IU in 4 ml	PILOT Oberhoff et al.	Registry/ 18	A–C	20	34	28 (24 wks)	0.61 ± 0.61		Catheter Cardiovasc Diagn 1998; **44**:267–74
InfusaSleeve	Heparin: 4000 IU	PAMI pilot	Registry/ 120	AMI	17	22	NA	NA	Low levels of target vessel revascularization seen	Catheter Cardiovasc Interv 1999; **47**:237–42
Micro- porous catheter	Nadro- parin	IMPRESS	RCT/250 LDD: 125 Control: 125	21 (LDD) 30 (Control)	10 (LDD) 13 (Con- trol)	10 (LDD) 11 (Control)	24 (LDD) 20 (Control)	0.88 ± 0.63 (LDD) 0.84 ± 0.62 (Control)	No reduction in restenosis or MACE with LDD	Eur Heart J 2000; **21**:1767–75
Infusa- Sleeve	Heparin: 5000 IU	HIPS	RCT/179 LDD: 91 Control: 88	15 (LDD) 34 (Control)	20 (LDD) 12 (Con- trol)	25 (LDD) 22 (Control)	12.5 (LDD) 12.7 (Control)	0.89 ± 0.46 (LDD) 0.83 ± 0.60 (Control)	No effect on clinical, angiographic, or IVUS endpoints of restenosis	Am Heart J 2000; **139**:1061–70

Table 3.9 *Continued*

Catheter name	Drug	Trial: Name or Acronym	Type of study/ number	Type of lesion: B2–C (%)	DM (%)	MACE (% at 6 mths)	Angiography: Binary restenosis rate (%)	Angiography: Late loss (mm)	Comment	Source
Transport catheter	Enoxaparin 10 mg	POLONIA	RCT/100 LDD: 50 Control: 50	A–B2	0	12 (LDD) 24 (control)	10 (LDD) 24 (control)	0.76 ± 0.42 (LDD) 1.07 ± 0.49 (control)	Reduced target vessel revascularization & angiographic restenosis	Circulation 2001; **103**:26–31
Dispatch catheter	VEGF plasmid/ liposomal gene transfer	Laitenen et al.	Controlled study not fully randomized/ 10	NA	NA	NA	10 (LDD)	0.15 (LDD) 0.03 (control)	nsd in angiographic restenosis	Hum Gene Ther 2000; **11**:263–70
Transport	Antisense oligo-nucleotide 10 mg	ITALICS	RCT/85 LDD: 42 Control: 43	A–C	10 (LDD) 9 (con-trol)	29 (LDD) 28 (control) at 210 days	34.2 (LDD) 38.5 (control) IVUS in-stent NI volume: 143 (LDD)/ 135 mm³ (control)	1.3 ± 0.2 (LDD) 1.2 ± 0.3 (control)	nsd in NIF or angiographic restenosis	J Am Coll Cardiol 2002; **39**:281–7

AMI, acute myocardial infarction; DM, diabetes mellitus; IVUS, intravascular ultrasound; MACE, major adverse cardiac event; RCT, randomized control trial; LDD, local drug delivery; POBA, plain old balloon angioplasty; NIA, neointimal area; NIF, neointimal formation; NI, neointimal; NA, not available; nsd, no significant difference.

Table 3.10 Clinical studies: inert stents

Stent name (Metal ± company)	Coating	Trial: Name or Acronym	Type of study/ number	Type of lesion: B2–C (%)	DM (%)	Follow-up (mths)	MACE (%)	Angiography: Binary restenosis rate (%)	Source
NIR (BSC)	Gold	NUGGET	RCT/165	55 (gold) 54 (control)	18 (gold) 18 (control)	6	12	NA	Circulation 2001; **104**:II–623
NIR (BSC)	Gold	Park et al.	RCT/216	52 (gold) 56 (control)	15 (gold) 17 (control)	9	23 (gold)/ 15 (control)	46.7 (gold)/ 26.4 (control)	Am J Cardiol 2002; **89**:872–5
Inflow (BSC)	Gold	Kastrati et al.	RCT/731	77 (gold) 80 (control)	21 (gold) 21 (control)	12	37 (gold)/ 27 (control)	49.7 (gold)/ 38 (control)	Circulation 2000; **101**:2478–83
Inflow (BSC)	Gold	Vom Dahl et al.	RCT/204	95 (gold) 96 (control)	37 (gold) 49 (control)	6	NA	36 (gold)/ 24 (control)	Am J Cardiol 2002; **89**:801–5
NIR/Inflow	Gold vs stainless steel	Hoffman et al.	Registry/311: 99 (Multilink)/ 73 (Inflow gold)/ 74 (Inflow)/ 12 (NIR gold)/ 12 (NIR)/ 41 (Palmaz-Schatz)	A–B2	21 (Multilink)/ 11 (Inflow gold)/ 19 (Inflow)/ 25 (NIR gold)/ 20 (NIR)/ 30 (Palmaz-Schatz)	6	NA	24 (all gold)/ 36 (all control) NI volume (IVUS) (mm^3) 47.3 (all gold)/ 40.9 (all steel)	Am J Cardiol 2002; **89**:1360–4
Tensum III (tantalum)	Silicon carbon	PSAAMI – POBA/ stent in AMI	Registry/44	66% B, 34% C (stent)/ 68% B, 32% C (POBA)	27 (stent) 21 (POBA)	35	23 (stent)	24 (stent)	Am J Med 2001; **110**:1–6

Table 3.10 *Continued*

Stent name (Metal ± company)	Coating	Trial: Name or Acronym	Type of study/number	Type of lesion: B2-C (%)	DM (%)	Follow-up (mths)	MACE (%)	Angiography: Binary restenosis rate (%)	Source
Tenax (Biotronik)	Silicon carbon	Carrie et al.	Registry/241	54	NA	12	17	20	J Interv Cardiol 2001; **14**:1–5
Tenax (Biotronik)	Silicon carbon	TRUST	RCT/485	Acute coronary syndromes	16 (Tenax) 13 (control)	6	10.1 (Tenax)/ 10.9 (control)	23.9 (Tenax) 23.7 (control)	Catheter Cardiovasc Interv 2003; **60**:375–81
Tenax (Biotronik)	Silicon carbon	BET: direct stenting (DS)/ predilatation (PD)	RCT/338	31 (DS) 19 (PD)	20 (DS) 24 (PD)	6	5 (DS) 11 (PD)	NA	Am J Cardiol 2001; **87**:693–8
Tenax (Biotronik)	Silicon carbon	Hanekamp et al.	Registry/174	NA	5	15	18	17	Int J Cardiovasc Intervent 1998; **1**:81–5
Tenax vs NIR	Silicon carbon/ Stainless steel (NIR)	TENISS-L	RCT/494	A–B2	22 (Tenax) 25 (NIR)	20	12 (Tenax) 14 (NIR)	NA	Am Heart J 2003; **145**:E17
Penchant	PC vs Stainless steel (Multilink)	DISTINCT	RCT/426	A–B2	21.4 (PC) 20.7 (control)	6	17 (PC) 14 (control)	19.9 (PC) 20.1 (control)	Not published
Penchant (Bio*divYsio*)	Phospho-rylcholine (PC)	Galli et al.	Registry/100	Acute MI	14	6	13	12	Catheter Cardiovasc Interv 2001; **53**:182–7

Table 3.10 *Continued*

Stent name (Metal ± company)	Coating	Trial: Name or Acronym	Type of study/ number	Type of lesion: B2–C (%)	DM (%)	Follow-up (mths)	MACE (%)	Angiography: Binary restenosis rate (%)	Source
Penchant (BiodivYsio)	PC	Galli et al.	Registry/218	59	14	6	13	NA	J Invasive Cardiol 2000; **12**:452–8
Penchant (BiodivYsio)	PC	Zheng et al.	Registry/224	62	15	6	9	6	J Invasive Cardiol 1999; **11**:608–14
Penchant (BiodivYsio)	PC	SOPHOS	Registry/425	50	13	9	13	18	Int J Cardiovasc Interv 2000; **3**:215–25
Carbostent (Sorin)	Turbo-stratic carbon	Antoniucci et al.	Registry/112	50	16	6	12	11	Am J Cardiol 2000; **85**:821–8
Carbostent (Sorin)	Turbo-stratic carbon	ANTARES	Registry/110	31	13	1	2 (1 mth)	NA	Catheter Cardiovasc Interv 2002; **55**:150–6
Helistent (Hexacath)	Titanium	Caussin et al.	Registry/133	71% B	21	6 (1 mth results available)	NA	NA	Am J Cardiol 2002;

DM, diabetes mellitus; MACE, major adverse cardiac event; RCT, randomized controled trial; IVUS, intravascular ultrasound; POBA, plain old balloon angioplasty; AMI, acute myocardial infarction; TLR, total lesion revascularization; NA, not available.

Table 3.11 Clinical studies: stent with immobilized heparin

Stent-type (Company)	Coating	Trial: Name or Acronym	Type of study/number	Type of lesion: B2–C (%)	DM (%)	Follow-up (mths)	MACE (%)	Angiography: Binary restenosis rate (%)	Source
Palmaz-Schatz (Cordis/J&J)	Polyethylene-imine & dextran sulfate (Carmeda)	Benestent II Pilot study	Registry/207	A–B2	8	6	13	13	Circulation 1996; **93**:412–22
Palmaz-Schatz (Cordis/J&J)	Polyethylene-imine & dextran sulfate (Carmeda)	Benestent II	RCT/824	55	13 (stent) 11 (POBA)	12	13 (stent) 19 (POBA)	16 (stent) 31 (POBA	Lancet 1998; **352**:673–81
Palmaz-Schatz (Cordis/J&J)	Polyethylene-imine & dextran sulfate (Carmeda)	TOSCA	RCT/410	Total occlusions	15 (stent) 18 (POBA)	6	23 (stent) 24 (POBA)	55 (stent) 70 (POBA)	Circulation 1999; **100**:236–42
Palmaz-Schatz (Cordis/J&J)	Polyethylene-imine & dextran sulfate (Carmeda)	Stent-PAMI	RCT/452	AMI	16 (stent) 14 (POBA)	6	13 (stent) 20 (POBA)	20 (stent) 34 (POBA)	N Engl J Med 1999; **341**:1949–56
Wiktor HepaMed (Medtronic)	Hepamed coating procedure	HEPACIS	Registry/105	ACS – STEMI (44)/UA (61)	NA	6	5.7	15.2	Am J Cardiol 2000; **86**:8
Wiktor Hepamed (Medtronic)	Hepamed coating procedure	MENTOR	Registry/132	32	10	12	15	22	Am J Cardiol 2000; **86**:385–9
Be-stent HepaMed (Medtronic)	Hepamed coating procedure	SISCA	RCT/145	42% B2 (stent)/ 30 (PTCA)	12 (stent) 14 (PTCA)	12	10 (stent) 24 (PTCA)	10 (stent) 19 (PTCA)	J Am Coll Cardiol 2001; **38**:1598–603

Table 3.11 *Continued*

Stent-type (Company)	Coating	Trial: Name or Acronym	Type of study/ number	Type of lesion: B2–C (%)	DM (%)	Follow-up (mths)	MACE (%)	Angiography: Binary restenosis rate (%)	Source
Wiktor Hepamed (Medtronic)	Hepamed coating procedure	Van Langenhove et al.	Registry/ 50	Saphenous vein grafts	14	6	10	22	Can J Cardiol 2000; **16**:473–80
Flexmaster Hepacoat (JoMed)	Inert polyamine layer	Shin et al.	Registry/ 102	AMI	NA	6	14	17	Catheter Cardiovasc Interv 2001; **52**:306–12
Flexmaster Hepacoat (JoMed)	Inert polyamine layer	COAST	RCT/ 588: coated stent/ control stent/ POBA	Small arteries (2–2.6 mm)	21 (coated) 18 (control)	6	11 (coated) 11 (control)	30 (coated)/ 26 (control)	Circulation 2003; **107**:1265–70
Flexmaster Hepacoat (JoMed)	Inert polyamine layer	ULM	RCT/278	30 (coated) 37 (control)	23 (coated) 17 (control)	6	25 (coated) 26 (control)	30 (coated)/ 33 (control)	Eur Heart J 2001; **22**:1808–16

DM, diabetes mellitus; MACE, major adverse cardiac event; POBA, plain old balloon angioplasty; AMI, acute myocardial infarction; ACS, acute coronary syndrome; STEMI, ST elevation myocardial infarction; UA, unstable angina; PTCA, percutaneous transluminal coronary angioplasty (without stent implantation); RCT, randomized control trial; NA, not available.

Table 3.12 Clinical studies: eluting stents

DES name (stainless steel stent name)	Coating	Drug used	Trial name or acronym	Type of study/ number	Type of lesion: B2–C (%)	DM (%)	Follow-up (months)	MACE (%)	Angiography: binary (>50%) restenosis rate (%)	Source
Tempo	Polyester amide	Tempamine (NO donor)	NOBLESSE I	Registry/ 47	37.8	ND	1, 4, 12	6.7 (4 m)	9.5 (4 m)	Eur Heart J 2003; **23** (suppl):86
Dexamet (BiodivYsio)	Phosphoryl- choline (PC)	Dexa- methasone 0.5 µg/mm²	STRIDE	Registry/ 71	31	0	6	3.3	13.3	Cath Cardiovasc Interv 2003; **60**:172–8
(BiodivYsio)	Phosphoryl- choline (PC)	17β-Estradiol 2.5 µg/mm²	EASTER	Registry/ 30	ND	10	6, 12	3.3 (12 m)	6.6 (6 m)	J Am Coll Cardiol 2003; **41** (Suppl A):
(BiodivYsio)	Phosphoryl- choline (PC)	Batimastat 2 µg/mm²	BRILLIANT	Registry/ 173	ND	13	6, 12	18 (6 m)	23 (6 m)	Eur Heart J 2003; **23** (suppl):268
Cypher (BxVelocity)	Poly(ethyl meth- acrylate)	Sirolimus 1.4 µg/mm² fast release (FR) slow release (SR)	FIM	Registry/ 30 FR:15 SR:15	31 (FR) 73 (SR)	26	4	0 (FR) 0 (SR)	0 (FR) 0 (SR)	Circulation 2001; **103**:192–5
Cypher (BxVelocity)	Poly(ethyl meth- acrylate)	Sirolimus 1.4 µg/mm² fast release (FR) slow release (SR)	FIM	Registry/ 45 FR: 15 SR: 30	A–B2	26	12	0 (FR) 0 (SR)	0 (FR) 0 (SR)	Circulation 2001; **104**:2007–11

Table 3.12 *Continued*

DES name (stainless steel stent name)	Coating	Drug used	Trial name or acronym	Type of study/ number	Type of lesion: B2–C (%)	DM (%)	Follow-up (months)	MACE (%)	Angiography: binary (>50%) restenosis rate (%)	Source
Cypher (BxVelocity)	Poly(ethyl methacrylate)	Sirolimus 1.4 μg/mm² fast release (FR) slow release (SR)	FIM	Registry/30 FR:15 SR:15	A–B2	26	24	3 (FR) 0 (SR)	0 (FR) 0 (SR)	Circulation 2003; **107**:381–3
Cypher (BxVelocity)	Poly(ethyl methacrylate)	Sirolimus SR: 1.4 μg/mm²	Rensing et al.	Registry/15	A–B2	NA	6	0	0	Eur Heart J 2001; **22**:2125–30
Cypher (BxVelocity)	Poly(ethyl methacrylate)	Sirolimus SR: 1.4 μg/mm²	Degertekin et al.	Registry/15	NA	26	24	20	0	Circulation 2002; **106**:1610–13
Cypher (BxVelocity)	Poly(ethyl methacrylate)	Sirolimus SR: 1.4 μg/mm²	RAVEL	RCT/238 SR: 120 Cont:118	54% B2 (SR)/ 61% B2 (control)	16 (SR) 21 (control)	12	6 (SR) 29 (control)	0 (SR) 27 (control)	N Engl J Med 2002; **346**:1773–80
Cypher (BxVelocity)	Poly(ethyl methacrylate)	Sirolimus SR: 1.4 μg/mm²	In-stent restenosis	Registry/25	In-stent restenosis	24	12	0	20	Circulation 2003; **107**:24–7
Cypher (BxVelocity)	Poly(ethyl methacrylate)	Sirolimus SR: 1.4 μg/mm²	SIRIUS	RCT/1058 SR: 533 Con: 525	59 (SR) 55 (control)	25 (SR) 28 (control)	8, 9	7.1 (SR) 18.9 (control) (9 m)	8.9 (SR) 36.3 (control) (8 m)	N Engl J Med 2003; **349**:1315–23

Table 3.12 *Continued*

DES name (stainless steel stent name)	Coating	Drug used	Trial name or acronym	Type of study/ number	Type of lesion: B2–C (%)	DM (%)	Follow-up (months)	MACE (%)	Angiography: binary (>50%) restenosis rate (%)	Source
Cypher (BxVelocity)	Poly(ethyl meth-acrylate)	Sirolimus SR: 1.4 µg/mm²	E-SIRIUS	RCT/352 SR: 175 Con: 177	62 (SR) 61 (control)	19 (SR) 27 (con-trol)	8, 9	8 (SR) 22.6 (control)	5.9 (SR) 42.3 (control)	Lancet 2003; **362**:1093–9
Cypher (BxVelocity)	Poly(ethyl meth-acrylate)	Sirolimus SR: 1.4 µg/mm²	C-SIRIUS	RCT/100 SR: 50 Con: 50	64 (SR) 54 (control)	24 (SR) 24 (con-trol)	8, 9	4 (SR) 18 (control)	2 (SR) 46 (control)	J Am Coll Cardiol 2003; **43**:1110–15
(Flex ceramic)	Aluminum oxide (ceramic)	Tacrolimus 0.4 µg/mm²	PRESENT I	RCT/44: Tac: 22 Cer: 20	NA	NA	6	Tac: 22 Cer: 20	NA	J Am Coll Cardiol 2004; **41** (Suppl A)
(Flex ceramic)	Aluminum oxide (ceramic)	Tacrolimus 1.7 µg/mm²	PRESENT II	RCT/30	NA	NA	6	32	NA	J Am Coll Cardiol 2003; **41** (Suppl A)
(Flex Progress)	None	Tacrolimus 1.7 µg/mm² 230 µg	PRESET	RCT/240: Tac: 120 Con: 120	NA	NA	6	NA	NA	2Q 2004 data available
Stent graft	ePTFE	Tacrolimus 2.2 µg/mm²	EVIDENT	Registry/ 32	NA	NA	6	NA	NA	TCT 2003 oral communi-cation
Challenge (S-stent)	Poly(D,L-lactide) polymer	Everolimus	FUTURE I	RCT/42: Eve: 27 Con: 15	Eve: 26 Con: 13	none	6	Eve: 7.7 Con: 7.7	Eve: 4 Con: 18.2	Eur Heart J 2003; **24** (Suppl):267 (abstract)

Table 3.12 *Continued*

DES name (stainless steel stent name)	Coating	Drug used	Trial name or acronym	Type of study/ number	Type of lesion: B2–C (%)	DM (%)	Follow-up (months)	MACE (%)	Angiography: binary (>50%) restenosis rate (%)	Source
Challenge (S-stent)	Poly(D,L-lactide) polymer	Everolimus	FUTURE II	RCT/64: Eve: 21 Con: 43	ND	yes	6	Eve: 4.8 Con: 17.5	Eve: 4.8 Con: 30.6	Eur Heart J 2003; **24** (Suppl):267 (abstract)
(Driver) Chrom-cobalt	Phosphoryl-choline (PC)	Abt 578	ENDEAVOR I	Registry/ 100	47	16	4, 12	5 (4 m)	2.1 (4 m)	TCT 2003 Oral communication
QuaDS-QP2	Polymer sleeve	7-hexanoyl-taxol 4 mg	BARDDS	Registry/ 32	A–B2	NA	11	0	0	Cath Cardiovasc Interv 2001; **53**:480–8
QuaDS-QP2	Polymer sleeve	7-hexanoyl-taxol	Honda et al.	Registry/ 20	ND	7	8	10	0	Circulation 2001; **104**:380–3
QuaDS-QP2 (QueST stent)	Polymer sleeve	7-hexanoyl-taxol	SCORE: IVUS subgroup	RCT/ 122: Qua: 66 Con: 56	ND	21 (Qua) 25 (control)	6	NA (IVUS only)	NVI: 0.79 (Qua)/ 2.48 (control)	Circulation 2002; **106**:1788–93
QuaDS-QP2	Polymer sleeve	7-hexanoyl-taxol	Liistro et al.	Registry/ 15	In-stent restenosis	30	12	87	62	Circulation 2002; **105**:1883–6
(Supra G stent)	None	Paclitaxel low dose (LD): 1.28 µg/mm²/high dose (HD): 3.1 µg/mm²	ASPECT	RCT/177	4 (LD) 7 (HD) 8 (control)	24 (LD) 18 (HD) 17 (control)	6	5 (LD) 4 (HD) 4 (control)	12 (LD) 4 (HD) 27 (control)	N Engl J Med 2003; **348**: 1537–45

Table 3.12 *Continued*

DES name (stainless steel stent name)	Coating	Drug used	Trial name or acronym	Type of study/ number	Type of lesion: B2–C (%)	DM (%)	Follow-up (months)	MACE (%)	Angiography: binary (>50%) restenosis rate (%)	Source
(Supra G stent)	None	Paclitaxel low dose (LD): 1.28 µg/mm²/high dose (HD): 3.1 µg/mm²	Paclitaxel low IVUS subgroup of ASPECT study	RCT/98	4% B2	18 (LD) 7 (HD) 16 (control)	6	5 (LD) 4 (HD) 4 (control)	12 (LD) 4 (HD) 27 (control)	Circulation 2003; **107**:517–20
(V-flex Plus)	None	Paclitaxel 0.2, 0.7, 1.4, 2.7 µg/mm²	ELUTES	RCT/192	9	11 (HD) 10 (control)	12	14 (HD) 18 (control)	3.1 (HD) 16 (control)	Circulation 2004; **109**:487–93
Achieve (Multi-link Rx Penta)	None	Paclitaxel (3 µg/mm²)	DELIVER	RCT/1041: Ach: 522 Con: 519	A–B2	30	6, 7	ND (Ach) ND (control) (7 m)	16.7 (Ach) 22.4 (Con) (6 m)	Am J Cardiol 2002; **90**:70 J Am Coll Cardiol 2003; **41** (Suppl A):
Achieve (Multi-link Rx Penta)	None	Paclitaxel 3 µg/mm²	DELIVER II	Registry/ 1533	A–C	NA	6	15.7	NA	ESC 2003 Late-Breaking Trials
Taxus (NIR)	Hydro-carbon-based polymer	Paclitaxel slow release SR: 1 µg/mm²	TAXUS I	RCT/61: SR: 31 Con: 30	29% B2 (SR)/ 43% B2 (control)	23 (SR) 13 (control)	6, 12	3 (SR) 10 (control) (12 m)	0 (SR) 10 (control) (6 m)	Circulation 2003; **107**:38–42

Table 3.12 *Continued*

DES name (stainless steel stent name)	Coating	Drug used	Trial name or acronym	Type of study/number	Type of lesion: B2-C (%)	DM (%)	Follow-up (months)	MACE (%)	Angiography: binary (>50%) restenosis rate (%)	Source
Taxus (NIR)	Hydro-carbon-based polymer	Paclitaxel SR: 1 µg/mm² MR: 1 µg/mm²	TAXUS II	RCT/536: SR: 131 Con: 136 MR: 135 Con: 134	A–B2	11 (SR) 16 (Con) 17 (MR) 14 (Con)	6, 12	10.9 (SR) 19.5 (Con) 7.8 (MR) 20 (Con) (12 m)	5.5 (SR) 20.1 (Con) 8.6 (MR) 23.8 (Con) (6 m)	Circulation 2003; **108**:788–94
(Taxus) NIR	Hydro-carbon-based polymer	Paclitaxel SR: 1 µg/mm²	TAXUS III In-stent restenosis	Registry/28	In-stent restenosis II–IV: 64%	14	6, 12	29 (12 m)	16 (6 m)	Circulation 2003; **107**:559–64
(Taxus) NIR	Hydro-carbon-based polymer	Paclitaxel SR: 1 µg/mm²	TAXUS IV	RCT/1314: SR: 662 Con: 652	NA	23.4 (SR) 25 (Con)	9	8.5 (SR) 15 (Con)	7.9 (SR) 26.6 (Con)	N Engl J Med 2004; **350**:221–31
(Taxus) NIR	Hydro-carbon-based polymer	Paclitaxel SR: 1 µg/mm²	TAXUS IV	RCT/1314: SR: 662 Con: 652	NA	23.4 (SR) 25 (Con)	12	10.8 (SR) 20 (Con)	NA	Circulation 2004; **109**:1942–7
Tetra		Actinomycin-D high dose (HD): 10 µg/mm² low-dose (LD): 2.5 µg/mm²	ACTION	RCT/360	NA	NA	NA	NA	NA	Stopped at 9 m due to increased restenosis with Actin-D (not published)

DM, diabetes mellitus; MACE, major adverse cardiac events; NVI, neointimal vclume index; STEMI, ST elevation myocardial infarction; UA, unstable angina; RCT, randomized controlled trial; NA, not available; angiography: binary (>50%) restenosis is given for in-segment analysis.

4

The ClearWay™ microporous balloon catheter

Geoffrey Moodie, Steve Grantz, and Paul Martakos

Introduction • **Drug delivery** • **Other potential applications** • **Conclusions**

INTRODUCTION

The Atrium Medical ClearWay™ microporous balloon catheter has been developed using expanded polytetrafluoroethylene (ePTFE) as a balloon material. This material has a porous architecture, as seen in Figure 4.1, with solid nodes connected by a series of fibrils. The fibril length between adjacent nodes is defined as internodal distance and one can select from a wide range of internodal distances by adjusting processing parameters.

Other catheters use a jetting action or microneedles to force drug deep into or, in some cases, through the medial layer of the vessel wall. Examples of jetting catheters include laser drilled angioplasty balloons, such as the Wolinsky Perforated Balloon,[1] and the microneedle approach is used by the Interventional Technologies Infiltrator Balloon Catheter.[2] The ClearWay™ catheter provides a less traumatic approach, using a low pressure system (<4 atm) to deploy drug to the intima of the vessel. This low pressure technique does not overextend or damage the vessel wall and it allows for treatment of native vessels, stented vessels, and synthetic grafts.

Infusate weeps out among the fibrils along the entire length of the balloon, ensuring a lubricating fluid layer over the whole surface as shown in Figure 4.2. The tortuous channels of ePTFE do not allow for a direct fluid path to the surface, and this prevents the damage-inducing 'jetting' effect. The rate of fluid flow can be controlled by the amount of pressure applied by the operator. Flow rates are plotted in Figure 4.3. Figure 4.4 shows infusate from the balloon coming through the wall of an ePTFE graft, indicating even coverage and sufficient pressure transmission to push the aqueous solution through the hydrophobic material. The material softness and the lack of fluid jetting action makes the Atrium

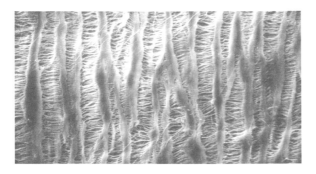

Fig. 4.1 The porous microarchitecture of expanded polytetrafluoroethylene (ePTFE).

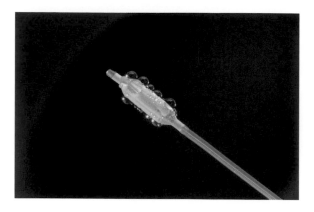

Fig. 4.2 Fluid weeping from ClearWay™ balloon.

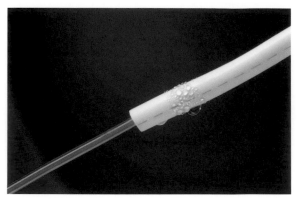

Fig. 4.4 Infusate from a ClearWay™ balloon passing through the wall of an ePTFE graft.

ClearWay™ balloon an ideal drug delivery system for intra-arterial use. The ePTFE balloon is designed to conform to the native vessel, deployed stent or any synthetic graft. Its conformability and pore design allow the Atrium ClearWay™ balloon to deliver complete circumferential treatment to the site.

Since the ClearWay™ requires very low pressure for delivery it can be used with standard hand syringes and does not require expensive or complex injection machines and pumps. When applicable, angioplasty inflation devices may also be used.

The infusate may be used to simply irrigate the vessel wall or it may incorporate one or more therapeutic substances (e.g. applying thrombolytic for thrombus removal in peripheral applications, see Figures 4.5 and 4.6).

The catheter is designed to be occlusive. It has been reported that stopping blood flow plays an important role in uptake of therapeutics into vessel walls,[3] and short periods of occlusion (30 sec–1 min) are commonly tolerated during percutaneous transluminal coronary angioplasty (PTCA) and stent deployment.

In addition to liquid formulations, the catheter can successfully deliver nanoparticles in suspension. This opens up possibilities for

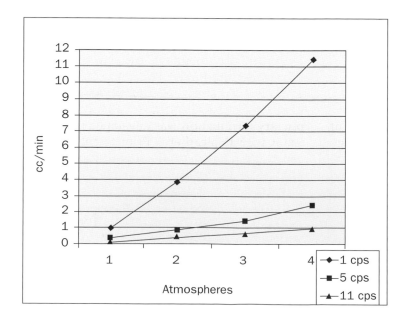

Fig. 4.3 Flow rates through the coronary ClearWay™ at several pressures and viscosities. cps, counts per second.

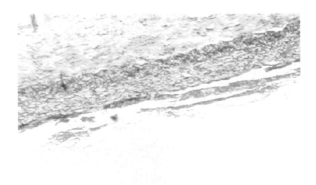

Fig. 4.5 Residual thrombus after thrombectomy with a latex balloon.

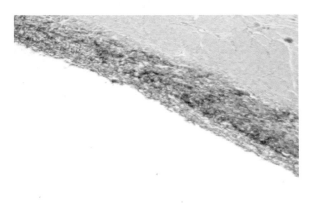

Fig. 4.6 Graft cleared of thrombus after ClearWay™ use with a thrombolytic.

administering insoluble compounds and controlled release systems.[4]

Over-the-wire peripheral models of this infusion catheter are commercially available for embolectomy, thrombectomy, and delivery of thrombolytics. Balloon sizes available range from 4.0–10.0 mm in diameter and 10–40 mm in length. A rapid exchange design is undergoing evaluation in a coronary model with balloon sizes from 2.5 mm to 4.0 mm in diameter and 10 mm to 50 mm in length.

DRUG DELIVERY

Staining experiments have been performed (in Dr Michael Buerke's laboratory at the Martin Luther University in Halle, Germany) using native rabbit femoral arteries. These determined that the ClearWay™ catheter primarily delivers to the intimal layer of the vessel, one to two cell layers deep at 2 atm and five layers deep at 6 atm. Infusion solutions may differ greatly from aqueous media in viscosity and/or chemical properties and this could significantly impact these numbers. Thus, solutions need to be tested on an individual basis. In addition, the efficacy and fate of any compound post delivery will be determined by its chemical stability, mechanism of action, metabolism, and physicochemical properties.[5] These are important points to consider when selecting compounds for use with the ClearWay™ or any other system.

Examples of drug delivery

Restenosis occurs after stenting as a response to injury. A neointima forms as smooth muscle cells change from the contractile to the synthetic phenotype, migrate into intima, proliferate, and secrete matrix. This neointima may grow to a point that the vessel once again becomes occluded. Occurrence ranges are reported to be 15–30%.[6] Recently, drug eluting stents have shown admirable results in reducing this problem; however, their high cost remains prohibitive and alternate, less expensive means to deliver drugs site-specifically could play a role.

Rapamycin, a drug known to suppress restenosis, was delivered through the ClearWay™ catheter at three dose levels to stented vessels. As this is a hydrophobic drug not conventionally administered intravenously, a proprietary formulation was developed in order to use it with this catheter. Prior to entering this experiment we confirmed using high performance liquid chromatography (HPLC) analysis that the drug was not filtered out by the ClearWay™ ePTFE balloon material.

In vivo studies were carried out in porcine coronary vessels. Atrium Flyer 3.0 mm × 16 mm stents were deployed without predilation in the left anterior descending and left circumflex coronary arteries at a 1.1:1 overstretch ratio. ClearWay™ catheters (3.0 mm ×

20 mm) were deployed into the stented segments. Drug-containing and control solutions easily passed through at the prescribed rate of 1 ml over 30 seconds.

The catheter tracked successfully into all stented areas. Balloon inflation and vessel occlusion were verified angiographically in several cases. The catheter could be rapidly deflated and removed after infusion was completed. In each case, angiography revealed the expected return of blood flow through the coronary segment.

The animals were sacrificed at 1 hour or 3 days and the hearts excised. In order to measure tissue rapamycin content the vessels surrounding the stents were cut free and flash frozen in liquid nitrogen. These were then homogenized and analysed via HPLC in Dr Napoli-Eaton's lab at the University of Texas, Houston.[7] A sample HPLC chroma-

togram for rapamycin can be seen in Figure 4.7. From these results we saw a dose-related deposition of rapamycin into the treated coronary artery segments (Figure 4.8).

The photograph in Figure 4.9 shows a stented left circumflex artery 3 days after catheter treatment. A portion of the stent can be seen through the tissue. From this image it can be seen that the surrounding tissues appear healthy and undamaged by stenting and balloon catheter infusion.

No evidence of vessel dissection ascribed to balloon inflation was apparent, even in unstented vessels, either angiographically or histologically. Figure 4.10 is a cross-section of an unstented vessel that had been treated. Note the intact internal elastic lamina. The stented vessels likewise showed no damage beyond that typically caused by stenting itself.

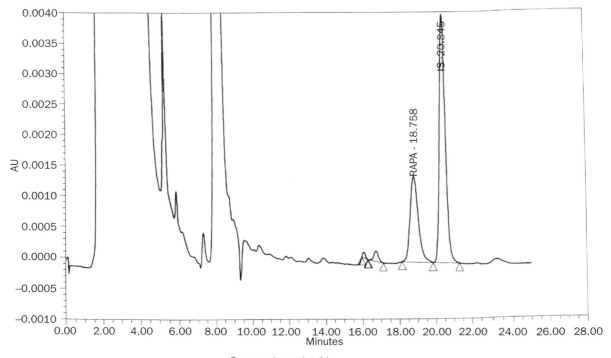

Rapamycin peak table

	Name	RT	Area	Height	Response	Amount	Units	AoverH
1	RAPA	18.758	42684	1396	0.3439	20.00	ng/ml	30.6
2	IS	20.345	91843	4058	4058.2263	1.00		22.6

Fig. 4.7 High performance liquid chromatogram (HPLC) for rapamycin.

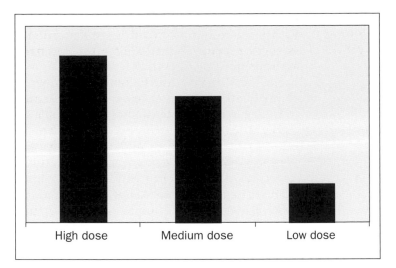

Fig. 4.8 Dose-related rapamycin loading of coronary vessel tissue.

High dose   Medium dose   Low dose

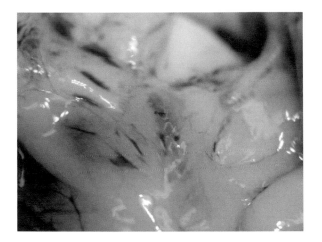

Fig. 4.9 Stented left circumflex artery 3 days after ClearWay™ treatment.

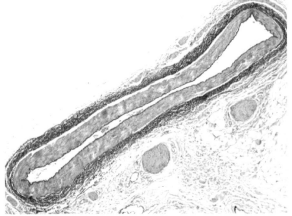

Fig. 4.10 Cross-section of the ClearWay™ treated vessel.

HPLC analysis of the stented segments showed tissue uptake of rapamycin similar to that seen with drug delivery stents.[6] The amount of tissue uptake could be controlled by the concentration of drug in the infusion solution dose-dependently. It remains to be tested whether or not this mode of delivery can have a long-term effect on stent-induced intimal hyperplasia.

OTHER POTENTIAL APPLICATIONS

Oncology

A known problem with many conventional oncology medications is systemic toxicity. By using the ClearWay™ we can infuse drugs directly into the tumor's vasculature, and its occlusive design may be used to stop blood flow to create a longer 'dwell time' for the medication.

Neurology

If a balloon is to be successful in a neurological application it must be very pliable and operate with minimal pressure due to the exceptionally delicate nature of the vessels in this area. The ClearWay's™ atraumatic nature offers potential here, and applications may include mechanical removal of clots, infusion of thrombolytics, and infusion of clotting media into aneurysms.

Urology

This technique may provide a way to deliver medications along the urinary tract using the minimally invasive ClearWay™ balloon catheter. Given the proper drug and delivery formulation characteristics this may provide a way to medicate the prostate.

Gene therapy

Similar to oncology applications, the ClearWay™ can be used to direct genes or antisense compounds to the point of vasculature where they are needed most. Stopping blood flow may also increase uptake of genes into the vessel wall.

Cosmetic surgery

This catheter may be used to clear debris from a wound bed without requiring a large incision. This would be advantageous for installation and removal of cosmetic implants.

CONCLUSIONS

The ClearWay™ catheter's flexibility, low profile, and balloon softness allow for it to be successfully tracked to a large range of deployment sites including the major vessels of the coronary vasculature. It is easily tracked angiographically with its radiopaque markers. Once in place the low pressure delivery and softness of the microporous ePTFE balloon catheter does not result in dissection of the target vessel wall. It has been shown that intimal delivery has been achieved, and rapamycin delivered through this catheter is taken up by the surrounding vessel at levels detectable by HPLC. This catheter holds promise for delivery of other drugs, such as thrombolytics, antineoplastics, and gene therapy. Future applications may include neurology, urology, oncology, cosmetic surgery, cardiology, and imaging technologies.

REFERENCES

1. McKay RG. Catheter-based techniques of local drug delivery. In Freed M, Grines C, Safian RD (eds), The New Manual of Interventional Cardiology. Physicians Press: Birmingham, MI 1996:645–60.
2. Kipshidze NN, Kim HS, Iverson P, et al. Intramural coronary delivery of advanced oligonucleotides reduces neointimal formation in the porcine stent restenosis model. J Am Coll Cardiol 2002; 39(10):1686–91.
3. Logeart D, Hatem S, Ruecker-Martin C, et al. Highly efficient adenovirus-mediated gene transfer to cardiac myocytes after single-pass coronary delivery. Hum Gene Ther 2000; 11:1015–22.
4. Atrium Medical (unpublished data).
5. Hwang CW, Wu D, Edelman ER. Physiological transport forces govern drug distribution for stent-based delivery. Circulation 2001; 104:600–5.
6. Suzuki T, Kopia G, Hayashi S, et al. Stent-based delivery of sirolimus reduces neointimal formation in a porcine coronary model. Circulation 2001; 104:1188–93.
7. Napoli KL, Kahan B. Sample clean-up and high-performance liquid chromatographic techniques for measurement of whole blood rapamycin concentrations. J Chromatog B 1994; 654:111–20.

5

The Dispatch® coronary infusion catheter

Wendy Naimark and James Barry

Introduction • Description • Drug delivery • Preclinical studies • Clinical studies
• Conclusions

INTRODUCTION

The Dispatch® catheter, also referred to as the coil catheter, is an endolumenal combination device with both infusion and continuous blood flow features. The balloon was designed so that a central conduit is formed on expansion to maintain distal coronary flow and allow for extended drug delivery within the coronary vasculature. The external coil is nondilatational and does not produce a high mechanical force against the vessel wall at nominal inflation pressures. Dispatch® catheter dwell times of up to 4 hours have been reported in clinical cases without hemodynamic compromise.[1]

The Food and Drug Administration (FDA) granted 510 K approval of the Dispatch catheter in 1996 for delivery of thrombolytic agents. Early clinical and preclinical studies conclusively demonstrated safety of the device for localized intracoronary delivery of heparin and urokinase.[2-4] To date, the Dispatch has been used to deliver a wide range of therapeutic agents in both preclinical and clinical studies.[2-15]

DESCRIPTION

The Dispatch coronary infusion catheter is a nondilatational, over-the-wire device designed for localized delivery of solutions through the openings located in the balloon segment (Figure 5.1). The device has a dual lumen shaft with a distally located 20 mm long inflation coil. The inflation coil, wrapped around a thin polyurethane sheath, may be inflated to further localize or isolate delivery to the vessel wall. The larger lumen of the shaft is used to transport solutions, as well as to house an inner tube

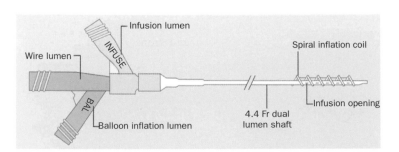

Fig. 5.1 Schematic of the Dispatch® coronary infusion catheter. The proximal portion of the catheter includes a manifold with two side ports, one for balloon inflation and one for infusion, and an end port for use with appropriately sized coronary guidewires.

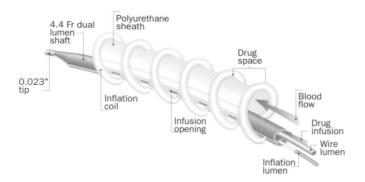

Fig. 5.2 Details of the Dispatch® catheter balloon design. The Dispatch® is an over-the-wire catheter that consists of a spiral inflation coil wrapped around a nonporous polyurethane sheath. When the spiral coil is inflated, it forms both an internal conduit that allows continued blood flow in the artery and a series of isolated drug spaces. Drugs are delivered through the infusion port and enter the delivery spaces through the isolated infusion openings on the balloon surface. The drug contacts the vessel wall and is isolated from blood flow during inflation of the spiral inflation coil.

positioned concentrically within the lumen. The inner tube permits use of a coronary guidewire (≤0.014 in/0.36 mm) to advance the device through the anatomy to the intended infusion site.

When the spiral coil is inflated it forms an internal conduit for continuous coronary flow and exposes a series of isolated pockets on the external surface between the balloon and the vessel wall (Figure 5.2). The coil exerts <2 atm of pressure against the wall enabling low uninterrupted pressure drug infusion over extended periods of time.[4] The drug is administered through an independent infusion port and delivered through slits on the balloon surface. The ports are positioned in the spaces between coil segments resulting in localized pockets of drug in contact with the artery wall. The distal tip is tapered to facilitate tracking of the device through the vasculature. A radiopaque marker runs the length of the inflation coil to assist in device placement.

DRUG DELIVERY

The Dispatch catheter has been used to deliver a wide variety of therapeutic agents in both preclinical and clinical studies. These agents include urokinase,[2,3] heparin,[4–6] L-arginine,[7,8]

various gene therapies,[9–13] recombinant tissue factor pathway inhibitor,[14] decoy oligonucleotides,[15] and endothelial cells.[16] (See Figure 5.3 for delivery features of the Dispatch catheter.)

PRECLINICAL STUDIES

Early preclinical studies focused on the feasibility of delivering the thrombolytic agent urokinase with the Dispatch catheter.[2,3] In studies spanning in vitro bench tests to clinical administration of urokinase, Mitchel and coworkers demonstrated the utility of local urokinase delivery.[2] Using an in vitro flow loop model, urokinase significantly reduced thrombus clot weight when compared with controls.[2] In vivo porcine coronary studies revealed that delivery efficiency of ^{123}I-urokinase with the Dispatch catheter was significantly higher than either systemic bolus or guiding catheter infusions (0.12% vs 0.0007% and 0.003%, respectively; $p<0.001$). Urokinase was detectable up to 5 hours post Dispatch infusion. In further preclinical studies, the relative efficacy of local versus systemic urokinase delivery in lysing intravascular thrombus was examined.[3] Urokinase infusion with the Dispatch catheter into porcine peripheral arteries resulted in a statistical increase in clot lysis in comparison

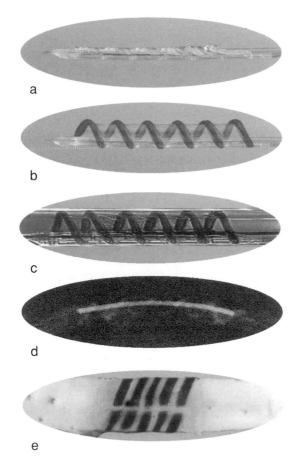

Fig. 5.3 Delivery features of the Dispatch® catheter. (a) The balloon has a low profile to facilitate lesion crossing. (b) Upon expansion the polyurethane sheath creates an open lumen for continued blood flow. (c) The inflated spiral inflation coil is infused with blue dye; the green dye shows isolation of infusate between the balloon surface and a simulated vessel wall; the red dye demonstrates the separation created between infusate and continued blood flow. (d) The radiopaque marker band runs through the entire spiral inflation coil. (e) The ex vivo porcine artery illustrates drug staining circumferentially across the artery.

with systemic and guiding catheter infusions (62.8% vs 8.8% and 20.8%, respectively; $p<0.05$). Consistent with these findings, intramural deposition of urokinase was significantly higher with the Dispatch catheter. Entrapment of the clot within the delivery pockets created between the sheath and vessel wall, in combi-

nation with mechanical disruption, are probable contributors to the effectiveness of this procedure.

Optimizing delivery parameters, including infusate volume, delivery time, and balloon design, are critical for successful delivery. The design of the Dispatch catheter allows for extended periods of distal flow and agent–vessel wall exposure. In comparison with the parameters established by McKay for the effective delivery of urokinase (30 min delivery time, 15 ml volume, 0.5 ml/min flow rate),[17] others have used significantly shorter delivery times of other agents without success. In particular, Baumbach and coworkers used the Dispatch to determine if local delivery of a high concentration of low molecular weight heparin (reviparin) would reduce neointimal formation.[6] While the device was found to be safe, and delivery feasible, a reduction in intimal hyperplasia was not observed. It is important to note that a volume of 4 ml (1000 IU/mg antifactor-Xa activity) was infused over 14 ± 4 sec (flow rate = 17 ml/min). In the Baumbach study, the lack of optimized delivery parameters makes it difficult to truly determine the reason for inconclusive results.

Arterial gene therapy approaches to reduce neointimal formation are challenged by inefficient gene transfer. As demonstrated by Palasis and coworkers diffusion appears to be a predominant mechanism of transport to the vessel wall using local delivery balloon catheters.[18] While longer incubation times have been shown to enhance transfection efficiency, most notably when the dwell delivery method is used,[19] the high risk of tissue ischemia and minimal clinical applicability limit the approach. The design of the Dispatch catheter, which allows for continuous distal flow, is suited for extended delivery times without the risk of inducing myocardial ischemia. The device has been used successfully to deliver a range of gene therapies.[9–13]

Tahlil and coworkers used the Dispatch catheter to localize an adenoviral vector encoding nuclear-targeted β-galactosidase (AdRSVβ-gal) to iliac arteries of normal and atheromatous rabbits.[9] A total of 300 μL of

AdRSVβ-gal (5×10^9 plaque forming units (pfu)) were infused and let dwell between the catheter pockets and vessel wall for 1 hour. Marked expression of the gene was detected in the endothelium ($16 \pm 8\%$/artery) without causing trauma to the vessel architecture or inducing myocardial ischemia. Superficial medial expression was detected and in several cases gene expression was observed deep into the media. Despite minimal evidence of medial expression, the fact that the Dispatch catheter preserves the endothelial layer and results in a high transduction rate in the endothelium clearly demonstrates that is well suited for gene therapy strategies targeting the endothelium.

In combination with endothelial denudation, the Dispatch catheter has been used to deliver adenovirus-mediated dominant negative mutant RasN17 (AdRasN17) to pig coronary arteries.[10] AdRasN17 targets smooth muscle cell proliferation by blocking the p21-ras mediated signal transduction pathway. The vessels were subjected to 1.5 times over-inflation with an angioplasty balloon followed by delivery of AdRasN17 via the Dispatch catheter. Each vessel was exposed to 5×10^9 pfu for 10 minutes; animals were sacrificed at 6 weeks. Transfer of AdRasN17 led to a significant decrease in neointimal formation (56%) and increase in lumen size (75%) in comparison with Adβgal transfected arteries. This study indicates that the Dispatch catheter can successfully target gene therapies to the media postendothelial denudation.

CLINICAL STUDIES

To assess feasibility and safety Camenzind and coworkers undertook an in-depth analysis of hemodynamic parameters immediately following heparin delivery and at 6 months follow up.[4] In a 22 patient study, infusion of approximately 15 ml of heparin (100 IU/ml) was delivered over 30 minutes. Device placement and depolyment was achieved in all patients without complication. Of the five patients who experienced anginal symptoms during placement, complications due to lesion severity and bifurcation branch blockage were implicated.

Signs of myocardial ischemia were used to evaluate the distal flow properties of the catheter. Hemodynamic parameters of relaxation and diastolic function did not change during coil placement relative to baseline. Overall, no significant changes in left ventricular function including ejection fraction and regional wall motion occurred during prolonged deployment. One asymptomatic patient died at 52 days after the procedure of congestive heart failure subsequent to blood transfusion for active ulcerative colitis. Neither myocardial infarction nor revascularization occurred in the 21 patient cohort at 7 months follow-up. Upon angiographic follow-up on 15 of 21 patients no evidence of aneurysmatic dilatation or an excessive restenosis rate at the treatment site was observed (restenosis was 7% as defined according to diameter stenosis >50%).

The Dispatch has been used to safely and feasibly deliver antithrombotics in combination with a number of interventional procedures including balloon angioplasty, directional atherectomy, stenting interventions, and treatment of thrombotic saphenous vein bypass grafts.[20–23] Treatment of intracoronary thrombus and thrombus-containing stenoses with local infusion of urokinase resulted in enhanced thrombolysis using drug concentrations that are significantly lower than used in standard intracoronary or systemic delivery. In a six patient study, infusion times of 30 minutes were well tolerated.[24] Angiographic analysis of coronary flow during Dispatch inflation demonstrated TIMI 3 in five of six patients treated. Distal flow was sufficient to prevent the development of chest pains and electrocardiographic changes. Distal embolization and no-reflow phenomena were not observed during further interventions with angioplasty or atherectomy. In a subsequent study, the Dispatch was used to deliver urokinase to a cohort of 19 patients presenting with thrombus-containing stenoses.[25] The clinical diagnoses of this group included unstable angina, acute myocardial infarction, and postinfarction angina. A reduction of thrombus-containing stenoses and complete disappearance of intracoronary thrombus was observed when 150 000 U of urokinase was locally delivered. All 19 patients treated had successful outcomes without evidence of abrupt closure, distal embolization or reflow.

The Dispatch catheter has been used to demonstrate the safety and feasibility of delivering gene therapies to human arteries.[11-13] Laitinen and coworkers first demonstrated that transgene expression could be detected using adenoviral mediated gene transfer of a reporter gene.[11] Patients who were suffering from chronic critical leg ischemia and scheduled to undergo limb amputation, were recruited for the trial. Replication-deficient adenovirus encoding the reporter gene β-galactosidase was infused at the area of critical stenosis following percutaneous transluminal coronary angioplasty (PTCA) over 10 minutes at a rate of 0.5 ml/min.[11] Gene transfer was successful in six of the eight patients treated with efficiency varying between 0.04% and 5.0% of all arterial cells. Transmural expression was detected out to the adventitia, however, distribution was not even and expression was not observed beneath advanced atherosclerotic lesions. Subsequently, both Laitinen and coworkers and Makinen and coworkers have evaluated the potential of local delivery of the gene encoding the angiogenic vascular endothelial growth factor protein (VEGF165), in both plasmid and adenoviral vector constructs, to human coronary and infrapopliteal arteries.[12,13] In two separate randomized double blinded placebo controlled studies, delivery of the gene encoding VEGF165 with the Dispatch catheter was shown to be safe and feasible. While intracoronary delivery of plasmid/liposome infusion resulted in a minimal transient increase in C-reactive protein at 2 days post procedure, no abnormalities in clinical biochemical parameters were seen as a result of cellular expression.[12] Neither VEGF plasmid nor recombinant VEFG protein was detected in the systemic circulation after transfer. Treatment of lower limb ischemia using local delivery of VEGF in both a plasmid/liposome formulation and in an adenoviral vector has also been shown to be safe.[13] The primary endpoint of increased vascularity was observed in both VEGF groups relative to controls. However, anti-adenovirus antibodies increased in 61% of the patients treated with adenovirus carrying VEGF. These studies highlight the importance of randomized double blinded placebo controlled trials to determine the efficacy of endovascular gene therapy strategies.

CONCLUSIONS

Developments in vascular and molecular biology, in addition to advancements in minimally invasive vascular medical device design, underscore the need to choose the correct device design and delivery parameters, in combination with the therapeutic agent, for efficient vessel targeting. The Dispatch catheter has proven safe and feasible for intracoronary delivery of a wide range of agents over extended periods. In specific cases, the coil pockets formed upon inflation have been shown to serve a dual purpose creating both isolated depots for site-specific agent delivery along with mechanical disruption of endolumenal blockages.

REFERENCES

1. Groh WC, Kurnik PB, Matthai WH, et al. Initial experience with an intracoronary flow support device providing localized drug infusion: The Scimed Dispatch Catheter. Catheter Cardiovasc Diagn 1995; 36:67–73.

2. Mitchel JF, Fram DB, Palme II DF, et al. Enhanced intracoronary thrombolysis with urokinase using a novel, local drug delivery system: In vitro, in vivo and clinical studies. Circulation 1995; 91:785–93.

3. Mitchel JF, Shwedick M, Alberghini TA, et al. Catheter-based local thrombolysis with urokinase: comparative efficacy of intraluminal clot lysis with conventional urokinase infusion techniques in an in vivo porcine thrombus model. Catheter Cardiovasc Diagn 1997; 41:293–302.

4. Carmenzind E, Kint P-P, Di Mario C, et al. Intracoronary heparin delivery in humans: acute feasibility and long-term results. Circulation 1995; 92:2463–72.

5. Kornowski R, Hong MK, Tio FO, et al. A randomized animal study evaluating the efficacies of locally delivered heparin and urokinase for reducing in-stent restenosis. Coron Artery Dis 1997; 8:293–8.

6. Baumbach A, Oberhoff M, Bohnet A, et al. Efficacy of low-molecular-weight heparin delivery with the Dispatch catheter following balloon angioplasty in the rabbit iliac artery. Catheter Cardiovasc Diagn 1997; 41:303–7.

7. Schwarzacher SP, Lim TT, Wang B, et al. Local intramural delivery of L-arginine enhances nitric oxide generation and inhibits lesion formation after balloon angioplasty. Circulation 1997; 95:1863–9.

8. Suzuki T, Hayase M, Hibi K, et al. Effect of local delivery of L-arginine on in-stent restenosis in humans. Am J Cardiol 2002; 89:363–7.

9. Tahlil O, Brami M, Feldman LJ, et al. The Dispatch™ catheter as a delivery tool for arterial gene transfer. Cardiovasc Res 1997; 33:181–7.

10. Wu CH, Lin CS, Hung JS, et al. Inhibition of neointimal formation in porcine coronary artery by a Ras mutant. J Surg Res 2001; 99:100–6.

11. Laitinen M, Makinen K, Manninen H, et al. Adenovirus-mediated gene transfer to lower limb artery of patients with chronic critical leg ischemia. Hum Gene Ther 1998; 9:1481–6.

12. Laitinen M, Hartikainen J, Hiltunen MO, et al. Catheter-mediated vascular endothelial growth factor gene transfer to human coronary arteries after angioplasty. Hum Gene Ther 2000; 11:263–70.

13. Makinen K, Manninen H, Hedman M, et al. Increased vascularity detected by digital subtraction angiography after VEGF gene transfer to human lower limb artery: a randomized, placebo-controlled, double-blinded phase II study. Mol Ther 2002; 6:127–33.

14. Yang LY, St Pierre J, Scherrer DE, et al. Comparison of methods for local delivery of tissue factor pathway inhibitor to balloon-injured arteries in rabbits. Coron Artery Dis 1999; 10:327–33.

15. Buchwald AB, Wagner AH, Webel C, Hecker M. Decoy oligodeoxynucleotide against activator protein-1 reduces neointimal proliferation after coronary angioplasty in hypercholesterolemic minipigs. J Am Coll Cardiol 2002; 39:732–8.

16. Dillavou E, Cupp P, Consigny PM. Delivery of endothelial cells to balloon-dilated rabbit arteries with use of a local delivery catheter. J Vasc Interv Radiol 2001; 12:601–5.

17. McKay RG. Site-specific, catheter-based thrombolysis: a new technique for treating intracoronary thrombus and thrombus-containing stenosis. J Invasive Cardiol 1995; 7:36E–43E.

18. Palasis M, Luo Z, Barry JJ, Walsh K. Analysis of adenoviral transport mechanisms in the vessel wall and optimization of gene transfer using local delivery catheters. Hum Gene Ther 2000; 11:237–46.

19. Flugelman MY, Jaklitsch MT, Newman KD, et al. Low level in vivo gene transfer into the arterial wall through a perforated balloon catheter. Circulation 1992; 85:1110–17.

20. Mitchel JF, McKay RG. Treatment of acute stent thrombosis with local urokinase therapy using catheter-based, drug delivery systems: a case report. Catheter Cardiovasc Diagn 1995; 34:149–54.

21. Glazier JJ, Kiernan FJ, Bauer HH, et al. Treatment of thrombotic saphenous vein bypass grafts using local urokinase infusion therapy with the Dispatch catheter. Catheter Cardiovasc Diagn 1997; 41:261–7.

22. Kerensy RA, Franco EA, Bertolet BD, et al. Lysis of intravascular thrombus prior to coronary stenting using the Dispatch infusion catheter. Catheter Cardiovasc Diagn 1996; 38:410–14.

23. Barsness GW, Ohman EM, Berdan LG, et al. Reduced thrombus burden with Abciximab delivered locally before percutaneous intervention in saphenous vein grafts. Am Heart J 2000; 139:824–9.

24. McKay RG, Fram DB, Hirst JA, et al. Treatment of intracoronary thrombus with local urokinase infusion using a new, site-specific drug delivery system: the Dispatch catheter. Catheter Cardiovasc Diagn 1994; 33:181–8.

25. Mitchel JF, Fram DB, Hirst JA, et al. Local dissolution of intracoronary thrombus with urokinase using the Dispatch catheter. J Am Coll Cardiol 1995; 25:348A.

6

The Remedy™ PTCA dilatation infusion catheter

Wendy Naimark and James Barry

Introduction • Description • Drug delivery • Conclusions

INTRODUCTION

The Remedy™ balloon catheter, also known as the channeled or multichannel balloon catheter, is a dual-purpose angioplasty and drug delivery catheter. The noncompliant dilatation balloon allows for high pressure angioplasty and is decoupled from the infusion lumen allowing simultaneous low pressure delivery of therapeutic agents. This design eliminates the problems observed with earlier porous infusion balloons which produced jet streams during high pressure delivery and ultimately caused vessel dissection and damage.[1]

The Remedy™ catheter received pre-market approval from the Food and Drug Administration (FDA) in 1999. The intended use was for clinically approved agents, such as heparinized saline and thrombolytic agents. Initial preclinical animal studies were conducted with heparin and proteins.[2–4] The Remedy™ has since been used for preclinical and clinical endolumenal gene delivery.[4–14] Most recently the device has been used in clinical trials to demonstrate that gene transfer of vascular endothelial growth factor (VEGF) for lower limb ischemia is well tolerated.[13]

DESCRIPTION

The Remedy percutaneous transluminal coronary angioplasty (PTCA) dilatation infusion catheter is an over-the-wire, triple lumen catheter with a channeled balloon at the distal tip. One lumen is used for the inflation of the balloon, therapeutic agents are delivered through a second lumen, and the third lumen allows use of a guidewire (≤0.014 in/0.36 mm) to facilitate advancement of the catheter to and through the stenosis to be dilated (Figure 6.1). The drug delivery lumen was designed with a low dead space (0.3–0.5 mL) to minimize agent loss during catheter preparation.

The balloon design consists of 18 channels embedded in the wall that run lengthwise on the balloon (Figure 6.2). The noncompliant polyethylene terephthalate balloon provides an inflatable segment of known diameter and length at recommended inflation pressures. The drug infusion mechanism is independent of the balloon inflation pressure and can be used to achieve low-to-moderate infusion pressures (0–3 atm). Each of the 18 longitudinal channels has one exterior pore that contains clusters of 30–35 μm holes per channel for

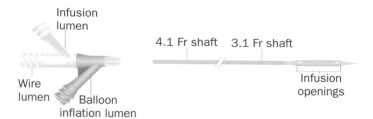

Fig. 6.1 Schematic of the Remedy™ balloon catheter. The proximal portion of the catheter includes a manifold with two side ports, one for balloon inflation and one for infusion, and an end port for use with appropriately sized coronary guidewires.

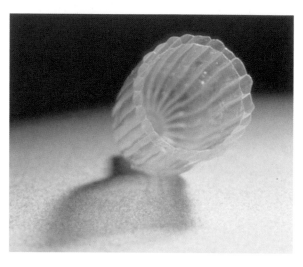

Fig. 6.2 The balloon cross-section. The agent travels through the channels and out the micropores. The low infusion lumen volume minimizes the amount of infusate required to prep the system (0.3–0.5 mL required).

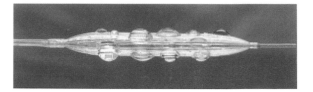

Fig. 6.3 Demonstration of infusate delivery. The agent appears to 'sweat' over the balloon from the micropores spirally configured over the exterior surface of the channels.

The Remedy catheter comes in four sizes (2.5–4.0 mm diameter × 20 mm length). The catheter has also been developed for peripheral delivery applications. The Agent™ catheter, a larger balloon version of the Remedy catheter, was designed for the treatment of lesions at or below the superficial femoral artery; however, the device is no longer being produced. The device was provided in a range of diameters and lengths (3–8 mm × 20, 40, and 100 mm lengths).

DRUG DELIVERY

Preclinical overview

The Remedy catheter has been tested with multiple agents to examine distribution and retention within the targeted vessel wall. In a series of early experiments, Hong and coworkers examined feasibility and efficiency of delivery with a range of agents.[2–4] Using three ex vivo canine peripheral arteries 2 ml of 0.1% methylene blue was infused over 1 min at 2 atm during simultaneous PTCA at 6 atm. The dye was observed to localize within the inner one third of the media.[2] Subsequently, tritiated heparin was used to estimate acute delivery efficiency. Infusions of 2 mL over 1 min at 2 atm or 4 atm during angioplasty (6 atm)

agent infusion. A spiral pattern of pores is uniformly distributed along the entire 20 mm dilatation zone of the balloon to achieve homogeneous local delivery. Solutions are delivered locally by infusion through the channels and out the clusters of holes. The low infusate pressures used for delivery cause the agent to 'sweat' or 'weep' from the external surface (Figure 6.3), as opposed to the jet streaming observed with early porous device designs.[1]

Under fluoroscopy, two radiopaque markers located at the distal and proximal ends of the balloon, aid in the placement of the balloon segment. The mid balloon profile of a wrapped 3.0 mm balloon measures 1.12 mm and the balloon can be rewrapped to a similar low profile after inflation. The device is effective for drug delivery alone or for infusion at PTCA site before or following coronary angioplasty.

resulted in delivery efficiencies from 24 to 48% (calculations were based on the assumption of a theoretical expected delivery).[2] These studies led to an acute in vivo rabbit experiment in which iliac arteries were infused with horse-radish peroxidase and iodonated insulin using the same delivery parameters as above. In this case, delivery zones appeared as both focal and transmural deposits in the excised rabbit iliac arteries.[2] To further characterize device delivery, microspheres were infused into atherosclerotic human necropsy arteries and into atheratomatous rabbit peripheral arteries. Microspheres were detected in all ex vivo arteries and 13 of 17 in vivo arteries at acute harvest. At 24 hours, sacrifice markers were detected in 50% of the arteries; microspheres tended to preferentially distribute within angioplasty-induced dissection planes.[3]

Postangioplasty delivery of the nitric oxide donor, molsidomine, has been shown to improve hemodynamics, wall mechanics, and histomorphometry when delivered locally with the larger diameter channeled balloons of sufficient size for peripheral arterial vessels.[16] Using an atherosclerotic porcine model, molsidomine was delivered to the superficial femoral artery (SFA) subsequent to angioplasty; the agent (2 mg/mL) was delivered over 2 min at a flow rate of 1 mL/min. No acute complications occurred during intra-SFA insertion, deployment infusion or balloon retrieval. In comparison with placebo controls, treatment with molsidomine prevented late lumen loss (mean lumenal diameter: 3.4 ± 0.3 mm vs 2.6 ± 0.3), increased compliance (66 ± 9 vs 11 ± 4 mL/mmHg), and lowered impedance (0.11 ± 0.05 vs 0.45 ± 0.14 mmHg/mL/min) ($p<0.05$ for all comparisons) at 5 months.

Gene therapy preclinical studies

Localized gene therapy for the treatment of vascular disease is a highly active area of study. The design of the Remedy catheter which includes: (1) low deadspace volume to minimize agent loss; (2) low infusion pressures to prevent vessel injury; and (3) spatially homogeneous distribution of infusate makes it a suitable delivery device for this approach. The catheter has been used in a wide range of pre-clinical and clinical gene delivery studies.[5–15]

Adenoviral vectors constructed with either reporter or therapeutic genes have been used to study delivery feasibility, efficiency, and distribution, in addition to efficacy. To understand the parameters influencing adenovirus-mediated gene delivery, Palasis and coworkers undertook a systematic analysis of delivery pressure, time, volume, and adenovirus concentration.[10] The study concluded that viral particle transport into the vessel wall is predominantly a diffusion-dependent event. Consistent with this mechanism, viral concentration was shown to be the key variable for viral transport. To demonstrate this, the Remedy catheter was used to deliver an applied concentration gradient of an adenoviral vector encoding nuclear-targeted β-galactosidase (AdCMVLacZ) in vivo to rabbit iliac arteries. After delivering 500 μL of AdCMVLacZ at three concentrations, 1.7×10^{10}, 5.6×10^{10}, and 1.7×10^{11} plaque forming units (pfu)/mL under 0.1 atm infusion pressure over 2 min, transduction was observed to increase in direct proportion to the increase in viral concentration ($1.8\% \pm 0.04\%$ to $17.8\% \pm 3.2\%$). Histology revealed progressively deeper and greater transfection of the media with the higher concentration of delivered virus (Figure 6.4). Additionally, there was no adverse effect of high virus concentration on cellular density nor were cellular infiltrates detectable upon analysis of hematoxylin and eosin-stained sections.

A number of rabbit and porcine models have been used to demonstrate gene transfer feasibility with the Remedy. Using a porcine coronary model, Varenne and coworkers have reported expression of the luciferase reporter gene after adenovirus-mediated transfection. Transgene expression following infusion from the Remedy catheter was shown to be significantly lower in comparison with other delivery devices.[6] Interestingly, the degree of injury was found to correlate with the level of expression, and may partially account for the differences between groups. Overall, the lowest balloon-to-artery ratios were reported for the Remedy arm of the study.

Yang and coworkers have studied delivery of gadolinium and lentivirus encoding green

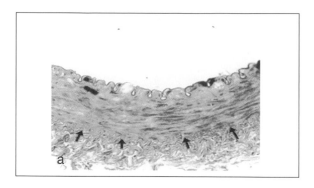

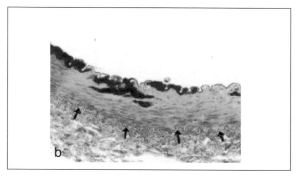

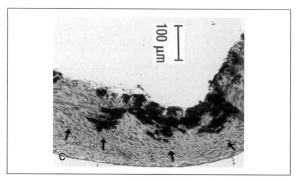

Fig. 6.4 Concentration dependence of gene transfer efficiency. Representative micrographs showing adenovirus-mediated transfer of the β-galactosidase gene as a function of virus concentration after staining with 5-bromo-4-chloro-3-indolyl-β-D-galactopyranoside. (a) 1.7×10^{10} pfu/ml delivered. (b) 5.6×10^{10} pfu/ml delivered. (c) 1.7×10^{11} pfu/ml delivered. β-Galactosidase activity is observed deeper into the media at the higher concentrations of delivered virus relative to the lower concentration. (Reproduced with permission from Palasis et al. Hum Gene Ther 2000; 11:237–46.[14])

fluorescent protein (GFP) under high resolution magnetic resonance imaging (MRI) in porcine femoral and iliac arteries.[9] Using the Remedy catheter outfitted with a 0.014 in intravascular MRI guidewire, a combination of gadolinium and GFP lentivirus was delivered over 10–15 min (10 mL/h). The gadolinium was visualized throughout the vessel and corresponded with GPF expression across the vessel wall.

Adenoviral-mediated transfection of the gene encoding β-galactosidase has been demonstrated in both normal and atherosclerotic rabbit iliac arteries using the Remedy catheter.[4] In normal arteries transgene expression was present in both superficial and deeper cell layers constituting 2% expression efficiency of the medial cells, while only 0.2% was reported for the atherosclerotic vessels. However, since β-galactosidase expression has been previously shown to underestimate transduction efficiency in vivo it is unclear how these findings correlate with efficacious outcomes.[15] Indeed, gene delivery using the Remedy catheter has proven efficacious in a number of animal models.[7,8,10,11] Hiltunen and coworkers have used the catheter to study the effect of adenovirus-mediated transfer of vascular endothelial growth factor (VEGF)-C on intimal thickening in balloon-denuded rabbit aorta.[7] Following a 2 ml delivery of 1.15×10^{10} pfu at 6 atm for 10 min (0.2 ml/min) the VEGF-C group was observed to have significantly less intimal thickness compared with the AdCMVLacZ control group at 2 weeks (Intima/media ratio: 0.38 ± 0.02, VEGF-C vs 0.57 ± 0.04, LacZ) ($p>0.05$). Palasis and coworkers have demonstrated the effectiveness of delivering herpes virus thymidine kinase (TK) using an in-stent restenosis pig femoral artery model.[10] Adenovirus-mediated TK (AdTK) was delivered with the Remedy catheter (5×10^{12} viral particles) followed by stent placement and ganciclovir treatment for 6 days. Vessels were analysed at 21 days and the AdTK group was found to have a significantly lower intima to media area ratio in comparison with the control group (0.29 ± 0.11, AdTK; 0.59 ± 0.01, control); ($p<0.05$).[10]

Atheromatous rabbit iliac models have been used to determine the efficacy of gene-mediated therapies to reduce neointimal formation after stent implantation.[5,8,12] Following angioplasty replication-defective adenovirus encoding the growth arrest homeobox gene (AdCMVGax) was delivered to atherosclerotic vessels using the Remedy catheter.[8] Stents were subsequently deployed at the site of delivery and the vessels were explanted at 1 month. In comparison with saline and adenoviral reporter gene control deliveries, the Gax treated arteries exhibited significantly less neointimal hyperplasia and lumen loss. Using a similar model, Cejna and coworkers have demonstrated adenovirus-mediated delivery and subsequent expression of the antiinflammatory protein IkBa, an inhibitor of nuclear factor kB (NF-kB) reduces neointimal formation following stent placement.[12] Reduction in the levels of systemic expression was reported and further demonstration of the efficacious potential of this approach may be improved with lower volumes of concentrated viral preparations.

Gene therapy clinical studies

In a phase II randomized, placebo-controlled, double blinded study, Makinen et al. used the larger diameter peripheral sized channeled balloon catheters to treat patients with peripheral artery occlusive disease.[13] Patients were divided into three groups receiving either: (1) AdVEGF 165 (2×10^{10} pfu); (2) plasmid-VEGF165/liposome (2 mg VEGF: 2 ml DOTMA: DOPE); or (3) Ringer's lactate. Following angioplasty of femoropopliteal lesions, the catheter was used to deliver the infusate over 10 min (0.5 ml/min). The primary endpoint, digital subtraction angiography, demonstrated that VEGF gene transfer increased vascularity for both groups treated with VEFG at 3 month follow-up. In addition, catheter delivery proved safe and well tolerated with only mild transient edema observed in a few patients in both control and treatment groups. Anti-adenovirus antibodies increased in 61% of the patients treated with AdVEGF. However, no tumors were observed and basic laboratory tests did not reveal any marked differences among the groups.

CONCLUSIONS

The Remedy catheter incorporates a novel combination of safety and delivery performance features. Enhanced intramural safety is achieved by uncoupling high pressure inflation from low pressure drug infusion to prevent vessel wall damage. The dilatation balloon can be inflated to perform coronary angioplasty and post-delivery expansion of balloon expandable stents. The reduced dead space within the lumen minimizes agent loss, particularly important when handling biological therapies. In addition, the spiral patterning of pores over the balloon surface facilitates homogeneous solution distribution against the vessel wall. The channel balloon catheter design has been shown to effectively deliver agents in both coronary and peripheral vascular applications.

REFERENCES

1. Camenzind E, Kutryk JB, Serruys PW. Use of locally delivered conventional drug therapies. Semin Interv Cardiol 1996; 1:67–76.
2. Hong MK, Wong SC, Farb A, et al. Feasibility and drug delivery efficiency of a new balloon angioplasty catheter capable of performing simultaneous local drug delivery. Coron Artery Dis 1993; 4:1023–7.
3. Hong MK, Wong SC, Farb A, et al. Localized drug delivery in atherosclerotic arteries via a new balloon angioplasty catheter with intramural channels for simultaneous local drug delivery. Catheter Cardiovasc Diagn 1995; 34:263–70.
4. Hong MK, Barry JJ, Leon MB. Multichannel balloon catheter. Semin Interv Cardiol 1996; 1:34–5.
5. Feldman LJ, Steg PG, Zheng LP, et al. Low-efficiency of percutaneous adenovirus-mediated arterial gene transfer in the atherosclerotic rabbit. J Clin Invest 1995; 95:2662–71.
6. Varenne O, Gerard RD, Sinnaeve P, et al. Percutaneous adenoviral gene transfer into

porcine coronary arteries: is catheter-based gene delivery adapted to coronary circulation? Hum Gene Ther 1999; 10:1105–15.

7. Hiltunen MO, Laitinen M, Turunen MP, et al. Intravascular adenovirus-mediated VEGF-C gene transfer reduces neointima formation in balloon-denuded rabbit aorta. Circulation 2000; 102:2262–8.

8. Maillard L, Van Belle E, Tio FO, et al. Effect of percutaneous adenovirus-mediated Gax gene delivery to the arterial wall in double-injured atheromatous stented rabbit iliac arteries. Gene Ther 2000; 7:1353–61.

9. Yang X, Atalar E, Dechun L, et al. Magnetic resonance imaging permits in vivo monitoring of catheter-based vascular gene delivery. Circulation 2001; 104:1588–90.

10. Palasis M, Akyurek L, San H, et al. Effective treatment of in-stent restenosis with TkciteGK vectors. Mol Ther 2001; 3:S297.

11. Luo Z, Garron T, Palasis M, et al. Enhancement of Fas ligand-induced inhibition of neointimal formation in rabbit femoral and iliac arteries by coexpression of p35. Hum Gene Ther 2001; 12:2191–202.

12. Cejna M, Breuss JM, Bergmeister H, et al. Inhibition of neointimal formation after stent placement with adenovirus-mediated gene transfer of IkBa in the hypercholesterolemic rabbit model: initial results. Radiology 2002; 223:702–8.

13. Makinen K, Manninen H, Hedman M, et al. Increased vascularity detected by digital subtraction angiography after VEGF gene transfer to human lower limb artery: a randomized, placebo-controlled, double-blinded phase II study. Mol Ther 2002; 6:127–33.

14. Palasis M, Luo Z, Barry JJ, Walsh K. Analysis of adenoviral transport mechanisms in the vessel wall and optimization of gene transfer using local delivery catheters. Hum Gene Ther 2000; 11:237–46.

15. Sata M, Perlman H, Murvue DA, et al. Fas ligand gene transfer to the vessel wall inhibits neointima formation and overrides the adenovirus-mediated T cell response. Proc Natl Acad Sci USA 1998; 95:1213–17.

16. Rolland PH, Bartoli JM, Piquet Ph, et al. Local delivery of NO-donor molsidomine post-PTA improves hemodynamics, wall mechanics and histomorphometry in atherosclerotic porcine SFA. Eur J Vasc Endovasc Surg 2002; 23:226–33.

7

The Infiltrator™ angioplasty balloon catheter

Alexander Popov, Gabor Matos, Herbert Radisch, and Peter Barath

Description • Delivery • Ongoing studies

DESCRIPTION

The Infiltrator™ angioplasty balloon catheter (IABC) consists of a noncompliant positioning balloon and an independently operated infiltration system. The infiltration system built on the balloon surface as three longitudinal channels spaced at 120 degree angles. The articulated roof of the channels consists of a row of seven (0.75 mm × 0.5 mm) individual stainless steel plates embedded in plastic. Each plate has an individual miniature injection nipple with a height of 0.25 mm connected to the channels and eventually, to a common delivery port located at the proximal end of the balloon catheter (Figs 7.1 and 7.2). Upon the inflation of the balloon to 2 atm, the injection nipples penetrate the media of the vessel. At that point, 0.4 ml of fluid can be slowly infiltrated directly into the vessel wall with hand injection.[1]

Technical information

- Manufacturer: Boston Scientific, Inc., San Diego, CA.
- Balloon type: noncompliant over-the-wire or rapid exchange.
- Balloon size (mm): 2.0–4.0 mm with 0.5 mm increment.
- Crossing profile (mm): 0.135.

- Balloon working length (mm): 15.
- Positioning radiopaque markers.
- Shaft diameter (Fr): 4.2.
- Shaft length (cm): 127.
- Recommended inflation pressure (atm): 2.
- Recommended balloon/artery ratio: 1:1, or minimally oversized.
- Injection nipple height (mm): 0.25.

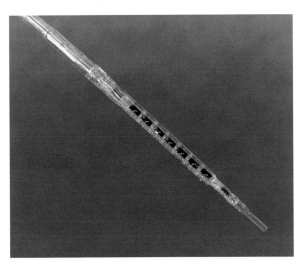

Fig. 7.1 A deflated Infiltrator™ angioplasty balloon catheter (IABC). Note two radiopaque markers and seven individual plates with miniature infiltration nipples. The individual plates are embedded in plastic to form the roof of three delivery channels.

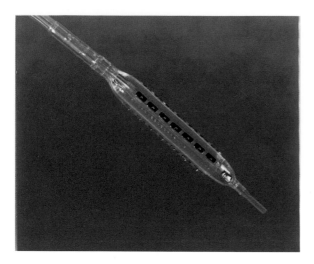

Fig. 7.2 An inflated Infiltrator™. The three delivery channels with the three rows of the delivery nipples are visible on the balloon surface.

- Recommended delivery method/amount (ml): slow hand infiltration/0.4.
- Regulatory status: EC Mark, master file with the Food and Drug Administration (FDA).

DELIVERY

Procedure

The recommended 0.4 ml of fluid represents the approximate volume of a 15 mm long infiltrated vessel wall segment. Delivering this amount of fluid does not cause significant histological damage or subacute intimal proliferation in pigs,[1,3] rabbit,[4] or angiographic changes in human.[2] The fluid is homogenously distributed in the infiltrated segment within 10 minutes as detected histologically after rhodamine tracer infiltration in pigs,[1] or with intravascular ultrasound after ethanol infiltration in human.[5] Occasionally, transient intramural fluid accumulation (hematoma?) was detected if the infiltrated fluid amount was doubled with IVUS.[5]

Efficiency

The device delivers the fluid directly into the media with high specificity and achieved 88.2% delivery efficiency as defined as the percentage of the delivered activity detectable by gamma camera immediately after infiltration of technetium-99 (^{99}Tc)-labeled sulfurcolloid.[1] In a comparative study, the delivery efficiency was found 50 times over that of the hydrogel balloon.[6] Without a proper carrier, however, the infiltrated fluid diffuses into the perivascular region and later, into the circulation.[1] On the other hand, if a proper carrier is used (e.g. hexamethyl propylenamine oxime – Ceretec) after a 15-min washout period in which about 30% of the original activity is lost, there is no further loss of the injected fluid for hours as detected with ^{99}Tc-labeled Ceretec.[7]

Site-specific delivery in animals and humans

The device is successfully used for high efficiency delivery of low molecular weight

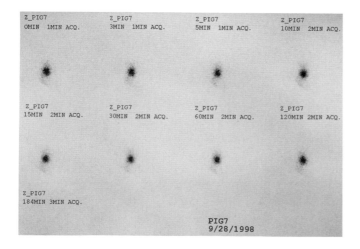

Fig. 7.3 An experiment in which 500 μCi of ^{99}Tc-labeled Ceretec was infiltrated into the coronary artery of a pig. The activity was detected with a gamma camera over the closed chest at 0, 3, 5, 10, 15, 30, 60, 120, and 180 min (scintigram shown starting at 15 min). Since the Ceretec is bound to the smooth muscle cells of the vessel wall within 10 min, there is only minimal decrease in the activity after the 15 min washout period.

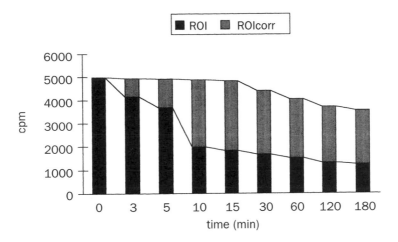

Fig. 7.4 Changes of the counts per minute (cpm) by time as detected with gamma camera in the experiment shown in Fig. 7.3 after infiltration of 500 μCi of ^{99}Tc-labeled Ceretec in the region of interest (ROI). The total height of each bar shows the expected activity corrected to the half-life of ^{99}Tc without washout effect (ROIcorr). The black segment of the bar shows the actual cpm. Note the early fast decrease in the activity due to the washout but after 15 minutes the expected and actual cpm become parallel suggesting that the activity loss is due to the decay of the isotope and not to further washout.

Table 7.1 Half-life corrected residual activity in the vessel wall*

Time (min)	Total (%)	Roi (%)
0	100	100
5	89	72 ± 9
15	80	58 ± 13
30	75	53 ± 12
60	72	50 ± 13
120	67	46 ± 14
180	65	45 ± 13

* In percentage of the original counts per minute (cpm) in the total detected area (Total %) and in the region of interest (ROI %). The averages of 15 pig experiments show the rapid early decrease of the cpm (washout) and the flattened cpm (specific binding after IABC infiltration into the vessel wall).

heparin,[2] heparin,[6] genes,[3,4,7,8] as well as natriuretic peptide in animals.[9] With an activity of 2 mCi of ^{99}Tc using the Ceretec system, the IABC is able to deliver an absorbed radiation dose of 28 Gy that is considered effective in preventing restenosis (Figs 7.3, 7.4, and Table 7.1).[7] In humans, 15–20% ethanol infiltration seems to be promising in preventing in-stent restenosis but larger randomized trials did not support the effectiveness of alcohol.[5,10]

Recent animal and human studies

Nitric oxide synthase (NOS) gene delivery experiments with the Infiltrator: Using a liposome carrier, the NOS gene significantly reduced the plaque area in an in-stent femoral artery (from 40.85 to 24.69 mm², $p=0.03$) and in an in-stent coronary artery model (by 45% from 4.0 to 2.2 mm², $p<0.01$).[11] Using an adenovirus carrier, also significantly reduced neointimal formation in a porcine coronary artery in-stent model (from 3.41 to 1.12 mm², p<0.05).[12]

The apolipoprotein A-IMilano/phospholipid complex ETC-216 delivered by the Infiltrator increased the lumen area from 2.1 (control) to 3.7 mm² (treated) in a in-stent coronary artery model.[13]

The advanced antisense c-*myc* oligonucleotide (Resten-NG) delivered without carrier from the Infiltrator reduced the neointima formation in a dose-dependent way: 3.88 mm² (control), 2.01 mm² and 1.95 mm² (5 and 10 mg, respectively), in a porcine coron-ary in-stent model.[14] In a recent multicenter human trial with the Infiltrator using the same antisense probe (AVI-4126) the target vessel revascularization at 6 month was 33.3 in the control and 7.1% in the 10 mg dose group; the binary restenosis rate was reduced from 33.3 and 8.3%, respectively.[15]

REFERENCES

1. Barath P, Popov A, Dillehay GL, et al. Infiltrator angioplasty balloon catheter: a device for combined angioplasty and intramural site-specific treatment. Catheter Cardiovasc Diagn 1997; 41:333–41.

2. Pavlides GS, Barath P, Maginas A, et al. Intramural drug delivery by direct injection within the arterial wall: first clinical experience with a novel intracoronary delivery – infiltrator system. Catheter Cardiovasc Diagn 1997; 41:287–92.

3. Varenne O, Gerard RD, Sinnaeve P, et al. Percutaneous adenoviral gene transfer into porcine coronary arteries: is catheter-based gene delivery adapted to coronary circulation? Hum Gene Ther 1999; 10:1105–15.

4. Teiger E, Deprez I, Dupouy P, et al. Local gene delivery within the media of rabbit iliac arteries by using the Infiltrator intramural delivery device. J Cardiovasc Pharmacol 1999; 33:726–32.

5. Liu MW, Alred D, Maehara A, et al. Safety study of coronary intramural ethyl alcohol delivery in reduction intimal hyperplasia after successful coronary stenting. Am J Cardiol 2000; 86(suppl 8A):25.

6. Mitchel JF, Fram DB, Gillam LD, et al. Enhanced local intracoronary delivery of heparin with the Infiltrator catheter: a comparative study. J Invasive Cardiol 1999; 11:463–70.

7. Barath P, Popov A, Gerlach J, et al. Uptake, retention dynamics and absorbed doses of 99m Technetium labeled hexamethyl propylenamine oxime (Ceretec) after intramural delivery with the Infiltrator/Irradiator Angioplasty Balloon Catheter. Circulation 1999; 100 (suppl I):306.

8. Varenne O, Pislaru S, Gillijns H, et al. Local adenovirus-mediated transfer of human endothelial nitric oxide synthetase reduces luminal narrowing after coronary angioplasty in pigs. Circulation 1998; 98:919–26.

9. Morishige K, Shimokawa H, Yamawaki T, et al. Local adenovirus-mediated transfer of C-type natriuretic peptide suppresses vascular remodeling in porcine coronary arteries in vivo. J Am Coll Cardiol 2000; 35:1040–7.

10. Fry JA, Michael J, Curran MJ, et al. Local drug delivery of intramural ethyl alcohol for treatment of diffuse in-stent restenosis: the Beaumont Alcohol Restenosis Study (BARS). JACC 2001; 86:Abstract.

11. Muhs A, Heublein B, Schletter J et al. Preclinical evaluation of inducible nitric oxide synthase lipoplex gene therapy for inhibition of stent-induced vascular neointimal lesion formation. Hum Gene Ther 2003; 14:375–83.

12. Wang K, Kessler PD, Zhou Z et al. Local adenoviral-mediated inducible nitric oxide synthase gene transfer inhibits neointimal formation in the porcine coronary stented model. Mol Ther 2003; 5:597–603.

13. Kaul S, Rushkin V, Santos R et al. Intramural delivery of recombinant apolipoprotein A-Imilano/phospholipid complex (ETC-216) inhibits in-stent stenosis in porcine coronary arteries. Circulation 2003; 107:2551–4.

14. Kipshidze NN, Kim HS, Iversen P et al. Intramural coronary delivery of advanced antisense oligonucleotides reduces neointimal formation in the porcine stent restenosis model. J Am Coll Cardiol 2002; 39:1686–91.

15. Kipshidze NN for AVAIL Study group: First human experience with local delivery on novel antisense AVI-4126 with Infiltrator Catheter in de novo native and restenotic coronary arteries: six month clinical and angiographic follow-up from AVAIL Study. Circulation 2004; 110 (suppl 17):pp757.

8

The Infiltrator™ local drug delivery catheter

Peter Sinnaeve and Stefan Janssens

Introduction • Drug delivery • Gene therapy • Future perspectives

INTRODUCTION

The Infiltrator™ delivery catheter takes a unique place among various types of local drug delivery catheters. It is a mechanical, intramural delivery catheter, in contrast to the majority of delivery catheters, which are in nature diffusion catheters. Whereas several other local drug delivery catheters are capable of delivering a substance intramurally or transmurally,[1] the Infiltrator™ has the unique feature to also serve as an angioplasty balloon catheter. The Infiltrator™ device consists of a delivery port and a 15 mm noncompliant balloon with an independent inflation port, and with a rated burst pressure of 8 atm. Because the crossing profile is 0.064 inches, an 8 Fr guiding catheter is required. The delivery port is connected through three U-shaped troughs with three metallic strips spaced at 120 degree angles on the surface of the balloon, each comprising seven injector nipples. Upon inflation of the balloon to a support pressure of 2 atm, the nipples extend radially and penetrate the medial layer of the vessel wall, allowing precise and direct injection of a substance in the vessel wall. The catheter's dead space needs to be preloaded with approximately 0.7 mL of infusate. The balloon can then be positioned over the target lesion, inflated to 2 atm after which 0.2 to 0.4 mL infusate can be delivered manually over 10 to 30 seconds.

DRUG DELIVERY

First developed by Barath,[2] the Infiltrator catheter has been successfully used and tested in porcine,[2] and human,[3] coronary arteries. In preclinical trials, the feasibility and safety of the catheter was tested in 117 normal porcine coronary arteries. Efficiency of local intramural delivery of technetium-99 (^{99}Tc)-labeled heparin was shown to be one order of magnitude higher than that of conventional diffusion-based or convection-based catheters.[4] In porcine coronary arteries, fluorescein-labeled heparin was detected throughout the vessel wall after delivery with the Infiltrator, with higher levels at the site of injection ports.[5]

In a first feasibility trial in 17 patients, low molecular weight heparin was injected intramurally using the Infiltrator after conventional balloon angioplasty.[3] In 10 of these patients, local drug delivery was followed by stenting because of suboptimal results after angioplasty. Residual stenosis was obviously not significantly altered by the local drug injection in this small study, but the hospital course was uneventful for all patients.

Subsequently, the Infiltrator catheter has been used for delivery of a variety of agents, mainly in protocols aimed at preventing restenosis after angioplasty. Local drug delivery of long-acting steroids followed by coronary stenting did not reduce the angiographic restenosis rate and the incidence of target lesion revascularization in 36 lesions in 24 patients.[6] In this study the investigators were unable to cross the lesions on four occasions (4 out of 40 lesions). In another study in 18 patients, varying concentrations of alcohol solutions (5%, 10%, 15%) were injected after balloon dilatation of de novo lesions, followed by stent deployment. Local delivery of alcohol resulted in a dose-dependent decrease in in-stent neointimal area as measured by intracoronary ultrasound.[7] All the above protocols are uncontrolled, small scale studies and warrant larger placebo-controlled randomized trials to identify potential clinical benefit.

The Infiltrator catheter has also been used for intramural delivery of radioisotopes,[8] an approach for which the device was temporarily referred to as the 'Irradiator catheter'. Intramural or 'intratissular' radiation with radioactive oligonucleotides resulted in a significant reduction of neointima formation after balloon injury in porcine coronary arteries.[9] Although initial results are encouraging, the variability of delivery efficiency and the potential systemic delivery of radioactive substances warranted further assessment of safety of this delivery modality.

Finally, the Infiltrator catheter was also used to locally deliver small amounts of thrombolytic drug to recanalize deep venous thrombosis in porcine iliac veins. Residual thrombus burden was significantly lower using the Infiltrator catheter compared to local infusion using a multisideport-wire.[10] This approach might be a valuable alternative for severe or refractory deep vein thromboses.

GENE THERAPY

Gene therapy, in principle, is an attractive alternative treatment for vasculoproliferative diseases, because it allows direct molecular interventions of complex restenotic processes and therefore may provide a biological solution to an in essence biological problem. However, local gene delivery at the very site of injury via conventional interventional techniques remains the Achilles' heel of vascular gene therapy because of low transfection efficacy. The Infiltrator catheter has been used in various local vascular gene transfer protocols because it allows rapid delivery without additional excessive injury to the target lesion. Furthermore, unlike diffusion catheters, the Infiltrator catheter can target the complete vascular wall including the adventitia. Preflushing with a serum albumin solution might be necessary to avoid inactivation of adenovirus vector infectivity.[11]

In a comparative study, the Infiltrator catheter was compared with three intramural pressure-driven catheters in a porcine coronary artery balloon angioplasty model.[12] Expression levels of the reporter gene encoding firefly luciferase and the distribution pattern of transgene products using the Infiltrator catheter compared favorably to results obtained with diffusion-type catheters. Using the Infiltrator catheter, local adenovirus-mediated overexpression of endothelial nitric oxide synthase (NOS3) or C-type natriuretic peptide (CNP), both vasodilators and inhibitors of vascular smooth muscle cell proliferation and migration, were shown to significantly reduce neointima formation after percutaneous transluminal coronary angioplasty (PTCA) in porcine coronary arteries.[13,14] The Infiltrator catheter was subsequently used to compare different genetic strategies to reduce intimal proliferation in the same animal model. Local gene transfer of NOS3 and thymidine kinase, but not of plasminogen activator inhibitor 1, resulted in significantly less neointima formation.[15] In this study, no acute systemic toxicity or viral shedding was observed, underscoring the *local* nature of gene transfer using a mechanical intramural delivery device, such as the Infiltrator. Finally, the Infiltrator catheter was also successfully used for local gene delivery in the prevention of in-stent stenosis.[16] Whether the current profile of this catheter will allow safe and effective gene transfer in in-stent neointima remains to be determined.

FUTURE PERSPECTIVES

The Infiltrator catheter has several characteristics that may provide a promising platform for local drug or gene delivery. In contrast with many other drug delivery devices, the vascular occlusion time is very short and the delivery volumes are small, thus reducing inadvertent distal spreading of genes and gene transfer vectors. Furthermore, in experimental studies, the catheter does not appear to cause additional injury to the targeted lesions. Several protocols also suggest that its use is both feasible and safe in patients. However, further refinement of the catheter's profile seems warranted to optimize its application in a broader spectrum of coronary lesions. In this respect, feasibility and safety of drug or gene delivery using the Infiltrator catheter to target in-stent neointimal hyperplasia remains to be demonstrated.

REFERENCES

1. Gonschior P, Goetz AE, Huehns TY, Hofling B. A new catheter for prolonged local drug application. Coron Artery Dis 1995; 6(4):329–34.
2. Barath P, Popov A, Dillehay GL, Matos G, et al. Infiltrator angioplasty balloon catheter: a device for combined angioplasty and intramural site-specific treatment. Catheter Cardiovasc Diagn 1997; 41(3):333–41.
3. Pavlides GS, Barath P, Maginas A, et al. Intramural drug delivery by direct injection within the arterial wall: first clinical experience with a novel intracoronary delivery-Infiltrator system. Catheter Cardiovasc Diagn 1997; 41(3):287–92.
4. Camenzind E, Bakker W, Van Harskamp E, et al. First quantification of intramural heparin delivery in man using the nipple catheter

(Infiltrator) following coronary balloon angioplasty. Circulation 1997; 96(8):I–527.
5. Mitchel JF, Fram DB, Gillam LD, et al. Enhanced local intracoronary delivery of heparin with the Infiltrator catheter: a comparative study. J Invasive Cardiol 1999; 11(8):463–70.
6. Reimers B, Moussa I, Akiyama T, et al. Persistent high restenosis after local intrawall delivery of long-acting steroids before coronary stent implantation. J Invase Cardiol 1998; 10:323–31.
7. Liu M, Alred D, Maehara A, et al. Safety study of coronary intramural ethyl alcohol delivery in reducing intimal hyperplasia after successful coronary stenting. Am J Cardiol 2000; 86(8A):25i.
8. Waksman R, Chan RC, Kim W, et al. Injection of radionuclides to the coronary arterial wall: 'hot arteries' a novel vascular brachytherapy approach to reduce restenosis. Circulation 1998; 98(17):I–652.
9. Fareh J, St-Jacques P, Martel R, Leclerc G. Combining local drug delivery and radiation therapy: efficacy of intratissular delivery of a radiopharmaceutical agent to prevent restenosis after balloon angioplasty in the swine. International LDDR 2001; 1(suppl):11.
10. Roy S, Laerum F, Brosstad F, et al. Selective venous thrombolysis with the nipple-balloon catheter: a comparative evaluation in vivo. JVIR 1999; 10:817–24.
11. Marshall DJ, Palasis M, Lepore JJ, Leiden JM. Biocompatibility of cardiovascular gene delivery catheters with adenovirus vectors: an important determinant of the efficiency of cardiovascular gene transfer. Mol Ther 2000; 1 (5 pt 1):423–9.
12. Varenne O, Gerard R, Sinnaeve P, et al. Percutaneous adenoviral gene transfer into porcine coronary arteries: is catheter-based gene delivery adapted to coronary circulation? Hum Gene Ther 1999; 10(7):1105–15.
13. Morishige K, Shimokawa H, Yamawaki T, et al. Local adenovirus-mediated transfer of C-type natriuretic peptide suppresses vascular remodeling in porcine coronary arteries in vivo. J Am Coll Cardiol 2000; 35(4):1040–7.
14. Varenne O, Pislaru S, Gillijns H, et al. Local adenovirus-mediated transfer of human endothelial

nitric oxide synthase reduces luminal narrowing after coronary angioplasty in pigs. Circulation 1998; 98(9):919–26.

15. Varenne O, Sinnaeve P, Gillijns H, et al. Percutaneous gene therapy using recombinant adenoviruses encoding human herpes simplex virus thymidine kinase, human PAI-1, and human NOS3 in balloon-injured porcine coronary arteries. Hum Gene Ther 2000; 11(9):1329–39.

16. Varenne O, Sinnaeve P, Gillijns H, et al. Adenoviral mediated NOS3 gene transfer in porcine coronary arteries reduces in stent restenosis. J Am Coll Cardiol 1999; 33(2)(suppl A):59A (abstract).

9

The needle catheter

Sigrid Nikol, Berthold Höfling, Juan Granada, Klaus Pels, and Tanya Y Huehns

Introduction • Description • Distribution of drugs • Safety • Delivery of therapy
• Atherosclerotic plaques • Conclusions • Acknowledgment

INTRODUCTION

In this chapter, we describe the needle catheter, an arterial delivery catheter developed in collaboration with a local company (Bavaria Medizin Technologie, Oberpfaffenhofen, Germany).[1]

The aim of designing a catheter from first principles was to achieve local delivery within the artery wall with minimal systemic delivery. The catheter was specifically created to deliver agents to the perivascular tissue, in the hope that this would circumvent some of the technical problems of previously designed local drug delivery catheters, where low local drug concentration and a large systemic leak were disadvantages.[2]

Mechanical delivery of drugs or gene therapy through the arterial wall is an elegant method of depositing active substances perivascularly. Such an approach avoids many of the difficulties encountered with prototype local drug delivery devices developed from standard angioplasty balloons. Increasing evidence of the pathophysiological role of the adventitia and perivascular tissue in restenosis supports the need to target this space.[3,4] Adventitial delivery is therefore a novel form of delivery with the added benefit of creating a local depot of active agent.

DESCRIPTION

The needle catheter has a 4.5 Fr shaft diameter (Figure 9.1). The shaft material is a braided polyimide, with a flexible polyamide portion at the distal end. The shaft is marked for accurate placement within the artery and has a usable length of 135 cm. There are three needles inside the catheter which can be expanded by pushing a stepped piston at the proximal end. The angle between the needles is 120 degrees, therefore, a circumferential treatment is possible. The needles each have an overall diameter of 250 μm and a maximum expansion diameter of 10 mm. The diameter of each needle is thus smaller than that of the smallest insulin needle. The needle catheter has a rapid exchange design, which allows the catheter to run on a 0.014 inch guidewire. This catheter may therefore be used for both peripheral and coronary applications.

For insertion of the catheter into an artery, the needles remain completely enclosed within a metal housing at the distal, or injection, end of the catheter. When the catheter tip is at the site for delivery, the needles can be extended from their position within the metal housing and penetrate the arterial wall. The needles are preshaped and bevelled for ease of entry. The

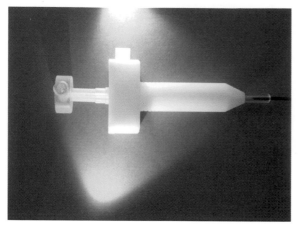

a

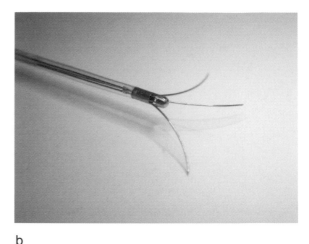

b

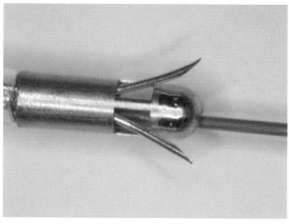

c

Fig. 9.1 The needle injection local delivery catheter. (a) Apparatus for needle extension. A syringe is connected for drug delivery at the circular port situated on the left at the distal end. (b) The catheter tip at the right-hand side of the catheter. Three needles are extended. The needles can be extended by a mechanism operated step-wise outside the body at the distal end. (c) Close up of the catheter tip with the three bevelled needles extended around a central guidewire. Each needle is 31 G, which is smaller in diameter than the smallest needles used for insulin injection. (Reproduced courtesy of Bavaria Medizin Technlogie, Oberpfaffenhofen, Germany.)

needles are extended by the operator who uses a handle mechanism at the other, proximal, end of the catheter.

The needles are prefilled with the drug or other material until this drips from the needles. When the needles are extended and are in place for injection, a syringe with the agent is connected by the operator to the injection port sited at the distal end, outside the body. While the needles remain within the tissue, the operator slowly injects the drug, or other material being tested, into the three needles, so that the drug is injected into perivascular tissue. After local delivery, the operator allows the needles to return to the housing fully and the catheter can be withdrawn without further damaging the artery.

DISTRIBUTION OF DRUGS

The needle catheter has been tested in vivo in porcine arteries. Lipids, dyes, photosensitive substances, drugs, and genes have all been used to locate deposited agents after needle catheter delivery. These studies show that the delivered substance can be located in all vessel layers and surrounding tissues three weeks after injection and in some segments up to five months.[5–11] There is gradual redistribution of a drug from the adventitia to the media and intima. Successful delivery of expression vector plasmids, and expression of the transferred genes at the messenger RNA and protein synthesis levels can be demonstrated after liposome-mediated gene delivery.[7–11]

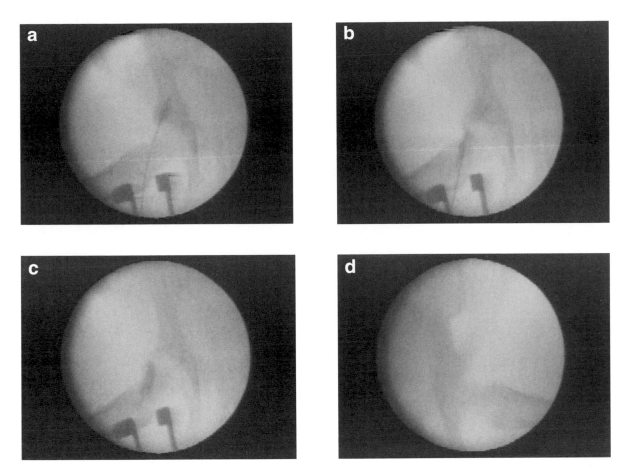

Fig. 9.2 Distribution of contrast injected into perivascular tissue with the needle catheter from within the iliac artery. (a) The needle catheter has been inserted via an opening in the femoral artery under direct vision, and passed proximally 7 cm into the iliac artery. Radio-opaque contrast has been injected into perivascular tissue via the needle catheter. It shows up in an oval measuring about 2.5 cm × 1.5 cm. (b) The needle catheter has been withdrawn 3.5 cm and contrast has been injected again at a second more distal injection site. (c) Picture taken at 60 min following injection. The contrast remains around the artery at one site. (d) No contrast is seen on the contralateral control side at 60 min or at any time after injection. (From Huehns et al., unpublished data.)

In iliac and coronary arteries, delivery of a dye or radio-opaque contrast shows that the infusion reaches local perivascular tissue up to about 1.5 cm from the injection site (Figure 9.2).[5,6] Between 3% and 10% of a radiolabeled dose of carvedilol remains after 30 minutes in the perivascular tissue and there are significant counts in the artery up to 4 hours after injection.[12]

SAFETY

Previously described local drug delivery devices have commonly been shown to create their own additional injury through the delivery process. It was particularly important to examine this question for the needle catheter, as the needles clearly must penetrate the arterial wall for delivery.

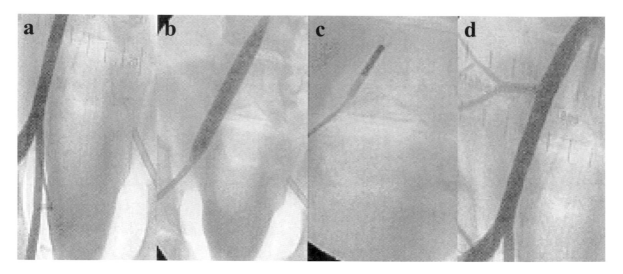

Fig. 9.3 Contrast studies to examine the patency of the iliac artery after balloon injury and needle catheter injection. This study was carried out in a normal pig. The femoral artery was exposed on the right-hand side. (a) Contrast injected via a catheter placed in a surgically created opening in the distal femoral artery. The artery is smooth-walled and clearly outlined by the contrast, visualized by the image intensifier. (b) The balloon catheter is inserted through the femoral artery opening, directed into the iliac artery and filled with contrast to expand it to the injury pressure. (c) After withdrawal of the balloon catheter, the needle catheter is inserted through the same opening. The needles are extended, penetrating the arterial wall. (d) The needle catheter is withdrawn. Contrast is injected via a catheter in the distal femoral artery as in (a). The artery remains smooth-walled. There is no evidence of any local dissection, thrombus or leakage from the needle holes. (Reproduced with permission from Gene Ther 1999; **6**: 637–48.[7])

Angiograms taken immediately following needle injection show no leakage of contrast through the site of the needle holes and no local thrombus, dissection or hematoma (Figure 9.3). There is no evidence of long-term damage, and there is healing without detectable scarring or intimal hyperplasia. The lack of local effects related to the needles is a result of the extremely ultra-thin fine, sharp needles employed, so that the holes are atraumatic and presumably rapidly plugged by blood products.

Following needle catheter reporter gene delivery, no plasmid or gene product is found in untransfected organs (Figure 9.4), and no plasmid can be measured in blood samples (Figure 9.5). In contrast, the same dose of a reporter gene injected directly into the systemic circulation via a peripheral vein resulted in plasmid detection in the blood after administration (Figure 9.5).[7]

DELIVERY OF THERAPY

Photodynamic therapy may work to prevent restenosis by producing free radicals. A photosensitizer delivered with the needle catheter, followed by a locally delivered activating light source, reduces intimal hyperplasia in a porcine model.[13]

Local gene therapy might be one way of targeting restenosis in a site-specific manner.[7–9,14–17] A reporter gene delivered with the needle catheter can transfect smooth muscle cells in the arterial wall after balloon injury, with individual transfected cells in all arterial wall layers, including the newly formed intimal hyperplasia. Local gene therapy might also be another way to induce therapeutic angiogenesis in a percutaneous transluminal fashion as an alternative to the widely used intramuscular delivery.[10,11,18]

Several studies have investigated the use of the needle catheter to deliver potentially

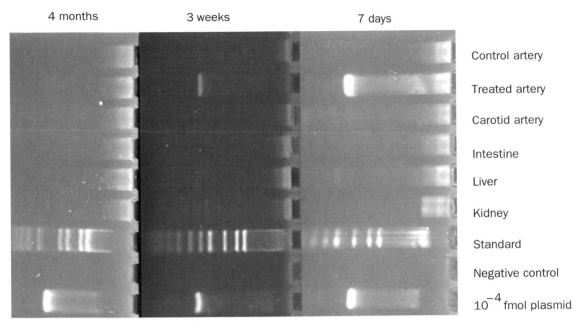

Fig. 9.4 Detection of plasmid DNA in arterial tissue and other organs. Results are from polymerase chain reaction (PCR) on homogenized tissue segments. Total DNA was isolated from arterial segments and organs or blood obtained from pigs 7 days, 21 days or 4 months after treatment with the gene for pre-pro-cecropin A or control. Only the treated artery shows the presence of plasmid DNA at 7 days, 21 days, and 4 months. No organs or untreated arteries indicate the presence of plasmid DNA. (Reproduced with permission from Gene Ther 1999; **6**:637–48.[7])

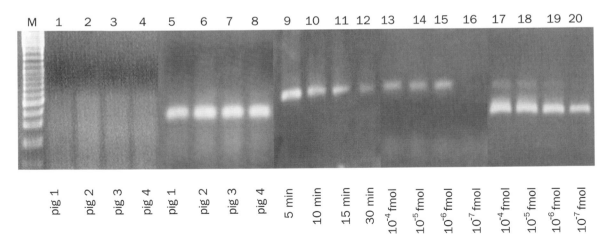

Fig. 9.5 Detection of plasmid DNA in peripheral blood samples after local or systemic gene delivery. Blood samples were analysed by polymerase chain reaction (PCR) after the same dose of plasmid had been administered locally via the needle catheter or systemically into a vein. *Local delivery* did not demonstrate contamination of blood with plasmid at 5, 10, 15 or 30 min after administration (lanes 1–4). In the same DNA preparations, a 398 base pair (bp) DNA fragment corresponding to the sequence for GAPDH (a control sequence always present) could be amplified (lanes 5–8). *Systemic delivery* demonstrated contamination of blood with a PCR product of 647 bp, corresponding to the administered plasmid, at each of the same time points (lanes 9–12). In the same samples, the 398 bp DNA fragment corresponding to the sequence for GAPDH was consistently seen after amplification (lanes 17–20). Control plasmid was added to blood samples in vitro in defined amounts (10^{-4}–10^{-7} fmol) to establish detectable levels (lanes 13–16). (M, 100 bp ladder.) (Reproduced with permission from Gene Ther 1999; **6**:637–48.[7])

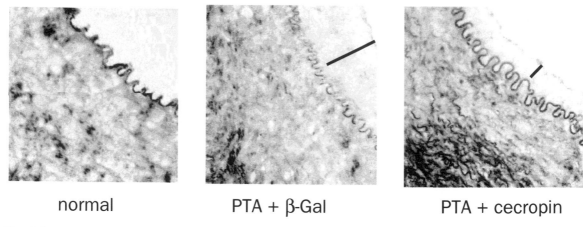

normal   PTA + β-Gal   PTA + cecropin

Fig. 9.6 Inhibition of restenosis formation following periarterial gene transfer. Formation of neointima was significantly reduced folowing application of the cecropin gene via the needle catheter. Results after 3 weeks. *Left*: normal control. *Centre*: control using the β-galactosidase reporter gene. *Right*: use of the therapeutic cecropin gene. Note the bar indicating neointima formation after 21 days. (Reproduced with permission from Gene Ther 1999; **6**:637–48.[7])

therapeutic genes to injured arteries in vivo. Increasing proteins that activate the cell cycle and therefore increase cell proliferation achieved a biological effect. This was attained by administration of the antisense to a gene for a negatively regulating protein, SDI-1 (Senescent cell-Derived Inhibitor-1), which increased cell proliferation in transfected cells.[8]

Intimal hyperplasia after injury was attenuated with the gene for the homeobox growth arrest protein Gax (Growth Arrest-specific homeoboX),[6] and was significantly reduced with the gene for the immature form of a cytostatic peptide, Cecropin A, a protein with a bystander effect (Figure 9.6).[7] This effect was more prominent when plasmid DNA was complexed with novel liposomes under optimized conditions, with comparable results to viral gene transfer.[9,16,17]

Following the establishment of an interventional occlusion model,[19] the catheter has been used to induce angiogenesis at the site of vessel occlusion through local gene delivery. A tenth of the vascular endothelial growth factor (VEGF) plasmid DNA dose used in clinical trials with intramuscular delivery was sufficient to achieve increases in collateralization (Figures 9.7–9.10).[10,11,18] The local approach makes unwanted side effects less likely.

The needle injection catheter has been also used to study the safety of angiogenic gene therapy in an established porcine coronary balloon angioplasty model. The effect of local (peri)adventitial transfer of the $VEGF_{165}$ gene was investigated under conditions comparable to those used in primarily successful human angiogenic gene therapy trials: following the induction of mechanical coronary lesions and susequent gene transfer, intima and media lesion formation and microvessel angiogenesis were evaluated. The results demonstrated that $VEGF_{165}$ gene transfer into the outer compartments of coronary arteries induces adventitial angiogenesis but does not promote intima and media microvessel angiogenesis nor accelerates vascular thickening/ intima and media growth (Figure 9.11).[20] Moreover, Pels et al. demonstrated that local (peri)adventitial $VEGF_{165}$ gene transfer after coronary artery angioplasty induces positive remodeling associated with an increase of neoadventitial vascularization (unpublished data).

ATHEROSCLEROTIC PLAQUES

High risk non-stenotic atherosclerotic plaques have become a clinical target for the practicing

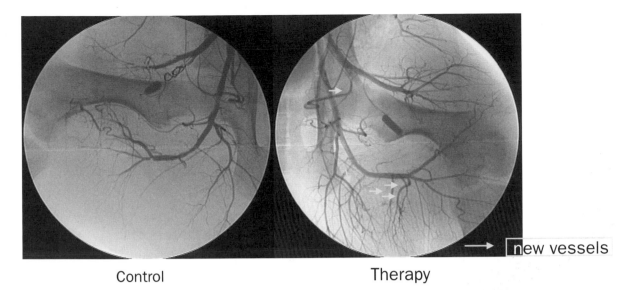

Control   Therapy

Fig. 9.7 Periarterial gene delivery of pVEGF$_{165}$. Gene delivery in pigs: application of 2 ml, 133 μg DNA complexed 1:10 with DOCSPER liposomes following interventional occlusion of the superficial femoral artery. Angiogram 5 months following delivery. *Left*: control using the β-galactosidase gene. *Right*: therapeutic delivery using the VEGF$_{165}$ plasmid. Arrow marks newly formed vessels. (Reproduced with permission from J Endovasc Ther 2002; 9:842–54[11] © International Society of Endovascular Specialists.)

VEGF   pCMVß (control)

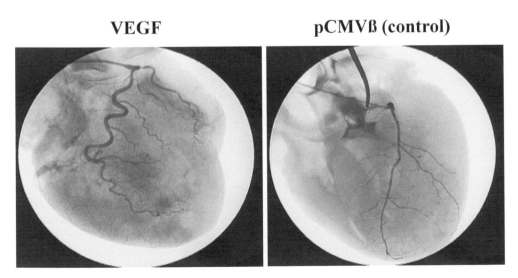

Fig. 9.8 Pericoronary gene delivery of pVEGF$_{165}$. Gene delivery in pigs: Application of 2 ml, 133 μg DNA complexed 1:10 with DOCSPER liposomes following interventional occlusion of the circumflex coronary artery. Angiogram 5 months following delivery. *Left*: control using the β-galactosidase gene. *Right*: theraptic delivery using the VEGF$_{165}$ plasmid. Note the elongation and enlargement of the remaining coronary artery (LAD). (Reproduced with permission from J Endovasc Ther 2002; **9**:842–54[11] © International Society of Endovascular Specialists.)

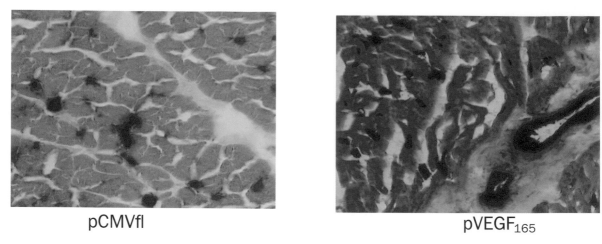

Fig. 9.9 Capillary density following adventitial coronary application of pVEGF$_{165}$. Using alkaline phosphatase staining, there was a marked increase in capillary density in the myocardium following pVEGF$_{165}$ application via the needle catheter 5 months following adventitial gene transfer. *Left*: control using the β-galactosidase gene. *Right*: transfer of the VEGF$_{165}$ gene. Capillaries are dark stained. (Reproduced with permission from J Endovasc Ther 2002; **9**:842–54[11] © International Society of Endovascular Specialists.)

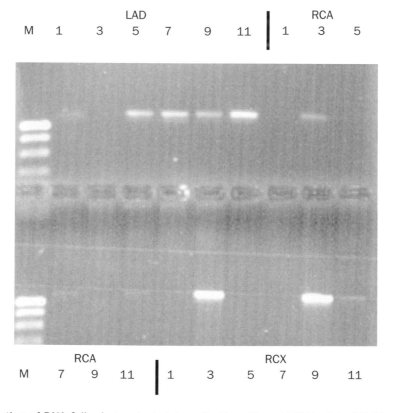

Fig. 9.10 Detection of DNA following periarterial application. Plasmid DNA of the VEGF$_{165}$ gene applied via the needle catheter was detectable for at least 5 months surrounding coronary arteries. (Reproduced with permission from J Endovasc Ther 2002; **9**:842–54[11] © International Society of Endovascular Specialists.)

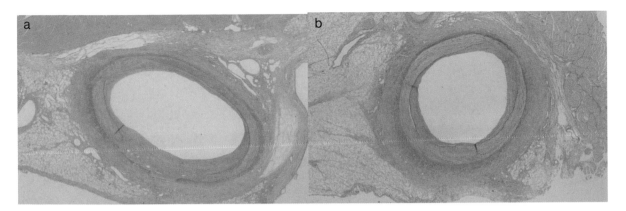

Fig. 9.11 Histomorphology of VEGF$_{165}$ and control gene (LacZ) transfected coronary arteries. Representative photomicrographs 28 days after coronary angioplasty and VEGF$_{165}$ (a) or LacZ (b) gene transfer using the needle injection catheter showing the intima plus media lesion development/vascular thickening. Both sections were stained with Elastica van Gieson (magnification ×20).

cardiologist. The field still lacks from a coronary in vivo experimental model that will allow systematic and reproducible testing for emerging diagnostic and therapeutic alternatives. Intramural delivery *without* balloon injury of atherogenic material into normal coronary arteries in large animals may be a valuable alternative to develop this model. Therefore, the local percutaneous intramural delivery of atherogenic material using the needle catheter was tested to develop complex vascular lesions in normal swine.[21]

Needles were deployed to the target coronary and iliac sites and approximately 130 μL containing cholesterol esters were injected in three vascular segments of each artery. After intervention, a high cholesterol diet was started and continued for 4 weeks. Intravascular ultrasound (IVUS) of lesion formation was performed in vivo at 2 and 4 weeks (Figure 9.12). IVUS confirmed lesion formation with mixed density similar to in vivo human lesions in the majority of the segments (Figure 9.13). Histological evaluation was also

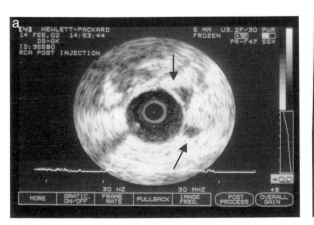
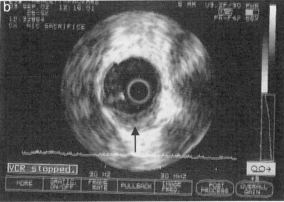

Fig. 9.12 Intravascular ultrasound (IVUS). Appearance following after injection (a) and 4 weeks later (b) in two different coronary arteries. (From Granada et al., unpublished data.)

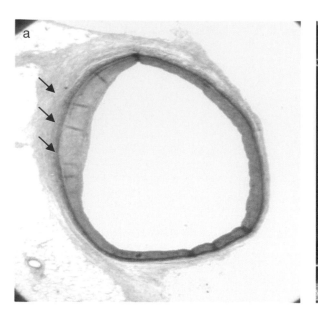 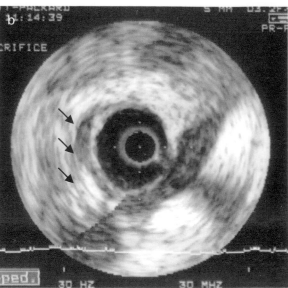

Fig. 9.13 Lesion formation. (a) a coronary artery lesion (arrows) formed after 4 weeks of cholesteryl linoleate deposition with the needle catheter (b) a corresponding IVUS image of the same site obtained immediately prior to sacrifice. (From Granada et al., unpublished data.)

encouraging, resembling complex atherosclerotic lesions (Figure 9.14). At 2 weeks, high lipid content was retained in all vascular layers, especially in the adventitia with extracellular matrix formation and foam cell formation. At 4 weeks, immunostains confirmed the presence of smooth muscle cells and macrophages, a characteristic feature of human atherosclerosis. With several modifications already implemented in the current model protocol, it is hoped that this model may offer insight into the physiopathology of plaque disruption and serves as a model for the evaluation of plaque detection technologies and therapies.

CONCLUSIONS

The needle catheter is a safe method of delivering agents to perivascular tissue. Delivery of lipids, photodynamic agents, drugs, and gene therapy with the needle catheter have effects on local intimal hyperplasia formation and on collateralization. For therapeutic approaches, the needle catheter permits the use of much lower doses than might be needed systemically.

ACKNOWLEDGMENT

We would like to thank Mrs Bien-Hung Pham for her editorial help.

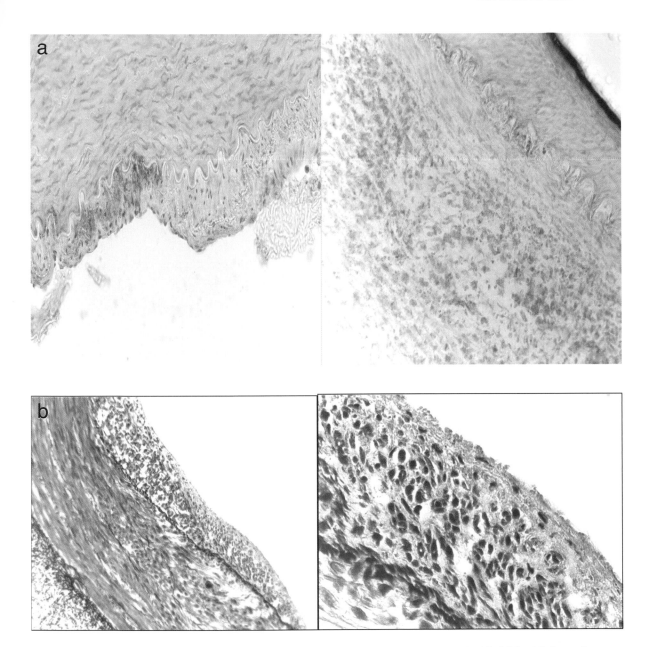

Fig. 9.14 Histology. (a) Frozen section of two different coronary arteries stained with Oil-Red-O 2 weeks after cholesteryl linoleate injection. *Left* (×10): high lipid retention after 2 weeks in the intima. *Right* (×10): retention also in all three layers of the vessel. (b) Histologic details of vascular lesions formed 4 weeks after intramural cholesteryl linoleate injections. *Left* (×20): an eccentric coronary lesion. There is eccentric medial thickening with a neointima infiltrated with mononuclear cells. *Right* (×100): part of the media and thickened intima infiltrated with monocytes. (From Granada et al., unpublished data.)

REFERENCES

1. Höfling B, Huehns TY, Gonschior P. The needle injection catheter. Semin Interv Cardiol 1995; 1:44–5.
2. Höfling B, Huehns TY. Intravascular local drug delivery after angioplasty. Eur Heart J 1995; 16:437–40.
3. Huehns TY, Gonschior P, Höfling B. Adventitia as a target for intravascular local drug delivery. Heart 1996; 75:437–8.
4. Shi Y, O'Brien JE, Fard A, et al. Adventitial myofibroblasts contribute to neointimal formation in injured porcine coronary arteries. Circulation 1996; 94:1655–64.
5. Gonschior P, Pahl C, Huehns TY, et al. Comparison of local intravascular drug-delivery catheter systems. Am Heart J 1995; 130:1174–81.
6. Huehns TY. Gene therapy strategies for restenosis delivered with a needle catheter. DM thesis, University of Nottingham 2000.
7. Nikol S, Huehns TY, Krausz E, et al. Needle injection catheter delivery of the gene for an antibacterial agent inhibits neointimal formation. Gene Ther 1999; 6:737–48.
8. Huehns TY, Krausz E, Mrochen S, et al. Neointimal formation following transluminal gene delivery to adventitial cells. Atherosclerosis 1999; 444:135–50.
9. Nikol S, Pelisek J, Engelmann MG, et al. Prevention of restenosis using the gene for cecropin complexed with DOCSPER liposomes under optimized conditions. Int J Angiol 2000; 9:87–94.
10. Nikol S, Engelmann MG, Pelisek J, et al. Local perivascular application of low amounts of a plasmid encoding for vascular endothelial growth factor (VEGF$_{165}$) is efficient for therapeutic angiogenesis in pigs. Acta Physiol Scand 2002; 176:151–9.
11. Nikol S, Pelisek J, Engelmann MG, et al. Vascular endothelial growth factor (VEGF$_{165}$) appears to have a district-specific influence on arteries of distinct developmental origin result-

ing in angiogenesis versus arteriogenesis in different vascular beds. J Endovasc Ther 2002; 9:842–54.
12. Gonschior P, Backfisch G, Muth G, et al. Local drug delivery via transvascular injection. J Invasive Cardiol 1999; 11:600–7.
13. Gonschior P, Gerheuser F, Fleuhaus M, et al. Local photodynamic therapy to obviate tissue hyperplasia in an experimental restenosis model. Photochem Photobiol 1996; 64:758–63.
14. Huehns TY, Höfling B, Nikol S. Gene therapy for restenosis – principles and potential. Intervent Cardiol Monit 1996; 3:33–9.
15. Nikol S, Maier A, Krausz E, et al. Current biotechnological approaches to the prevention of restenosis. BioDrugs 1998; 9:376–88.
16. Armeanu S, Pelisek J, Krausz E, et al. Optimization of non-viral gene transfer of vascular smooth muscle cells in vitro and in vivo. Mol Ther 2000; 1:366–75.
17. Pelisek J, Engelmann MG, Golda A, et al. Optimisation of non-viral transfection: variables influencing liposome-mediated gene transfer in proliferating versus quiescent cells in culture and *in vivo* using a porcine restenosis model. J Mol Medicine 2002; 80:724–36.
18. Pelisek J, Fuchs A, Engelmann MG, et al. Vascular endothelial growth factor response in porcine coronary and peripheral arteries using non-surgical occlusion model, local delivery and liposome-mediated gene transfer. Endothelium 2003; 10: 247–55.
19. Nikol S, Armeanu S, Engelmann MG, Pelisek J, et al. Evaluation of endovascular techniques to create a porcine femoral artery occlusion model. J Endovasc Ther 2001; 8:401–7.
20. Pels K, Deiner C, Coupland SE, et al. Effect of adventitial VEGF165 gene transfer on vascular thickening after coronary artery balloon injury, Cardiovasc Res 2003; 60: 664–72.
21. Granada J, Other applications of the needle injection catheter: development of a porcine model of complex vascular lesions. (in prep).

10

Stent-mediated local drug delivery

Yanming Huang and Ivan K De Scheerder

Introduction • Thromboresistant stents • Heparin-coated stents
• Drug eluting thromboresistant stents • Drug eluting stents to decrease neointimal hyperplasia
• Endothelial cell seeding and gene transfer • Conclusions • Summary

INTRODUCTION

Compared with plain coronary angioplasty, coronary stent implantation could dramatically decrease in-hospital events and improve long-term patency in some subsets of lesions. Early stent thrombosis remains, however, a problem; furthermore, increased arterial wall injury caused by stent deployment initiates a multi-factorial process that leads to neointimal hyperplasia and restenosis, especially in smaller arteries and longer lesions. Coating with different kinds of polymers has been suggested in order to improve the biocompatibility of metal stents. Drug loaded polymer-coated stents, that serve as a drug reservoir for sustained local drug delivery, have been proposed as a potential solution for subacute thrombosis and restenosis.

THROMBORESISTANT STENTS

With new antiplatelet therapeutic approaches and optimal stent implantation, thrombotic complications have decreased significantly. Thrombogenicity remains, however, a challenge in some vessels and lesions. As an initial and unavoidable event during stent implantation, thrombosis is also involved in the development of neointimal hyperplasia. Stents showing flow restriction have shown significantly greater neointimal formation in comparison with unrestricted stents in a canine femoral artery model. Furthermore, the neointima resulted from replacement of stent thrombosis.[1] Thromboresistant stents may therefore have potential benefits in both the inhibition of thrombosis and neointimal formation. Thromboresistant stents can be divided into stents with an inert thromboresistant surface, such as those with phosphorylcholine (PC) coating, gold coating, and silver coating, and heparin-coated stents and thromboresistant drug eluting stents.

HEPARIN-COATED STENTS (Table 10.1)

Heparin is an antithrombin III factor. It can be attached to a metallic surface either chemically or physically. Endpoint covalent attachment of heparin to a polymer-coated surface is stable and efficient. The immobilized heparin interacts with circulating antithrombin III. In vitro and in vivo experiments showed that heparin-coated stents can decrease platelet aggregation and thrombogenic events.[2–6,10–16,18,19,21] Also, using Duraflo II heparin coating in a rat arteriovenous shunt model, the thrombus weight,

Table 10.1 Heparin-coated stents

Source (1st author)	Year	Type of stent	Polymer	Model	Control	Thrombosis reduction	Neointimal reduction
In vitro studies							
Kocsis[2]	1996	P-S	Carmeda	In vitro	Bare stent	Yes	–
Chronos[3]	1996	P-S	Carmeda	Baboon A-V	Bare stent	Yes	–
Blezer[4]	1998	Tantalum	NA	In vitro	Bare stent	Yes	–
Christensen[5]	1998	Stent-graft	PTFE	In vitro	Bare stent	Yes	–
Beythien[6]	1999	NA	NA	Pulsed floating	Bare stent	Yes	–
In vivo studies							
Bonan[7]	1991	Zig-zag	NA	Dog coronary art	Bare stent	No	No
Zidar[8,9]	1992	Cordis	NA	Dog coronary art	Bare stent	No	No
Bailey[10]	1992	P-S	NA	Rabbit iliac art	Bare stent	Yes	–
Stradienko[11]	1993	P-S	NA	Rabbit iliac art	Bare stent	Yes	–
van der Giessen[12]	1994	P-S	NA	Pig coronary art	Bare stent	Yes	No
Jeong[13]	1995	Wallstent	NA	Pig carotid art	Bare stent	Yes	–
Sheth[14]	1995	Harts	SPUU-PEO	Rabbit carotid art	Bare stent	Yes	–
Chronos[15]	1995	Cordis	Hepamed	Baboon carotid	Bare stent	Yes	Yes
Wilczek[16]	1996	Copper	PUR	Pig coronary art	Bare stent	Yes	No
Gao[17]	1996	Biodegradable	CL+LA	Pig carotid art	–	–	–
Hardhammer[18]	1996	P-S	Carmeda	Pig coronary art	Bare stent	Yes	No
De Scheerder[19]	1997	Self-designed	Duraflo II	Rat A-V shunt pig coronary art	Bare stent	Yes	No

Table 10.1 *Continued*

Source (1st author)	Year	Type of stent	Polymer	Model	Control	Thrombosis reduction	Neointimal reduction
In vivo studies (continued)							
Schurmann[20]	1997	Cragg	Dacron	Sheep iliac art	Bare stent	–	No
Ahn[21]	1999	Wiktor	Hepamed	Pig coronary art	Bare stent	Yes	Yes
Goodwin[22]	2000	Collagen stent-graft	Collagen	Pig peripheral art	–	No	No
Clinical studies							
Serruys[23]	1996	P-S	Carmeda	Human coronary art	–	Yes	–
Vrolix[24]	1997	Wiktor	Hepamed	Human coronary art	–	–	–
Serruys[25]	1998	P-S	Carmeda	Human coronary art	PTCA	Yes	Yes
Wöhrle[26]	1999	Jomed	Corline	Human coronary art	Bare stent	No	No
Vrolix[27]	2000	Wiktor	Hepamed	Human coronary art	–	Yes	–
Van Langenhove[28]	2000	Wiktor	Hepamed	Human coronary saphenous vein bypass	–	–	Yes
Degertekin[29]	2000	Jomed	Corline	Human coronary art	Bare stent	–	No
Degertekin[30]	2000	Jomed	Corline	Human coronary art (CTO)	PTCA	–	Yes
Shin[31]	2000	Jomed	Corline	Human coronary art (AMI)	–	Yes	–

art, artery; A-V, arteriovenous; NA, not available; CTO, chronic total occlusion; PTCA, percutaneous transluminal coronary angioplasty; P-S, Palmaz-Schatz; PUR, polyurethane; SPUU-PEO, segmented polyurethaneurea-polyethylene oxide; CL, caprolactone; LA, D,L-lactide; PTFE, polytetrafluoroethylene.

radiolabeled platelet, and fibrinogen were significantly reduced after 30 min.[19] For neointimal hyperplasia, controversial results have been published.[7–9,12,15,16,18–22] Most studies showed that heparin-coated stents have a limited effect on neointimal hyperplasia. In one study, histomorphometric analysis after 4 weeks showed a significant increase in neointimal thickness with the highest heparin activity, although no significant difference was observed at 12 weeks follow-up.[18] Heparin also interacts with several growth factors and other glycoproteins. Thus, the heparin coating could hamper endothelial cell coverage of the coated stents. Modifying the structure of heparin to retain its anticoagulant activity and to eliminate other side effects has been proposed.

Heparin-coated Palmaz-Schatz (P-S), Wiktor, and Jomed are currently available for clinical use. Compared to balloon angioplasty, heparin-coated stents could significantly reduce the rate of subacute stent thrombosis and late restenosis.[25,30] However, no significant difference in restenosis was observed between the heparin-coated stent and the bare stent control.[26,29]

DRUG ELUTING THROMBORESISTANT STENTS
(Table 10.2)

Drug eluting stents to reduce thrombotic complications have also been evaluated. It has been known that a final common pathway for platelet aggregation exists. Platelet aggregation is mediated through glycoprotein IIb/IIIa (GPIIb/IIIa) receptors on the platelet membrane. Stents loaded with different kinds of GPIIb/IIIa inhibitors have been investigated. Results showed that GPIIb/IIIa inhibitor loaded stents could significantly decrease thrombus formation in different models, even compared to polymer-coated controls.[38,39,43–45,47,51] However, no significant effect on neointimal hyperplasia was demonstrated.[44] The use of specific GP IIb/IIIa inhibitors and a possible insufficient dose were the possible reasons.

Hirudin, a specific and direct thrombin inhibitor, does not require a cofactor to antagonize thrombin activity. It has, however, no direct effects on platelets. Prostacyclin is a potent inhibitor of platelet aggregation. Stent coatings impregnated with hirudin and prostacyclin analogs have been investigated. Incorporation of a polyethyleneglycol (PEG)-hirudin and a prostaglandin I_2 (PGI$_2$) analog in a polylactic acid stent coating showed initial exponential release characteristic of PEG-hirudin and a slow release of PGI$_2$.[33,34,37] These release properties could allow a fast and prolonged antithrombotic effect after stent implantation. PEG-hirudin and PGI$_2$ analog-loaded stent coatings have a significant inhibitive effect on both platelet activation and blood coagulation in a human shunt model.[35,37] Furthermore, in a sheep and pig coronary artery model, favorable effects on neointimal formation were observed.[46,52]

Other antithrombotic loaded stents, such as activated protein C and forskolin, have also been studied.[36,40,41,49,50]

DRUG ELUTING STENTS TO DECREASE NEOINTIMAL HYPERPLASIA (Table 10.3)

The process of neointimal formation consists of thrombosis, inflammatory reaction, smooth muscle cell migration, and proliferation. Mural thrombi may serve as scaffold for subsequent cell proliferation and undergo organization. However, early thrombus formation alone is not responsible for development of neointimal hyperplasia. A linear correlation has been reported between the number of monocytes per artery and the extent of arterial intimal growth.[74] Furthermore, a positive correlation between inflammatory reaction and restenosis has been observed.[75] Perivasculitis, caused by stent deployment, also participates in neointimal formation.[76] Corticosteroid, as an anti-inflammatory agent, has been evaluated. Methylprednisolone (MP) loaded stents with different doses showed a positive dose-related effect on neointimal hyperplasia.[56,64] Dexamethasone also showed an inhibitive effect on neointimal hyperplasia.[60,70] For other types of drugs with antiinflammatory characteristics, such as ibuprofen and colchicine,[55,64] no favorable effects on neointimal hyperplasia were observed.

Table 10.2 Thromboresistant drug eluting stents

Source (1st author)	Year	Type of stent	Polymer	Model	Drug	Dose	Release kinetics	Control stent	Thr-R	Neo-R
In vitro studies										
Baron[32]	1997	NA	NA	In vitro	C7E3 Fab	466 ng/cm wire	46.5% in 12 d	–	–	–
Schmidmaier[33,34]	1997	NA	PLLA	In vitro	5% PEG-hirudin 1% PGI$_2$	10 µg 2 µg	52.8% in 30 d 11.8% in 30 d	–	–	–
Schmidmaier[35]	1997	NA	PLLA	Human stasis	5% PEG-hirudin 1% PGI$_2$	NA	NA	Bare	Yes	–
Foo[36]	1998	NA	NA	In vitro	Activated protein C	NA	NA	Bare Polymer	Yes Yes	– –
Herrmann[37]	1999	InFlow	PLLA	Human stasis ex vivo	5% PEG-hirudin 1% iloprost	10 µg 2 µg	60% in 90 d 10% in 90 d	Bare	Yes	–
Baron[38,39]	2000	Cook GR II	CHC	In vitro	C7E3 Fab	1146 ng/cm wire	47% in 12 d	Bare	Yes	–
In vivo studies										
Lambert[40]	1994	Harts	PUR	Rabbit carotid art	Forskolin	1.58 mg	95% in 24 h	–	Yes	–
Dev[41]	1995	Nitinol	PUR	Rabbit carotid art	Forskolin Etidronate	1.5 mg 2.8 mg	95% in 24 h 50.5% in 72 h	–	–	–
Baker[42]	1996	PEAK	FIB	Rabbit iliac art	RGD	NA	NA	Bare	–	Yes
Tanguay[43]	1996	NA	NA	Dog coronary art	GPIIb/IIIa inhibitor	NA	NA	Bare	Yes	–

Table 10.2 *Continued*

Source (1st author)	Year	Type of stent	Polymer	Model	Drug	Dose	Release kinetics	Control stent	Thr-R	Neo-R
In vivo studies (*continued*)										
Aggarwal[44]	1996	Cook	CEL	Rabbit iliac art	GPIIb/IIIa inhibitor	1.15 µg	60% in 14 d	CEL	Yes	No
Aggarwal[45]	1997	NA	CEL	Rabbit iliac art	GPIIb/IIIa inhibitor+UK	–	–	CEL	Yes	–
Alt[46]	1997	P-S	PLLA	Sheep coronary art	PEG-hirudin PGI$_2$	10 µg / 2 µg	NA / NA	Bare	–	Yes
Santos[47]	1998	NA	NA	Dog coronary art	L703,081	40w%	18% in 2 h / 50% in 24 h / >90% in 89 h	Bare	Yes	–
Kruse[48]	1999	NA	NA	Pig coronary art	Argatroban	NA	NA	Bare	Yes	–
Foo[49,50]	1999	Cook	CEL	In vitro	Activated protein C	67.5 µg	74.1% in 24 h	Bare	Yes	–
	2000			Rabbit iliac art				CEL Albumin loaded	Yes / Yes	– / –
Jeong[51]	2000	ReoPro-coated stent	NA	Pig coronary art	GPIIb/IIIa inhibitor	NA	NA	Bare	Yes	Yes
Alt[52]	2000	P-S	PLLA	Pig coronary art	5%r-PEG-hirudin	NA	NA	Bare	–	Yes
				Sheep coronary art	1% iloprost	NA	NA			

CEL, cellulose; PLLA(PLA), poly-l-lactic acid; CHC, chlorohydrocarbon; RGD, arginine-glycine-aspartic acid; UK, urokinase; Thr-R, thrombosis reduction; Neo-R, neointimal reduction. Other abbreviations in Table 10.1.

Table 10.3   Drug eluting stents for decreasing neointimal hyperplasia

Source (1st author)	Year	Type of stent	Polymer	Model	Drug	Dose	Release kinetics	Control stent	Thr-R	Neo-R
In vitro studies										
Swanson[53]	2000	BiodivYsio	PC	In vitro	Paclitaxel	127 µg	86.6% in 24 h 96.2% in 48 h	–	–	–
In vivo studies										
Cox[54]	1992	Cook	CEL	Pig coronary art	Heparin –Metho Heparin +Metho	NA	>21 d	Bare	–	No
Eccleston[55]	1995	Tantalum	PLLA	Pig coronary art	Colchicine	3.96 mg 0.99 mg	34.3% in 28 d 2.1% in 28 d	–	–	No
De Scheerder[56]	1996	Wiktor	POP	Pig coronary art	MP	300 µg	96% in 24 h	POP	–	Yes
De Scheerder[57]	1996	Wiktor	POP	Pig coronary art	Angiopeptin	250 µg	91% in 24 h	POP	–	Yes
Lincoff[58]	1997	Wiktor	PLLA	Pig coronary art	DXM	0.8 mg	>50% in 2–3 d	PLLA Bare	– –	No No
Farb[59]	1997	NA	CSG	Rabbit iliac art	Paclitaxel	42 µg 8.6 µg 1.5 µg	–	Bare CSG	– – –	Yes No No
Strecker[60]	1998	Strecker	dl-PLA or PLA-co-TMC	Dog femoral art	DXM	8 mg	20% in 24 h 100% in 40 d	Bare	–	Yes

Table 10.3 *Continued*

Source (1st author)	Year	Type of stent	Polymer	Model	Drug	Dose	Release kinetics	Control stent	Thr-R	Neo-R
In vivo studies (*continued*)										
Drachman[61]	1998	NA	NA	Rabbit iliac art	Paclitaxel	NA	NA	Bare Polymer	– –	Yes Yes
Yamawaki[62]	1998	PLLA biodegradable	PLLA	Pig coronary art	ST638	0.8 mg	>60% in 21 d PLLA		–	Yes
Armstrong[63]	1999	Bio*divYsio*	PC	Pig coronary art	Angiopeptin	8.3 µg	1% in 30 min 57% in 7 d	–	–	–
De Scheerder[64]	2000	Self-designed	PFM-P75	Pig coronary art	MP	Dipcoating: 10–15 µg in 5% (g/g) 20–25 µg in 10% (g/g) Spraycoating: 100–150 µg in 9% (g/g) 400–450 µg in 33% (g/g) 700–1000 µg in 50% (g/g)	20% in 1 h 100% in 48 h 20% in 48 h 50% in 48 h 80% in 48 h	PFM-P75 PFM-P75	–	Yes Yes
De Scheerder[64]	2000	Self-designed	PFM-P75	Pig coronary art	Ibuprofen Valsartan	10–15 µg in 5% (g/g) 20–25 µg in 10% (g/g)	100% in 1 h >72 h	PFM-P75 PFM-P75	– –	No No
De Scheerder[64]	2000	Self-designed	PFM-P75	Pig coronary art	Trapidil	92 µg in 10% (g/g)	100% in 24 h	PFM-P75	–	No

Table 10.3 Continued

Source (1st author)	Year	Type of stent	Polymer	Model	Drug	Dose	Release kinetics	Control stent	Thr-R	Neo-R
In vivo studies (continued)										
Drachman[65]	2000	NIR	PLA/pCL	Rabbit iliac art	Paclitaxel	200 μg	36% in 24 h 55% in 7 d 63% in 14 d 78% in 30 d 91% in 56 d	Bare Polymer	– –	Yes Yes
Rogers[66]	2000	NIR	NA	Pig coronary art	Paclitaxel	NA	NA	Bare	–	Yes
Carter[67]	2000	NA	NA	Pig coronary art	Rapamycin	NA	NA	Bare Polymer	– –	Yes Yes
Klugherz[68]	2000	BX Velocity	NA	Rabbit iliac art	Rapamycin	64 μg 196 μg	NA NA	Bare Polymer	– –	Yes Yes
Klugherz[69]	2000	BX Velocity	NA	Pig coronary art	Rapamycin	NA	68% in 28 d	–	–	–
De Scheerder[70]	2001	BiodivYsio	PC	Pig coronary art	MP DXM	269 μg 95 μg 265 μg	16% in 15 min 100% in 20 h	Bare	– –	Yes No Yes
Heldma[71]	2001	P-S	–	Pig coronary art	Paclitaxel	0.2 μg 15 μg 187 μg	–	Bare	– – –	No No Yes

Table 10.3 Continued

Source (1st author)	Year	Type of stent	Polymer	Model	Drug	Dose	Release kinetics	Control stent	Thr-R	Neo-R
Clinical studies										
Sousa[72]	2000	BX Velocity	NA	Human coronary art	Rapamycin	140 μg/cm²	<15 d ≥28 d	–	–	–
Grube[73]	2000	Q-DL	NA	Human coronary art	Paclitaxel	NA	>180 d	Q-M	–	Yes

DXM, dexamethasone; MP, methylprednisolone; Metho, methotrexate; POP, polyorganophosphazene; FIB, fibrin; PC, phosphorylcholine; CSG, chondroitin sulfate and gelatin; PFM-P75, polyfluoroalkoxyphosphazene; Q-DL, Quanam drug eluting stent; Q-M, quanam metal stent. Other abbreviations in Table 10.1 and 10.2.

Histologic analysis of in-stent restenosis showed that smooth muscle cells and activated smooth muscle cells comprised, respectively, 59% and 25% of all cells.[77] Interference with smooth muscle cell proliferation could inhibit neointimal formation. Different classes of drugs with antiproliferative properties have been tested. Angiopeptin, paclitaxel, rapamycin, and ST638 all showed a beneficial effect on neointimal hyperplasia.[57,59,61,62,65–69,71] Based on experimental studies, clinical evaluation of dexamethasone, paclitaxel, and rapamycin loaded stents is under investigation. Unlike other antiproliferation agents, paclitaxel can easily pass through the cell membrane and have a long lasting antiproliferative action.[78]

ENDOTHELIAL CELL SEEDING AND GENE TRANSFER (Table 10.4)

Endothelial regeneration after stent implantation can also influence vascular thrombogenicity and neointimal hyperplasia. Endothelial cell seeding on stents or locally delivered endothelium-derived relaxing factors has been proposed for inhibiting the restenosis process. Genetically modified endothelial cells can be seeded on stents.[79,80,83] Vascular endothelial growth factor (VEGF) loaded stents can significantly decrease the thrombus formation and neointimal hyperplasia.[81,88] Nitric oxide (NO) loaded stents showed decreased thrombosis, although controversial results on neointimal formation were observed.[84,85,90]

Gene therapy has been proposed to transfer a desired gene from the stent coating to the cells of the arterial wall. Naked DNA, viral vector containing DNA, and antisense oligonucleotides have been evaluated. Using DNA-coated stents as gene carriers, transgene expression was observed.

Until now, endothelial cell seeding and gene therapy are in early stages of development, which is hampered by technical difficulties and potential complications.

CONCLUSIONS

As shown in Tables 10.1–10.4, both biodegradable and nonbiodegradable polymers have been used as matrices for local drug delivery. The most important consideration in selecting polymers for drug eluting stents is biocompatibility. Increased thrombogenicity and inflammatory reactions induced by the polymer coating can counteract the beneficial effect of local stent-mediated drug delivery. As most synthetic polymer coatings induced an inflammatory response, biological polymers, such as fibrin and phosphorycholine (PC), have been evaluated for coating stents for local drug delivery. Biological polymers have the advantages, in theory, of low thrombogenicity and minimizing inflammatory response. Studies have demonstrated that PC coating did not provoke increased arterial neointimal hyperplasia in rabbit iliac and porcine coronary artery models, although the coating did not reduce restenosis.[91,92]

Local drug concentration could influence the biological effect of polymers. The drug could be mixed with polymer, then applied to the stent surface by dipcoating or spraycoating for local delivery. The drug could also be adsorbed in the polymer-coated surface. The property of the polymer, the concentration of the drug used, and the thickness of the coating could determine the amount of drug be loaded. However, the use of drug loaded polymer-coated stents is hampered by limited drug loading capacity.

Drug release is associated with passive diffusion from the polymer matrix or the rate of matrix degradation. Polymer matrix characteristics, loaded drug concentration, and the drug itself could influence the release process. The higher the amount of drug loaded, the faster the drug is released.[64] The release kinetics in current studies showed that most drugs had an initial rapid washout followed by a slower release. This release profile might have a desired effect by interfering in early thrombotic formation. However, to modulate neointimal hyperplasia, a prolonged and sufficient drug release is probably required to match the cascade of restenosis. The rapid drug release characteristics could be responsible for the failure of drug eluting stents to interfere with neointimal formation in some studies. To overcome the limited drug loading and the too

Table 10.4   Endothelial cell seeding and gene therapy

Source (1st author)	Year	Type of stent	Polymer	Model	Drug	Dose	Release kinetics	Control stent	Thr-R	Neo-R
In vitro studies										
Dichek[79]	1989	Johnson – Johnson	Fibronectin	In vitro	Sheep EC seeding	–	–	–	–	–
Flugeman[80]	1992	Johnson – Johnson	Fibronectin	Pulsatile flow	Sheep EC seeding	–	–	–	–	–
Armstrong[81]	2000	BiodivYsio	PC	Pig carotid art ex vivo	AS-ODN-c-myc	500 μg	81% in 1 h 98.7% in 6 h 99% in 12 h	–	–	–
Swanson[82]	2001	Cook	Hydro-cardon	In vitro	VEGF	–	80% in 9 d	Bare BSA	–	–
In vivo studies										
Scott[83]	1995	Cordis	–	In vitro Pig coronary art	Human EC seeding	–	–	–	–	–
Folts[84,85]	1995	P-S	PSNO-BSA	Pig carotid art	NO	NA	NA	Bare	Yes	Yes
Landau[86]	1995	PLLA/PCL biodegradable	PLLA/PCL	Rabbit carotid art	Recombinant adenovirus vectors	NA	80% in 15 min	–	–	–
Labhasetwar[87]	1998	DNA polymer-coated suture	NA	Rat skeletal muscle Dog atrial myocardium	Plasmid DNA	777.2 μg	9.3% in 24 h 84% in 26 d	–	–	–

Table 10.4 Continued

Source (1st author)	Year	Type of stent	Polymer	Model	Drug	Dose	Release kinetics	Control stent	Thr-R	Neo-R
In vivo studies (continued)										
Mir-Akbari[88]	1999	Cook	NA	Rabbit iliac art	phVEGF	–	–	Bare	–	Yes
Klugherz[89]	1999	Crown	NA	Pig coronary art	Plasmid DNA	NA	NA	–	–	–
Buergler[90]	2000	Cordis	PCL	Pig coronary art	NO	1 mg	>10 d	PCL	–	No

rapid release of the drug from the coating, a new local intraluminal medicine releasing system (ELUT™ stent) has been developed. ELUT™ stent contains laser-drilled holes in the stent struts. The holes can be filled with drug plus polymer. Then, the surface of the stent can be loaded with the same or a different drug loaded polymer. By using this system, two kinds of agents with antithrombotic and antiproliferative characteristics can be loaded at the same time. Furthermore, an increment of loaded drug and considerable prolongation of drug release can be achieved. ELUT™ stents and control stents dipcoated with 10% methylprednisolone (MP) impregnated in a PFM-P75 were studied. In vitro studies showed that the total methylprednisolone content of the ELUT™ stent was significantly increased compared to the control stents (823 ± 21 μg vs 22 ± 3 μg). In the control stents, 20% of the MP was released after 1 hour and all the MP was released within 48 hours. In the ELUT™ stents the MP release was significantly prolonged – 20% of the MP was released within 10 days and 80% of the MP was released within 100 days.[93] With this release profile, a favorable effect on neointimal hyperplasia can be expected.

SUMMARY

Although some progression with drug loaded stents has been made during the past decade, the limitations of the studies are apparent. Except for heparin-coated and rapamycin loaded stents, few drug loaded stents have been evaluated in clinical trials. It is not clear whether the beneficial results from animal models will translate to humans. Second, the normal coronary and peripheral arteries of animals have been used for local drug delivery in these studies. Atherosclerotic lesions in humans may respond differently to the stents with local drug release. Studies have shown that young rabbits have a greater proliferative response and luminal narrowing than older rabbits following balloon injury. In human arteries, a low rate of proliferation has been reported.[94] Third, most drug release kinetics have been carried out and analyzed in vitro. These may not reflect the behavior of local delivered drugs. At the target site, the state of the vessel and local metabolism could influence drug distribution and its biological activity. Finally, we are still lacking biocompatible polymers with an adequate drug loading capacity. By increasing the thickness of the applied coating, more drugs could be loaded on a stent. However, this might change the profile of the stent, and then enhance thrombogenicity and neointimal formation.

Local drug delivery with stents, as a promising solution for subacute thrombosis and neointima, needs to be investigated further.

REFERENCES

1. Richter GM, Palmaz JC, Noeldge G, et al. Blood flow and thrombus formation determine the development of stent neointima. J Long Term Eff Med Implants 2000; 10(1–2):69–77.
2. Kocsis JF, Lunn AC, Mohammad SF. Incomplete expansion of coronary stents: risk of thrombogenesis and protection provided by a heparin coating. J Am Coll Cardiol 1996; 27(suppl A): 84A (abstract).
3. Chronos N, Robinson K, White D, et al. Heparin coating dramatically reduces platelet deposition on incompletely deployed Plamaz-Schatz in the baboon A-V shunt. J Am Coll Cardiol 1996; 27:84A (abstract).
4. Blezer R, Cahalan l, Cahalan PT, et al. Heparin coating of tantalum coronary stents reduces surface thrombin generation but not factor Ixa generation. Blood Coagul Fibrinolysis 1998; 9(5):435–40.
5. Christensen K, Larsson A, Emanuelsson H, et al. The stent graft: modulation of platelet and coagulation activation with heparin coating. Eur Heart J 1998; 19(suppl):498 (abstract).
6. Beythien C, Gutensohn K, Bau J, et al. Influence of stent length and heparin coating on platelet activation: a flow cytometric analysis in a pulsed floating model. Thromb Res 1999; 94(2):79–86.
7. Bonan R, Bhat K, Lefevre T, et al. Coronary artery stenting after angioplasty with self-expanding parallel wire metallic stents. Am Heart J 1991; 121:1522–30.

8. Zidar I, Jackman J, Gmmon R, et al. Serial assessment of heparin coating on vascular response to a new tantalum stent (abstract). Circulation 1992; 89:I–185.

9. Zidar I, Virmani R, Culp S, et al. Quantitative histopathologic analysis of the vascular response to heparin coating of the Cordis stent. J Am Coll Cardiol 1993; 12:336A (abstract).

10. Baily SR, Paige S, Lunn A, et al. Heparin coating of endovascular stents decreases subacute thrombosis in a rabbit model. Circulation 1992; 86(suppl):I–186.

11. Stratienko A, Zhu D, Lambert C, et al. Improved thromboresistance of heparin coated Palmaz-Schatz coronary stents in an animal model. Circulation 1993; 88:I–596 (abstract).

12. van der Giessen WJ, Hardhammar PA, van Beusekom HMM, et al. Prevention of (sub)acute thrombosis using heparin-coated stents. Circulation 1994; 90(suppl):I–650.

13. Jeong M, Owen W, Staab M, et al. Does heparin release coating of the Wallstent limit thrombosis and platelet deposition?: Results in a porcine carotid injury model. Circulation 1995; 92:I–37 (abstract).

14. Sheth S, Dev V, Jacobs H, et al. Prevention of subacute stent thrombosis by polymer-polyethylene oxide-heparin coating in rabbit carotid artery. J Am Coll Cardiol 1995; 25:348A (abstract).

15. Chronos N, Robinson K, Kelly A, et al. Thrombogenicity of tantalum stents is decreased by surface heparin bonding: scintigraphy of antithrombin III in-platelet deposition in baboon carotid arteries. Circulation 1995; 92:I–490 (abstract).

16. Wilczek KL, De Scheerder IK, Wang K, et al. Implantation of balloon expandable copper stents in porcine coronary arteries. A model for testing the efficacy of stent coating in decreasing stent thrombogenicity. Eur Heart J 1996; 17(suppl):455 (abstract).

17. Gao R, Shi R, Qiao S, et al. A novel polymeric local heparin delivery stent: initial experimental study. J Am Coll Cardiol 1996; 27:85A (abstract).

18. Hardhammar P, Van Beusekom H, Emanuelsson H, et al. Reduction in thrombotic events with heparin-coated Palmaz-Schatz stents in normal coronary arteries. Circulation 1996; 93:423–30.

19. De Scheerder I, Wang K, Wilczek K, et al. Experimental study of thrombogenicity and foreign body reaction induced by heparin-coated coronary stents. Circulation 1997; 95:1549–53.

20. Schurmann K, Vorwerk D, Uppenkamp R, et al. Iliac arteries: plain and heparin-coated Dacron-covered stent-grafts compared with noncovered metal stents – an experimental study. Radiology 1997; 203(1):55–63.

21. Ahn YK, Jeong MH, Kim JW, et al. Preventive effects of the heparin-coated stent on restenosis in the porcine model. Catheter Cardiovasc Interv 1999; 48(3):324–330.

22. Goodwin SC, Yoon HC, Wong GC, et al. Percutaneous delivery of a heparin-impregnated collagen stent-graft in a porcine model of atherosclerotic disease. Invest Radiol 2000; 35(7):420–5.

23. Serruys P, Emanuelsson H, van der Giessen W, et al. Heparin-coated Palmaz-Schatz stents in human coronary arteries: early outcome of the Benestent-II pilot study. Circulation 1996; 93:412–22.

24. Vrolix M, Grollier G, Legrand V, et al. Heparin-coated wire coil (Wiktor) for elective stent placement – The MENTOR trial. Eur Heart J 1997; 18:155 (abstract).

25. Serruys P, Emanuelsson H, van der Giessen W, et al. Heparin-coated Palmaz-Schatz stents in human coronary arteries: early outcome of the Benestent-II pilot study. Circulation 1996; 93:412–22.

26. Wöhrle J, Grotzinger U, AI-Kayer I, et al. Comparison of the heparin-coated and the uncoated version of the JOMED stent with regards to stent thrombosis and restenosis rates. Eur Heart J 1999; 20(suppl):271 (abstract).

27. Vrolix M, Legrand V, Reiber JH, et al. Heparin-coated Wiktor stents in human coronary arteries. Am J Cardiol 2000; 86(4):385–9.

28. Van Langenhove G, Vermeersch P, Serrano P, et al. Saphenous vein graft disease treated with the Wiktor Hepamed stent: procedural outcome, in-hospital complications and six-month angiographic follow-up. Can J Cardiol 2000; 16(4):473–80.

29. Degertekin M, Gencbay M, Sonmez K, et al. Comparison of heparin-coated Jomed stents with uncoated stents in patients with coronary artery disease. *3rd International Congress*

on *Coronary Artery Disease*, Lyon, France, 2–5 October 2000:128.

30. Degertekin M, Sonmez K, Gencbay M, et al. Heparin-coated stent implantation in chronic total occlusion. *3rd International Congress on Coronary Artery Disease*, Lyon, France, 2–5 October 2000:67.

31. Shin EK, Sohn S, Son JW, et al. Efficacy of heparin-coated stent in the early setting of acute myocardial infarction. *3rd International Congress on Coronary Artery Disease*, Lyon, France, 2–5 October 2000:152.

32. Baron JH, Aggrawal R, de Bono D, Gershlick AH. Adsorption and elution of c7E3 Fab from polymer-coated stents in-vitro. Eur Heart J 1997; 18(suppl):503 (abstract).

33. Schmidmaier G, Stemberger A, Alt E, et al. Time release characteristics of a biodegradable stent coating with polylactic acid-releasing PEG-hirudin and PGI$_2$-analog. J Am Coll Cardiol 1997; 29:94A (abstract).

34. Schmidmaier G, Stemberger A, Alt E, et al. Non-liner time release characteristics of a biodegradable polylactic acid coating releasing PEG hirudin and a PGI$_2$ analog. Eur Heart J 1997; 18(suppl):571 (abstract).

35. Schmidmaier G, Stemberger A, Alt E, et al. A new biodegradable polylactic acid coronary stent-coating, releasing PEG-Hirudin and a prostacycline analog, reduces both platelet activation and plasmatic coagulation. J Am Coll Cardiol 1997; 29:354A (abstract).

36. Foo RS, Hogrefe K, Baron JH, et al. Activated protein C adsorbed on a stent reduces its thrombogenicity. Circulation 1998; 17(suppl):I–855 (abstract).

37. Herrmann R, Schmidmaier G, Markl B, et al. Antithrombogenic coating of stents using a biodegradable drug delivery technology. Thromb Haemost 1999; 82(1):51–7.

38. Baron JH, Gershlick AH, Hogrefe K, et al. In vitro evaluation of c7E3-Fab (ReoPro) eluting polymer-coated coronary stents. Cardiovasc Res 2000; 46(3):585–94.

39. Baron JH, Aggarwal RK, Azrin MA, et al. Development of c7E3 Fab (abciximab) eluting stents for local drug delivery: effect of sterilization and storage. Circulation 1998; 98:17(suppl): I–855(abstract).

40. Lambert T, Dev V, Rechavia E, et al. Localized arterial wall drug delivery from a polymer-coated removable metallic stent: kinetics, distribution, and bioactivity of forskolin. Circulation 1994; 90:1003–11.

41. Dev V, Eigler N, Sheth S, et al. Kinetics of drug delivery to the arterial wall via polyurethane-coated removable nitinol stent: comparative study of two drugs. Catheter Cardiovasc Diagn 1995; 34:272–8.

42. Baker J, Nikolaychik V, Zulich A, et al. Fibrin coated stents as depot to deliver RGD peptide inhibit vascular reaction in atherosclerosis rabbit model. J Am Coll Cardiol 1996; 27:197A (abstract).

43. Tanguay JF, Santos RM, Kruse KR, et al. Local delivery of a potent GPIIb/IIIa inhibitor using a composite polymeric stent reduces platelet deposition. Eur Heart J 1996; 17(suppl):454 (abstract).

44. Aggarwal R, Ireland D, Azrin M, et al. Antithrombotic potential of polymer-coated stents eluting platelet glycoprotein IIb/IIIa receptor antibody. Circulation 1996; 94:3311–17.

45. Aggarwal R, Ireland D, Azrin M, et al. Reduction in thrombogenicity of cellulose polymer-coated stents by immobilisation of platelet-targeted urokinase. J Am Coll Cardiol 1997; 29:353A (abstract).

46. Alt E, Beilharz C, Preter G, et al. Biodegradable stent coating with polylactic acid, hirudin and prostacyclin reduces restenosis. J Am Coll Cardiol 1997; 29:238A (abstract).

47. Santos RM, Tanguay JF, Crowley JJ, et al. Local administration of L-703,081 using a composite polymeric stent reduces platelet deposition in canine coronary arteries. Am J Cardiol 1998; 82(5):673–5,A8.

48. Kruse KR, Crowley JJ, Tanguay JF, et al. Local drug delivery of argatroban from a polymeric-metallic composite stent reduces platelet deposition in a swine coronary model. Catheter Cardiovasc Interv 1999; 46(4):503–7.

49. Foo RS, Hogrefe K, Baron JH, et al. Activated protein C-eluting stent inhibits platelet deposition in an in vivo model. Eur Heart J 1999; 20(suppl):367(abstract).

50. Foo RS, Gershlick AH, Hogrefe K, et al. Inhibition of platelet thrombosis using an

activated protein C-loaded stent: in vitro and in vivo results. Thromb Haemost 2000; 83(3):496–502.

51. Jeong M, Ahn Y, Kang K, et al. ReoPro® coated stent inhibits porcine coronary stent thrombus and restenosis. Circulation 2000; 102(18):II–666 (abstract).

52. Alt E, Haehnel I, Beilharz C, et al. Inhibition of neointima formation after experimental coronary artery stenting: a new biodegradable stent coating releasing hirudin and the prostacyclin analogue iloprost. Circulation 2000; 101(12):1453–8.

53. Swanson N, Hogrefe K, Javed Q, et al. Drug-eluting stents – could drugs tailored to the patient be loaded in the cather lab? Eur Heart J 2000; 21(suppl):285 (abstract).

54. Cox D, Anderson P, Roubin G, et al. Effects of local delivery of heparin and methotrexate on neointimal proliferation in stented porcine coronary arteries. Coron Artery Dis 1992; 3:237–48.

55. Eccleston D, Lincoff A, Furst J. Administration of colchicine using a novel prolonged delivery stent produces a marked local biological effect within the porcine coronary artery. Circulation 1995; 92:I–87 (abstract).

56. De Scheerder I, Wang K, Wilczek K, et al. Local methylprednisolone inhibition of foreign body response to coated intracoronary stents. Coronary Artery Dis 1996; 7:161–6.

57. De Scheerder I, Wilczek K, Van Dorpe J, et al. Local angiopeptin delivery using coated stents reduces neointimal proliferation in over-stretched porcine coronary arteries. J Invasive Cardiol 1996; 8:215–22.

58. Lincoff A, Furst J, Ellis S, et al. Sustained local delivery of dexamethasone by a novel intravascular eluting stent to prevent restenosis in the porcine coronary injury model. J Am Coll Cardiol 1997; 29:808–16.

59. Farb A, Heller PF, Carter AJ, et al. Paclitaxel polymer-coated stents reduced neointima. Circulation 1997; 96:I–608 (abstract).

60. Strecker EP, Gabelmann A, Boos I, et al. Effect on intimal hyperplasia of dexamethasone released from coated metal stents compared with non-coated stents in canine femoral arteries. Cardiovasc Intervent Radiol 1998; 21:487–96.

61. Drachman DE, Edelman ER, Kamath KR, et al. Sustained stent-based delivery of paclitaxel arrests neointimal thickening and cell proliferation. Circulation 1998; 17(suppl):I–740 (abstract).

62. Yamawaki T, Shimokawa H, Kozai T, et al. Intramural delivery of a specific tyrosine kinase inhibitor with biodegradable stent suppresses the restenotic change of the coronary artery in pigs in vivo. J Am Coll Cardiol 1998; 32:780–6.

63. Armstrong J, Gunn J, Holt CM, et al. Local angiopeptin delivery from coronary stents in porcine coronary arteries. Eur Heart J 1999; 20(suppl):336 (abstract).

64. De Scheerder I, Huang Y, Schacht E. New concepts for drug eluting stents. *6th Local Drug Delivery Meeting and Cardiovascular Course on Radiation and Molecular Strategies*. Geneva, Switzerland, 27–29 January 2000.

65. Drachman DE, Edelman ER, Seifert P, et al. Neointimal thickening after stent delivery of paclitaxel: change in composition and arrest of growth over six months. J Am Coll Cardiol 2000; 36(7):2325–32.

66. Rogers C, Groothuis A, Toegel G, et al. Paclitaxel release from inert polymer material-coated stents curtails coronary in-stent restenosis in pigs. Circulation 2000; 102(18):II–566 (abstract).

67. Carter AJ, Bailey LR, Llanos G, et al. Stent based sirolimus delivery reduces neointimal proliferation in a porcine coronary model of restenosis. J Am Coll Cardiol 2000; 35(suppl A):13 (abstract).

68. Klugherz BD, Lianos G, Lieuallen W, et al. Dose-dependent inhibition of neointimal formation using a sirolimus-eluting stent. Eur Heart J 2000; 21(suppl):283 (abstract).

69. Klugherz BD, Lianos G, Lieuallen W, et al. Intramural kinetics of sirolimus eluting from an intracoronary stent. Circulation 2000; 102(18):II–733 (abstract).

70. De Scheerder I, Huang Y. Anti-inflammatory approach to restenosis. In Rothman MT (ed), *Restenosis: multiple strategies for stent drug delivery*. ReMEDICA: London 2001:13–31.

71. Heldman AW, Cheng L, Jenkins GM, et al. Paclitaxel stent coating inhibits neointimal hyperplasia at 4 weeks in a porcine model of coronary restenosis. Circulation 2001; 103(18):2289–95.

72. Sousa JE, Costa MA, Abizaid A, et al. Lack of neointimal proliferation after implantation of sirolimus-coated stents in human coronary arteries: a quantitative coronary angiography and three-dimensional intravascular ultrasound study. Circulation 2001; 103(2):192–5.

73. Grube E, Gerckens U, Rowold S, et al. Inhibition of in-stent restenosis by a drug eluting polymer stent: pilot trail with 18 month follow-up. Circulation 2000; 102(18):II–554 (abstract).

74. Rogers C, Welt FGP, Karnovsky MJ, et al. Monocyte recruitment and neointimal hyperplasia in rabbits: coupled inhibitory effect of heparin. Arterioscler Thromb Vasc Biol 1996; 16:1312–18.

75. Kornowski R, Hong MK, Tio FO, et al. In-stent restenosis: contributions of inflammatory response and arterial injury to neointimal hyperplasia. J Am Coll Cardiol 1998; 31:224–30.

76. De Scheerder I, Szilard M, Huang Y, et al. Evaluation of the effect of oversizing on vascular injury, thrombogenicity and neointimal hyperplasia using the Magic Wallstent™ in a porcine coronary model. J Am Coll Cardiol 2000; 35(2):70A (abstract).

77. Newby AC. Biological/pharmacological treatment and prevention. *XXIInd Congress of the European Society of Cardiology*, Amsterdam, The Netherlands, 27–30 August 2000.

78. Axel DI, Kunert W, Goggelmann C, et al. Paclitaxel inhibits arterial smooth muscle cell proliferation and migration in vitro and in vivo using local drug delivery. Circulation 1997; 96:636–45.

79. Dichek DA, Neville RF, Zwiebel JA, et al. Seeding of intravascular stents with genetically engineered endothelial cells. Circulation 1989; 80:1347–53.

80. Flugelman MY, Virmani R, Leon MB, et al. Genetically engineered endothelial cells remain adherent and viable after stent deployment and exposure to flow in vitro. Circ Res 1992; 70:348–54.

81. Amstrong J, Chan KH, Gunn J, et al. Antisense delivery from phosphorycholine (PC) coated stents. Eur Heart J 2000; 21(suppl):285.

82. Swanson N, Hogrefe K, Javed Q, et al. VEGF-Eluting stents stimulate endothelial cell growth in vitro. J Am Coll Cardiol 2001; 37:1A.

83. Scott NA, Candal FJ, Robinson KA, et al. Seeding of intracoronary stents with immortalized human microvascular endothelial cells. Am Heart J 1995; 129:860–6.

84. Folts J, Maalej N, Keaney J, Loscalzo J. Coating Palmaz-Schatz stents with a unique NO donor renders them much less thrombogenic when placed in pig carotid arteries. Circulation 1995; 92:I–670 (abstract).

85. Folts J, Maalej N, Keaney J, Loscalzo J. Palmaz-Schatz stents coated with a NO donor reduces reocclusion when placed in pig carotid arteries for 28 days. J Am Coll Cardiol 1996; 27:86A (abstract).

86. Landau C, Willard JE, Clagett GP, et al. Biodegradable stents function as vehicles for vascular delivery of recombinant adenovirus vectors. Circulation 1995; 92(8):I–670 (abstract).

87. Labhasetwar V, Bonadio J, Goldstein S, et al. A DNA controlled-release coating for gene transfer: transfection in skeletal and cardiac muscle. J Pharm Sci 1998; 87(11):1347–50.

88. Mir-Akbari H, Sylven C, Lindvall B, et al. phVEGF coated stent reduces restenosis intimal hyperplasia. Eur Heart J 1999; 20(suppl):275 (abstract).

89. Klugherz BD, Chen W, Jones PL, et al. Successful gene transfer to the arterial wall using a DNA-eluting polymer-coated intracoronary stent in swine. Eur Heart J 1999; 20:367 (abstract).

90. Buergler JM, Tio FO, Schulz DG, et al. Use of nitric-oxide-eluting polymer-coated coronary stents for prevention of restenosis in pigs. Coron Artery Dis 2000; 11(4):351–7.

91. Kuiper KK, Robinson KA, Chronos NA, et al. Phosphorylcholine-coated metallic stents in rabbit iliac and porcine coronary arteries. Scand Cardiovasc J 1998; 32(5):261–8.

92. Whelan DM, van der Giessen WJ, Krabbendam SC, et al. Biocompatibility of phosphorylcholine coated stents in normal porcine coronary arteries. Heart 2000; 83(3):338–45.

93. De Scheerder I, Huang Y, Qiang B, et al. Improved local drug delivery using the ELUT™ coronary stent. *3rd International Congress on Coronary Artery Disease*, Lyon, France, 2–5 October 2000:607.

94. Shroff S, Farb A, Virmani R, et al. Are current animal models representative of human vascular responses? Effect of aging on cellular proliferation and neointimal growth after balloon injury. Am J Cardiol 1999; 84(6A):64P (abstract).

11

Silicon carbide-coated stents

Bernd Heublein[†]

Introduction • Coating characteristics/biophysical principles

INTRODUCTION

Reducing the local thrombogenicity of an implanted stent remains an important and clinically significant goal (e.g. in cases of unstable angina, treatment following recanalization of an acute or chronic occlusion, primary stenting of type C lesions, venous grafts, and after brachytherapy). Aside from preventing thrombosis (early response), a primary reduction in local thrombogenicity can also be expected to have a positive influence on the late response by reducing mitogenic factors, including platelet-derived growth factor (PDGF).[1] Other known factors that influence early and late local responses can be traced back to the adhesion and activation of leukocytes.[2] Sawyer et al. studied the physical nature of contact activation of blood.[3] They demonstrated that the electrolysis of blood only causes clotting at the anode, and this was the first indication of the participation of electrons in the interaction between blood and metal surfaces. Subsequently, Baurschmidt and Schaldach described the biophysical principle of thrombogenesis on metallic surfaces as an electron transfer from fibrinogen to the metal.[4] This

knowledge was technologically applied in developing a new therapeutic principle, that of using hybrid materials made of a metallic substrate coated with a semiconducting layer.[5] Subsequently, as the result of a scientific development strategy, a novel and effective stent coating was derived from these biophysical descriptions – the silicon coating.[6] This principle is demonstrated in the Tenax[R] stent (Biotronik, Berlin, Germany), which was proven comprehensively in vitro,[7] and also clinically in a variety of patient groups.[8–11]

COATING CHARACTERISTICS/BIOPHYSICAL PRINCIPLES

Electron transfer processes are fundamental interactions between implant materials and proteins or cells. This is due to the fact that the basic physical structure of all proteins, which are dominated by the chain structure of interacting amino acids, is very similar. Proteins have the electronic properties of a semiconductor (Figure 11.1a). With the knowledge of the electronic structure of fibrinogen, and with the metallic surface as the reaction partner (the

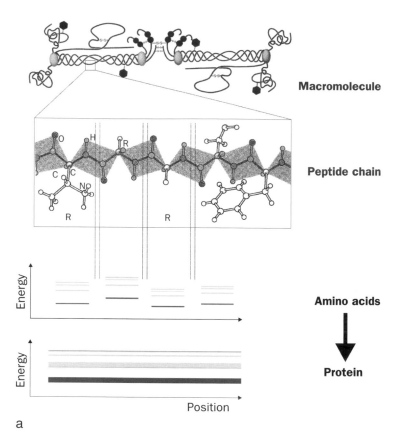

Macromolecule

Peptide chain

Amino acids

Protein

Fig. 11.1 (a) Electronic states in a macromolecule derive from atomic energy levels (orbitals). These levels may be shifted from their free atom values according to the chemical environment of each atom. Thus, in a macromolecule-like fibrinogen there is generally a 'band' of occupied and unoccupied orbitals. (b) Schematic density of electronic states in a metal (left) and a semiconductor (right) in contact with the blood protein, fibrinogen. The fraction of occupied and unoccupied states at an ambient temperature is indicated schematically. The metal provides unoccupied states where protein electrons may be transferred into, and thus cause fibrinogen degradation. Conversely, no such states are available in a semiconductor with a sufficiently large 'band gap' (right). No activation of the protein by an electron transfer is possible and fibrinogen degradation is prevented.

a

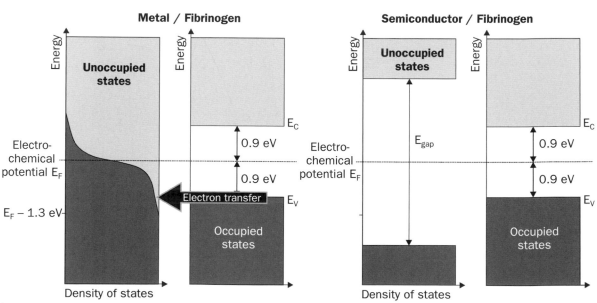

b

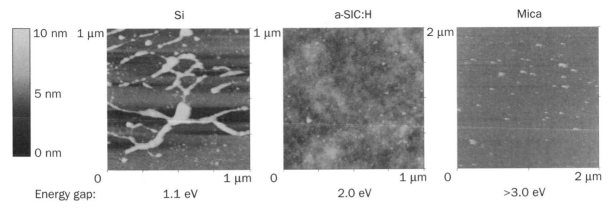

Fig. 11.2 Atomic force microscopy (AFM) images showing Si (left), a-SiC:H (center), and mica (right) surfaces incubated with fibrinogen solution (6 μg/ml). Wide fibrin networks are imaged on Si, while only single molecules and small clusters of fibrin are found on the materials with larger 'band gaps' (a-SiC:DH and mica), as expected from the electronic model of contact activation.

energy levels of the electrons), it is possible to define the physical parameters that lead to permanent surface passivation. Electron transfer, the basic mechanism for fibrinogen degradation, is prevented when the alloplastic material has an energy 'band gap' >1.4 eV and when the electric conductivity is higher than 10^{-5} S/cm.[5] An optimized (coating) material that meets these electronic requirements is amorphous hydrogen-rich phosphorus-doped silicon carbide (a-SiC:H) (Figure 11.1b). The behavior of a-SiC:H, the proof of this concept, can be verified by comparing materials with different electronic properties in a solution containing fibrinogen by using scanning force microscopy (SFM) (Figure 11.2). On silicon (Si), which has the smallest energy gap (E_{gap} = 1.1 eV), electron transfer is possible and conversion to fibrin occurs. In contrast, in the substrate's mica (E_{gap}>3 eV) and a-SiC:H (E_{gap} = 2.0 eV), the gaps are large enough to prevent the tunneling of electrons.[12] Because of the fundamental principles of the described interaction between proteins and alloplastic surfaces, similar behavior can be expected regarding the activation between the solids and the proteins of cell membranes of platelets and leukocytes. An example of results after 90 seconds contact between both silicon carbide-coated and un-

coated 316L stainless steel and a platelet-containing electrolyte (100 000 platelets/μl) is demonstrated in Figure 11.3.

Another potentially advantageous property is that the silicon carbide coating acts as a diffusion barrier for ions coming from the underlying substrate (in the case of 316L stainless steel, and especially chromium and nickel ions) (Figure 11.4).[13] The internal structure of a-SiC:H prevents this type of diffusion-related local toxic or allergic vessel response. In addition, this type of coating can be the basis for forming covalent bonds with biologically active molecules using carbon atoms (Figure 11.5). Depending on the type of spacer molecules, either stable bonding or slow release by biodegradation seems feasible.

By using a plasma-enhanced chemical vapor deposition process, it is possible to completely coat even complicated geometrical structures, such as stents, with a homogenous silicon carbide layer (Figure 11.6). Such a hybrid design, consisting of a stainless steel body and a surface coating, allows for the separation of the optimization process of stent mechanics and biocompatibility. Lower complication rates due to reclosure by acute or subacute stent thrombosis or exaggerated local cell proliferation (late lumen loss) can be expected.

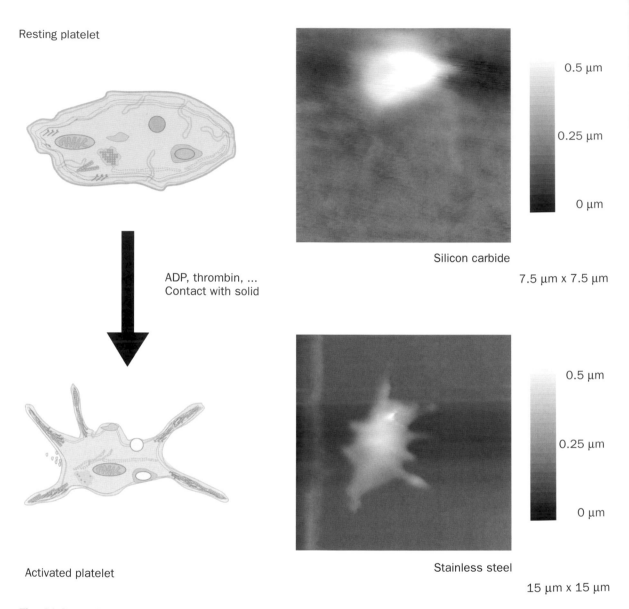

Resting platelet

ADP, thrombin, ...
Contact with solid

Activated platelet

Silicon carbide

7.5 μm x 7.5 μm

Stainless steel

15 μm x 15 μm

Fig. 11.3 *Left*: schematic changes in platelet morphology in response to external activation.
Right: observation of a platelet on an a-SiC:H-coated surface (top) and on a 316L medical steel surface
(bottom) by in vitro atomic force microscopy (AFM). Characteristic pseudopodia in the lower panel indicate
platelet activation by the metallic surface, while no activation is indicated on the semiconducting a-SiC:H
coating. ADP, adenosine diphosphate.

Fig. 11.5 The H-saturated 'dangling bonds' within the a-SiC:H coating allows attachment to biochemically
active macromolecules (e.g. heparin) to the surface by means of chemically stable covalent bonds. By
including a 'spacer' molecule in this link, the macromolecule's structural (and thereby, functional) degrees of
freedom are almost completely preserved in the attached state.

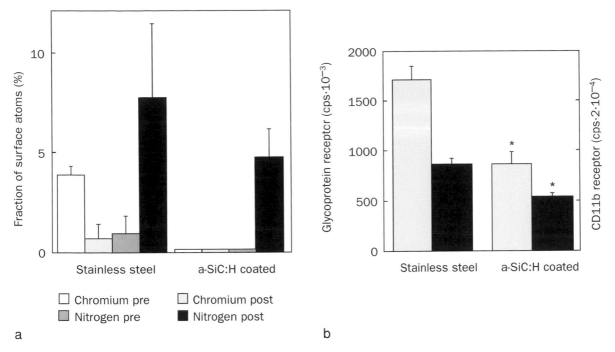

Fig. 11.4 (a) Elemental signals of a-SiC:H-coated and uncoated 316L medical steel surfaces before and after exposure to circulating blood, as measured by X-ray photoelectron spectroscopy (XPS). Chromium is found, before circulation, to be almost 4% at the surface, while a-SiC:H completely covers the chromium. After circulation, the exposed chromium concentration is reduced and replaced by an increasing nitrogen concentration, representing the deposition of proteins. On a-SiC:H nitrogen is also deposited, though to a lesser extent. (b) Platelet glycoprotein IIIa receptor antigen and granulocyte CD11b receptor antigen deposits are significantly higher on stainless steel stents than on a-SiC:H-coated stents ($p<0.05$).[13]

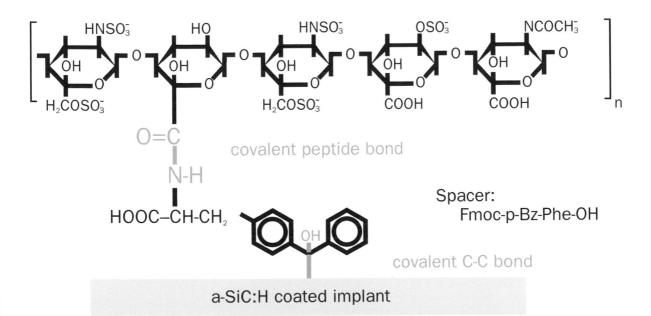

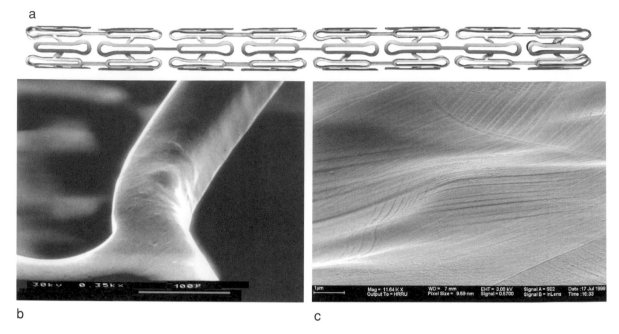

Fig. 11.6 (a) View of an a-SiC:H coated coronary stent (Tenax[R]; Biotronik, Berlin, Germany). (b) A scanning electron micrograph of a stent strut coated with a-SiC:H after dilatation in a region with high mechanical stress and deformation. (c) A scanning electron micrograph of a site with highly stressed a-SiC:H coating at high magnification.

REFERENCES

1. Chandrasekar B, Tanguay JF. Platelets and restenosis. JACC 2000; 35:555–62.

2. Miller DD, Karim MA, Edwards WD, Schwartz RS. Relationship of vascular thrombosis and inflammatory leukocyte infiltration to neointimal growth following porcine coronary artery stent placement. Atherosclerosis 1996; 124:145–55.

3. Sawyer PN, Brattain WH, Boddy PJ. *Electrochemical Criteria in the Choice of Materials used in Vascular Prostheses*. In Sawyer PH (ed.), Biophysical mechanism in vascular hemostasis and intravascular thrombosis. (Appleton-Century-Crofts: New York 1965:337–48.

4. Baurschmidt P, Schaldach M. The electrochemical aspects of the thrombogenicity of a material. J Bioeng 1977; 1:261–78.

5. Bolz A, Schaldach M. Amorphous silicon carbide: a semiconducting coating with superior hemocompatability. Artifi Organs 1991; 14:151–60.

6. Harder C, Rzany A, Schaldach M. Coating of vascular stents with antithrombogenic amorphous silicon carbide. Prog Biomed Res 1999; 1:71–7.

7. Monnink SHJ, van Boven AJ, Peels HJ, et al. Silicon-carbide-coated coronary stents have low platelet and leukocyte adhesion during platelet activation. J Investig Med 1999; 47:304–10.

8. Heublein B, Özbek C, Pethig K. Silicon-carbide-coated stents: Clinical experience in coronary lesions with increased thrombotic risk. J Endovasc Surg 1998; 5:32–6.

9. Carrie D, Khalife K, Hamon M, et al. Initial and follow-up results of the Tenax coronary stent. Prog Biomed Res 2000; 5:224–8.

10. Hannekamp CEE, Koolen JJ. Coated stents in small coronary vessels – a successful strategy? Prog Biomed Res 2000; 5:221–3.

11. Heublein B, Kreksch K, Pethig K, et al. Coronary stenting in cardiac allograft vasculopathy: The impact of silicon carbide coating on luminal re-obstruction. Prog Biomed Res 2000; 5:215–20.

12. Rzany A, Harder C, Schaldach DM. Silicon carbide as an anti-thrombogenic stent coating: an example of a science-based development strategy. Prog Biomed Res 2000; 5:168–78.

13. van Oeveren W. Reduced depositon of blood formed elements and fibrin onto amorphous silicon carbide coated stainless steel. Prog Biomed Res 1999; 4:78–83.

12

The Carbostent: a Carbofilm™-coated stent

Antonio L Bartorelli

Introduction • Design characteristics • Carbofilm™ coating • Preclinical evaluation

INTRODUCTION

In 1997, the Carbostent, a balloon-expandable, tubular slotted, coated stent was developed by Sorin Biomedica, Saluggia, Italy. (See Table 12.1 for technical details.)

DESIGN CHARACTERISTICS

The Sorin Carbostent is characterized by a complete set of original features aimed to address major procedural and long-term outcome issues (Table 12.1). The design is based on an homogeneous cellular architecture (Figure 12.1). The cell interconnection scheme provides longitudinal flexibility, avoids a fishscale effect consequent to bending during implantation, and obtains zero shortening of the stent upon expansion. Two radiopaque platinum markers positioned at the stent ends ensure excellent fluoroscopic visibility, while the low degree of Carbostent radiopacity does not interfere with the angiographic appearance and quantitative coronary angiography (QCA) analysis of the contrast-filled coronary lumen. The presence of radiopaque

markers, together with no shortening upon expansion, allows very precise positioning and safe postdilatation. Each cell of the Carbostent is designed to realize an ideal elastic matching between the stent and the vessel wall, in order to avoid stress concentration, which can stimulate neointimal proliferation and in-stent restenosis. To achieve this goal, the cell consists of different curved segments, each one characterized by a variable cross-section to optimize individual mechanical response to stent expansion, flexure, and torsion (Figure 12.1). The entire surface of the Carbostent is treated with electrochemical and diamond polishing, derived from Sorin's heart valve technology that provides round edges and a mirror-like surface (Figure 12.2a). The smooth surface enhances stent trackability, while stent rounded edges minimize the risk of vessel injury during stent advancement into the coronary arteries. The stent is available in a full range of sizes. The lengths are 9, 12, 15, 19, 25, and 32 mm. The diameters are 2.5 mm (4 cells configuration), 3.0–3.5 mm (5 cells), and 4.0 mm (6 cells). The characteristics of the Carbostent delivery system are summarized in Table 12.2.

Table 12.1   Carbostent technical specification

Material	316LVM (vacuum-melted) stainless steel
Technology	Laser micromachining of a seamless thin wall tube
Stent design	Multicellular architecture
Cell design	Curved segments with variable cross-sections
Surface finishing	Mirror-like
Coating	Permanent and integral thromboresistant film (0.3–0.5 μm) of turbostratic carbon (Carbofilm™)
Degree of radiopacity	Moderate/low
Radiopaque markers	Two terminal platinum markers (350 μm)
Ferromagnetism	None (MRI safe)
Longitudinal flexibility	High
Shortening upon expansion	0
Coverage area (expanded state)	12–17%
Degree of elastic recoil	3–6%
Strut thickness	0.075 mm (0.003 inch)
Strut width	0.075–0.125 mm (0.003–0.005 inch)
Currently available lengths	9, 12, 15, 19, 25, and 32 mm
Currently available diameters	2.5 mm (4 cells) 3.0–3.5 mm (5 cells) 4.0–4.5 mm (6 cells)

MRI, magnetic resonance imaging.

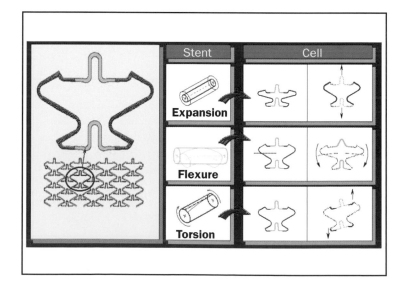

Fig. 12.1 Schematic drawing illustrating the cell functionality concept of the Carbostent. The stent cell (left panel) comprises curved segments designed with variable cross-sections that optimize mechanical response to stent expansion (blue segments), flexure (green segments), and torsion (red segments) (center and right panels).

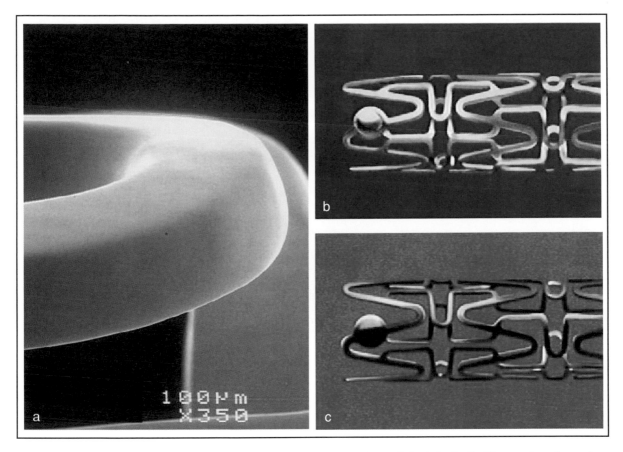

Fig. 12.2 (a) Scanning electron micrograph showing the mirror-like polished, Carbofilm™-coated surface of the Carbostent. Right: photographs of the Carbostent before (b) and after (c) Carbofilm™ coating.

CARBOFILM™ COATING

Pyrolytic carbon is an artificial carbon developed in the early 1960s for applications in the nuclear energy field. This material is characterized by a 'turbostratic' crystal structure, which is intermediate between diamond and graphite (Figure 12.3). Ideal properties for implantable prostheses in contact with blood were found to be associated with the turbostratic structure: chemical inertness, low density, compactness, elasticity, high strength,[1–3] considerable hardness, wear resistance,[4] and hemocompatibility. This last characteristic is largely dependent on atraumatic interaction with proteins that form a layer adhering to the material surface without alteration of their structure.[5–8] Thanks to these properties, pyrolytic carbon has been used worldwide for more than 30 years in the produc-

tion of the most critical cardiovascular prostheses, the mechanical heart valves. The excellent clinical results observed in more than a million pyrolytic carbon valves offer the best evidence of the advantages and quality of this material.[9]

The high temperature involved in the manufacturing process, which precludes the possibility of coating most materials, including stainless steel, limits an extensive application of pyrolytic carbon. In 1982, Sorin Biomedica's laboratories developed an original physical vapor deposition (PVD) process which allows the transfer of atoms from a pyrolytic carbon target to the substrate to be coated. The process parameters can be tuned in order to perform the transfer even at room temperature. Therefore, turbostratic carbon (Carbofilm™) can be deposited on a variety of heat-sensitive

Table 12.2   Carbostent delivery system

Deployment mechanism	Balloon expandable	Balloon protrusion	0.6 mm
Premounted	Yes	Radiopaque markers	2 on proximal and distal balloon ends
Protective sheath/ cover	No	Balloon rated burst pressure	16 atm (average 22 atm)
Delivery catheter	Rapid-exchange balloon catheter	Guidewire compatibility	0.014 inch (0.36 mm)
Balloon characteristics	Semicompliant, trifolding balloon	Minimum recommended guide catheter	5 Fr
Balloon material	Polyamide		

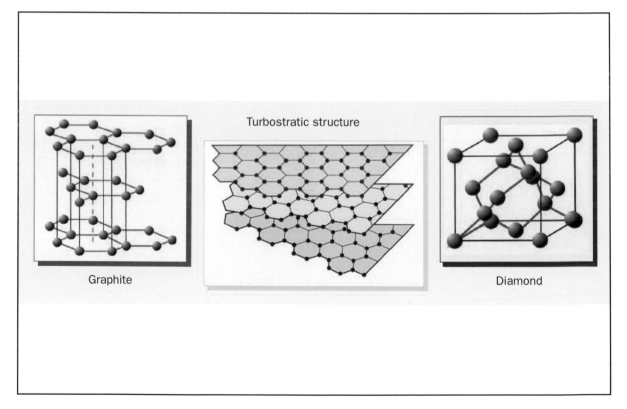

Fig. 12.3   Crystal structure of graphite, pyrolytic carbon, and diamond.

substrates (e.g. metals, polymers). This is done in high vacuum to prevent chemical reactions, to preserve the purity of the deposited material, and to retain all chemical, physical and biological properties of pyrolytic carbon.[10] The PVD technique obtains intrinsically stable bonds, resulting in permanent adhesion of the coating to the substrate – even after very long exposure to blood – and provides an extremely thin film (0.3–0.5 μm), which does not alter the

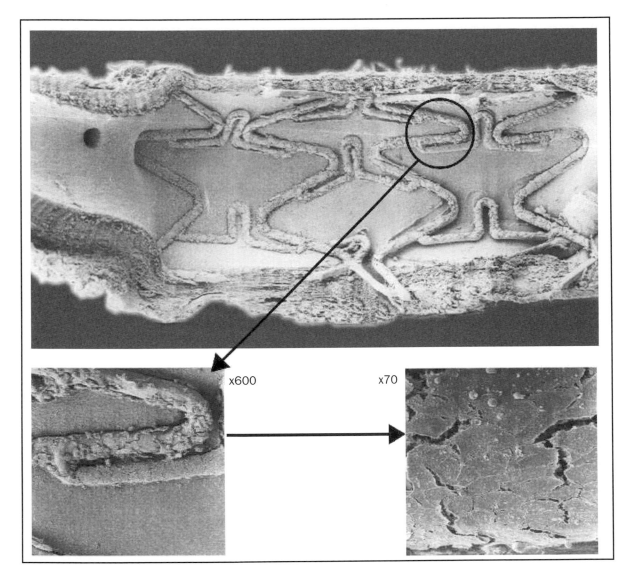

Fig. 12.4   Scanning electron micrograph (SEM) images of a pig coronary artery 4 days after Carbostent implantation. The lumen is widely patent and the stent is well apposed to the vessel wall. High magnification shows large areas of spindle and polygonal-shaped endothelial cells growing on fibrin and cellular thrombus.

morphologic and physical characteristics of the coated substrate. Extensive laboratory and in vivo studies conducted on Carbofilm™-coated vascular prostheses have shown reduced thrombus formation, platelet adhesion, and activation.[11–14] Moreover, a tissue reaction characterized by a well-organized neointima, devoid of foreign body giant cells and significantly thinner than controls, has consistently been observed.[15] The flexibility of Sorin's coating technique allowed the Carbofilm™ to

be applied to a variety of materials currently used for implantable devices: titanium alloy for valve housings, polyester fabric for vascular grafts, silicone rubber for pacemaker leads, and, more recently, stainless steel for the Carbostent (Figure 12.2b,c).

PRECLINICAL EVALUATION

Tissue response and biocompatibility of the Carbostent were evaluated in the coronary

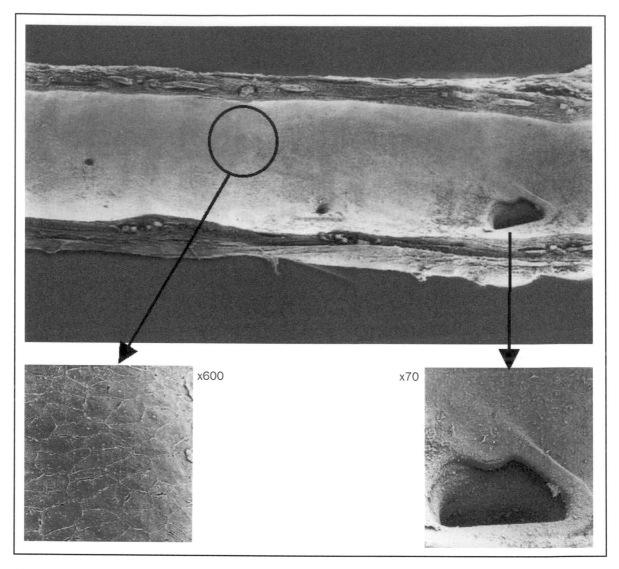

Fig. 12.5 Scanning electron micrograph (SEM) images of a pig coronary artery 180 days after Carbostent implantation. The lumen surface is smooth and completely lined with a well-formed endothelial layer of polygonal-shaped cells with prominent tight junctions. Note the small branch ostium, which remained patent within the neointimal layer.

arteries of non-atherosclerotic minipigs (30–45 kg).[16] Thirty Carbostent (3.0 mm diameter, 15 mm length) were implanted in the LAD, LCx, and RCA of 27 minipigs that were pretreated with aspirin monotherapy for 3 days. Aspirin was continued for 7 days only following implantation. No adverse event was observed and all stents were angiographically patent before animal sacrifice. Histology evalu-

ation at 72 hours revealed minimal covering of the stent surface by platelets with few neutrophils and monocytes. Scanning electron micrograph (SEM) studies showed that the stent surface was completely covered by fibrin and cellular thrombus with large areas of endothelium composed by spindle and polygonal-shaped endothelial cells (Figure 12.4). At 30–60 days, mild neointimal formation was observed, consisting of smooth muscle cells embedded within a proteoglycan matrix with the lumen surface fully covered by endothelial cells. It is noteworthy that no significant chronic inflammatory response was present and the vessel wall injury was minimal. At longer follow-up (>180 days), the neointimal thickness decreased with fewer smooth muscle cells in a collagen matrix. At SEM, the lumen surface was completely lined with well-formed endothelial layer of polygonal-shaped cells with prominent tight junctions (Figure 12.5).

REFERENCES

1. Kaae JL, Gulden TD. Structure and mechanical properties of co-deposited pyrolytic C-SiC alloys. J Am Ceram Soc 1971; 54:605–9.
2. Bokros JC. Variation in the crystallinity of carbon deposited in fluidized beds. Carbon 1965; 3:201–11.
3. Shim HS. The behavior of isotropic pyrolytic carbon under cyclic loading. Biomater Med Dev Art Org 1974; 2:55–65.
4. Shim HS. The wear of titanium alloy, and UHMW polyethylene caused by LTI carbon stellite 21. J Bioeng 1977; 1:223–9.
5. Bokros JC. Carbon biomedical devices. Carbon 1977; 15:355–71.
6. Haubold AD. Blood/carbon interaction. ASAIO J 1983; 6:88–92.
7. Benson J. Elemental carbon as a biomaterial. J Biomed Mater Res Symposium 1971; 2:41–7.
8. Haubold AD, Shim HS, Bokros JC. Biocompatibility of clinical implant materials. In Williams DF (ed), *Carbon in Medical Devices?*: Boca Raton: CRC Press, 1981: 325–31.
9. Borman JB, Brands WGB, Camilleri L, et al. Bicarbon valve – European multicenter clinical evaluation. Eur J Cardiothorac Surg 1998; 13:685–93.
10. Paccagnella C, Majni G, Ottaviani G, et al. Properties of a new carbon film for biomedical applications. J Artif Org 1986; 9:115–18.
11. Sbarbati R, Giannessi D, Cenni MC, et al. Pyrolytic carbon coating enhances Teflon and Dacron fabric compatibility with endothelial cell growth. Int J Artif Organs 1991; 14:491–8.
12. Cenni E, Granchi D, Arciola CR, et al. Platelet and coagulation factor variations induced in vitro by polyethylene terephtalate (Dacron) coated with pyrolytic carbon. Biomaterials 1995; 16:973–6.
13. Cenni E, Granchi D, Arciola CR, et al. Adhesive protein expression on endothelial cells after contact in vitro with polyethylene terephtalate coated with pyrolytic carbon. Biomaterials 1995; 16:1223–7.
14. Cenni E, Granchi D, Ciapetti G, et al. In vitro complement activation after contact with pyrolytic carbon-coated and uncoated polyethylene terephtalate. J Mater Sci: Mater Med 1997; 8:771–4.
15. Aebischer P, Goodard M, Hunter TJ, et al. Tissue reaction to fabrics coated with turbostratic carbon: subcutaneous versus vascular implants. Biomaterials 1998; 9:80–5.
16. Virmani R, Santarelli A, Galloni M, et al. Tissue response and biocompatibility of the Sorin Carbostent: experimental results in porcine coronary arteries. Am J Cardiol 1998; 82(Suppl 7A):65 (abstract).

13

The PC-coated Bio*divYsio*™ stent

Andrew Lewis and Julian Gunn

Introduction • **Mechanical properties** • **Non-thrombogenicity** • **Non-inflammatory reaction** • **Long-term stability in vivo** • **Clinical data** • **Summary**

INTRODUCTION

The Bio*divYsio*™ family of coronary stents (AS, OC, and SV: see Figure 13.1) is characterized by the presence of an ultra-thin coating of a phosphorylcholine (PC) polymer. The PC coating is a synthetic copy of the predominant phospholipid that comprises the outside of the red blood cell membrane (Figure 13.2).[1] The surface of devices coated with this material therefore mimic the body's own chemistry, and any response to the foreign implant is lessened. The PC coating on coronary stents has been shown to be non-thrombogenic, non-inflammatory, and stable for over 6 months when implanted.

MECHANICAL PROPERTIES

In addition to the PC portion for biocompatibility, the coating polymer has been designed with several other components included for other specific purposes (see Figure 13.3a). A hydrophobic lauryl alkyl chain component aids in the initial adhesion and film formation of the polymer on to the stainless steel stent substrate. Other groups allow thermally induced cross-linking both within the polymer to form a water-swellable elastic network, and also with

metal oxide groups on the stent surface to achieve firm anchorage.

The polymer can be sterilized by conventional methods. In addition, the mechanical properties of the coating can be further enhanced by a gamma-irradiation step that is used to fully cross-link the coating (Figure 13.3b). Atomic force microscopy (AFM) and nanoindentation studies have shown that the coating is tenaciously adhered to the stent and can survive balloon expansion without damage.[2]

NON-THROMBOGENICITY

There have been a plethora of in vitro experiments performed on PC coatings to show that they resist protein adsorption, do not activate complement, and reduce both platelet adhesion and activation.[3]

Evidence such as that from coated stents used in the ex vivo baboon shunt model (Figure 13.4a), in vivo baboon brachial implants (Figure 13.4b), and clinical usage of guidewires (Figures 13.4c,d) show that the coatings have excellent resistance against thrombus formation. This is reflected in a zero incidence of subacute thrombosis in the

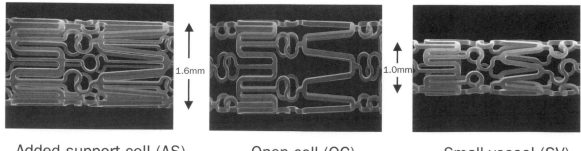

Added support cell (AS)
8 mm
11 mm
15 mm

- Higher metal-to-surface ratio gives greater paving function for lesions where additional support is required

Open cell (OC)
8 mm 11 mm
15 mm 18 mm
22 mm 28 mm

- Improved side branch access
- Increased flexibility

Small vessel (SV)
7 mm 10 mm
15 mm 18 mm

- 2.0 mm, 2.25mm, and 2.5mm diameter
- Specifically designed for small vessels
- Increased flexibility

Figure 13.1 The Bio*divYsio* range of stents.

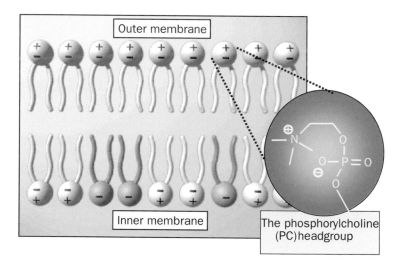

Figure 13.2 Schematic of the red blood cell membrane.

DISTINCT trial and a very low occurrence in other clinical trials using these coated stents.[4]

NON-INFLAMMATORY REACTION

Previous studies on polymer-coated stents have raised concerns about excessive inflammatory response to the coating materials.[5] During wound healing, the PC coating has been shown to illicit a similar tissue reaction to the non-coated stent, with no additional adverse inflammation (Figure 13.5 shows results from 6 month implantation in pig coronary arteries: Palmaz-Schatz 153 vs Bio*divYsio* 15 mm AS). In the porcine model, the coating was also shown not to interfere with endothelialization of the stent.[6]

LONG-TERM STABILITY IN VIVO

The coating on the stent is approximately 50–100 nm in thickness, as determined by atomic force microscopy (AFM). This method not only enables the thickness to be determined, but also measures the force required to remove it from the stent. A similar evaluation

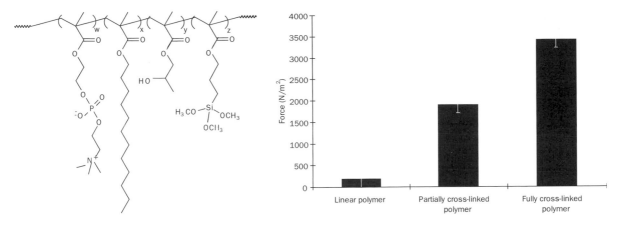

Figure 13.3 (a) Generalized structure of the PC polymer. (b) Force to remove uncured, partially cured, and fully cured PC coatings from a stent.

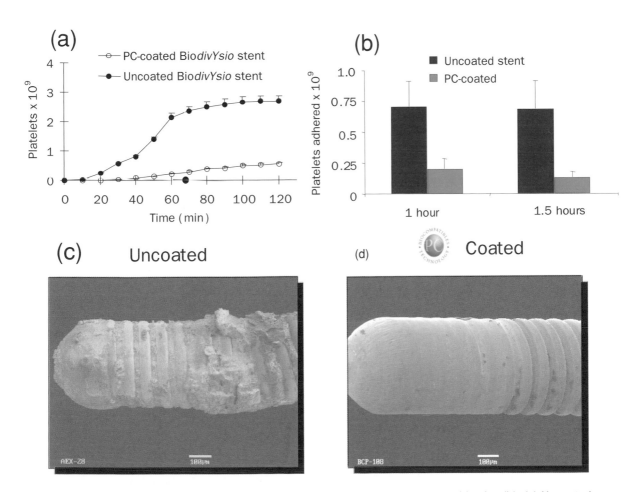

Figure 13.4 (a) Platelet adhesion to PC-coated and uncoated stents ex vivo and in vivo (b). (c) Uncoated guidewire after 28mm procedure. (d) PC-coated guidewire after 108mm procedure.

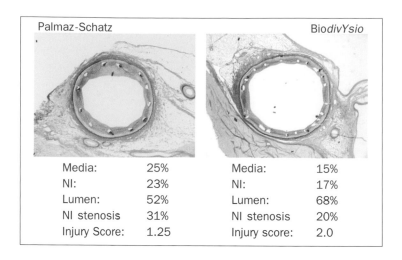

Figure 13.5 Comparison of histological sections of a Palmaz-Schatz and Bio*divYsio* stented artery. NI, neointima.

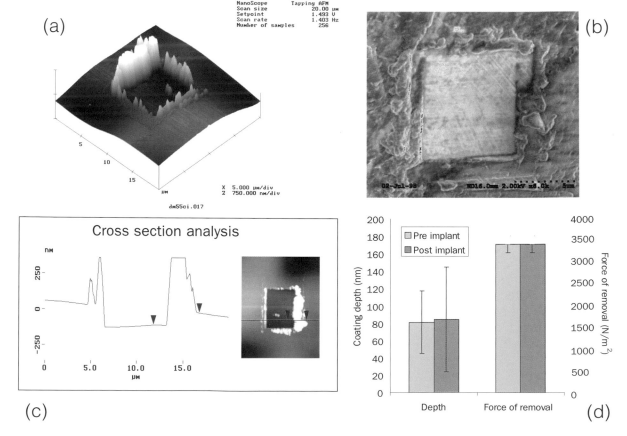

Figure 13.6 (a) AFM and (b) SEM of the surface after hole excavation. (c) Cross-section analysis. (d) Depth and force of removal comparison pre and post implantation. ATM, atomic microscopy; SEM, scanning electron microscopy.

Table 13.1 Summary of DISTINCT data

Key outcome	BiodivYsio AS (n = 313)	Multilink duet (n = 309)
Binary restenosis at 6 mths	19.7	20.1
TVF at 6 mths	8.3	7.4
SAT (<30 days)	0	0.6
Single stent binary restenosis rate		
Binary restenosis at 6 mths	17.8	22.2

TVF, target vessel failure
SAT, (Sub)acute arterial thrombosis.

Table 13.2 Summary of European trials

	SOPHOS		CE mark	Open registry
Arm:	A	B		
Death	0.5	0	0	0.7
MI	5.0	2.7	2.0	6.4
CABG	2.5	1.3	1.3	0.7
Re-PTCA	8.0	6.7	5.3	6.4
Total MACE	16.0	10.7	8.6	14.2
Binary restenosis	17	NA	NA	NA

A, angiographic follow-up at 6 months; B, clinical follow-up only; MI, myocardial infarction; CABG, coronary artery bypass graft; PTCA, percutaneous transluminal coronary bypass graft; MACE, major adverse coronary event.

has been made 6 months post implantation in a porcine model and has shown the force of removal and coating depth to be equivalent to that prior to implantation (Figure 13.6).[7] The PC coating is therefore not affected over this time scale by the vessel environment.

CLINICAL DATA

The BioDIvYsio Stent IN controlled Clinical Trial (DISTINCT) study was a 622 patient multicenter randomized trial designed to show equivalence with the Multilink Duet with respect to target vessel failure (TVF) at 6 months. The main findings of the study are summarized in Table 13.1 and show equivalent TVF rates and binary restenosis at 6 months, although analysis of single stent patients favors the BiodivYsio stent. A summary of selected European clinical outcomes at 6 months is also shown (Table 13.2).

SUMMARY

The biocompatibility and stability of the PC coating make it an ideal candidate as a system for local drug delivery. The coating has been modified for this purpose, which is described fully in Chapter 16 on drug delivery PC coatings.

REFERENCES

1. Lewis AL. Phosphorylcholine-based polymers and their use in the prevention of biofouling. Coll Surf B: Biointerfaces 2000; 18:261–75.
2. Lewis AL, Cumming ZC, Goreish HH, Kirkwood LC, Tolhurst LA, Stratford PW. Crosslinkable coatings from phosphorylcholine-based polymers. Biomaterials 2001; 22:99–111.
3. Campbell EJ, O'Byrne V, Stratford PW, et al. Biocompatible surfaces using methacryloylphosphorylcholine laurylmethacrylate copolymers. ASAIO Journal 1994; 40:853–7.
5. van der Giessen WJ, Lincoff AM, Schwartz RS, et al. Marked inflammatory sequelae to implantation of biodegradable and nonbiodegradable polymers in porcine coronary arteries. Circulation 1996; 94:1690–7.
6. Whelan DM, van der Giessen WJ, Krabbendam SC, et al. Biocompatibility of phosphorylcholine coated stents in normal porcine coronary arteries. Heart 2000; 83:338–45.
7. Lewis AL, Tolhurst LA, Stratford PW. Analysis of a phosphorylcholine-based polymer coating on a coronary stent pre- and post-implantation. Biomaterials 2002; 23:1697–06.

14

PTFE-covered stents

Richard R. Heuser, Lisa M. Kelly

Treatment for heart disease has changed considerably over the last several decades. One of the most important advances has been the advent of catheter-based techniques that allow minimally invasive solutions for treating ischemic heart disease. After Charles Dotter introduced transluminal angioplasty in the 1960s, coronary angioplasty was pioneered by Andreas Gruentzig following development of his balloon catheter in 1974. More recently, stents and covered stents have proven to be important adjuncts to Gruentzig's original procedure.

Dilatation of an artery with balloon angioplasty may injure the arterial lumen and produce a rough, irregular surface with small areas of dissection. The current theory of restenosis suggests a myoproliferative response to this injury causes subsequent intimal hyperplasia and a rapid cellular proliferation that leads to stenosis. Stenting may prevent injury to the lumen and reduce the potential for hyperplasia and restenosis; the likelihood of plaque disruption and embolization may also be decreased.

The introduction of stents has impacted the fields of cardiology and vascular surgery substantially by expanding therapeutic options for the treatment of cardiac and blood vessel disease. Stenting has been used with great success to improve luminal diameter and restore flow in occluded arteries; results have proved far superior to those seen with laser and atherectomy procedures. When compared with coronary balloon angioplasty, coronary stenting has been shown to reduce angiographic and clinical restenosis rates in patients with de novo lesions in a single coronary artery,[1–5] and/or vein graft.[6] A meta-analysis of the BENESTENT, STRESS, and START trials indicates that stenting reduced restenosis by 31% as compared to angioplasty ($p < 0.0001$) and decreased the risk of further need for a revascularization procedure by 35% ($p < 0.0001$).[5] The mechanism by which a stent reduces restenosis is thought to be its ability to safely enlarge the vessel lumen at the obstructive coronary lesion,[2,7,8] and prevent acute coronary recoil and long-term vascular contraction.[9]

While stents have reduced restenosis as compared to angioplasty, they have not obliterated the problem. The role of covered stents (also known as endoluminal grafts) as a treatment modality for both occlusive and aneurysmal disease is under study worldwide. The use of endovascular grafts for treatment of abdominal aortic aneurysm (AAA) was introduced by Parodi in 1991,[10] and since that time, a number of investigators have described the successful use of covered stents or endoluminal grafting in these procedures. Comparison of open repair and endovascular intervention in the general population indicates that endovascular treatment of AAA is associated with significant reductions in blood loss and transfusions.[11,12]

Covered stents may offer a measure of protection against intimal hyperplasia and restenosis because their internal surface inhibits neointimal formation. Much of the work to date has employed polytetrafluoroethylene (PTFE) tube grafts fixated by Palmaz stents. In the 1930s, researchers at Dupont were studying chlorofluorocarbons and inadvertently developed PTFE, which is much better known by the trade name, Teflon®. PTFE does not attract oils, fats, or proteins, and it resists to some of the most corrosive chemicals we know. The latter property made it ideal for use in the atomic bomb, where it protected gaskets and other mechanisms from uranium hexafluoride. In 1969, Bob Gore, of WL Gore and Associates, discovered that PTFE could be stretched to form a strong material and expanded its uses under the trade name, Gore-Tex®. PTFE material is a natural for grafts and stent coverings; it is inert, biocompatible, resists corrosion, and conforms to a variety of shapes. The inhibition of neointimal formation with PTFE is related to the electronegativity and porosity of the expanded polymer.

Since 1995, when our group first noted the importance of providing complete PTFE coverage in an endoluminal graft used to exclude an aneurysm in an aortocoronary saphenous vein graft,[13] a variety of investigators have made similar observations about PTFE's success in reducing intimal hyperplasia and restenosis in coronary and peripheral interventions.[14–17] While many investigators have fashioned covered stents themselves, there are several commercial grafts available or coming to market.

The commercial devices we are seeing today are lower in profile and easier to deliver than the prototypes used in the mid to late 1990s. In general, these new PTFE-covered devices incorporate self-expanding stents, which are well suited for use in large vessels, but can be difficult to place accurately in small vessels. One stent-graft system (Jomed, Helsingbord, Sweden) designed for use in the coronaries comprises a balloon expandable stent, which can be placed directly at the site of the lesion. The graft itself is constructed using a 'sandwich' technology – ultra-thin PTFE is placed between two stents. The material stays fixed longitudinally as the graft is expanded so that stent-graft shortening is minimized and complete PTFE coverage is provided. The design of the Jomed device represents a considerable advance over the early prototype devices. Likewise, a new device by SciMed (Symbiot, SciMed/Boston Scientific, Maple Grove, MN) that has not yet been approved in the United

States, incorporates a self-expanding nitinol stent and uses a similar PTFE 'sandwich' that minimizes shortening. The device is deployed distal rather than proximal to the lesion, with the idea that this may reduce the risk of embolic phenomena. As yet, this theory has not been proven in actual practice.

Recently, Stoerger and colleagues have reported their results with 70 Jomed grafts in 62 patients with degenerated saphenous vein grafts.[18] Acute technical success was 99%, and the binary restenosis rate was 22%. The authors concluded that the grafts were a safe and effective treatment; however, restenosis rates were similar to those obtained with conventional stents in these difficult lesions – this despite the use of aspirin and ticlopidine in all patients and the addition of glycoprotein IIb/IIIa inhibitors in 26 patients. Clearly, the relative effectiveness of covered stents in these lesions has generated the need for further study. The Randomized Evaluation of polytetrafluoroethylene COVERed stent in Saphenous vein grafts (RECOVERS) trial considered the usefulness of a PTFE covered stent compared with a stainless steel (SS) stent for the prevention of restenosis and major adverse cardiac events (MACE) in patients undergoing saphenous vein graft (SVG) treatment. The study demonstrated that the incidence of 30-day MACE was higher in the PTFE group (10.9% versus 4.1%, $P=0.047$) and was attributed to MI (10.3% versus 3.4% $P=0.037$). The primary end point, the restenosis rate at 6-month follow-up, was similar between the two groups (24.2% versus 24.8% $P=0.237$). The authors concluded no difference in restenosis rates and 6-month clinical outcome between PTFE-covered stent and the SS stent for treatment of SVG lesions.[19] Similar findings were demonstrated in the randomized trail of polytetrafluoroethylene-membrane-covered stents compared with conventional stents in aortocoronary saphenous vein grafts or the STent IN Graft (STING) trial which considered conventional stent to a PTFE-membrane covered stent (Jostent Stentgraft). Investigators determined that the controlled trial did not indicate a superiority of the PTFE-covered Stentgraft compared with a conventional stent with respect to acute results, restenosis or clinical event rates.[20] Most recently the SYM-BIOTT III trial demonstrated similar results. The 8-month study enrolled 400 patients with up to two de novo lesions or restenotic lesions in a single SVG. Overall MACE occurred in 30.6% of the PTFE Symbiot group and in 26.6% of the bare metal control (*P*=0.43) Buchbinder and colleagues concluded the Symbiot and bare metal control outcomes were comparable. The PTFE covered Symbiot stent did not provide an additional advantage compared to the bared metal stent with regard to restenosis and did not appear to reduce intimal hyperplasia.[21]

Our own experience with covered stents (Figures 14.1–14.4) includes their use in saphenous vein grafts, enlarging aneurysms and pseudoaneurysms, as well as in the exclusion of arteriovenous fistulas. In general, our results have been encouraging, but we have yet to determine the long-term success of these interventions. Results of the STents And Radiation Therapy (START) trial (*n* = 476) – the largest in-stent radiation trial – indicate that beta radiation may play an important role in reducing in-stent restenosis without the risk of acute or chronic thrombosis. Studying combination

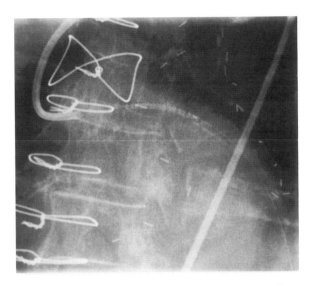

Fig. 14.2 Fluoroscopic image of placement of a Jomed covered stent.

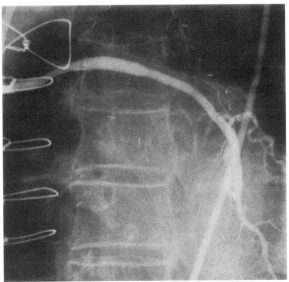

Fig. 14.3 Arteriogram after placement of a Jomed covered stent showing obliteration of the aneurysm.

therapies that incorporate multiple modalities for preventing restenosis is a logical next step for research in percutaneous intervention strategies.

Promising results have emerged in two randomized clinical trails comparing sirolimus-eluting stent to bare stent for in-stent restenosis. The RAVEL trial examined the impact of

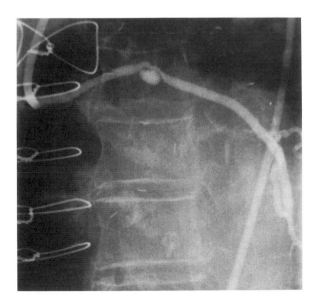

Fig. 14.1 Arteriogram of saphenous vein graft in a 70-year-old woman with severe angina pectoris. There is a complicated mid vessel aneurysmal lesion with a tight stenosis.

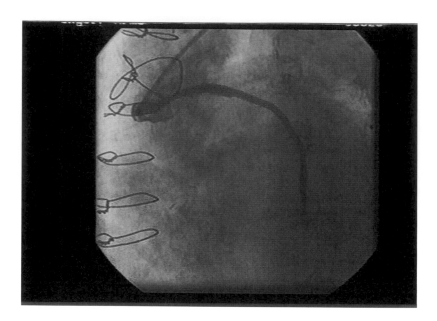

Fig. 14.4 Arteriogram at 8-month follow-up showing continued patency of the saphenous vein graft with no stenosis.

sirolimus-eluting stent (SES) on outcomes in diabetic patients. The RAVEL study randomized 238 patients to treatment with SES or bare metal stent. Forty-four patients were diabetics; 19 received SES and 25 were treated with bare metal stents. Six-month follow-up angiography revealed the in-stent late lumen loss was significantly lower for diabetics with SES than the bare metal group (0.07+/−0.2 versus 0.82+/−0.5mm; $P<0.001$) and similar to that in non-diabetic patients (-0.03+/−0.27mm) There was zero restenosis in the SES groups, both diabetic and non-diabetic compared to a 42% restenosis rate in the diabetic population assigned to bare metal stents ($P=0.001$). The results demonstrated diabetics treated with SES experienced a virtual abolition of neointimal proliferation and low event rates at long-term follow-up.[22] The SIRIUS Trial assessed the l-year clinical outcome in 1058 patients enrolled in a randomized trial of a sirolimus-eluting stent versus a control bare stent in patients at high risk for coronary restenosis. Holmes and colleagues demonstrated at 9 months, the target-lesion revascularization rate for the sirolimus-eluting stent was 4.1% versus 16.6% in the control bare metal stent ($P<0.001$). At 12 months the differences had widened to 4.9% versus 20.0% ($P<0.001$). The trial demonstrated

the even in high-risk subsets, there was a 70%–80% relative reduction in restenosis at 12 months with the sirolimus-eluting stent.[23]

REFERENCES

1. Nobuyoshi M, Kimura T, Nosaka H, et al. Restenosis after successful percutaneous transluminal angioplasty: serial angiographic follow-up of 229 patients. J Am Coll Cardiol 1988; 12:616–23.
2. Hirshfeld JW Jr, Schwartz JS, Jugo R, et al. Restenosis after coronary angioplasty: a multivariate statistical model to relate lesion and procedure variables to restenosis. J Am Coll Cardiol 1991; 18:647–56.
3. Fischman DL, Leon M, Baim D, et al. A randomized comparison of coronary-stent placement and balloon angioplasty in the treatment of coronary artery disease. Stent Restenosis Study Investigators. N Engl J Med 1994; 331:496–501.
4. Serruys PW, de Jaegere P, Kiemenij F, et al. A comparison of balloon-expandable stent implantation with balloon angioplasty in patients with coronary artery disease. Benestent Study group. N Engl J Med 1994; 331:489–95.
5. Masotti M, Serra A, Betriu A. Stents and de novo coronary lesions. Meta-analysis. Rev Esp Cardiol 1997; 50(suppl):3–9.

6. Savage MP, Douglas JS, Fischman DL, et al. Stent placement compared with balloon angioplasty for obstructed coronary bypass grafts. Saphenous Vein De Novo Trial Investigators. N Engl J Med 1997; 337:740–7.

7. Kuntz RE, Safian RD, Levine MJ, et al. Novel approach to the analysis of restenosis after the use of three new coronary devices. J Am Coll Cardiol 1993; 19:1493–9.

8. Kuntz RE, Gibson CM, Nobuyoshi M, et al. Generalized model of restenosis after conventional balloon angioplasty, stenting, and directional atherectomy. J Am Coll Cardiol 1993; 21:15–25.

9. Mintz GS, Popma JJ, Hong MK, et al. Intravascular ultrasound to discern device specific effects and mechanisms of restenosis. Am J Cardiol 1996; 78(3A):18–22.

10. Parodi JC, Palmaz JC, Barone HD. Transfemoral intraluminal graft implantation for abdominal aortic aneurysm. Ann Vasc Surg 1991; 5(6):491–9.

11. May J, White GH, Yu W, et al. Concurrent comparison of endoluminal versus open repair in the treatment of abdominal aortic aneurysm: analysis of 303 patients by life table method. J Vasc Surg 1998; 27(2):213–20.

12. Zarins KZ, Rodney AW, Schwarten D, et al. AneuRx stent graft versus open surgical repair of abdominal aortic aneurysm: Multicenter prospective clinical trial. J Vasc Surg 1999; 29(2):292–308.

13. Heuser RR, Reynolds GT, Papazoglou C, Diethrich EB. Endoluminal grafting for percutaneous aneurysm exclusion in an aortocoronary saphenous vein graft: the first clinical experience. J Endovasc Surg 1995; 2:81–8.

14. Marin ML, Veith FJ, Cynamon J, et al. Effect of polytetrafluoroethylene covering of Palmaz stents on the development of intimal hyperplasia in human iliac arteries. J Vasc Interv Radiol 1996; 7:651–6.

15. Heuser RR, Woodfield S, Lopez A. Obliteration of a coronary artery aneurysm with a PTFE-covered stent: endoluminal graft for coronary disease revisited. Catheter Cardiovasc Interv 1999; 64:113–6.

16. Lukito G, Vandergoten P, Jaspers L, et al. Six months clinical angiographic, and IVUS follow-up after PTFE graft stent implantation in native coronary arteries. Acta Cardiol 2000; 55:255–60.

17. Baldus S, Koster R, Elsner M, et al. Treatment of aortocoronary vein graft lesions with membrane-covered stents: a multicenter surveillance trial. Circulation 2000; 102:2024–7.

18. Stoerger H, Haase J, Hofmann M, Schwarz F. Implantation of coronary PTFE-grafts in degenerated saphenous vein grafts: acute and intermediate term results. Circulation 2000; 102(suppl):2642 (abstract).

19. Stankovic G, Colombo A, Presbitero P, et al. The Randomized Evaluation of Polytetrafluoroethylene COVERed stent in Saphenous vein grafts (RECOVERS) Trial. Circulation 2003; 108:37–42.

20. Schächinger V, Hamm C, Münzel T, et al. A randomized trial of polytetrafluoroethylene-membrane-covered stents compared with conventional stents in aortocoronary saphenous vein grafts. J Am Coll Cardiol 2003; 42:1360–9.

21. Buchbinder, M. SYMBIOT III: ePTFE-covered Nitinol Stent Does Not Reduce Intimal Hyperplasia in SVG Interventions. TCT 2004.

22. Abizaid A, Costa M, Blanchard D, et al. Sirolimus-eluting stents inhibit neointimal hyperplasia in diabetic patients. Insights from the RAVEL Trial. Eur Heart J 2004; 25:107–12.

23. Holmes D, Leon M, Moses J, et al. Analysis of 1-year clinical outcomes in the SIRIUS trail: A randomized trial of a sirolimus-eluting stent versus a standard stent in patients at high risk for coronary restenosis. Circulation 2004; 109:634–40.

15

Overview of drug delivery coatings

Michael Kuehler and B. BRAUN MELSUNGEN AG

Introduction • **Drug release mechanisms** • **Release profiles** • **Materials for drug delivery**

INTRODUCTION

Implant surfaces are coated with drugs for several reasons. These agents can be permanently bonded to an implant (e.g. covalent like heparin or temporary like rapamycin for coronary stents). However, covalent fixed coatings only allow the action of biological processes very close to the implant surface, and a drug carrier from the implant surface to specific cell sites is frequently required. In order to fulfill the need for optimal drug delivery, several important issues need to be considered.

If the drug is eluted over a defined time period a drug carrier is often necessary and should be able to deliver an incorporated drug. Therefore, the release mechanism of the carrier material must be coordinated with the characteristics of the drug itself (e.g. the permeability of the carrier with the molecular weight of the drug). Furthermore, the carrier should allow an adequate release rate, profile, and support drug transport to specific cells.

Another issue is to ensure that there is a sufficient amount of the agent on the implant surface. This is especially the case for small implants, such as stents, where the surface area is limited. When developing a drug eluting surface, the structure of the implant and drug–tissue pharmacokinetics also have to be considered.[1]

In this chapter an overview of drug release mechanisms for coated implants is discussed.

DRUG RELEASE MECHANISMS

Implant drug delivery systems generally can be classified into those with an additional carrier material (and without additional carrier material) (Figure 15.1). In systems without an additional carrier diffusion of the agent will be controlled by the implant's surface topography (e.g. with holes, pores etc. on the surface hydrophobicity of the drug and drug dispersion). Combinations of both groups are possible. Coating-based release systems can be separated into three groups:

1. Diffusion controlled release
2. Swelling controlled release, and
3. Biodegradable systems.

Diffusion controlled release systems

In the diffusion controlled system, the drug is dissolved or dispersed in the matrix (Figure 15.2). When it comes into contact with the implant site the agent will diffuse from the carrier coating. Two release systems can be differentiated:

1. Matrix systems (Figure 15.2a) have a release rate that decreases over the time. But

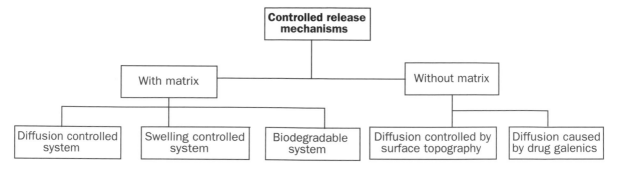

Fig. 15.1   Overview of different drug release mechanisms.

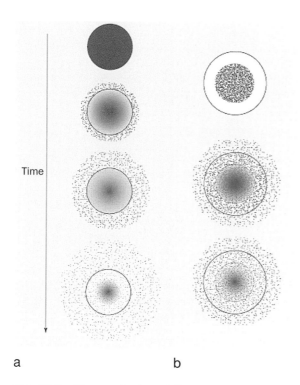

a   b

Fig. 15.2   The matrix drug delivery system (a), and reservoir system (b).[2]

continuous or so-called zero release profiles are often required.

2. Reservoir systems (Figure 15.2b) have a fairly stable diffusion rate. They comprise a core that contains the concentrated agent within a polymer matrix and a shell, whereas the shell is made of a rate controlling

material. With regard to a stent strut this is equivalent to a two-layer system with a drug in the first layer and a barrier coating in the second layer.

Diffusion is driven by the concentration gradient between the core and the outside of the shell or barrier coating.

Swelling controlled release systems[2]

Another option for drug release is the use of swelling controlled materials. The material in the drug is compact in the dry state but swells during contact with liquids. Caused by the swelling, which is often combined with a diffusion process, the incorporated drug is released. Again, differences between matrix and reservoir systems can be differentiated.

Most of the compounds used in swelling controlled release systems are based on hydrogels. These are polymers that can absorb a large amount of water without dissolving. For some polymers, this property can be triggered by a change in the environment surrounding the implant. If there is a change in pH, temperature or ionic strength, the system can either shrink or swell (Figure 15.3).

Biodegradable release systems

When the carrier is biologically degraded the drug is released from the matrix. Depending on the type and mesh size of the carrier, diffusion

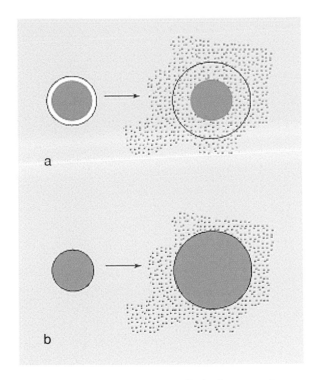

Fig. 15.3 The swelling controlled release system: (a) reservoir (b) matrix.[2]

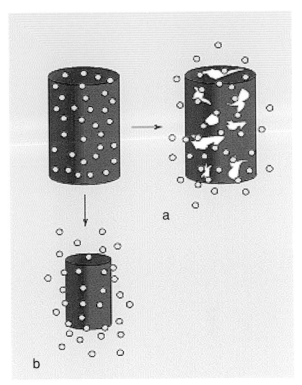

Fig. 15.4 Biodegradable system: (a) bulk and (b) surface erosion.[2]

also plays a role. Depending on the type of degradation, the systems are differentiated into bulk and surface degradable systems (Figure 15.4). Surface degradable systems are favorable for drug delivery systems in blood vessels because the risk of bulk fragments in the blood stream, and therefore the risk of thrombosis caused by fragments is minimized.

RELEASE PROFILES

With conventional release systems like pills, considerable changes in drug concentration occur, whereas the drug level varies between ineffective and toxic. Controlled drug release coatings can deliver a drug continuously during a desired time frame. Very often, a zero order pattern is desirable (Figure 15.5).

Coatings based on matrix systems will have a Fickian order for a constant source (dispersed drug) or a mixed Fickian and first order release for a non-constant source (only dissolved drug).

Reservoir systems that have a constant source (pure liquid drug or dispersed drug) provide a zero order release rate. A non-constant source (dissolved drug in solution) provides a first order release rate.

MATERIALS FOR DRUG DELIVERY

Drug carriers can be made from lipids and, of course, polymers, which can be loosely differentiated into permanent and degradable (Figure 15.6).

Lipids and liposomes[3,4]

Lipids are amphipathic molecules (e.g. fatty acids, fats, and phospholipids). Lipids have a dual structure that comprises a hydrophilic and a hydrophobic region. They are soluble in organic solvents and form clusters in aqueous solutions. Monolayer, micelles, and liposomes are the favored forms in aqueous solutions.

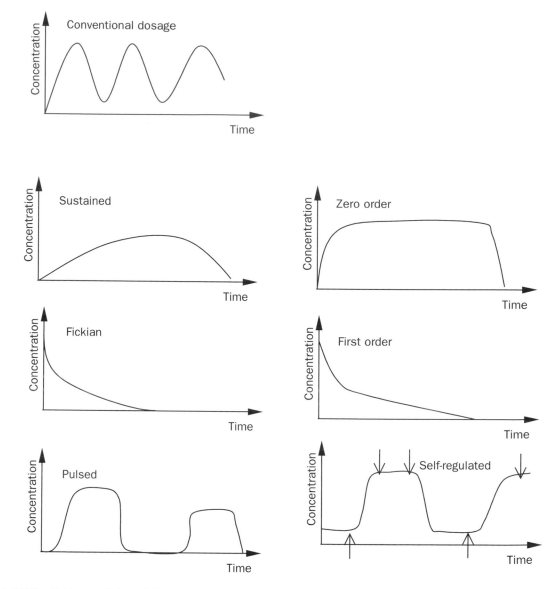

Fig. 15.5 Patterns of drug delivery.

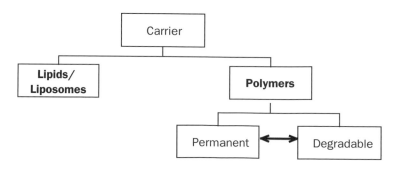

Fig. 15.6 Potential carrier materials for drug delivery.

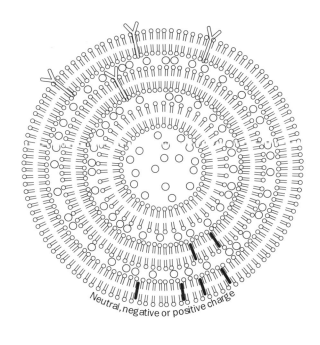

Neutral, negative or positive charge

○ Water-soluble molecules

▌ Lipid-soluble molecules

Υ Water-soluble molecules with hydrophobic moiety penetrating lipid phase

Fig. 15.7 Diagrammatic representation of a liposome in which three phospholipid bilayers alternate with aqueous compartments.[3]

Liposomes are spherical lipid clusters consisting of one or more lipid bilayers enclosing one or more aqueous compartments (Figure 15.7). They can mimic several properties of cell membranes (e.g. respond to osmotic forces, have a permeability barrier). Liposomes are a suitable environment responsive system for drug delivery. Several chemical and physical triggers for drug release exist (e.g. pH, heat, magnetic field, light, polyelectrolytes).

In the aqueous layers of the liposome, water-soluble drugs can be entrapped by intercalation while lipid-soluble drugs can be made soluble within the hydrocarbon interiors of the lipid bilayers.

Polymers

Many polymers are known to have the potential for drug delivery coatings. Figure 15.8

shows some of the most common permanent polymers. If a polymer is degradable or not depends on some chemical characteristics, such as molecular weight and hydrophobicity. In reality, everything degrades but the question is how fast it degrades. For drug delivery applications, degradation in the human time scale is important.

Depending on the implantation site additional biocompatibility characteristics have to be considered for polymers. For example, some of them may cause inflammation (e.g. in blood vessels) but are well tolerated in other parts of the body. Other potential disadvantages of polymer coatings are difficulties with mechanical behavior after sterilization, and expansion if the implant undergoes high plastic deformations (e.g. like stents).

Permanent polymers[4]

A number of more or less stable polymers with a potential for drug delivery are known (Figure 15.8). Whereas hydrophobic or less hydrophilic polymers are suitable for diffusion controlled coatings, very hydrophilic polymers, known as hydrogels, will form swelling controlled coatings and are a group of polymers often used as drug delivery matrices.

If a drug is mixed uniformly with the polymer the drug are dispersed in a homogenous polymer matrix (matrix system). Some of the drug molecules dissolve into and saturate the polymer matrix. These dissolved molecules can diffuse through the matrix into the surrounding medium. The saturation of the matrix is lost and the dispersed molecules have to re-dissolve to re-saturate the polymer matrix. After the drug is diffused out of the polymer, pores remain and become filled with aqueous medium. The drug release through the matrix and the pores is thus facilitated. Due to osmotic pressure generated by the drug particles the polymer may fracture.

Depending on the hydrophobicity of the drug, the use of hydrophilic and hydrophobic polymers or polymer blends allows the tailoring of release behavior.

A disadvantage of permanent polymers is that a rest content of the drug will remain

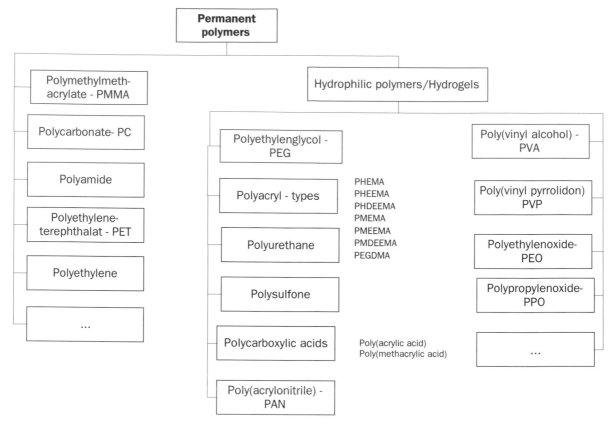

Fig. 15.8 Permanent polymers.

in the polymer. Depending on the type of polymer, the mesh size and the size of the drug molecule, a variable amount of drug will be encapsulated permanently. Late burst effects due to a long term instability of the polymer could occur.

Hydrophilic polymers[5,6]
Hydrophilic polymers are soluble in and compatible with water. A wide range of applications is known, such as in food, cosmetics, and medical implants.

Most hydrophilic polymers are based on acrylated and methacrylated composites. As well as other monomeric species they possess polar dependent groups in the vinyl position.

The side chain groups on the other carbon atoms contribute to the overall properties of the hydrophilic polymer and they also create a large amount of free volume between neighboring polymer molecules because of their size and flexibility. Their generally poor mechanical properties can be enhanced by cross-linking them.

Hydrogels
Some materials, when placed in water, swell very rapidly and retain up to a multiple of their own weight of aqueous fluid. These hydrogels usually comprise hydrophilic polymer molecules that are cross-linked by chemical bonds or other cohesion forces, such as ionic interaction, hydrogen bonding or hydrophobic interaction.

Because of their unique bulk and surface properties, hydrogels have favorable biocompatibility and are ideal for several drug delivery applications. They have no interfacial tension with surrounding biological fluids and tissue, which minimizes the driving force of

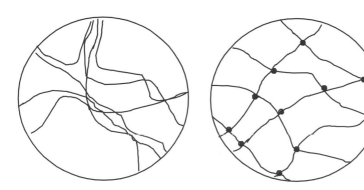

Fig. 15.9 General structure of physical (left) and chemical (right) gels.

protein adsorption and cell adhesion. Furthermore, hydrogels simulate hydrodynamic properties of natural biological gels, cells, and tissue in many ways.

Types of hydrogels

The three-dimensional network of a hydrogel is held together by physical or chemical bonds (Figure 15.9) and can be divided into two major categories: the physical hydrogels and the chemical hydrogels.

Physical gel networks comprise an amorphous hydrophilic polymer phase, held together by highly ordered aggregates of polymer chain segments arising from secondary molecular forces in conjunction with other types of molecular interaction. They are soluble in water or solvents and can be melted by heat.

Chemical gels are formed by the introduction of primary covalent cross-links. They do not dissolve in water or organic solvents even on heating.

If two or more monomeric species are interwoven an interpenetrating network (IPN) (Figure 15.10) is formed. They are used to modify properties that hydrogels normally lack. If one or both phases are biodegradable the IPN can be used for drug delivery applications. Semi-IPNs are IPNs with one cross-linked phase to immobilize the non-crosslinked phase. This technique is useful for implant coatings or drug release systems. Through modification of the boundary conditions it is possible to alter the release characteristics. In particular chemical configurations of some hydrogels are biodegradable.

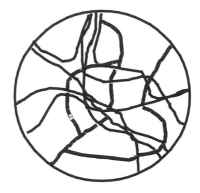

Fig. 15.10 An interpenetrating network (IPN) with two components.

Biodegradable polymers[4,7]

Biodegradable polymers have become increasingly important in the development of drug delivery systems because they do not require removal after drugs are depleted.

Biodegradation can occur in many different structural levels (i.e. molecular, macromolecular, microscopic, and macroscopic) depending on the mechanism. The polymers become less complex through biodegradation; this occurs through four different mechanisms: (1) solubilization, (2) charge formation followed dissolution, (3) hydrolysis, and (4) enzyme-catalyzed degradation. In polymers, biodegradation undergoes four stages: (i) hydration, (ii) strength loss, (iii) loss of mass integrity, and (iv) mass loss.

The evaluation of the biocompatibility of a degradable polymer also requires an evaluation of the degradation products. A biocompatible polymer can degrade into toxic degradation products. The number and size of fragments must be therefore specified.

Degradable polymers can undergo bulk or surface erosion. The nature of erosion depends on the diffusion of water inside the matrix, the degradation rate of the polymer's functional groups, and matrix dimensions. For the matrix, a critical device dimension $L_{critical}$ can be calculated. The polymer will undergo surface erosion if the matrix is larger than $L_{critical}$, if not it will undergo bulk erosion.[7]

If the polymer degrades in bulk, the rate of water penetration into the matrix is faster than the rate of the polymer degradation. If the degradation rate occurs at a uniform rate throughout the polymer matrix this process is homogeneous.

For a polymer that undergoes surface degradation, the rate of water penetration into the matrix is slower than the rate of degradation. A heterogeneous process with degradation of only a thin surface layer occurs.

Drug delivery matrices can be categorized in four different groups (Figure 15.11): (1) cross-linked polymer network, (2) cleavable linear polymer, (3) insoluble linear polymer, and (4) drug-conjugated polymer. The release of the drugs follows the mechanisms (i) diffusion, (ii) polymer degradation, (iii) osmosis, and (iv) labile covalent bonds cleavage between drug and polymer.

The biodegradable polymers can be categorized as those with synthetic origins and those with natural origins (Figures 15.12 and 15.13).

The degree of polymer degradability depends on different properties:

- The higher the cristallinity of the polymer the slower the degradation.
- The type of degradable bonds present on the polymer determines the rate of degradation. It follows: Anhydride→Esters→Amides.

- Hydrophilics degrade faster than hydrophobic polymers.
- Polymers with a high molecular weight degrade slower than polymers with a low molecular weight.

Biodegradable polymers with synthetic roots
Biodegradable synthetic polymers often have advantages over the natural polymers with regard to controlled release (e.g. they can be tailored for specific needs). In addition, crystallinity, degradability, solubility, hydrophobicity, glass transition, and melting temperature can be easily changed by the synthesis and recipe and condition.

Figure 15.12 presents some of the most common synthetic biodegradable polymers. Each polymer possesses different crystallinity, degradability, solubility, processibility, and stability.

A large group of polymers for drug delivery matrices are the polyesters. Poly(lactide acid), poly(glycolic acid), poly(lactic-co-glycolic acid), poly(ε-caprolactone), and poly(lactid acid-co-ε-caprolactone) are very common in controlled release systems. The lactic/glycolic acid polymers have been extensively investigated for their potential as a drug-containing matrix. Generally, they show little inflammatory response or other harmful side effects, and the degradation products are non-toxic.

Degradable polymers with natural roots
The use of natural biodegradable polymers is limited by their lack of versatility: only modification rather than synthesis of these is possible. Until now the modification is limited to the effect that the resulting products may not meet controlled release requirements.

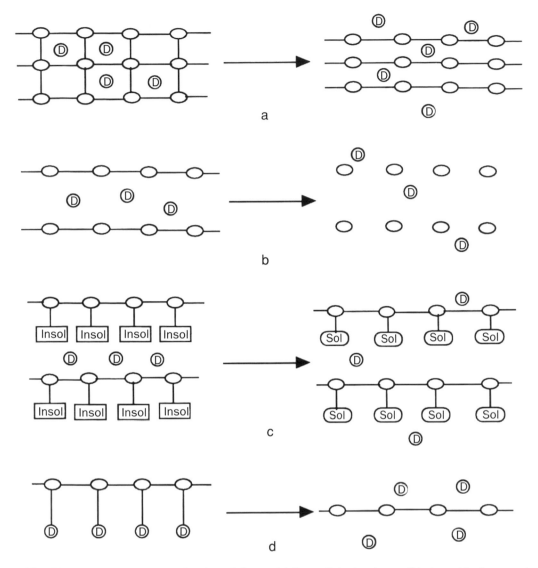

Fig. 15.11 Biodegradable polymers for drug delivery. (a) Cross-linked polymer, (b) cleavable linear polymer, (c) insoluble linear polymer, and (d) drug-conjugated polymer. (D, drug).[4]

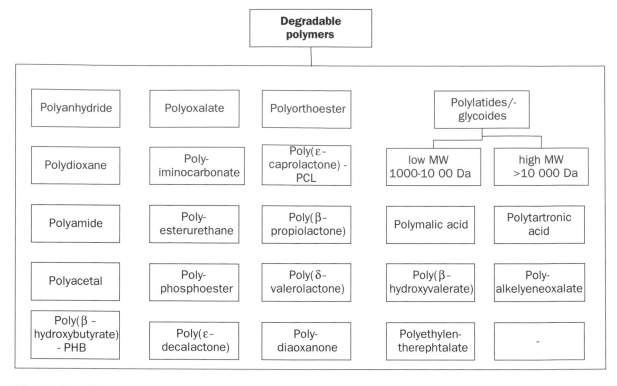

Fig. 15.12 Biodegradable polymers with synthetic roots.

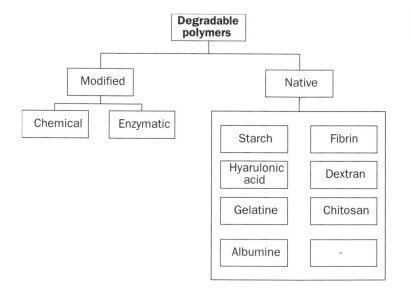

Fig. 15.13 Biodegradable polymers with natural roots.

REFERENCES

1. Hwang Chao-Wei AB, Wu D, Edelman ER. Physiological transport forces govern drug distribution for stent-based delivery. Circulation 2001; 104:600–5.

2. Brannon-Pepas L. 'Polymers in Controlled Drug delivery'. Medical Plastics and Biomedical Magazine archive 1997: www.devicelink.com/mpb/archive/97/11/003.html

3. Davis 'Colloidal drug delivery' University of Nottingham, Faculty of Science 2001: www.nottingham.ac.uk/~paz51/fage.html

4. Wu Xue Shen. Controlled drug delivery systems. Technomic: Lancaster, PA 1996.

5. Park K, Shalaby WSW. Park H. Biodegradable hydrogels for drug delivery. Technomic: Lancaster, PA 1993.

6. LaPorte RJ. Hydrophilic polymer coatings for medical devices. Technomic: Lancaster, PA 1997.

7. Burkersroda F von, Schedl L, Gopferich A. Why degradable polymers undergo surface erosion or bulk erosion. Biomaterials 2002; 23:4421–31.

16

Phosphorylcholine (PC Technology™) coated stents as a drug delivery platform

Ivan De Scheerder, Andrew Lewis, and Anthony Collias

Introduction • Non-thrombogenicity • Non-inflammatory response • Long-term stability in vivo
• Clinical performance • A flexible drug delivery platform • Designed for drug delivery
• A strategy for tackling restenosis

INTRODUCTION

The Bio*divYsio*® family of coronary stents is characterized by the presence of a phosphoryl-choline (PC) polymer coating. The PC coating is a synthetic copy of the predominant phospholipid that comprises the outside of the red blood cell membrane.[1] The surface of devices coated with this material therefore mimics the body's own chemistry, and any response to the foreign implant is lessened. The data reviewed in this chapter demonstrate that PC Technology™ is well suited as a platform for stent-mediated drug delivery because PC coatings are:

- non-thrombogenic
- non-inflammatory
- have physicomechanical properties to enable them to survive the rigors of stent placement and expansion
- are non-detrimental to critical stent mechanics
- have long-term stability within the body
- are able to deliver a range of therapeutic agents in a controlled fashion for a sustained period
- have proven long-term clinical experience.

There are two PC-coated drug delivery coronary stent formats currently available (Bio*divYsio*™ Matrix LO and Bio*divYsio*™ Matrix HI) that, unlike all other stent drug delivery systems, *do not possess a preselected drug on the stent*. They can be loaded with any one of a variety of compounds by simple immersion of the stent in a solution of the drug at the appropriate concentration for a short period of time. This self-loading approach has been specifically developed to offer physicians total flexibility in their choice of therapeutic option. These stents are thus tools in the quest for an antirestenotic treatment with the most appropriate balance between efficacy and patient safety. The Bio*divYsio*™ Matrix LO coronary stent is suitable for many compounds that possess a molecular weight less than 1200 daltons, whereas Bio*divYsio*™ Matrix HI has been developed with gene therapy in mind, being suitable for the delivery of higher molecular weight species which possess a net negative charge (such as heparin, oligonucleotides or DNA fragments).

In addition to the PC portion for biocompatibility, the coating polymers have been designed with several other components included for

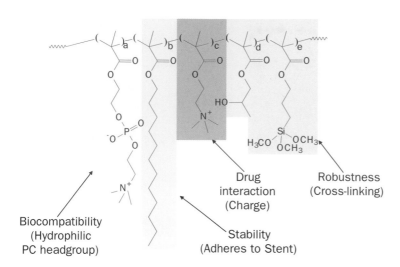

Fig. 16.1 Generic structure for phosphorylcholine (PC) polymer coatings.

Biocompatibility
(Hydrophilic
PC headgroup)

Drug
interaction
(Charge)

Robustness
(Cross-linking)

Stability
(Adheres to Stent)

other specific purposes (Figure 16.1). A hydrophobic lauryl alkyl chain component aids in the initial adhesion and film formation of the polymers on to the stainless steel stent substrate. Other groups allow thermally induced cross-linking both within the polymer to form a water-swellable network, and also with metal oxide groups on the stent surface to achieve firm anchorage. It is the swollen polymer network that forms the vehicle into which therapeutic agents can be absorbed and released from the Bio*divYsio*™ Matrix LO stent, the 1200 dalton molecular weight cut-off in this system being a function of the size of the hydrated spaces that form within the network structure.[2] There are, however, a multitude of biological molecules that are of potential use in the treatment of restenosis that are simply too large to be absorbed into any ordinary polymeric coating. For this reason, the PC Technology™ coating has been modified so that it is capable of interacting with the negatively charged groups found in many of these biological molecules (such as gene fragments and antibodies). This has been achieved by the introduction of cationically charged groups into the basic polymer used for Bio*divYsio*™ Matrix LO stents (Figure 16.1). The introduction of such groups into a stent coating could have the potential to reduce both the blood and tissue compatibility of the polymer.[3] With the Bio*divYsio*™ Matrix HI coating, a carefully

balanced combination of the cationic centers with the PC technology ensures that a biologically inert platform has been maintained whilst enabling delivery of large molecular weight compounds. In this way, the drug has an affinity for the coating and is adsorbed to its surface, where it can be released into the tissue over time (Figure 16.2).

These polymers can be sterilized by conventional methods, and indeed the mechanical properties of the coatings are further enhanced by a γ-irradiation step that is used to fully cross-link the coating. Atomic force microscopy (AFM) and nanoindentation studies have thus shown that the coating is tenaciously adhered to the stent and can survive balloon expansion without damage.[4]

NON-THROMOBOGENICITY

There have been a plethora of in vitro experiments performed on PC coatings to show that they resist protein adsorption, do not activate complement, and reduce both platelet adhesion and activation.[5–8] The ex vivo non-human primate model,[7,9] offers one of the closest simulators of human hemostatic function. The PC coating has been evaluated using this model where the increase in radioactivity associated with the accumulation of indium (^{111}In)-labeled platelets was monitored over time. Figure 16.3(a) shows a comparison of the platelets adhering

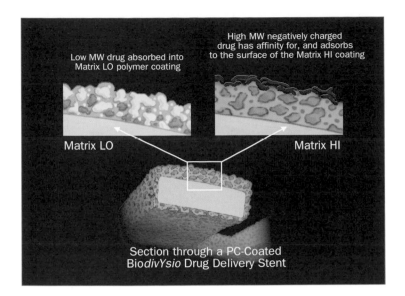

Fig. 16.2 Mode of loading for the Bio*divYsio* Matrix LO and HI stents.

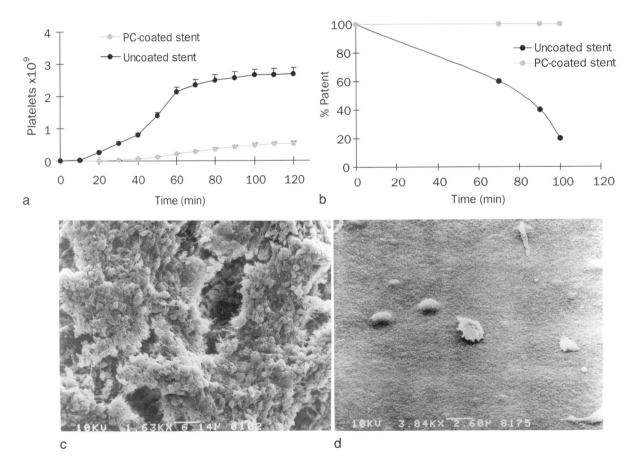

Fig. 16.3 (a) Platelet adhesion in the ex vivo shunt model. (b) Percent patency of the shunt over time. Scanning electron micrographs of the uncoated (c) and PC-coated (d) stent surfaces.

over a 2 hour period for a PC-coated versus an uncoated stent. Figure 16.3(b) shows the estimate of the extent of thrombus occlusion in the stented sections of the shunt over the same time period. The PC-coated stent showed minimal platelet adhesion over the test period (although some platelets adhered to the tubing and at the edges of the stent due to flow disturbance), whilst platelets rapidly adhered to the uncoated sample. Analysis of the stent surfaces by scanning electron microscopy (SEM) after the experiment was complete confirmed the build-up of significant thrombus on the uncoated stent surface (Figure 16.3c), whereas the PC-coated surface was free from any adhered protein or cells (Figure 16.3d).

Furthermore, in the human ex vivo flowing blood model used by Chronos et al. the PC coating significantly reduced the interaction of blood components with artificial surfaces, even in the absence of anticoagulant.[10] These experiments demonstrate a decrease of fibrinogen and platelet adsorption of up to 98%. Whilst in vitro and ex vivo experiments clearly support the non-thrombogenic and biocompatible nature of the PC coating, these data are limited in their predictive ability of clinical perform-

ance. Platelet adhesion has therefore been evaluated in vivo using implantation into the brachial arteries of non-human primates. As with the ex vivo shunt model, platelets were sampled and labeled with radioactive indium prior to implantation of the stents. Subsequent to stent deployment, platelet accumulation in the stented area was monitored by use of a gamma camera placed on the arm above the device location. Figure 16.4 shows the comparison of platelet number for PC-coated versus uncoated stents after the first 60 and 90 minutes. A significant reduction in platelet adhesion was noted relative to the uncoated control stents at each time point ($p<0.03$ in each case).

Other studies have involved the use of a baboon aorto-iliac model,[11] and observed markedly reduced thrombosis on PC-coated stents harvested at one month post placement (and interestingly, up to a one-third reduction in neointimal area compared to uncoated control stents). This accumulation of evidence to support the non-thrombogenicity of PC coatings is somewhat reflected in the clinical situation, with a zero incidence of subacute thrombosis recorded in the DISTINCT randomized trial (see Table 16.1) and very low

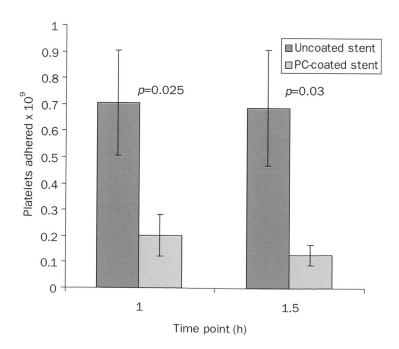

Fig. 16.4 Platelet adhesion in a baboon brachial implant model.

Table 16.1 The DISTINCT randomized trial single stent data		
DISTINCT *Single stent data*	*BiodivYsio AS* *stent*	*Guidant Multilink* *Duet*
6 month TVF	6.4%	8.6%
Binary angiographic restenosis rates	17.9%	22.2%

- No subacute thromboses occurred in the Bio*divYsio* stent arm
- Demonstration of safety of the Bio*divYsio* PC-coated stent at 12 months and equivalence to the ACS Multilink Duet stent

occurrence in other clinical trials with these coated stents.[12]

NON-INFLAMMATORY RESPONSE

Previous studies on polymer-coated stents have raised concerns about excessive inflammatory response to the coating materials.[3,13] During wound healing, the PC coating has been shown to illicit a similar tissue reaction to the non-coated stent, with no additional adverse inflammation. In initial studies reported by Kuiper,[14,15] arterial wall reaction to PC-coated stents was examined in rabbits and pigs. Compared to non-coated stents, no significant difference was found by angiography and histology. The PC coating did not provoke any additional neointimal formation or decreased lumen diameter, nor did it reduce restenosis in these models. A more detailed comparison of PC-coated and uncoated stents implanted in porcine coronary arteries has been made using angiographic, morphometric, light microscope (LM) and electron microscope (EM) techniques.[16] Forty stents (25 PC-coated, 15 uncoated) were implanted in the coronary arteries of 20 pigs; quantitative coronary angiography (QCA) was performed prestent and post implantation on 15 pigs at 28 days. No angiographically occlusive thrombosis occurred in any of the stents. LM at 5 days showed endothelialization of both coated and uncoated stents, which was confirmed by EM

at 14 days. QCA and morphometry showed no significant differences between the coated and uncoated stents. A few inflammatory cells were observed for both stent types at 5 days, with no inflammation or additional tissue reaction to the PC coating compared to uncoated at 28 days. This indicated that no adverse or specific histological changes were associated with the PC coating, a problem that has been reported on occasion with other polymeric stent coatings.[3,13] The biocompatibility of the coating was again confirmed in a baboon iliac artery study which compared histopathology of 15 mm uncoated and PC-coated Bio*divYsio* stents ($n = 5$ for each group) at 1, 3, and 6 months (Hanson et al. unpublished data). The vascular wall response was similar to that found in other preclinical coronary artery stent implant investigations (Figure 16.5). A well-defined neointima was present for all stents, with the greatest increase evident between the first and third month. The neointimal area for the PC-coated stents did not increase between the third and sixth month, but rather decreased slightly. For the uncoated stents, the neointima increased between 3 and 6 months. For all Bio*divYsio* stents, regardless of implant duration, the endothelial cell layer was intact. Stent struts, as shown in the following figures, were well deployed into the media, with variable amounts of compression noted. No evidence was observed of coating delamination from the PC-coated stents.

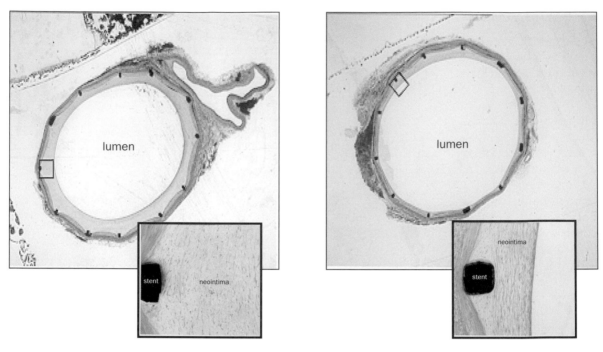

Fig. 16.5 Typical histological sections from porcine arteries stented with uncoated (left) and PC-coated (right) Bio*divYsio* stents.

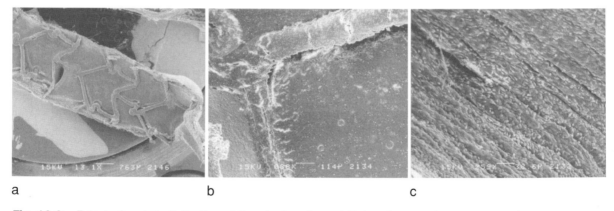

a   b   c

Fig. 16.6 Extent of endothelialization of the stent surface at 5 days in a porcine coronary artery demonstrating a confluent layer of cells: (a) at ×13.1, (b) ×88, and (c) ×259 magnification.

A similar assessment of the biocompatibility of the PC-coated stents was performed in a 25 pig study by Whelan et al.,[17,18] using 20 PC-coated and 21 uncoated stents, with assessments made at 5 days ($n = 6$), 4 weeks ($n = 7$) and 12 weeks ($n = 8$). Both uncoated and PC-coated stents were equally well endothelialized at 5 days (92% and 91%, respectively), again indi-cating that the PC coating did not impede cellular overgrowth of the stent (Figure 16.6), contrary to predictions from many in vitro findings.[1] At 4 and 12 weeks there was no difference in intimal thickening between coated and non-coated stents and at 12 weeks the PC coating was still discernible in the stent struts voids and was not associated with any adverse tissue reaction.

LONG-TERM STABILITY IN VIVO

The coating on the conventional non-drug delivery Bio*divYsio* stent is approximately 50–100 nm in thickness, compared to approximately 2 μm on the outer strut surface of the Bio*divYsio* Matrix LO and HI stents. These ultra-thin thicknesses can be determined by an atomic force microscopic technique (AFM), which also allows measurement of the force required to remove the coating from the stent.[4] A similar evaluation has been made on stents removed after a prolonged implantation time. Following 6 month implantation in porcine coronary arteries Bio*divYsio* stents have been examined using AFM and SEM techniques in order to determine whether the PC coating was still present.[8,19] The study showed the coating was present and that both its thickness, and the force required to remove the coating from the stent was largely unchanged (Figure 16.7). In a more recent study, portions of a stent were retrieved from a patient at 6 months as a result of a routine atherectomy.[20] Similar AFM and EM techniques were used to show that the thickness and force to remove the coating were once again unchanged. Additional AFM fingerprinting techniques were used to identify the layer on the stent as the original PC coating, and laser ablation high resolution inductively coupled plasma mass spectrometry was utilized to detect the tiny amounts of silicon present in the crosslinking groups of the PC coating (Figure 16.1). The PC coating is therefore not affected over this timescale by the vessel environment.

These data, together with the histological observations described in the previous sections, provide evidence that the PC coating is biocompatible, does not illicit an unfavorable biological reaction and hence is not subject to degradation within the body.

CLINICAL PERFORMANCE

There have been a number of interesting clinical studies evaluating the Bio*divYsio* stent, including an adhesion molecule study that showed reduced platelet activation without endothelial cell activation,[21] an evaluation of primary stenting in the treatment of acute myocardial infarction,[22] and an early mobilization study after protamine reversal of heparin,[23] all of which produced very positive outcomes for the PC-coated stent. There have been a number of open registries evaluating the clinical performance of the stent in well over 1000 patients,[24–28] including the large formal 425 patient Study Of PHosphorylcholine On Stents registry

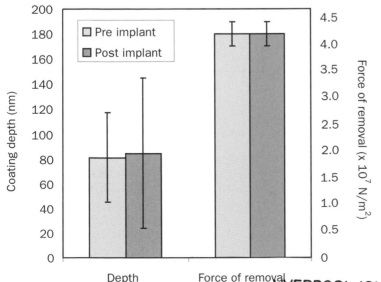

Fig. 16.7 Force of removal and PC coating depth preimplantation and 6 months postimplantation in porcine arteries.

(SOPHOS),[29] all of which support the safety and efficacy of the device and its use in a broad spectrum of indications. The Bio*DIvYsio* Stent IN controlled Clinical Trial (DISTINCT) study was a 622 patient multicenter randomized trial designed to show equivalence with the Multilink Duet with respect to target vessel failure (TVF) at 6 months.[13] The main findings of the study are summarized in Table 16.1 and show equivalent TVF rates and binary restenosis at 6 months, although analysis of single stent patients favors the Bio*divYsio* stent.

A FLEXIBLE DRUG DELIVERY PLATFORM

The swelling properties of the PC coatings have been fully characterized by spectroscopic ellipsometry and neutron diffraction and have shown that the majority of the coating hydrates within minutes of being placed within an aqueous environment.[30] This process is even faster in more effective solvents, such as lower alcohols. It is therefore possible to obtain a significant loading in the stent coating of a wide variety of compounds by immersion in an appropriate solution for just five minutes. The Bio*divYsio* Matrix LO/HI coatings are capable of loading compounds of varying molecular weight

and solubility, the extent of loading being mainly controlled by the concentration of the loading solution in which it is placed. This therefore provides flexibility in the amount of drug that can be loaded on to the stents by simply varying the concentration of drug solution. Release of the absorbed material takes place partly by simple diffusion out of the PC coating in a similar manner to the process used for absorption on to the stents. In vitro studies investigating the release of the selected drugs from Bio*divYsio* Matrix LO/HI drug delivery stents indicate essentially first order release profiles (Figure 16.8). This is somewhat reflective of the drug's solubility profile in aqueous media (below), but also with evidence of interaction with domains within the polymer for the more hydrophobic compounds.[2] This affords additional flexibility for tailoring the release profiles. Therefore, the more hydrophobic the drug the longer the time of elution and vice versa for water-soluble compounds. These results demonstrate the ability of the PC Technology™ to release, in a controlled and sustained manner, a range of different pharmaceutical compounds. PC coating is purely an inert matrix for drug delivery and no specific irreversible interactions exist between the polymer and drug.

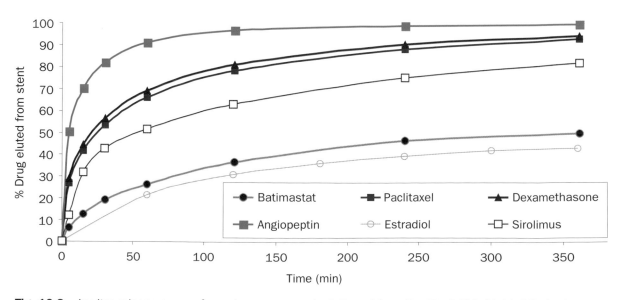

Fig. 16.8 In vitro release curves for various compounds delivered from the Bio*divYsio* Matrix LO stent.

DESIGNED FOR DRUG DELIVERY

The design of the Bio*divYsio* stent family has several features that make it particularly suitable as a device for intravascular drug delivery. The unique symmetrical cellular design ensures that once expanded against the arterial wall, there is an even strut spacing to allow more uniform deposition of the desired drug along the stented arterial segment (Figure 16.9a). This minimizes the occurrence of local areas of high and low drug concentration. Furthermore, for the Bio*divYsio* Matrix LO and HI stents, the PC coating has been engineered using a proprietary process, so that the coating thickness is significantly thicker on the outer (tissue) side of the stent strut compared to the inner (lumen) side (Figure 16.9b). These systems are loaded with drug with the stent crimped onto the delivery catheter. This, coupled with the targeted application of the coating on the outside of the struts, ensures that the majority of the drug loads on to the outside of the stent, max-imizing delivery directly to the vessel wall, and minimizing systemic loss via the bloodstream.

A STRATEGY FOR TACKLING RESTENOSIS

The fact that restenosis encompasses a complex series of interrelated steps means there are potentially multiple therapeutic targets that can be addressed to overcome its effects.[31] Much of the current focus is on 'bazooka-type' compounds, such as actinomycin D and paclitaxel. These compounds are highly potent inhibitors of the cell cycle, that interfere by various mechanisms with cell replication; hence, their mode of action is targeted completely in the proliferation phase of the restenosis process (see Figure 16.10).

However, there is some concern that these aggressive therapeutics may not be necessarily suitable for the treatment of all patient types. In particular, that low risk group that is only likely to have about a 15% chance of restenosis

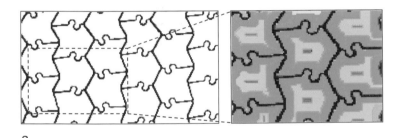

a

b

Fig. 16.9   (a) The uniform cell structure ensures even delivery to the vessel wall. (b) The targeted asymmetric application of the coating ensures maximized delivery to the vessel wall with minimal systemic loss.

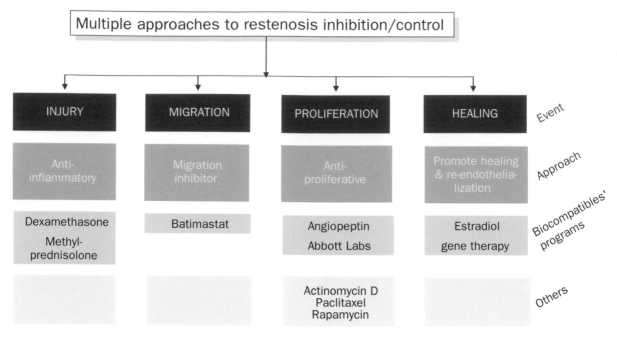

Fig. 16.10 The 'restenosis matrix': multiple approaches to control restenosis.

occurring anyway. Excellent short-term outcomes using brachytherapy to treat restenosis have been overshadowed by the occurrence of some adverse long-term events (late stent thrombosis) that are most likely a consequence of the inhibition of re-endothelialization of the stent.[32] These findings highlight a potential pitfall for late toxic effects from delivery of potent compounds such as these, which must be accounted for when constructing clinical studies.

The PC-coated stent platforms enable the study of a much wider range of active agents that may have effects in each of the other phases of the restenosis process (Figure 16.10). The 'restenosis matrix' is a strategy that is being pursued by Biocompatibles, which aims to identify the most appropriate therapeutic treatments for different patient subsets.[33] This is being achieved through a combination of company-sponsored and physician-led clinical studies, aimed at gathering valuable

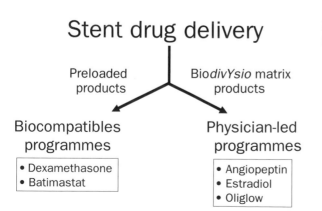

Fig. 16.11 Drug delivery programs utilizing the Bio*divYsio* Matrix stent platforms.

information on both the mechanistic aspects of the restenotic condition and the best therapeutic strategies for its prevention (Figure 16.11). Clearly, those patients who are at less risk from restenosis may require a more 'gentle' therapy (e.g. the antiinflammatory, dexamethasone), compared for instance with diabetics, who are known to be at much greater risk of restenosis occurring (which may therefore require a more potent antimigratory or antiproliferative compound). The drug delivery stent platforms described here are the enabling factors in this strategy, providing proven coatings with the flexibility to deliver a whole host of interesting pharmaceutics.

REFERENCES

1. Lewis AL. Phosphorylcholine-based polymers and their use in the prevention of biofouling. Coll Surf B: Biointerfaces 2000; 18:261–75.

2. Lewis AL, Vick TA, Collias AMC, et al. Phosphorylcholine-based polymer coatings for stent drug delivery. J Mat Chem: Mat Med 2001; 12: 865–70.

3. van der Giessen WJ, Lincoff AM, Schwartz RS, et al. Marked inflammatory sequelae to implantation of biodegradable and nonbiodegradable polymers in porcine coronary arteries. Circulation 1996; 94(7):1690–7.

4. Lewis AL, Cumming ZC, Goreish HH, et al. Crosslinkable coatings from phosphorylcholine-based polymers. Biomaterials 2001; 22:99–111.

5. Hall B, Pearce DJ, Campbell EJ, et al. Enzyme-linked immunoabsorbant assay for biocompatibility testing. In Lemm W (ed), The Reference Materials of the European Community: Results of Haemocompatibility Tests. Kluwer: London 1992: 147–55.

6. Campbell EJ, O'Byrne V, Stratford PW, et al. Biocompatible surfaces using mathacryloylphosphorylcholine laurylmethacrylate copolymers. ASAIO J 1994; 40(3):853–7.

7. Campbell EJ, Chronos NAF, Robinson KA, et al. Non-thrombogenic phosphorylcholine coatings for stainless steel. Trans Soc Biomaterials 1995; 18:15.

8. Lewis AL, Tolhurst LA, Stratford PW. Analysis of a phosphorylcholine-based polymer coating on a coronary stent pre- and post-implantation. Biomaterials 2002; 23:1697–706.

9. Chronos NAF, Robinson KA, Kelly AB, et al. Thromboresistant phosphorylcholine coating for coronary stents. Circulation 1995; 92(8):pl-685 (abstract).

10. Chronos N, Campbell EJ, Wilson DJ, et al. Improved haemocompatibility of artificial surfaces can be achieved by phosophorylcholine coating: a human ex-vivo flowing blood model. Eur Heart J 1994; 15:312, P1645.

11. Hanson SR, Chronos NAF. Cardiovascular device surface properties, thrombosis and healing. Trans Soc Biomaterials 1997; 20:16.

12. Moses JW, Aluka AO, Barbeau GR et al. The first clinical trial comparing a coated *versus* a non-coated coronary stent: The Biocompatibles Bio*divY*sio™ stent in randomised control trial (distinct). Circulation 2000; 102 (suppl 18).

13. Murphy JG, Schwartz RS, Edwards WD, et al. Percutaneous polymeric stents in porcine coronary arteries: initial experience with polyethylene terephthalate stents. Circulation 1992; 86:1596–604.

14. Kuiper KK, Robinson KA, Chronos NAF, et al. Implantation of metal phosphorylcholine-coated stents in rabbit iliac and porcine coronary arteries. Circulation 1997; 96(suppl 1):209.

15. Kuiper KK, Robinson KA, Chronos NAF, et al. Phosphorylcholine-coated stents in rabbit iliac and porcine coronary arteries. Scand Cardiovasc J 1998; 32:261–8.

16. Malik N, Gunn J, Shepherd L, et al. Phosphorylcholine-coated stents in porcine coronary arteries: in-vivo assessment of biocompatibility. J Invasive Cardiol 2001; 13:193–201.

17. van Beusekomm HMM, Whelan DM, Krabbendam SC, et al. Biocompatibility of phosphorylcholine coated stents in a coronary artery model. Circulation 1997; 96(suppl 1):29.

18. Whelan DM, van der Giessen WJ, Krabbendam SC, et al. Biocompatibility of phosphorylcholine coated stents in normal porcine coronary arteries. Heart 2000; 83(3):338–45.

19. Tolhurst LA. The analysis of post-implant phosphorylcholine coating on cardiovascular stents. The Spring Medical Device Technology Conference Proceedings 1999:427–41.

20. Lewis AL, Furze JD, Small S, et al. Long-term stability of a coronary stent coating post-implantation. J Biomed Mat Res: Appl Biomat 2002; 63:699–705.

21. Atalar E, Haznedaroğli I, Aytemir K, et al. Effects of stent coating on platelets and endothelial cells after intracoronary stent implantation. Clin Cardiol 2001; 24:159–64.

22. Galli M, Sommariva L, Prati F, et al. Acute and mid-term results of phosphorylcholine-coated stents in primary coronary stenting for acute myocardial infarction. Cathet Cardiovasc Interv 2001; 53:182–7.

23. Kuiper KKJ, Nordrehaug JE. Early mobilization after protamine reversal of heparin following implantation of phosphorylcholine coated stents in totally occluded coronary arteries. Am J Cardiol 2000; 85:698–706.

24. de Swart H, Bar F, et al. Long-term outcome and clinical results of the BiodivYsio PC-coated stent. Am J Cardiol 1998; 84(suppl 6A):4S.

25. Cumberland D, Bonnier H, Columbo A, et al. Phosphorylcholine (PC) coated divYsio stent – initial clinical experience from an open registry. JACC 1998; 10:407C.

26. Zheng H, Barragan P, Corcos T, et al. Clinical experience with a new biocompatible phospho-rylcholine-coated coronary stent. J Invasive Cardiol 1999; 11:608–14.

27. Corcos T, Barragan P, Zheng H, et al. Clinical evaluation of a biocompatible phosphoryl-choline-coated coronary stent. Eur Heart J 1999; 20(abstract suppl):P1521.

28. Galli M, Bartorelli A, Bedogni F, et al. Italian BiodivYsio open registry (BiodivYsio PC-coated stent): study of clinical outcomes of the implant of a PC-coated coronary stent. J Invasive Cardiol 2000; 12:452–8.

29. Boland JL, Corbeij HAM, van der Giessen, et al. Multicentre evaluation of the phosphoryl-choline-coated BiodivYsio stent in short de novo coronary lesions: The SOPHOS study. Int J Cardiol Interv 2000; 3:215–25.

30. Tang Y, Lu JR, Lewis AL, et al. Swelling of zwit-terionic polymer films characterised by spectro-scopic ellipsometry. Macromolecules 2001; 34:8768–76.

31. Edelman E, Rogers C. Pathobiologic responses to stenting. Am J Cardiol 1998; 81(7A):4E–6E.

32. Waksman R. Late thrombosis after radiation. Circulation 1999; 100:780–2.

33. Rothman, MT. Restenosis, past, present and future. In Rothman MT (ed), Restenosis: Multiple Strategies for Stent Drug Delivery. London: ReMedica 2001:1–10. (ISBN 1 901 346 36 6).

17

Direct stent coating: an alternative for polymers?

Koen J Salu, Johan M Bosmans, Hidde Bult, and Chris J Vrints

Introduction • **Immobilized drugs** • **Conclusions**

INTRODUCTION

The use of intracoronary stents has become the first choice of therapy in interventional cardiology. In most centers in the United States and Europe, stents are used in 70–80% of percutaneous coronary interventions.[1,2] Although coronary stents reduce the incidence of restenosis compared to balloon angioplasty alone by opposing elastic recoil and late remodeling of the vessel,[3,4] an excessive neointimal hyperplasia still induces in-stent restenosis in 10–30% of the patients.[1] In-stent restenosis is a local, chronic response of the vessel wall to a foreign body, which involves a cascade of thrombotic, proliferative, and inflammatory phases.[5] Many different cell types are recruited to play a pivotal role in this wound healing phenomenon: platelets, smooth muscle cells (SMCs), myofibroblasts, endothelial cells, and inflammatory cells (macrophages, lymphocytes, granulocytes, neutrophils). These cells release all kinds of growth factors which again stimulate the fibromuscular proliferative response of the vessel wall. The problem of in-stent restenosis is thus complex and therefore difficult to solve.

Systemic administration of several drugs acting on one component of this entire cascade – heparin, abciximab, angiotensin-converting enzyme (ACE)-inhibitors, hirudin, angiopeptin, tranilast, nitric oxide donors – showed good potency in animal studies, but all failed in the clinic.[6,7] This was probably due to inefficient local drug concentrations and an inappropriate knowledge of the complex restenosis pathophysiology in humans at that time. Also, local intracoronary radiation therapy, which acts by inhibiting the proliferation of SMCs, showed initially encouraging results, but now several deleterious effects, such as delayed intimal thickening and re-endothelization, late total occlusions, and exaggerated tissue proliferation at the edges of the stent (the so-called 'candy wrapper'), are emerging.[8–10] Therefore, the combination of a stent together with the addition of a local application of a wide acting pharmacological agent on its surface, could become a potential alternative for the prevention of in-stent restenosis. Already in the early 1990s, the first studies appeared using polymer-coated stents as carriers for numerous agents in the prevention of in-stent restenosis, with very promising results.[11–13] Later, however, several studies were published showing that both biodegradable (e.g. poly(organo)phosphazene, polyglycolic acid/polylactic – PLGA) and non-biodegradable polymers (e.g. polyurethane, polyethylene terephthalate) could induce marked detrimental inflammatory responses, even when they were impregnated with antithrombotic or antiproliferative drugs.[14–20] Recently developed new stent technologies, however, produced more biocompatible polymers carrying various agents or genes, showing promising results both in animal studies,[21–26] and in clinical trials (RAVEL, SCORE, TAXUS I).[27–29]

To prevent inflammatory responses of the vessel wall, alternatives for the use of polymers were developed. This chapter discusses the so-called 'direct stent coating' technology. Direct stent coating includes the direct loading of drugs on top of the stent surface, without using synthetic polymers, to reduce neointimal hyperplasia. We first will discuss some animal data using this technology and then give an overview of the preliminary clinical data.

IMMOBILIZED DRUGS

Preclinical data

Animal data concerning direct stent coating are very limited. Only short-term (4 weeks) porcine data using the microtubule stabilizer, paclitaxel, have been published.[30] Paclitaxel alters the dynamic equilibrium between microtubules and α- and β-tubulin by favoring the formation of abnormal stable microtubules.[31] This leads to multiple effects: the inhibition of cell division and migration, intracellular signaling and protein secretion. In vitro, growth factor-stimulated smooth muscle cell proliferation and migration were inhibited by paclitaxel, supported by in vivo rat data showing a decrease in intimal hyperplasia by the local application of paclitaxel by means of microporous balloons.[32] Heldman et al. used direct coated stents, by dipping them in a volatile solvent (ethanol). Evaporation of the solvent leaves a fine residue of paclitaxel that adheres to the metallic surface of the stent. It allows immediate contact of paclitaxel with the vessel, favoring, in theory, a rapid accumulation by

arterial tissue. This is especially interesting for hydrophobic, lipophilic agents, such as paclitaxel, which stick to the metallic stent surface when introduced in the systemic circulation and rapidly enter the cell. Heldman et al. showed that using the direct coating technique, even 68% of a 187 μg paclitaxel-coated stent could be recovered from the stent surface after 15 minutes of implantation in a porcine coronary artery. With a 15 μg coating, this percentage decreased to 34%. So the hydrophobic and lipophilic character of the molecule is probably an important prerequisite for optimal success. If a drug has the opposite characterization (i.e. hydrophilic and lipophobic), most of the drug will even be lost before reaching the target vessel, due to the first contact with the systemic circulation. Additional drug loss can occur during ex vivo manipulation of the stent, by simple handling of the stent before mounting (<5%), and during the brief exposure to the coronary circulation before deployment (<5%). Nevertheless, this strategy for local drug delivery resembles short-term irradiation by optimizing the conditions for blocking the earliest cellular events triggered by injury.[5,30]

In the experiments of Heldman et al., Palmaz-Schatz stents (Johnson & Johnson) with four different paclitaxel doses (0, 0.2, 15, and 187 μg/stent) were implanted in the left anterior descending coronary artery of 41 minipigs. The follow-up period was 4 weeks and quantification was performed using quantitative coronary analysis (QCA) and morphometry. The 4 week angiograms showed a graded effect of paclitaxel with a late loss index of 0.352 in the control group towards 0.055 (an 84% decline) in the highest dose group ($p<0.05$). Also the mean luminal diameter at follow-up rose to 146% of the control group in the highest dose group ($p<0.05$). Morphometry at 4 weeks showed a dose-dependent response, with a significant 39% decrease in intimal area ($p<0.05$) and 55% decrease in neointimal thickness ($p<0.05$) in the highest dose group and a significant 190% increase in their luminal area when compared to the control group ($p<0.05$) (Figure 17.1). This meant that not only the decrease in neointima counted for this luminal

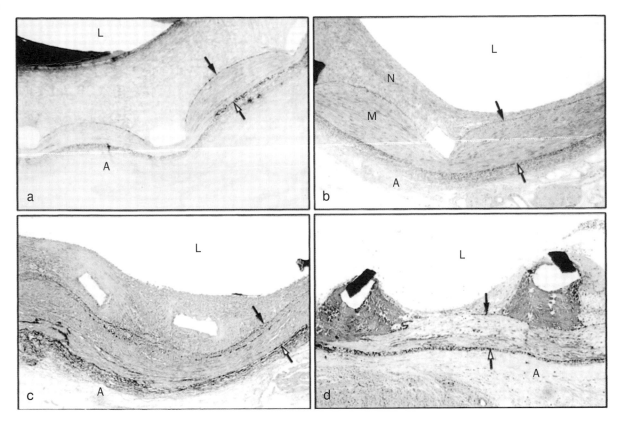

Fig. 17.1 Photomicrographs of stented LAD cross-sections (×40). (a) No paclitaxel (control); (b) low dose paclitaxel (0.2 μg/stent); (c) intermediate dose paclitaxel (15 μg/stent); (d) high dose paclitaxel (187 μg/stent). Solid and open arrows indicate boundaries formed by internal and external elastic laminae, respectively. L, lumen; N, neointima; M, media; A, tunica adventitia. (Reproduced from Heldman et al. Circulation 2001; 103:2289–95.[30])

increase. Also, a wall dilatation relative to the stent was seen in the highest dose, accounting for 42% of the luminal increase, and moreover, a trend (26%) toward reduction in medial wall thickness ($p = 0.09$) in the highest dose group compared to the control group. This loss of quiescent, non-dividing SMCs in the medial wall suggests some local cytotoxic effect of the high paclitaxel dose. Moreover, although the stent circumference and the vascular injury scores were similar in all groups, higher incidences of focal neointimal and medial hemorrhages, tissue necrosis, acellular material or calcified deposits were seen in the highest dose group. However, inflammatory cells and re-endothelization were similar in all treatment groups. Nevertheless, long-term studies will be required to evaluate whether adequate tissue

levels of paclitaxel can be maintained to prevent neointimal proliferation over longer periods of time and also whether complications (aneurysm, wall rupture, delayed healing) can be overcome. In conclusion, direct paclitaxel stent coating is technically feasible with good short-term results.

Our group evaluated with the same technique whether also actin-skeleton inhibitors could achieve the same results in a porcine coronary in-stent restenosis model. This group of drugs works very specifically on another component of the cytoskeleton, namely, the actin filaments, and therefore share some similar effects as paclitaxel, which is a stabilizer of the microtubuli. The cytochalasins are the best known participants of this class of drugs, together with the recently discovered latrunculins. Although their mode of action is different (the cytochalasins bind with the fast growing actin filaments, while the latrunculins bind monomeric actin), they share some similar effects on various cell types which play a role in the restenosis pathophysiology. They block cell proliferation,[33–36] inhibit protein and DNA synthesis[35,37] reduce cell migration,[38–40] inhibit phagocytosis by macrophages,[38,41–43] induce apoptosis,[44–46] and prevent SMC differentiation.[47,48] Finally, as well as their high specificity in blocking actin polymerization, they are also both very lipophilic and hydrophobic. These important characteristics allow their adherence to the metallic stent surface during passage through the systemic circulation, and they also favor their rapid transport through the cell membrane. Thus, their chemical characteristics and cellular effects make these drugs very suitable as potential candidates for the prevention of in-stent restenosis with the use of the direct coating technique.

Although local cytochalasin D delivery using a perivascular approach failed to prevent intimal hyperplasia, it did inhibit SMC migration in vitro and in vivo and also migration of inflammatory macrophages and T-cells into the vessel wall was diminished.[40] In vitro, cytochalasin D also reduced SMC proliferation dose-dependently, both by counting cells as using bromodeoxyuridin-labeling (Salu et al., unpublished data). Therefore, we evaluated a direct stent coating approach on a porcine coronary in-stent restenosis model, placing randomly 12 cytochalasin D coated stents and 12 control (ethanol dipped only) stents in the right or left coronary artery.[49] Direct coating involved dipping the coronary stents in an ethanolic 1 mg/ml cytochalasin D solution for 1 minute and then air-drying. The dipcoating technique allows the drug to have immediate contact with the vessel wall, favoring rapid uptake by the arterial tissue, and does not have the possible inflammatory responses as seen with the use of polymers.[30] When 2 µg cytochalasin D was applied directly on a stent, it disappeared within 2 hours during in vitro incubation (Figure 17.2). Nevertheless, this fast in vitro release, angiographical analysis at 6 weeks follow-up showed a decreased late lumen loss

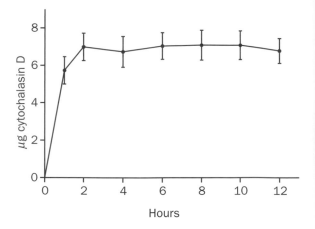

Fig. 17.2 Release kinetics of 7 µg direct cytochalasin D-coated stents ($n = 3$). Measurements were performed in wells containing 1 ml NaCl at 37°C using ultraviolet spectrophotometry (absorbance at 205 nm). After every time point, the stents were placed in new well of 1 ml NaCl.

in cytochalasin D-treated vessels (0.05 ± 0.04 vs 0.19 ± 0.05 mm, $p = 0.05$) compared to control segments. Morphometry also showed favorable results: decreased intimal area (0.93 ± 0.09 vs 1.29 ± 0.14 mm^2, $p<0.05$), intimal thickness (200 ± 15 vs 264 ± 27 µm, $p<0.05$), percentage stenosis (14 ± 1 vs $21 \pm 3\%$, $p<0.005$), and larger luminal area (5.91 ± 0.24 vs 5.40 ± 28 mm^2, $p<0.05$) in cytochalasin D-treated vessels compared to control segments (Figure 17.3). Moreover, histological analysis showed, in addition similar injury scores (1.48 ± 0.05 vs 1.53 ± 0.07, $p = 0.58$),[50] a favorable trend toward less inflammatory response, as shown by a reduced inflammation score in the cytochalasin D-coated stents (0.07 ± 0.03 vs 0.20 ± 0.09, $p = 0.12$).[51] No edge effects or thromboses were seen, and the stents were completely covered by endothelium. Thus, as well as influencing SMC migration, SMC proliferation was also inhibited by cytochalasin D in vitro, resulting in reduced intimal hyperplasia in a porcine in-stent restenosis model in vivo. In conclusion, this study proved that local drug delivery of cytochalasins using a stent platform can be an interesting approach to inhibit restenosis. Further studies are, however, necessary to investigate for optimized doses, toxicity, and

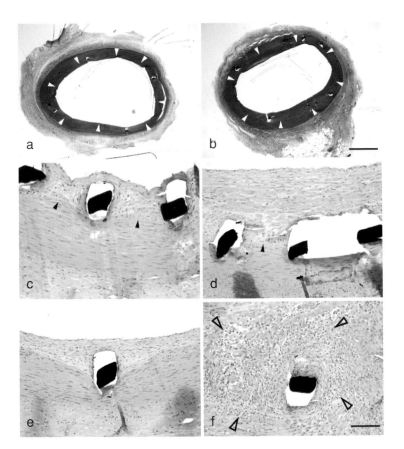

Fig. 17.3 Photomicrographs of stented LAD cross-sections (a, b ×2; c–f ×40). (a, c, e) 2 μg cytochalasin D-coated stents. (b, d, f) Control stents. Arrowheads indicate an influx of inflammatory cells.

the pharmacokinetics of cytochalasins in the vascular wall. Also, longer follow-up studies and more controlled release forms, such as polymers, should be evaluated in the future before clinical studies of cytochalasin D-coated stents can even be considered.

Using the same direct coating technique in the same model, we also evaluated whether latrunculin A could be used for the prevention of in-stent restenosis. In vitro, SMC proliferation was also dose-dependently inhibited by latrunculin A, with complete inhibition with 10^{-6} M (Salu et al., unpublished data). Latrunculin A (1.5 μg) was applied to coronary stents, showing complete release after 4 hours in vitro. At 6 weeks follow-up, quantitative angiographic analysis showed a reduced late lumen loss (-0.03 ± 0.20 vs 0.23 ± 0.029 mm, $p<0.05$) and percentage stenosis (15 ± 5 vs $30 \pm 14\%$, $p<0.005$) in latrunculin A-treated segments ($n = 11$) compared to control vessels

($n = 11$). However, morphometry analysis showed similar intimal areas (1.50 ± 0.79 vs 1.60 ± 1.09 mm^2, $p = 0.68$) in both groups, but an increased injury-score in the latrunculin A group (1.44 ± 0.46 vs 1.16 ± 0.28, $p<0.01$) compared to control segments. This resulted in a reduced intima/injury value (1.0 ± 0.4 vs 1.3 ± 0.8 mm^2, $p = 0.08$) in the latrunculin A group. No edge effects or thromboses were seen, and vWF immunostaining showed complete re-endothelialization at 6 weeks in both groups. Thus, the applied dose of latrunculin A, although showing the same inhibition of SMC proliferation in vitro and being, in previous studies, 10–20 times more potent than the cytochalasins,[36,52] was insufficient for the inhibition of in-stent restenosis in a porcine coronary model. Moreover, higher injury scores were seen, suggesting that using the direct coating technique, latrunculin can be toxic in the vessel wall, even in this low dose, which was equivalent to cytochalasin D. Therefore, controlled release forms need to be evaluated in larger animal studies and also the toxicity and pharmacokinetics of the latrunculins need to be studied in the future.

Clinical applications

The clinical efficacy of direct stent coating has recently been shown by the results of two prospective, multicenter, randomized, triple blinded, dose-finding studies, namely, the ELUTES (EvaLUation of pacliTaxel-Eluting Stent) and the ASPECT (ASian Paclitaxel-coated stEnt Clinical Trial) trials. Both studies used direct, 'sugared' paclitaxel-coated stents, by spraying the stents with a paclitaxel containing ethanol solution, leaving a fine layer of paclitaxel directly on the metallic surface. Thus, they do not use polymers, binding agents, overcoatings or any other possible carrier. The ELUTES trial was conducted to evaluate the safety and efficacy of this technique, using the V-Flex Plus™ coronary stent coated with 4 progressive doses of paclitaxel treatment groups (0.2, 0.7, 1.4, and 2.7 $\mu g/mm^2$) and one control group (uncoated) in patients with single de novo lesions. Exclusion criteria were severe lesion calcification, left main lesion and multiple lesions in the target vessel. Primary study endpoints included percentage diameter stenosis and late loss at 6 months measured by quantitative coronary angiographic (QCA) analysis, and major adverse cardiac events (MACE, i.e. death, Q-wave myocardial infarction (MI), coronary artery bypass graft (CABG), subacute arterial thrombosis (SAT), and non-Q-MI) at 1 and 6 months. Patients received aspirin plus clopidogrel (300 mg bolus, followed by 75 mg od) for 3 months. The study had independent core lab QCA analysis, clinical events adjudication, and data safety monitoring. Finally, 192 patients were included. No difference in baseline patient and lesion characteristics were noted in either group. Also baseline and poststent QCA findings were identical in the five groups. However, follow-up QCA in 110 patients revealed a dose-related reduction in diameter stenosis. The latter

ranged from 14% for the study arm that received the most densely coated stent (2.7 $\mu g/mm^2$) to 34% in the placebo arm ($p<0.01$). Also, the late loss decreased dose-dependently, with 0.10 mm in the highest group and 0.73 in the control group ($p<0.002$). Finally, in-stent binary restenosis figures amounted to 20.6% in the control group, while the highest dose only represented 3.1% ($p = 0.055$). In addition, in two high risk subgroups, namely, diabetics and patients with small vessels (<2.5 mm), these results persisted. At 1 month one death, one SAT, and one non-Q-MI occurred in the highest dose group, with a total of 92% of the patients remaining event-free. This was no different from the control group, with only one SAT, leaving 97% of the patients event-free ($p = 0.55$). The events in the highest dose group were all related to complications with non-trial stents placed in the same patients. At 6 months, an additional one target lesion revascularization (TLR) occurred in the highest dose group, one TLR in the 1.4 μg group, one non-Q-MI and one TLR in the 0.7 μg group, 2 TLR in the 0.2 μg group and 3 TLR in the control group. Thus, 89% of the patients were event-free in the high dose, 97% in the 1.4 μg, 95% in the 0.7 μg, 95% in the 0.2 μg, and 89% in the control group.[53,54]

The ASPECT trial showed similar results. This study evaluated the safety and the efficacy of direct coated paclitaxel Supra-G™ stents (Cook). The same coating technology, spraying of a paclitaxel containing ethanol solution on the stent surface with subsequent air drying, was used. A total of 177 patients were enrolled and randomly divided in three study arms: a high dose 3.1 $\mu g/mm^2$ ($n = 60$), a low dose 1.3 $\mu g/mm^2$ ($n = 58$), and a control (uncoated) group ($n = 59$). As the Supra-G™ stent has a larger stent surface (42 mm^2) compared to the V-Flex™ (22 mm^2), the total delivered maximal dose in this trial was 130 μg compared to 60 μg in the ELUTES trial. However, the same angiographic and clinical endpoints were assessed in this trial, analyzed by an independent core angiographic laboratory and clinical events committee. The diameter stenosis at 6 month follow-up was 38% in the control group, 24% in the low dose, and only 12% in the high dose group ($p<0.01$). Of the 60 patients in the high dose group, 98% had a diameter stenosis of less than 50% at follow-up. Forty-six percent of the patients in the combined paclitaxel groups presented at follow-up with diameter stenosis of less than 50%, compared to only 9% in the control group ($p<0.0001$). Also, the binary restenosis figures were impressive, amounting to 27% in the control group, 12% in the low dose, and only 4% in the high dose group ($p<0.05$). An intravascular ultrasound (IVUS) analyzed substudy found that neointimal hyperplasia volumes decreased dose-dependently from 31 ± 22 mm^3 in the control group, towards 18 ± 15 mm^3 in the low dose, and 13 ± 14 mm^3 in the high dose group ($p<0.0001$). These results were accompanied by an excellent safety profile, with 96% of the patients with conventional antiplatelet therapy being event-free in all study arms. No late thrombotic events were seen.[55–57]

Using this technology, the ELUTES and ASPECT trials also began an in-stent restenosis arm. This was developed to evaluate the safety and efficacy of treating recurrent in-stent restenosis lesions (which had repeatedly undergone multiple conventional angioplasties) with a direct coated paclitaxel stent. The in-stent ELUTES is a large prospective, blinded, randomized, multicenter (15 European centers) trial with 450 patients enrolled, all with refractory in-stent lesions treated with multiple devices – balloon dilatation, cutting balloon (no brachytherapy!), ... These will be divided into three study arms: no additional treatment ($n = 150$), a low dose arm ($n = 150$), and a high dose arm ($n = 150$). A single center pilot study (UZ Leuven) has already shown promising results.[58,59] This study included 21 patients who had undergone between 4 and 9 previous procedures to cure their in-stent restenosis lesion (mean: 5.3). The 3 µg/mm^2 paclitaxel-coated stents were 16 mm V-Flex™ coronary stents (total dose: 60 µg per stent, Cook) and predilatation occurred with a cutting balloon to optimize the predilatation and to minimize the injured zone. Patients received ticlopidine or clopidogrel for at least 3 months. In 12 patients,

the entire injured zone was not completely covered by the coated stent, leaving an uncovered visual dissection in five patients. From these 12 patients with a mismatch between the injured zone and the paclitaxel stent, three developed a significant restenosis in 6 months. From the nine patients with optimal paclitaxel stent coverage, the restenosis rate was 0%. There was one in-hospital thrombotic stent occlusion, and two late subacute arterial thrombosis (SAT) events, one after 14 days under ticlopidine and one after 4 months when ticlopidine treatment had stopped 3 weeks previously. One of these patients had prior brachytherapy. Therefore, the results of this pilot study suggest that implantation of a paclitaxel-coated stent is also feasible and safe in patients who are refractory to multiple prior interventions. Clinical and angiographic results are very promising, but optimal coverage of the injured zone with the paclitaxel stent seems mandatory. Also, prolonged antiplatelet (6–12 months) therapy seems mandatory in order to avoid late thrombotic stent occlusions, especially in patients with prior brachytherapy.

In conclusion, the ELUTES and ASPECT trials have shown that, based on the lipophilic nature of paclitaxel and avoiding as such the use of polymers, direct coated paclitaxel stents reduce in-stent restenosis dose-dependently, without short-term side effects. The clinical minimum effective dose density appeared to be approximately 3 µg/mm^2. This dose reduced in-stent restenosis rates by 5%. However, long-term effects and effects on more challenging lesions remain to be determined. Therefore, multiple trials are now ongoing to answer some pertinent questions. The DELIVER trial (USA) evaluates the safety and efficacy of direct 3 µg/mm^2 paclitaxel-coated MULTI-LINK Penta™ stents (also called the ACHIEVE™ stent design, Guidant) in coronary de novo native lesions of ≤25 mm length in vessels with a 2.5–4.0 mm diameter. They use the same coating technology as the ELUTES and ASPECT trials, with the 3 µg/mm^2 paclitaxel directly applied to the abluminal metallic surface of the stent, without using polymers or other carriers. It is a prospective, randomized, single blinded, parallel group (two arms), multicenter clinical trial, with 1043 patients enrolled at 61 participating clinical sites in the USA. The primary endpoint is target vessel failure at 270 days, defined as the composite of death, both Q- as non-Q-wave myocardial infarction (MI) and both target vessel as lesion as vessel revascularization by coronary artery bypass graft (CABG) or percutaneous coronary intervention (PCI). Secondary endpoints are angiographic percentage diameter stenosis and binary restenosis and clinical major adverse clinical events (MACE). Patients will receive clopidogrel for 3 months and the follow-up period is 5 years. Another large trial that will be started to support US product development, is the US PATENCY trial, using the same parameters as the DELIVER trial, thus evaluating only a single dose (3 µg/mm²) in small vessels (2.5–4.0 mm diameter). Also, an in-stent arm will be conducted in this trial.

CONCLUSIONS

Direct stent coating, by dipping coronary metallic stents into a solution of drugs dissolved in pure ethanol and then air-dried, proved to be effective in animal models. Although direct stent coating has a drawback in that the period of drug delivery is generally shorter as compared to controlled release types, this appeared to be not a major limitation in either animal studies or clinical trials. This suggests that inhibitory effects on the early vascular events immediately after stent implantation are sufficient to translate into a prolonged suppression of restenosis in the subsequent weeks and months. Moreover, direct stent coating has the advantage that it prevents possible inflammatory reactions by not using polymers as controlled release platforms. Short-term results are very promising, but attention should be made regarding potential toxic effects, such as delayed healing or increased inflammatory response due to inappropriate doses. Translating this technique into the clinic has shown preliminary beneficial results so far. Paclitaxel direct coating in the ELUTES and ASPECT trials showed 6 month restenosis figures of <5%. Longer follow-up studies are now being instigated, with the DELIVER and PATENCY trials. Studies are also being developed for the prevention of in-stent restenosis. Finally, other candidates as well as paclitaxel, which show the same chemical characteristics as the microtubule stabilizer, are also being investigated. Within one or two years, we will know if this technique has its place in daily clinical practice. Until then, the race to obtain drugs to inhibit in-stent restenosis remains a quest for the Holy Grail.

REFERENCES

1. Hoffmann R, Mintz GS. Coronary in-stent restenosis – predictors, treatment and prevention. Eur Heart J 2000; 21:1739–49.
2. Hofma SH, van Beusekom HM, Serruys PW, et al. Recent developments in coated stents. Curr Interv Cardiol Rep 2001; 3:28–36.
3. Serruys PW, de Jaegere P, Kiemeneij F, et al. A comparison of balloon-expandable-stent implantation with balloon angioplasty in patients with coronary artery disease. Benestent Study Group. N Engl J Med 1994; 331:489–95.
4. Fischman DL, Leon MB, Baim DS, et al. A randomized comparison of coronary-stent placement and balloon angioplasty in the treatment of coronary artery disease. Stent Restenosis Study Investigators. N Engl J Med 1994; 331:496–501.
5. Virmani R, Farb A. Pathology of in-stent restenosis. Curr Opin Lipidol 1999; 10:499–506.
6. Bult H. Restenosis: a challenge for pharmacology. Trends Pharmacol Sci 2000; 21:274–9.
7. Gruberg L, Waksman R, Satler LF, et al. Novel approaches for the prevention of restenosis. Expert Opin Investig Drugs 2000; 9:2555–78.
8. Costa MA, Sabat M, van der Giessen WJ, et al. Late coronary occlusion after intracoronary brachytherapy. Circulation 1999; 100:789–92.
9. Albiero R, Nishida T, Adamian M, et al. Edge restenosis after implantation of high activity (32)P radioactive beta-emitting stents. Circulation 2000; 101:2454–7.
10. Verin V, Popowski Y, de Bruyne B, et al. Endoluminal beta-radiation therapy for the prevention of coronary restenosis after balloon angioplasty. N Engl J Med 2001; 344:243–9.

11. Lambert TL, Dev V, Rechavia E, et al. Localized arterial wall drug delivery from a polymer-coated removable metallic stent. Kinetics, distribution, and bioactivity of forskolin. Circulation 1994; 90:1003–11.

12. Fontaine AB, Koelling K, Clay J, et al. Decreased platelet adherence of polymer-coated tantalum stents. J Vasc Interv Radiol 1994; 5:567 72.

13. Aggarwal RK, Ireland DC, Azrin MA, et al. Antithrombotic potential of polymer-coated stents eluting platelet glycoprotein IIb/IIIa receptor antibody. Circulation 1996; 94:3311–17.

14. Murphy JG, Schwartz RS, Edwards WD, et al. Percutaneous polymeric stents in porcine coronary arteries. Initial experience with polyethylene terephthalate stents. Circulation 1992; 86:1596–604.

15. Holmes DR, Camrud AR, Jorgenson MA, et al. Polymeric stenting in the porcine coronary artery model: differential outcome of exogenous fibrin sleeves versus polyurethane-coated stents. J Am Coll Cardiol 1994; 24:525–31.

16. De Scheerder IK, Wilczek KL, Verbeken EV, et al. Biocompatibility of polymer-coated oversized metallic stents implanted in normal porcine coronary arteries. Atherosclerosis 1995; 114:105–14.

17. De Scheerder I, Wilczek K, Van Dorpe J, et al. Local angiopeptin delivery using coated stents reduces neointimal proliferation in overstretched porcine coronary arteries. J Invasive Cardiol 1996; 8:215–22.

18. van der Giessen WJ, Lincoff AM, Schwartz RS, et al. Marked inflammatory sequelae to implantation of biodegradable and nonbiodegradable polymers in porcine coronary arteries. Circulation 1996; 94:1690–7.

19. Rechavia E, Litvack F, Fishbien MC, et al. Biocompatibility of polyurethane-coated stents: tissue and vascular aspects. Cathet Cardiovasc Diagn 1998; 45:202–7.

20. van Beusekom HM, Schwartz RS, van der Giessen WJ. Synthetic polymers. Semin Interv Cardiol 1998; 3:145–8.

21. Klugherz BD, Jones PL, Cui X, et al. Gene delivery from a DNA controlled-release stent in porcine coronary arteries. Nat Biotechnol 2000; 18:1181–4.

22. Bär FW, van der Veen FH, Benzina A, et al. New biocompatible polymer surface coating for stents results in a low neointimal response. J Biomed Mater Res 1999; 52:193–8.

23. Ganaha F, Doo YS, Elkins CJ, et al. Efficient inhibition of in-stent restenosis by controlled hybrid stent-based local release of nitric oxide. Circulation 2001; 104:II-506 (abstract).

24. Su S-H, Landau C, Chao RYN, et al. Expandable, bioresorbable endovascular stent with anti-platelet and anti-inflammation treatments. Circulation 2001; 104:II-507 (abstract).

25. Huang Y, Wang L, Vermeire I, et al. Methylprednisolone coated stents decrease neointimal hyperplasia in a porcine coronary model. Circulation 2001; 104:II-665 (abstract).

26. Rohde R, Heublein B, Ohse S, et al. Stent covering using insolubilized degradable biopolymers based on cross-linked hyaluronan or chitosan – response to stent injury in coronary arteries of pigs. Circulation 2001; 104:II-666–II-667 (abstract).

27. Sousa JE, Costa MA, Abizaid AC, et al. Sustained suppression of neointimal proliferation by sirolimus-eluting stents: one-year angiographic and intravascular ultrasound follow-up. Circulation 2001; 104:2007–11.

28. Honda Y, Grube E, de La Fuente LM, et al. Novel drug-delivery stent: intravascular ultrasound observations from the first human experience with the QP2-eluting polymer stent system. Circulation 2001; 104:380–3.

29. Grube E, Silber SM, Hauptmann KE. Taxus I: prospective, randomized, double-blind comparison of NIR$_x$™ stents coated with paclitaxel in a polymer carrier in de-novo coronary lesions compared with uncoated controls. Circulation 2001; 104:II-463 (abstract).

30. Heldman AW, Cheng L, Jenkins GM, et al. Paclitaxel stent coating inhibits neointimal hyperplasia at 4 weeks in a porcine model of coronary restenosis. Circulation 2001; 103:2289–95.

31. Rowinsky EK, Donehower RC. Paclitaxel (taxol). N Engl J Med 1995; 332:1004–1014.

32. Axel DI, Kunert W, Goggelmann C, et al. Paclitaxel inhibits arterial smooth muscle cell proliferation and migration in vitro and in vivo using local drug delivery. Circulation 1997; 96:636–45.

33. Carter SB. Effects of cytochalasins on mammalian cells. Nature 1967; 213:261–4.

34. Aubin JE, Osborn M, Weber K. Inhibition of cytokinesis and altered contractile ring morphology induced by cytochalasins in synchronized PtK2 cells. Exp Cell Res 1981; 136:63–79.

35. Iwig M, Czeslick E, Muller A, et al. Growth regulation by cell shape alteration and organization of the cytoskeleton. Eur J Cell Biol 1995; 67:145–57.

36. Spector I, Shochet NR, Blasberger D, et al. Latrunculins – novel marine macrolides that disrupt microfilament organization and affect cell growth: I. Comparison with cytochalasin D. Cell Motil Cytoskeleton 1989; 13:127–44.

37. Ornelles DA, Fey EG, Penman S. Cytochalasin releases mRNA from the cytoskeletal framework and inhibits protein synthesis. Mol Cell Biol 1986; 6:1650–62.

38. Klaus GG. Cytochalasin B. Dissociation of pinocytosis and phagocytosis by peritoneal macrophages. Exp Cell Res 1973; 79:73–8.

39. Kielbassa K, Schmitz C, Gerke V. Disruption of endothelial microfilaments selectively reduces the transendothelial migration of monocytes. Exp Cell Res 1998; 243:129–41.

40. Bruijns RH, Bult H. Effects of local cytochalasin D delivery on smooth muscle cell migration and on collar-induced intimal hyperplasia in the rabbit carotid artery. Br J Pharmacol 2001; 134:473–83.

41. Zigmond SH, Hirsch JG. Effects of cytochalasin B on polymorphonuclear leucocyte locomotion, phagocytosis and glycolysis. Exp Cell Res 1972; 73:383–93.

42. de Oliveira CA, Mantovani B. Latrunculin A is a potent inhibitor of phagocytosis by macrophages. Life Sci 1988; 43:1825–30.

43. DeFife KM, Jenney CR, Colton E, et al. Disruption of filamentous actin inhibits human macrophage fusion. FASEB J 1999; 13:823–32.

44. Kolber MA, Broschat KO, Landa-Gonzalez B. Cytochalasin B induces cellular DNA fragmentation. FASEB J 1990; 4:3021–7.

45. Rubtsova SN, Kondratov RV, Kopnin PB, et al. Disruption of actin microfilaments by cytochalasin D leads to activation of p53. FEBS Lett 1998; 430:353–7.

46. Suria H, Chau LA, Negrou E, et al. Cytoskeletal disruption induces T cell apoptosis by a caspase-3 mediated mechanism. Life Sci 1999; 65:2697–707.

47. Sotiropoulos A, Gineitis D, Copeland J, et al. Signal-regulated activation of serum response factor is mediated by changes in actin dynamics. Cell 1999; 98:159–69.

48. Mack CP, Somlyo AV, Hautmann M, et al. Smooth muscle differentiation marker gene expression is regulated by RhoA-mediated actin polymerization. J Biol Chem 2001; 276:341–7.

49. Salu KJ, Yanming H, Bosmans JM, et al. Direct cytochalasin D stent coating inhibits neointimal formation in a porcine coronary model. Circulation 2001; 104:II-506 (abstract).

50. Schwartz RS, Huber KC, Murphy JG, et al. Restenosis and the proportional neointimal response to coronary artery injury: results in a porcine model. J Am Coll Cardiol 1992; 19:267–74.

51. Kornowski R, Hong MK, Tio FO, et al. In-stent restenosis: contributions of inflammatory responses and arterial injury to neointimal hyperplasia. J Am Coll Cardiol 1998; 31:224–30.

52. Spector I, Shochet NR, Kashman Y, et al. Latrunculins: novel marine toxins that disrupt microfilament organization in cultured cells. Science 1983; 219:493–5.

53. Gershlick AH, Descheerder I, Chevalier B, et al. Local drug delivery to inhibit coronary artery restenosis. Data from the ELUTES (EvaLUation of pacliTaxel Eluting Stent) clinical trial. Circulation 2001; 104:II-416 (abstract).

54. Chevalier B, De Scheerder I, Gershlick A, et al. Effect on restenosis with a paclitaxel eluting stent: factors associated with inhibition in the elutes clinical study. J Am Coll Cardiol 2002; 6 March:59A (abstract).

55. Park S-J, Shim WH, Ho DS, et al. The clinical effectiveness of paclitaxel-coated coronary stents for the reduction of restenosis in the ASPECT trial. Circulation 2001; 104:II-464 (abstract).

56. Kaluza GL, Raizner AE, Park S-J, et al. Dramatic inhibition of neointimal proliferation by the paclitaxel-eluting stents showing radiation-like results without radiation: insights from the QCA core laboratory. J Am Coll Cardiol 2002; 6 March:26A (abstract).

57. Hong M-K, Mintz GS, Park S-W, et al. Paclitaxel coating reduces in-stent restenosis: a serial volumetric intravascular ultrasound analysis. J Am Coll Cardiol 2002; 6 March:38A (abstract).

58. De Scheerder I, Huang Y, Dens J, et al. Treatment of in-stent restenosis using paclitaxel eluting stents: a single centre pilot trial. Circulation 2001; 104:II-742 (abstract).

59. De Scheerder I, Huang Y, Dens J, et al. Treatment of in-stent restenosis using paclitaxel eluting stents: results from the Leuven pilot trial. J Am Coll Cardiol 2002; 6 March:59A–60A (abstract).

18

Radioactive stents

Christoph Hehrlein

Introduction • Processes of stent activation • Dosimetry • Vascular biology of stent-based irradiation • Clinical pilot trials with radioisotope stents • New concepts • Conclusions • Summary

INTRODUCTION

Despite the benefits of stenting to treat coronary artery disease, in-stent restenosis remains a significant problem, particularly in long lesions and smaller diameter vessels.[1] Experimental and clinical data have demonstrated that in-stent restenosis is principally caused by neointimal formation.[2] Radiation therapy is known to be effective in reducing benign dermatosis, keloid formation or heterotopic bone formation.[3] Studies systematically evaluating the effects of radiation on atherosclerotic arteries began in 1965.[4] Later, cell culture studies showed that both migration and proliferation of vascular cells are inhibited by the application of ionizing radiation.[5–7] However, depite an obvious therapeutic benefit, many studies showed that ionizing radiation can induce damage to the skin and nearby vascular structures.[8] The late effect of, for instance, high volume external beam irradiation is fibrosis, which can cause severe carotid or coronary artery stenosis.[9,10] Recently, however, endovascular irradiation has been shown to be a highly effective method of reducing neointimal formation and, thus, preventing restenosis, with excellent midterm results.[11,12]

Catheter-based irradiation using an ^{192}Ir and a ^{90}Sr/Y source has been effective in reducing neointimal formation after balloon injury, both in a porcine restenosis model and clinically.[13,14] An alternative and perhaps simpler approach is the use of a stent as the platform for local radiation delivery as a means to prevent restenosis. Experimental studies have demonstrated that stents ion-implanted with ^{32}P reduce neointimal formation at activities as low as 0.5 μCi.[15–17]

PROCESSES OF STENT ACTIVATION

There are at least three methods for the fabrication of a radioisotope stent. These include, but are not limited to:

- bombardment of metallic stents with charged particles (i.e. deuterons or protons)
- direct ion implantation of stents with radioisotopes
- chemical methods for radioisotope incorporation into the metallic stents or stent coatings.

Stents can be placed in a cyclotron and bombarded with charged particles.[18] Furthermore, it is technically possible to selectively implant a single type of radioisotope (i.e. ^{32}P or ^{103}Pd) into the stent surface. ^{32}P is a 'pure' β-particle emitter with a half-life of 14.3 days and maximum energy of 1.71 MeV. The portion of bremsstrahlung produced by a stent incorporating ^{32}P decays into the stable isotope ^{32}S. After 5 months, the radiation essentially disappears. The maximum penetration depth of the radiation from ^{32}P in tissue is 8.3 mm. In tissue, the dose decrease is very steep with ^{32}P. An alternative isotope, ^{103}Pd, is a weak γ-emitter with a longer radial and transverse penetration depth and with a maximum energy of 21 keV and a half-life of 17 days.

Finally, chemical methods using radioactive polymer films coated on to the stent surface (electrochemical deposition) provide alternative, and possibly more cost-effective, means for fabrication of radioisotope stents using ^{32}P or ^{103}Pd, or other potentially valuable isotopes.

DOSIMETRY

Radioisotope stents are permanent implants and deliver radiation continuously according to initial activity and half-life of the isotope. Despite low dose rates and very low activities compared with catheter-based irradiation devices, the near-field cumulative dose can be quite high with stents in the higher activity ranges. The dosimetry of a ^{32}P stent has previously been described in detail. Janicki et al. characterized the near-field dose of a 1.0 μCi, 15 mm long Palmaz-Schatz stent (Cordis, Miami, FL, USA) using a modification of the dose-point kernel method.[19] Using mathematical modeling, modification of the dose distribution around a uniform cylinder of ^{32}P to account for the geometry of a tubular, slotted Palmaz-Schatz stent allowed construction of three-dimensional dose maps. The non-uniformity of dosing, reflective of the stent geometry, decreases at distances of 1–2 mm from the surface. The dosimetry predicted by the dose calculations correlated well with the measured dose using radiochromic film. However, the accuracy of the dosimetry may be improved with methods other than radiochromic film. While dosimetry data provide an in vitro analysis of dosing from a radioactive stent, the actual dose distribution is affected by variations in atherosclerotic plaque morphology and symmetry of stent expansion.

Because the cumulative radiation doses to the subendothelium are quite high (i.e. several hundred grays for 6–48 μCi ^{32}P stents), radioisotope stents impregnated with radiosensitizers may reduce radiotoxicity and improve long-term results. Stent design appears to be an important denominator of dose perturbations by vascular irradiation. If stents are irradiated by β-particles from endovascular radiation sources, thicker struts with high atomic numbers induce 'cold' spots in the dose distribution adjacent to the wires.[20] In addition, the cell size of the stents significantly influences dose homogeneity in the near field.

VASCULAR BIOLOGY OF STENT-BASED IRRADIATION

Stent-based vessel irradiation causes localized inhibition of smooth muscle cell (SMC) migration and proliferation.[7] In addition, radiation-induced apoptosis appears to play a role in the shrinkage of the newly formed neointimal layer after stent implantation.[21] Interestingly, both in rabbit and porcine restenosis models, neointimal lesion formation after stent-based vessel irradiation consists predominantly of excessive extracellular matrix formation.[15,22] Excessive matrix formation after stent implantation and vessel irradiation appears to be dose-dependent to a greater extent at high radiation doses.[23] Largely unexplained but probably the result of proteoglycan accumulation is the occurrence of the so-called 'black hole', a process of lumen narrowing which is difficult to detect by conventional intravascular ultrasound (IVUS) techniques. The morphology of this 'black hole' most likely corresponds with a specific array of the glycoprotein decorin assembled in the newly formed bulk of extracellular matrix.[15]

CLINICAL PILOT TRIALS WITH RADIOISOTOPE STENTS

American studies

The initial clinical experience with β-particle emitting stents was gained in the USA beginning in October 1996. The Phase 1 Isostent for

Restenosis Intervention Study (IRIS) IA and IB trials were non-randomized trials designed to evaluate the safety of implanting very low activity (0.5–1.5 μCi) ^{32}P, 15 mm long Palmaz-Schatz coronary stents in patients with symptomatic de novo or restenotic native coronary lesions.[24,25]

Stent placement was successful in all patients. The mean stent activity at the time of implant in the IRIS trials was 0.7 μCi. There were no cases of acute or subacute stent thrombosis, target lesion revascularization, death or other major cardiac events within the first 30 days (primary safety endpoint), thus demonstrating acceptable early event-free survival. At 6 month follow-up there was a binary restenosis rate of 31% (10/32) and a clinically driven target vessel revascularization (TVR) rate of 21%. Interestingly, there was only one restenosis (proximal to stent) in the 10 patients treated for restenosis lesions (10%) and only an 18% rate for patients receiving stents >0.75 μCi. There were no further TVR events between 6 and 12 months after intervention. A significant amount of diffuse disease was detected by IVUS, since a mean of 41% cross-sectional area (CSA) stenosis was found in reference vessels at the time of stent implantation. Optimal stent implantation, assessed by IVUS, was achieved in only 56% of cases, mainly due to high plaque burden preventing an optimal ratio of stent CSA to reference-vessel CSA. Quantitative angiographic follow-up at 6 months demonstrated a lesion late loss of 0.94 mm for the group as a whole and 0.70 mm for the restenosis subgroup.[24]

European studies

A small pilot feasibility trial using 1.5–3 μCi, 15-mm-long, ^{32}P Palmaz-Schatz stents started in June 1997 in Heidelberg, Germany. Eleven stents were implanted successfully in patients with coronary artery restenosis.

Optimal stent deployment was controlled by IVUS guidance. The patients received ticlopidine for a period of 2 months after stent implantation. There were no major adverse cardiac events (death, myocardial infarction, coronary artery bypass grafting) noted at the 30 day safety endpoint and after 6 months. However, the study was terminated early because angiographic restenosis rates were high (54%) due to edge effects occurring at, in particular, the bridging strut of the Palmaz-Schatz stent.[26] After this trial, only radioactive stents without an articulation (BX stents [Cordis, Miami, Fl, USA]) were used in further studies. Twenty-six patients with coronary ^{32}P stents with activity levels of 0.75–1.5 μCi were studied in a non-randomized fashion. The clinical results were different to those from the IRIS trials. In contrast to American studies with coronary ^{32}P stents of the same activity range, restenosis rates were low (i.e. in-stent restenosis occurred in 17% of the patients and 13% had repeat revascularization). No restenosis was observed at the stent edges. However, the angiographic late loss of 0.99 ± 0.59 and loss index of 0.53 ± 0.35 were comparable to data from the IRIS trials and known results of conventional stent implantation.[27] In a series of 42 patients receiving 6–12 μCi ^{32}P stents, two uneventful vessel closures occurred in the follow-up period. All other vessels remained patent after 6 months and had no in-stent restenosis, although the rate of edge restenosis was 44%. In this study, one non-Q-wave acute myocardial infarction (MI) was noted due to transient thrombotic closure of the coronary artery. The group in Rotterdam is currently studying a series of patients in which radio-isotope stents with 'hot' and 'cold' ends have been implanted into the coronary arteries.

Albiero et al. recently reported on a cohort of 122 patients studied after implantation of three groups of ^{32}P coronary stents in the activity range 0.75–12 μCi.[28] At 6 month follow-up, no deaths had occurred and only one patient had stent thrombosis. The intrastent restenosis rate was 16% for stents with activities of 0.75–3 μCi (group 1), 3% for stents with activities of 3–6 μCi (group 2), and 0% for stents with activities of 6–12 μCi (group 3). However, the intralesion restenosis rate was 52% in group 1, 41% in group 2, and 50% in group 3, due to restenosis at the stent edges. The authors concluded that an 'aggressive' approach to stenting, in combination with a dose fall-off at the stent end below therapeutic levels, was responsible for the results of this procedure. In a subsequent study of only moderate to high activity stents (3–12 μCi), the authors reported a rate of edge restenosis (persistent intrastent restenosis) of 24–38%.[28] The edge restenosis process appears to occur independently of the activity levels used in the study. These findings with 3–12 μCi ^{32}P stents were made despite a 'gentle' implantation technique using stent deployment pressures of only 8–10 atm, and despite a postdilatation technique using a shorter balloon inside the stent to avoid mechanical damage (barotrauma) at the stent ends.[29–31]

NEW CONCEPTS

The unsolved problem of edge restenosis after radioisotope stenting initiated the intense search for better stent-based radiation sources. Because the dose falls off by 50% at the ends of a homogeneously coated ^{32}P stent, stents were manufactured with increasing activity levels at the edges ('hot-ends') to prevent edge restenosis. Higher activities at the stent ends could counteract a 'stimulatory effect' of low-dose radiation for smooth muscle cell (SMC) proliferation. The concept of 'cold-end' radioactive stents is based on the assumption that hyperproliferative neointimal SMCs piling up at the stent ends are allowed to migrate into the stent ends to 'smooth out edge restenosis'. In theory, migration of SMCs occurs from the stent ends into the stent until it is stopped by the radioactive portion of the stent body (electron fence hypothesis). Another hypothesis related to the 'candy wrapper problem' is that the radioactivity at the stent ends induces constrictive vascular remodeling. The solution here could also be a non-radioactive stent end. These two concepts ('hot' and 'cold' ends for radioactive stents) have been tested clinically in small pilot trials in Rotterdam and Milan, however, edge effects were not reduced (PW Serruys, pers. comm.).

Several new concepts are at a pre-clinical testing phase:

- Balloon expandable γ-emitting stents (^{103}Pd) or mixed β- and γ-emitting stents (i.e. with the isotopes ^{32}P and ^{103}Pd) that provide higher longitudinal penetration depth and could theoretically prevent edge restenosis.
- Self-expanding radioisotope stents that potentially eliminate balloon barotrauma beyond the stent edges because they lack a balloon delivery system.
- Balloon expandable radioisotope stents with drug eluting stent ends providing antiproliferative drug effects beyond the stent ends.

Apart from these new concepts, there are design strategies to improve stent delivery balloons aimed at reducing edge effects, ranging from minimal balloon overhang and square-shouldered balloons to temporarily placed radioactive stents.

Animal studies using pig and rabbit restenosis models studying the ^{32}P self-expanding stent and the ^{103}Pd balloon expandable stent have been recently completed. The results of the ^{103}Pd balloon expandable stents indicate that the occurrence of edge restenosis correlates with the extent of vessel injury at the stent ends (i.e. it is more pronounced at distal stent ends where the vessel tapers).[32] This finding suggests that a gentle implantation technique may improve clinical results, but only if the vessel does not taper too much. However, even ^{103}Pd-impregnated stents show a steep transversal dose fall-off at the stent ends. In other words, even γ-emitting stents may not prevent edge effects if vascular injury occurs in the dose fall-off zone of the radioactive stent end (Figures 18.1a, b).[32] In Japan, another γ-emitting stent using the isotope ^{133}Xe was successfully tested in a preclinical study.[33] Therefore, whether a higher longitudinal penetration depth of the radiation compared with ^{32}P stents sufficiently prevents edge restenosis is subject to further trials.

Self-expanding radioisotope stents have been successfully tested in preliminary animal studies.[34] Findings in a small group of pigs in whom self-expanding ^{32}P stents were implanted showed that neointimal hyperplasia at the stent edges is reduced (Figures 18.2 and 18.3). Whether this new and promising technology can be implemented in a clinical application remains to be seen.

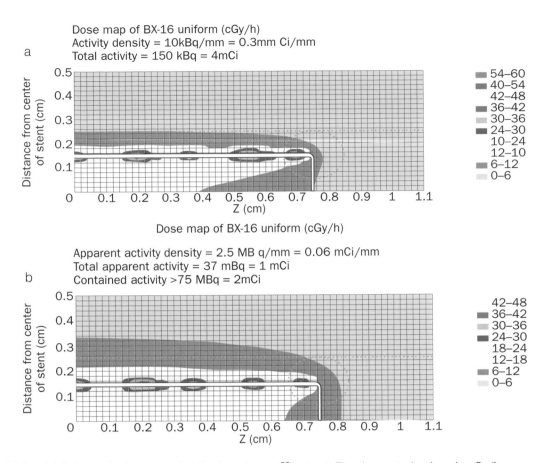

a

Dose map of BX-16 uniform (cGy/h)
Activity density = 10kBq/mm = 0.3mm Ci/mm
Total activity = 150 kBq = 4mCi

Legend (a):
- 54–60
- 40–54
- 42–48
- 36–42
- 30–36
- 24–30
- 10–24
- 12–10
- 6–12
- 0–6

Dose map of BX-16 uniform (cGy/h)

Apparent activity density = 2.5 MB q/mm = 0.06 mCi/mm
Total apparent activity = 37 mBq = 1 mCi
Contained activity >75 MBq = 2mCi

b

Legend (b):
- 42–48
- 36–42
- 30–36
- 24–30
- 18–24
- 12–18
- 6–12
- 0–6

Fig. 18.1 (a) Schematic dose rate distribution along a ^{32}P stent. The dose rate is given in cGy/h. (b) Schematic dose rate distribution along a ^{103}Pd stent. Note that distance of dose penetration axially away from the ^{103}Pd stent edge is only slightly higher as compared to the ^{32}P stent for comparative dose rates. (The dose calculations were performed by Klaus Schloesser, PhD, Forschungszentrum Karlsruhe, Germany.)

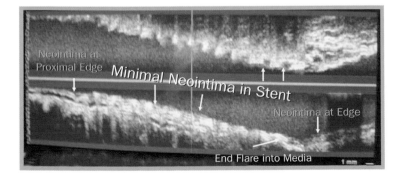

Fig. 18.2 Longitudinal intravascular ultrasound (IVUS) image of a self-expanding nitinol stent (control) implanted into the iliac artery of the pig. The image shows neointimal coverage of the struts within the stent and at the edges of the stent.

CONCLUSIONS

Vascular brachytherapy with catheter-based systems can potently inhibit restenosis. Late coronary thrombosis after stent-based irradiation is rare, but edge restenosis after implanta-tion of radioisotope stents is a serious problem. The major research topics are now related to the interaction of dose in the radiation fall-off zone at the stent ends and vascular injury (barotrau-ma) after stent delivery, and efforts to improve

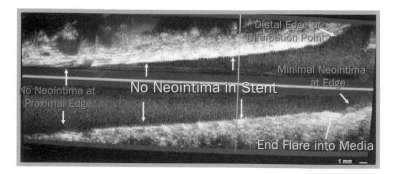

Fig. 18.3 Longitudinal intravascular ultrasound (IVUS) image of a self-expanding ^{32}P-impregnated nitinol stent implanted into the iliac artery of the pig. The image shows no neointima formation within the stent and minimal neointimal formation at the stent edges (arrows).

results include optimizing stent platforms and delivery techniques. By improving stent delivery systems, minimizing barotrauma at the stent ends, and applying sufficient radiation doses (i.e. perhaps including means of eluting antiproliferative drugs or radiosensitizers), it may be possible to overcome the edge problem currently observed with radioisotope stents.

SUMMARY

Worldwide clinical studies with more than 400 implants of balloon expandable radioisotope coronary stents have demonstrated safety of the technology with acceptable procedural and event-free survival. The studies uniformly show that restenosis rates are markedly decreased in a dose-dependent fashion within the bodies of radioisotope stents. According to clinical pilot trials, major adverse cardiac events (MACE), including thrombotic occlusion of the coronary artery after stent-based coronary irradiation, are rare events. However, the major problem of balloon expandable radioisotope stents is excessive restenosis at the stent edges, leading to revascularization rates similar to those observed after conventional stenting. The typical angiographic pattern of restenosis after implantation of radioisotope stents is luminal narrowing at the proximal and distal stent edges, which is called an 'edge effect'. The reasons for edge restenosis are most likely multifactorial. Low radiation doses in the fall-off zone, for instance, interact with variable degrees of vascular injury (barotrauma) at the stent ends depending on the means of stent delivery and pre- and postdilation procedures. With improving stent delivery

balloons minimizing balloon barotrauma at the stent ends, it may be possible to reduce the rates of edge restenosis. Recent studies comparing stent-based β- and γ-irradiation indicate that the steep longitudinal dose fall-off at the stent edges results in edge effects if the stents are implanted by delivery balloons with a balloon 'overhang' of 1–2 mm. Eluting radiosensitizers at the stent ends may be alternative strategies or self-expanding stent platforms are currently evaluated in preclinical trials. In summary, although radioisotope stents inhibit within stent restenosis and coronary thrombosis or aneurysm formation are rare events, the causes of edge effects need to be eliminated before further clinical studies commence.

REFERENCES

1. Serruys PW, de Jaegere P, Kiemeneij F, et al. A comparison of balloon-expandable-stent implantation with balloon angioplasty in patients with coronary artery disease. Benestent Study Group. N Engl J Med 1994; 331:489–95.
2. Schwartz RS, Edwards WD, Bailey KR, et al. Differential neointimal response to coronary artery injury in pigs and dogs. Implications for restenosis models. Arterioscler Thromb 1994; 14:395–400.
3. Escarmant P, Zimmermann S, Amar A, et al. The treatment of 783 keloid scars by iridium 192 interstitial irradiation after surgical excision. Int J Radiat Oncol Biol Phys 1993; 26:245–51.
4. Friedman M, Byers SO. Effects of iridium 192 radiation on thromboatherosclerotic plaque in the rabbit aorta. Arch Pathol 1965; 80:285–91.
5. Ootsuyama A, Tanooka H. Threshold-like dose of local beta irradiation repeated throughout the

life span of mice for induction of skin and bone tumors. Radiat Res 1991; 125:98–101.

6. Maity A, McKenna WG, Muschel RJ. The molecular basis for cell cycle delays following ionizing radiation: A review. Radiother Oncol 1994; 31:1–13.

7. Fischell TA, Kharma BK, Fischell DR, et al. Low-dose, beta-particle emission from 'stent' wire results in complete, localized inhibition of smooth muscle cell proliferation. Circulation 1994; 90:2956–63.

8. Hopewell JW, Sieber VK, Heryet JC, et al. Dose- and source-size-related changes in the late response of pig skin to irradiation with single doses of beta radiation from sources of differing energy. Radiat Res 1993; 133:303–11.

9. Silverberg GD, Britt RH, Goffinet DR. Radiation-induced carotid artery disease. Cancer 1978; 41:130–7.

10. Brosius FC, Waller BF, Roberts WC. Radiation heart disease. Analysis of 16 young (aged 15 to 33 years) necropsy patients who received over 3,500 rads to the heart. Am J Med 1981; 70:519–30.

11. Tierstein PS, Massullo V, Popma JJ, et al. Catheter-based radiotherapy to inhibit restenosis after coronary stenting. N Engl J Med 1997; 336:1697–703.

12. Condado JA, Waksman R, Gurdiel O, et al. Long-term angiographic and clinical outcome after percutaneous transluminal coronary angioplasty and intracoronary radiation therapy in humans. Circulation 1997; 96:727–32.

13. Wiedermann JG, Marboe C, Amols H, et al. Intracoronary irradiation markedly reduces restenosis after balloon angioplasty in a porcine model. J Am Coll Cardiol 1994; 23:1491–8.

14. Waksman R, Robinson KA, Crocker IR, et al. Intracoronary low-dose beta-irradiation inhibits neointima formation after coronary artery balloon injury in the swine restenosis model. Circulation 1995; 92:3025–31.

15. Hehrlein C, Gollan C, Dönges K, et al. Low-dose radioactive endovascular stents prevent smooth muscle cell proliferation and neointimal hyperplasia in rabbits. Circulation 1995; 92:1570–5.

16. Hehrlein C, Stintz M, Kinscherf R, et al. Pure beta-particle-emitting stents inhibit neointima formation in rabbits. Circulation 1996; 93:641–5.

17. Carter AJ, Laird JR, Bailey LR, et al. Effects of endovascular radiation from a beta-particle-emitting stent in a porcine coronary restenosis model. A dose–response study. Circulation 1996; 94:2364–8.

18. Fehsenfeld P, Golombeck M, Kleinrahm A, et al. On the production of radioactive stents. Sem Interv Cardiol 1998; 3:157–61.

19. Janicki C, Duggan DM, Coffey CW, et al. Radiation dose from a phosphorus-32 impregnated wire mesh vascular stent. Med Phys 1997; 24:437–45.

20. Amols HI, Trichter F, Weinberger J. Intracoronary radiation for prevention of restenosis. Dose perturbations caused by stents. Circulation 2000; 98:2024–9.

21. Hehrlein C, Kollum M, Arab A, et al. Increased apoptotic cell death in the neointima after stent-based vascular irradiation. Role of radiation-induced apoptosis for restenosis reduction. J Interv Cardiol 1999; 12:299–305.

22. Carter AJ, Douglas S, Bailey L, et al. Dose-response effects of ^{32}P radioactive stents in an atherosclerotic porcine coronary model. Circulation 1999; 100:1548–54.

23. Hehrlein C, Kaiser S, Riessen R, et al. External beam radiation increases neointimal hyperplasia by augmenting smooth muscle cell proliferation and extracellular matrix accumulation. J Am Coll Cardiol 1999; 34:561–6.

24. Fischell TA, Hehrlein C. The radioisotope stent for the prevention of restenosis. Herz 1998; 23:373–9.

25. Hehrlein C, Fischell TA. History of the radioisotope stent. Vasc Radiotherapy Mon 1999; 1:66–9.

26. Hehrlein C, Hardt S, Brachmann J, et al. P32 stents for the prevention of restenosis. Results from the Heidelberg safety trial using the Palmaz–Schatz stent design at moderate activity levels in patients with restenosis after PTCA. Circulation 1998; 98(suppl I):I-780 (abstract).

27. Wardeh AJ, Kay IP, Sabate M, et al. Beta-particle emitting radioactive stent implantation: A safety and feasibility study. Circulation 1999; 100:1684–9.

28. Albiero R, Adamian M, Kobayashi N, et al. Short- and intermediate-term results of ^{32}P radioactive β-emitting stent implantation in

patients with coronary artery disease. Circulation 2000; 101:18–26.

29. Albiero R, Nishida T, Adamian M, et al. Edge restenosis after implantation of high activity ^{32}P radioactive β-emitting stents. Circulation 2000; 101:2454–60.

30. Serruys PW, Kay IP. I like the candy, I hate the wrapper. The ^{32}P radioactive stent. Circulation 2000; 101:3–7.

31. Wardeh AJ, Kook AHM, Kay IP, et al. Clinical and angiographic follow-up after implantation of 6–12 μCi radioactive stent in patients

with coronary artery disease. Eur Heart J 2001; 22:669–75.

32. Hehrlein C, DeVries JJ, Arab A, et al. Failure of a novel balloon expandable gamma emitting (Pd103) stent to prevent edge effects. Circulation 2001; 104:2358–62.

33. Watanabe S, Osa A, Sekine T, et al. Production of radioactive endovascular stents by implantation of ^{133}Xe ions. Appl Radiat Isot 1999; 51:197–202.

34. Lauer MA, DeVries JJ, Haller SD, et al. Initial results with a P32 self-expanding nitinol stent. Circulation 2000; 102:II-424 (abstract).

19

Overview of potential drugs to inhibit in-stent restenosis

Ivan K De Scheerder

To select appropriate drugs to inhibit in-stent restenosis, one must understand the pathophysiological cascade leading to neointimal hyperplasia and in-stent restenosis. Implantation of a stent results in deep vascular wall injury. This results in a thrombogenic surface-inducing activation of the thrombus cascade and platelet activation. Deep vessel injury, together with the implantation of a foreign body, results in an aspecific inflammatory response causing activation of nuclear factor kappa B (NF-κB) and stimulation of cell dedifferentiation, proliferation, and migration. Drugs to inhibit neointimal hyperplasia will have to act on one or more steps of this cascade.

Antiplatelet and antithrombotic drugs may decrease (sub)acute thrombotic complication after stent implantation. However, they do not seem to play a major role in inhibiting in-stent restenosis.

The use of antioxidants to scavenge free oxygen radicals released by inflammatory cells is a novel concept but has failed so far to inhibit significantly neointimal hyperplasia following stent implantation.

Most popular, so far, are antiproliferative and immunosuppressive agents. Both paclitaxel and sirolimus have been shown to be very effective in blocking in-stent restenosis in large double blind randomized trials. Also, both drugs have a significant effect on inflammation, and therefore act on the three critical levels of the neointimal hyperplasia cascade.

Antimigratory agents, such as batimastat, did not show any significant benefit in clinical trials.

Agents that promote endothelial cell regrowth and vascular healing are also a possibility, however, these are less effective compared to antiinflammatory/immunosuppressive/antiproliferative drugs. (See Table 19.1 for a summary of drugs that could be used for inhibition of restenosis.)

Table 19.1 Multiple approaches for restenosis inhibition

Antithrombotic	Antioxidants	Antiinflammatory Immunomodulator	Antiproliferative	Migration inhibitor ECM-modulator	Promote healing and re-endothelialization
Hirudin	Omega 3 fatty acids	Dexamethasone	QP-2, Taxol	Batimastat	BCP671
Glycoprotein IIb/IIIa	Vitamin E	M-prednisolone	Actinomycine	Prolyl hydroxylase inhibitors	VEGF
Heparin	Melatonin	Interferon-γ1b	Methothrexate	Halofuginone	Estrogen?
	Tempamine	Leflunomide	Angiopeptin	C-proteinase inhibitors	
		Sirolimus	Vincristine	Probucol	
		Tacrolimus?	Mitomycine		
		Everolimus?	Statins?		
		Mycophenolic acid?	c-myc antisense		
		Mizoribine	Abbott ABT-578?		
		Cyclosporine	RestenASE		
		Tranilast	2-chloro-deoxyadenosine		
			PCNA ribozyme		

ECM, extracellular matrix; VEGF, vascular endothelial growth factor.

20

Direct antithrombins

Vincenzo Toschi

The role of thrombin in arterial thrombosis and restenosis • **Direct thrombin inhibitors**

THE ROLE OF THROMBIN IN ARTERIAL THROMBOSIS AND RESTENOSIS

Arterial thrombus formation occurs on a fissured or ulcerated atherosclerotic plaque upon exposure to flowing blood of its inner components.[1] We demonstrated that the thrombogenicity of atherosclerotic lesions is closely related to their tissue factor (TF) content which is highest in the lipid-rich core.[2] TF is able to activate the coagulation cascade by binding factors VII/VIIa which activate factors IX and X leading to the generation of thrombin that, in turn, mediates fibrin deposition and platelet recruitment.[3] Thrombin is the fastest and most powerful activator of platelets and platelet-rich thrombus formation on severely injured vessel wall (such as that resulting after plaque rupture or percutaneous transluminal coronary angioplasty – PTCA) is highly dependent on local thrombin generation.[4–6] Clot-bound thrombin is also responsible for the high thrombogenicity of mural thrombus that may persist after reperfusion by thrombolysis or PTCA.[7–9] PTCA is associated with severe local vascular damage, which may cause thrombin generation and mural thrombus formation immediately after the procedure.[10] Thrombin is also able to mediate the secretion of a series of growth factors at the site of vascular lesion, such as platelet-derived growth factor (PDGF)

and transforming growth factor-beta (TGF-β),[13] and to directly stimulate smooth muscle cell migration and proliferation,[14] thus playing a crucial role in neointima formation and restenosis.

DIRECT THROMBIN INHIBITORS

The introduction of direct thrombin inhibitors in the clinical setting has revealed a new scenario for the treatment of arterial thrombosis. Direct thrombin inhibitors are a class of antithrombotic agents that specifically and directly block thrombin thus antagonizing its biologic action independently of the action of antithrombin that is a necessary cofactor for indirect antithrombin drugs, such as unfractionated (UFH) and low molecular weight heparins (LMWH). UFH may also be neutralized by some plasma proteins, has a low bioavailability (30%) and a relative high incidence of thrombocytopenia. LMWHs have a better bioavailability (>90%), can induce less frequently thrombocytopenia, but share with UFH the inability to bind fibrin-bound thrombin,[15] which acts as a protected ongoing source of thrombogenesis. Direct thrombin inhibitors, as well as their independence from antithrombin, do not cause thrombocytopenia, are not neutralized by plasma proteins, and most importantly, potently and specifically inactivate fibrin-bound thrombin.[15,16] The prototypic thrombin inhibitor is the naturally occurring *hirudin*, which is still the most powerful and specific inhibitor of thrombin.[16] Initially isolated from leech saliva it is now produced as a recombinant-type molecule. Recombinant hirudin (r-hirudin, desirudin, lepirudin) is a 65 amino acid polypeptide with a molecular weight of about 7000 daltons. The hirudins have two distinct domains: a NH_2-terminal region and a COOH-terminal tail. Inactivation of thrombin by hirudins involves both the N-terminal domain that binds and inhibits the active catalytic site of thrombin, and the carboxy-terminal region that binds to the fibrin recognition region site.[17] Hirudin inactivates thrombin after forming an almost irreversible 1:1 stoichiometric complex. *Hirugen* is a synthetic dodecapeptide derivative that consists of the terminal 12 COOH amino acid residues of hirudin, and its binding to thrombin is therefore similar to that of the C-terminal of hirudin.[18] The antithrombotic activity of hirugen is lower than that of hirudin or hirulog and the drug has not been tested in clinical studies. *Bivalirudin (hirulog)* are a group of synthetic peptides having an amino acid sequence at the N-terminus with a high specificity for thrombin's active center, linked to the hirudin C-terminal peptide.[19] Like hirudin, these molecules are therefore able to block both the active catalytic site and the fibrin recognition region of thrombin and are potent thrombin inhibitors. Their binding affinity for thrombin is, however, lower than that of r-hirudin and reversible thus explaining some of the pharmacologic differences between hirudin and hirulog.[18,19]

Hirudin is able to block all the biologic actions of thrombin. It inhibits fibrin formation and prevents activation of factors V, VIII, IX, and X. It also inhibits thrombin-mediated platelet aggregation and the release reaction, and the exposure of glycoprotein IIb/IIIa receptors on platelets.[16] Experimental studies have also clearly demonstrated that hirudin is markedly superior to heparin in reducing platelet-rich thrombus formation on deeply injured arterial wall at high and low shear rates both in carotid and coronary artery thrombosis, and that it is also able to prevent venous thrombosis.[4–6,20] Moreover, hirudin was shown to totally block growth of thrombus on fresh mural thrombus by inhibition of clot-bound thrombin,[9] thus being superior to high dose heparin or heparin plus aspirin, and indicating the relative inability of heparin–antithrombin complexes to reach clot-bound thrombin. Hirudin is also able to accelerate thrombolysis,[4,9,21,22] to sustain coronary recanalization with streptokinase and rt-PA,[22] and to minimize residual thrombus after thrombolysis.[22] Moreover, the potential activity of hirudin in reducing restenosis after PTCA is clearly demonstrated by the significant reduction in neointimal formation after balloon angioplasty in the femoral arteries of atherosclerotic rabbits,[23] and more recently, after coronary angioplasty in a pig model.[24,25] Finally, the results of several recent clinical trials demonstrate that hirudin may be effective in the prevention of venous thromboembolism and in the treatment of patients with acute coronary syndromes.[26,27]

The synthetic direct antithrombin agent D-*Phe-Pro-Arg chloromethyl ketone* (or *PPACK*) is a tripeptide with a structure similar to a fibrinogen cleavage region. It acts as an irreversible thrombin antagonist inactivating both soluble and thrombus-bound thrombin. PPACK has proved to be effective in preventing growth of platelet-rich, aspirin- and heparin-resistant thrombi on Dacron vascular grafts and vascular stents after systemic infusion.[28–30] Transient (1 hour) intravenous infusion of this drug induces lasting interruption of platelet deposition at sites of surgical atherectomy by irreversibly inactivating thrombin bound to, and generated by, fresh mural thrombus.[28] However, optimal dosage and toxicity of PPACK in humans still need to be adequately investigated.

Argatroban is a synthetic arginine derivative, with potent direct antithrombin activity. It binds thrombin at a site adjacent to the active catalytic site, thus blocking it. However, unlike PPACK, argatroban is a competitive antagonist of thrombin and has a short half-life.[31] Argatroban was able to accelerate and to prevent reocclusion of arterial thrombi treated with rt-PA in dog and rabbit models,[32] was more potent than heparin in inhibiting arterial thrombus formation in rabbits,[33] and showed antithrombotic activity in arterial and venous thrombosis in a rat model.[34]

Other potent active-site thrombin inhibitors, include *melagatran* and *ximelagatran*. Ximelagatran is the orally absorbed prodrug of the active compound melagatran, which is a dipeptide specifically inhibiting thrombin-active sites. Its inhibitory activity is related to its structural homology to the portion of fibrinopeptide-A that interacts with the active site of thrombin. After intestinal absorption ximelagatran it is rapidly converted to melagatran through two intermediate metabolites and is excreted by the kidney.[35] In vitro studies demonstrate that melagatran is able to prolong prothrombin time and partial thromboplastin time and to inhibit thrombin-induced platelet aggregation at very low concentrations.[36] Moreover, this drug effectively increased the fibrinolytic activity of t-PA in a canine model of coronary thrombosis.[37] Finally, results of recent clinical studies suggest that melagatran/ximelagatran may be promising in both prevention and treatment of venous thrombosis and in the prevention of arterial embolism in patients with atrial fibrillation.[26]

REFERENCES

1. Fuster V. Mechanisms leading to myocardial infarction: insights from studies of vascular biology. Lewis A Conner Memorial Lecture. Circulation 1994; 90:2126–46.
2. Toschi V, Gallo R, Lettino M, et al. Tissue factor modulates the thrombogenicity of human atherosclerotic plaques. Circulation 1997; 95:594–9.
3. Nemerson Y. Tissue factor and hemostasis. Blood 1988; 71:1–8.
4. Heras M, Chesebro JH, Penny WJ, et al. Effects of thrombin inhibition on the development of acute platelet-thrombus deposition during angioplasty in pigs: Heparin versus recombinant hirudin, a specific thrombin inhibitor. Circulation 1989; 79:657–65.
5. Heras M, Chesebro JH, Webster MWI, et al. Hirudin, heparin, and placebo during deep arterial injury in the pig: In vivo role of thrombin in platelet-mediated thrombosis. Circulation 1990; 82:1476–84.
6. Badimon L, Badimon JJ, Lassila R, et al. Thrombin regulation of platelet interaction with damaged vessel wall and isolated collagen type I at arterial flow conditions in a porcine model: Effects of hirudin, heparin, and calcium chelation. Blood 1991; 78:423–34.
7. Weitz JI, Hudoba M, Massel D, Maraganore J, et al. Clot-bound thrombin is protected from inhibition by heparin-antithrombin III but is susceptible to inactivation by antithrombin III-independent inhibitors. J Clin Invest 1990; 86:385–91.
8. Kumar R, Béguin S, Hemker HC. The influence of fibrinogen and fibrin on thrombin generation – Evidence for feedback activation of the clotting system by clot bound thrombin. Thromb Haemost 1994; 72:713–21.
9. Meyer BJ, Badimon JJ, Mailhac A, et al. Inhibition of growth of thrombus on fresh mural thrombus: Targeting optimal therapy. Circulation 1994; 90:2432–8.
10. Marmur JD, Merlini PA, Sharma SK, et al. Thrombin generation in human coronary arteries after percutaneous transluminal angioplasty. J Am Coll Cardiol 1994; 24:1484–91.
11. McNamara CA, Sarembock I, Gimple L, et al. Thrombin stimulates proliferation of cultured rat aortic SMC by a proteolytically activated receptor. J Clin Invest 1993; 91:94–8.
12. Ip JH, Fuster V, Israel D, et al. The role of platelets, thrombin and hyperplasia in restenosis after coronary angioplasty. J Am Coll Cardiol 1991; 17:77B–88B.
13. Ross R. The pathogenesis of atherosclerosis: A perspective for the 1990s. Nature 1993; 362:801–9.
14. Libby P, Schwartz D, Brogi E, et al. A cascade model of restenosis. A special case of atherosclerosis progression. Circulation 1992; 86(suppl):III47–III52.
15. Hirsh J, Raschke R, Warkentin TE, et al. Heparin: Mechanism of action pharmacokinetics,

dosing consideration, monitoring, efficacy, and safety. Chest 1995; 8(suppl):259–75.

16. Toschi V, Lettino M, Gallo R, et al. Biochemistry and biology of hirudin. Coron Artery Dis 1996; 7:420–8.

17. Marki WE, Grossenbacher H, Grutter MG, et al. Recombinant hirudin: Genetic engineering and structure analysis. Semin Thromb Hemost 1991; 17:88–93.

18. Skrzypczak-Jankun E, Carperos VE, Ravichandran KG, et al. Structure of hirugen and hirulog 1 complexes of α-thrombin. J Mol Biol 1991; 221:1379–93.

19. Maraganore JM, Bourdon P, Jablonski J, et al. Design and characterization of hirulogs: A novel class of bivalent peptide inhibitors of thrombin. Biochemistry 1990; 29:7095–101.

20. Bossavy JP, Sakariassen KS, Rübsamen K, et al. Comparison of the antithrombotic effect of PEG-hirudin and heparin in a human ex vivo model of arterial thrombosis. Arterioscler Thromb Vasc Biol 1999; 19:1348–53.

21. Rigel KF, Olson RW, Lappe RW. Comparison of hirudin and heparin as adjuncts to streptokinase thrombolysis in a canine model of coronary thrombosis. Circ Res 1993; 72:1091–102.

22. Mruk JS, Zoldhelyi P, Webster MWI, et al. Does antithrombotic therapy influence residual thrombus after thrombolysis of platelets-rich thrombus? Effects of recombinant hirudin, heparin, or aspirin. Circulation 1996; 93:792–9.

23. Sarembock IJ, Gertz SD, Gimple LW, et al. Effectiveness of recombinant desulphatohirudin in reducing restenosis after balloon angioplasty of atherosclerotic femoral arteries in rabbits. Circulation 1991; 84:232–43.

24. Gallo R, Padurean A, Toschi V, et al. Prolonged thrombin inhibition reduces restenosis after balloon angioplasty in porcine coronary arteries. Circulation 1998; 97:581–8.

25. Mayer BJ, Fernandez-Ortiz A, Mailhac A, et al. Local delivery of r-hirudin by double-balloon perfusion catheter prevents mural thrombus and minimizes platelet deposition after angioplasty. Circulation 1994; 90:2474–80.

26. Weitz JI, Crowther M. Direct thrombin inhibitors. Thromb Res 2002; 106:V275–84.

27. Eikelboom J, White H, Yusuf S. The evolving role of direct thrombin inhibitors in acute coronary syndromes. J Am Coll Cardiol 2003; 41:70S–78S.

28. Lumsden AB, Kelly AB, Schneider PA, et al. Lasting safe interruption of endoarterectomy thrombosis by transiently infused antithrombin peptide D-Phe-Pro-ArgCH2Cl in baboons. Blood 1993; 81:1762–70.

29. Hanson SR, Harker LA. Interruption of acute platelet-dependent thrombosis by the synthetic antithrombin D-phenylalanyl-L-prolyl-L-arginyl chloromethylketone. Proc Natl Acad Sci USA 1988; 85:3184–8.

30. Krupski WC, Bass A, Kelly AB, et al. Heparin-resistant thrombus formation by endovascular stents in baboons: Interruption by a synthetic antithrombin. Circulation 1990; 82:570–7.

31. Kikumoto R, Tamao Y, Tezuka T, et al. Selective inhibition of thrombin by (2R,4R)-4-methyl-1-[N2-[(3-methyl-1,2,3,4-tetrahydro-8-quino-linyl+++)sulfolnyl]-l-arginyl)]-2-piperidinecarboxylic acid. Biochemistry 1984; 23:85–90.

32. Gold HK, Yasuda T, Jang IK, et al. Animal models for arterial thrombolysis and prevention of reocclusion. Erythrocyte-rich versus platelet-rich thrombus. Circulation 1991; 83:IV26–IV40.

33. Berry CN, Girard D, Girardot C, et al. Anti-thrombotic activity of argatroban in experimental thrombosis in the rabbit. Semin Thromb Hemost 1996; 22:233–41.

34. Schumacher WA, Heran CL, Steinbacher TE. Low-molecular-weight heparin (fragmin) and thrombin active-site inhibitor (argatroban) compared in experimental arterial and venous thrombosis and bleeding time. J Cardiovasc Pharmacol 1996; 28:19–25.

35. Gustafsson D, Nystrom J-E, Carlsson S, et al. The direct thrombin inhibitor melagatran and its oral prodrug H 376/95: intestinal absorption properties, biochemical and pharmacodynamic effects. Thromb Res 2001; 101:171–81.

36. Gustafsson D, Antonsson T, Bylund R, et al. Effects of melagatran, a new low-molecular-weight thrombin inhibitor, on thrombin and fibrinolytic enzymes. Thromb Haemost 1998; 79:110–18.

37. Mattsson C, Bjorkman JA, Abrahamsson T, et al. Local proCPU (TAFI) activation during thrombolytic treatment in a dog model of coronary artery thrombosis can be inhibited with a direct, small molecule thrombin inhibitor (melagatran). Thromb Haemost 2002; 87:557–62.

21

Tissue factor inhibitors

Maddalena Lettino, Vincenzo Toschi, and Juan Jose Badimon

Introduction • Tissue factor pathway inhibitor • Synthetic inhibitors of the TF-FVIIa complex

INTRODUCTION

Tissue factor (TF) is considered to be a major regulator of coagulation and thrombosis. It is a membrane-bound glycoprotein synthesized by almost all the cells present in the atherosclerotic lesions; it is also particularly abundant in the relatively acellular lipid core of the atherosclerotic plaque. TF exposed to flowing blood rapidly forms a high affinity complex with factor VII/VIIa, which in turn catalyzes the activation of factors IX and X, leading to thrombin generation.[1] The consequent platelet activation and fibrin deposition are the main events leading to acute thrombosis.

It is well known that arterial injury after percutaneous transluminal coronary angioplasty (PTCA) triggers acute thrombus formation. Restenosis may be considered a reparative process activated in response to injury: mural thrombus formation occurs immediately and is followed by smooth muscle cell (SMC) activation, migration, proliferation, and increased extracellular matrix deposition.[2] Since the TF content of human atherosclerotic plaques correlates with their thrombogenicity in an ex vivo perfusion system,[3] blockade of TF activity may reduce thrombosis.

TISSUE FACTOR PATHWAY INHIBITOR

The major physiological inhibitor of TF is the tissue factor pathway inhibitor (TFPI). It is mainly found in the endothelial cells and also circulates in association with plasma lipoproteins and platelets.[4] The structure of TFPI consists of an acidic N-terminal region followed by three repeated Kunitz-type domains and a highly basic C-terminal region. TFPI acts by initially forming a complex with factor Xa, which then forms a quaternary complex with TF-FVIIa. The initial binding of factor Xa by the second Kunitz domain potentiates inhibition of the TF-FVIIa complex by the first Kunitz-type domain. Human TFPI commonly used in research is produced by recombinant technology.[5]

In a previous study using an ex vivo perfusion system with porcine blood flowing on disrupted human atherosclerotic plaques, TF activity was inhibited by recombinant TFPI (rTFPI); the results have shown a significant reduction of plaque thrombogenicity as demonstrated by the inhibition of both platelets and fibrin deposition.[6]

Therapeutic strategies with TFPI have also been proven beneficial in preventing arterial reocclusion after fibrinolysis.[7]

Some experimental studies have highlighted the key role that the coagulation cascade activation plays in restenosis and the opportunity of an early anti-TF treatment in case of percutaneous procedures causing arterial damage. TFPI administered to minipigs fed an atherogenic diet and submitted to the experimental injury of one of the carotid arteries has been demonstrated to be particularly effective in attenuating subsequent neointimal formation and stenosis.[8] In the atherosclerotic rabbit arterial injury model intravenous injection of TFPI reduced angiographic restenosis and decreased neointimal hyperplasia, when compared with controls.[9]

Roque et al. reported the results of TFPI treatment in Yorkshire albino swine submitted to multivessel coronary angioplasty.[10] In this study, inhibition of TF activity by rTFPI abolished acute thrombus formation. The association of rTFPI with heparin had a synergistic anticoagulant effect but resulted in a high incidence of bleeding in the injured areas, suggesting the opportunity to keep heparin at a minimal dose to ensure adequate anticoagulation without bleeding complications during and immediately after PTCA. The authors have also evaluated coronary specimens harvested 4 weeks after angioplasty from animals which had received continuous intravenous infusion of rTFPI for 14 days. In these specimens, they found a significant reduction in the neointimal proliferation in comparison with the no-treatment controls. Recombinant TFPI, administered for several days after coronary angioplasty, inhibits the formation of a platelet-rich thrombus at the site of vascular injury, which might serve as a matrix for smooth muscle cell (SMC) migration and proliferation, and may directly inhibit SMC. Both actions may be explained by thrombin blockade since this molecule is a powerful platelet agonist and also acts as a growth factor for SMC.

To further define the mechanism of action of rTFPI the in vitro effects of this protein on cultured human aortic SMC have also been studied. Recombinant TFPI did not inhibit SMC growth but was able to reduce platelet-derived growth factor (PDGF)-inducible SMC migration in a dose-dependent fashion. Thus, a lesser degree of restenosis obtained in the animals treated with the TF-inhibitor might be the consequence of the combined antithrombotic and anti-SMC migration effect. Since TFPI does not interact directly with PDGF or its receptors, it has been hypothesized that the inhibition of SMC migration is due to the interaction between TFPI and TF, suggesting the possibility that the binding of TFPI to TF transduces an intracellular signal. Experimental evidence shows that the TF-FVIIa complex induces migration of aortic smooth muscle cells,[11] and therefore it cannot be excluded that SMC migration might be regulated by a product of TF catalytic activity such as thrombin or factor Xa and, consequently, that it might be altered by TF activity inhibition.

Tissue factor, mRNA, and protein are rapidly induced in human aortic and coronary arterial SMC by PDGF and thrombin, as a consequence of an increase in TF transcription. Surface TF activity seems to increase transiently, peaking 4–6 hours after agonist stimulation and returning to baseline within 16 hours.[12] Moreover, active TF is present not only on SMC surfaces after growth factor stimulation; taking into account that surface TF is only about 20% of total activity measured in cell lysates, the remainder being intracellular (about 30%) and as latent surface protein (about 50%).

It is possible to argue that the migratory effect of PDGF on SMC is mediated through the synthesis of TF. In fact, under the experimental conditions of the study previously reported by Roque et al.,[10] SMC were exposed to PDGF for 6 hours, well within the time frame for the surface expression of newly synthesized TF.

SMC are the major cellular component of the arterial wall and are found in abundance in human atherosclerotic plaques. After acute arterial injury SMC are often exposed to circulating blood and subjected to any PDGF isoform stimulation with consequent induction of TF surface activity. In addition, as SMC contain pools of intracellular and latent surface TF, even more TF activity might be available in the presence of severe injuries associated with extensive cell damage. Consistently enhanced TF activity might therefore account for both the potent thrombogenic stimulus evoked after coronary angioplasty and for the upregulation of SMC migration with subsequent neointimal proliferation. Therefore, in addition to its antithrombotic effect, rTFPI may also exert an inhibitory effect on intimal hyperplasia by impairing SMC migration, thus appearing as a novel therapeutic approach to limit the complications associated with percutaneous coronary interventions in terms of acute thrombosis and restenosis.

SYNTHETIC INHIBITORS OF THE TF-FVIIa COMPLEX

Taking into account the importance of the TF-FVIIa complex in atherosclerotic plaque thrombosis and in restenosis after PTCA, as well as in physiological hemostasis, a number of artificial antagonists of TF-FVIIa complex formation other than rTFPI have been recently developed. The first of these compounds, AP-1, is a rabbit anti-TF monoclonal antibody. This antibody has been proven to potently inhibit TF-mediated carotid artery thrombosis in a rabbit model,[13] and to accelerate the thrombolytic activity of t-PA and to prevent reocclusion in the same experimental model.[14] Another potent anti-TF-FVIIa complex inhibitor, NAPc2, has been cloned from hookworms.[15] The recombinant protein (rNAPc2) is an 85 amino acid polypeptide which requires binding to circulating factor Xa as prerequisite to form a binary complex prior to its interaction and inhibition of membrane-bound FVIIa-TF. The binding of rNAPc2 to factor X results in a prolonged half-life (>50 hours) following either subcutaneous or intravenous administration.[16] Recombinant NAPc2 has proven clinically effective in the prevention of venous thromboembolism after total knee replacement,[17] and it was also shown to suppress thrombin generation in patients undergoing elective coronary angioplasty in combination with aspirin, clopidogrel, and unfractionated heparin, as assessed by the measurement of the prothrombin fragment 1 + 2.[18]

Another interesting powerful anti-TF-FVIIa complex inhibitor is factor VIIai. It consists of human recombinant factor VIIa in which the active site is covalently blocked with an inhibitor, such as chloromethylchetone.[19] The rationale for the use of this compound is based on the same affinity for TF as the wild-type factor VIIa, but having the active site blocked, it cannot activate factors IX and X into their active forms, and consequently inhibits the activation of the coagulation cascade at its initial step. This compound has been shown to effectively prevent rabbit carotid artery thrombosis and to reduce the occurrence of myocardial injury during postischemic reperfusion of rabbit hearts in terms of reduction in both infarct size and no-reflow area.[20] This suggests that TF-dependent reduction in coronary blood flow might contribute to reperfusion injury and that recombinant factor VIIai might be beneficial in patients with acute myocardial infarction undergoing reperfusion therapies.

REFERENCES

1. Nemerson Y. Tissue factor and haemostasis. Blood 1988; 71:1–8.
2. Fuster V, Falk-E, Fallon JT, et al. The three processes leading to post PTCA restenosis: dependence on the lesion substrate. Thromb Hemost 1995; 14:552–9.
3. Toschi V, Gallo R, Lettino M, et al. Tissue factor modulates the thrombogenicity of human atherosclerotic plaques. Circulation 1997; 95:594–9.
4. Broze GJ. Tissue factor pathway inhibitor and the revised hypothesis of blood coagulation. Trends Cardiovasc Med 1992; 2:72–7.
5. Diaz-Collier JA, Palmier MO, Kretzmer K, et al. Refold and characterization of TFPI expressed in E. coli. Thromb Haemost 1994; 71:339–46.
6. Badimon JJ, Lettino M, Toschi V, et al. Local inhibition of tissue factor reduces the thrombogenicity of disrupted human atherosclerotic plaques. Effects of tissue factor pathway inhibitor on plaque thrombogenicity under flow conditions. Circulation 1999; 99:1780–7.
7. Abendschein DR, Meng YY, Torr-Brown S, Sobel BE. Maintenance of coronary patency after

fibrinolysis with tissue factor pathway inhibitor. Circulation 1995; 92:944–9.

8. Oltrona L, Speidel CM, Recchia D, et al. Inhibition of tissue factor-mediated coagulation markedly attenuates stenosis after balloon-induced arterial injury in minipigs. Circulation 1997; 96:646–52.

9. Jang Y, Guzman LA, Lincoff AM, et al. Influence of blockade at specific levels of the coagulation cascade on restenosis in a rabbit atherosclerotic femoral artery injury model. Circulation 1995; 92:3041–50.

10. Roque M, Reis ED, Fuster V, et al. Inhibition of tissue factor reduces thrombus formation and intimal hyperplasia after porcine coronary angioplasty. J Am Coll Cardiol 2000; 36:2303–10.

11. Sato Y, Asada Y, Marutsuka K, et al. Tissue factor induces migration of cultured aortic smooth muscle cells. Thromb Haemost 1996; 75:389–92.

12. Schecter AD, Giesen PLA, Taby O, et al. Tissue factor expression in human arterial smooth muscle cells. J Clin Invest 1997; 100:2276–85.

13. Pawashe AB, Golino P, Ambrosio G, et al. A monoclonal antibody against rabbit tissue factor inhibits thrombus formation in stenotic injured rabbit carotid arteries. Circ Res 1994; 74:56–63.

14. Ragni M, Cirillo P, Pascucci I, et al. Monoclonal antibody against tissue factor shortens tissue plasminogen activator lysis time and prevents reocclusion in a rabbit model of carotid artery thrombosis. Circulation 1996; 93:1913–18.

15. Stassen JM, Lambeir AM, Vreys I, et al. Characterisation of a novel series of aprotinin-derived anticoagulants: II. Comparative antithrombotic effects on primary thrombus formation in vivo. Thromb Haemost 1995; 74:655–9.

16. Lee AY, Vlasuk GP. Recombinant nematode anticoagulant protein c2 and other inhibitors targeting blood coagulation factor VIIa/tissue factor. J Intern Med 2003; 254:313–21.

17. Lee A, Agnelli G, Buller H, et al. Dose-response study of recombinant factor VIIa/tissue factor inhibitor recombinant nematode anticoagulant protein c2 in prevention of postoperative venous thromboembolism in patients undergoing total knee replacement. Circulation 2001; 104:74–8.

18. Moons AH, Peters RJ, Bijsterveld NR, et al. Recombinant nematode anticoagulant protein c2, an inhibitor of the tissue factor/factor VIIa complex, in patients undergoing elective coronary angioplasty. J Am Coll Cardiol 2003; 41:2147–53.

19. Golino P. The inhibitors of the tissue factor: factor VII pathway. Thromb Res 2002; 106:V257–V265.

20. Golino P, Ragni M, Cirillo P, et al. Effects of recombinant active site-blocked activated factor VII in rabbit models of carotid stenosis and myocardial infarction. Blood Coagul Fibrinolysis 2000; (suppl 1):S149–S158.

22

Nitric oxide-related interventions and restenosis

Hidde Bult, Koen Salu, and Guido RY De Meyer

Introduction • **Expression of nitric oxide synthases after vascular injury** • **Donors of nitric oxide**
• **Systemic treatment with NO donors and intimal hyperplasia** • **Local treatment with NO donors**
• **Systemic treatment with ʟ-arginine** • **Local treatment with ʟ-arginine**
• **Nitric oxide-related gene therapy** • **Discussion** • **Summary** • **Acknowledgments**

INTRODUCTION

Since the late 1970s percutaneous transluminal coronary angioplasty (PTCA) has found widespread application in the therapy of coronary artery stenosis. Although the immediate success rate of PTCA has increased to more than 95%, long-term success remains limited by significant renarrowing of the artery (restenosis) in 20–50% of patients within 6 months of intervention. Finding effective therapies to combat restenosis has been difficult.[1–3] At first, research was focused on inhibition of intimal thickening, often referred to as neointima formation. Commonly studied models involve gentle withdrawal of an inflated low pressure Fogarty balloon along normal rat carotid or rabbit femoral arteries to create a modest injury of smooth muscle cells (SMCs) in the media.[4] The SMCs start to proliferate and migrate to the intima, where cell division continues and matrix components are deposited. This healing process leads to formation of a neointima that replaces the original intima consisting solely of a monolayer of endothelial cells.

It is now appreciated that acute elastic recoil, incorporation of mural thrombi, and constrictive vascular remodelling may be equally important or dominant to determine the final lumen caliber.[5] The significance of acute elastic recoil and late constrictive remodeling is illustrated by a 25 to 32% lower frequency of angiographic restenosis in patients receiving coronary stents than in patients treated with conventional angioplasty.[2] Intravascular ultrasound (IVUS) results indicate that the stent effectively opposes acute elastic recoil and late arterial shrinking. Although the stent elicits more pronounced neointima formation, the net result at 6 months remains better than with standard PTCA. Stent restenosis develops in 20–30% of patients and might be more sensitive to therapies directed at inhibition of intimal thickening than restenosis after standard PTCA. With 50% or more of the coronary interventions involving stents,[2] prevention of neointima formation remains an important therapeutic target. The gentle denudation models lack the thrombotic and remodeling features of clinical restenosis, but these aspects can be mimicked by repeated inflation of an oversized angioplasty balloon in arteries of rabbits or pigs.

EXPRESSION OF NITRIC OXIDE SYNTHASES AFTER VASCULAR INJURY

Nitric oxide is produced from the amino acid L-arginine by different isoforms of the enzyme NOS. In normal arteries the constitutive, calcium-dependent isoform in endothelial cells (eNOS or NOS-III) is an important physiological regulator of vasomotor tone in response to chemical (e.g. 5-hydroxytryptamine, bradykinin) and physical (shear stress, stretching) stimuli. Balloon angioplasty of lesion-free rabbit arteries creates extensive vascular injury with a concomitant loss of endothelial cells and eNOS activity. Although the endothelial cells regenerate quickly after angioplasty – which differs from models employing denudation injury – the eNOS pathway remains dysfunctional. The delay of functional recovery is related to the degree of overstretching during balloon dilatation.[6–10]

In vitro studies demonstrated that NO, in addition to its vasomotor effects, may exert pleiotropic anti-restenosis activities.[3,11,12] NO may interfere with oxidative processes, the activity of the superoxide anion forming enzymes xanthine oxidase,[13–15] and NADPH oxidase,[14] the expression of adhesion molecules,[16,17] and of monocyte chemotactic protein-1,[18] the adhesion and recruitment of leukocytes,[19,20] the adhesion and aggregation of blood platelets,[21] and the migration of SMCs.[22–24] Vascular SMC migration is facilitated by matrix metalloproteinases (MMPs), which degrade the basement membrane and extracellular matrix. NO inhibits interleukin-1β-stimulated MMP-9 induction by inhibiting superoxide generation and subsequent activation of extracellular signal-regulated kinase (ERK).[25] Furthermore, high concentrations of NO may exert modest antiproliferative effects on SMCs,[24,26–29] fibroblasts,[30] and T-lymphocytes.[31–33] The inhibition of SMC migration and proliferation are both mediated by cyclic GMP.

Studies in eNOS-deficient mice indeed suggest that NO generated from eNOS promotes compensatory vascular remodeling,[34] and inhibits SMC proliferation and intimal hyperplasia in response to the placement of a rigid collar around the femoral arteries.[35]

During inflammatory conditions, an inducible isoform of NOS (iNOS, NOS-II) may come to expression in macrophages, vascular SMCs, and other cell types under the influence of cytokines (interleukin-1, interferon-γ, tumor necrosis factor-α) or mechanical injury of vascular SMCs.[36] Unlike eNOS, iNOS is not calcium-dependent and expressional regulation represents the main mechanism of activation of iNOS. In advanced atherosclerotic plaques, which are the substrate of percutaneous interventions, the activity of iNOS,[37] and the expression of its mRNA and protein have been documented in humans and in rabbits.[38–41] The immunohistochemical detection of iNOS using polyclonal antibodies is strongly complicated by unexpected immunoreactivities in several cell populations, including vascular SMCs.[42] To exclude false positive findings, it is therefore essential to confirm immunohistochemical findings by means of functional or biochemical tests of the activity of iNOS or an analysis of the expression of iNOS mRNA.

Functional and immunohistochemical studies pointed to iNOS induction after denudation of the rat carotid artery.[43–46] In that model, iNOS mRNA became apparent within 24 h post injury, and in situ hybridization located iNOS mRNA in neointimal SMCs, particularly at the luminal side of the vessel, conferring a non-thrombogenic surface.[45] On the other hand, the balloon injury leads to a loss of guanylate cyclase activity in the medial SMCs. As a consequence both the basal cyclic GMP levels and the response to application of exogenous NO donors diminish in the vasculature after denudation injury.[24]

Neither iNOS expression nor activity of iNOS could be detected in the media or intima of collared rabbit arteries after positioning a soft silicone collar that induces intimal thickening.[47,48] An immunohistochemical study that suggested that iNOS is expressed in the intima of collared rabbit arteries suffered from a lack of specificity. However, the perivascular collar induces the expression of iNOS mRNA and protein in the adventitia,[47] but the modest vascular injury created by the flexible collar is apparently not sufficient to invoke iNOS expression in media or intima. By contrast, the placement of a rigid collar around murine arteries, an intervention that creates more pronounced vascular injury and even leads to a complete and sustained loss of the endothelial cells, is associated with the induction of iNOS in the SMCs of the media.[36] Furthermore, both functional,[9] and immunohistochemical[49] studies documented that the profound and extensive injury of the media created by repeated inflation of an angioplasty balloon leads to the induction of iNOS in rabbit carotid arteries as well, where it is mainly found in macrophages.

The impact of the induction of iNOS on the development of intimal hyperplasia is unclear and could depend on the extent of the vascular injury and the concomitant formation of reactive oxygen species at the site. At low concentrations iNOS may exert anti-restenosis effects, as mentioned for eNOS (see below). Indeed, it has been proposed that iNOS induction confers a non-thrombogenic surface to the vascular SMCs after gentle endothelial denudation of the rat carotid artery.[45] However, under conditions with increased vascular superoxide anion generation NO may activate processes that promote restenosis. Superoxide combines with NO to form the stronger oxidants peroxynitrite ($ONOO^-$) and its decomposition product the hydroxyl radical.[50–52] The rate of peroxynitrite formation appears to be critically dependent on the concentrations of NO, superoxide, and iron.[53] In the absence of iron, equimolar fluxes of NO and superoxide interact to yield potent oxidants, such as peroxynitrite, which oxidize organic compounds. Excess production of either radical remarkably inhibits these oxidative reactions. In the presence of redox-active iron complexes, NO may enhance or inhibit superoxide-dependent oxidation and hydroxylation reactions depending on their relative fluxes.[53] The concept that peroxynitrite formation occurs in response to vascular injury is supported by the immunohistochemical demonstration of nitration of protein tyrosines in rabbits.[48] Excessive NO synthesis and peroxynitrite formation have been implicated in cytotoxic effects in endothelial cells, SMCs, and macrophages.[51,54–57] Cell damage results from the inhibition of mitochondrial respiration, aconitase activity, and DNA synthesis, as well as from iron loss,[58] and induction of oxidative DNA damage.[59]

The impact of iNOS on intimal thickening appears to be different among animal models. In mice, the expression of iNOS, unlike eNOS, promotes intimal thickening in response to the extensive injury evoked by a rigid perivascular collar.[36] In contrast, local infusion of the selective iNOS inhibitor L-N(6)-(1-iminoethyl)-lysine-HCl (L-NIL) to inhibit the activity of iNOS in adventitial macrophages and T-cells, reduced the nitrotyrosine residue formation, but augmented the intimal hyperplasia induced by a soft and flexible collar placed around the rabbit carotid artery.[48] Also in the rabbit abdominal aorta, NOS blockade with nitro-L-arginine augmented intimal thickening within but not proximal to the stent.[60]

DONORS OF NITRIC OXIDE

In view of the anti-restenosis activities of NO the impact of both the NOS substrate L-arginine (see below) and various NO donors have been studied in models of intimal hyperplasia. Because of the short half-life of NO in vivo and the limited utility of authentic NO gas, several classes of compounds that have the capability to release NO have been developed. Since the enzymatic or non-enzymatic mechanisms of the NO formation, the kinetics of NO release, and the pharmacokinetic properties differ greatly among these classes,[61–63] they are briefly discussed.

Organic nitrates

The classic organic nitrate esters, including glyceryl trinitrate (nitroglycerin), isosorbide dinitrate, and isosorbide 5-mononitrate, have been used for decades as a form of NO-replacement therapy for patients with ischemic heart disease. These compounds are all pro-drugs requiring biotransformation to release NO, and thiols potentiate their action. The metabolic pathways leading to NO generation are still not fully resolved, but probably involve the cytochrome P-450 system, gluthathione-S-transferase,[63] and mitochondrial aldehyde dehydrogenase activities.[64] In the vascular SMCs, NO stimulates cyclic GMP formation, affecting both calcium regulation and contractile proteins. The effectiveness of NO in angina is due partly to peripheral venous and arterial dilatation leading to a reduction of cardiac load, partly to dilatation of atherosclerotic and collateral coronary arteries, thereby increasing cardiac oxygenation.

The clinical use of the classic NO donors is hampered by the development of tolerance on long-term treatment. The mechanisms underlying nitrate tolerance are multifactorial, and probably involve neurohormonal counter-regulatory systems, impaired biotransformation, and changes in the function of vascular endothelial cells and SMCs.[65,66] Recent evidence supports a role of increased vascular superoxide production in nitrate-induced tolerance.[67,68] The superoxide anion combines with NO, either derived from the NO donor or from eNOS, to produce peroxynitrite, thereby limiting the vasodilator and antiplatelet activity of NO. Moreover, peroxynitrite may promote the oxidation of the NOS cofactor tetrahydrobiopterin,[69] or the NOS substrate L-arginine.[70] Depletion of intracellular tetrahydrobiopterin or of L-arginine have both been shown to uncouple NOS isoforms. This means the NOS activity switches from NO generation to superoxide anion production, thereby further increasing vascular oxidative stress and reducing NO bioavailability. Furthermore, peroxynitrite exerts inhibitory effects on soluble guanylate cyclase, the downstream target of NO,[71] and tolerance is associated with downregulation of type 1 cyclic GMP-dependent protein kinase.[72] In addition superoxide may activate protein kinase C. In vascular smooth muscle this second messenger enzyme raises the sensitivity to vasoconstrictors, such as angiotensin II and

endothelin I,[67,73] while in the endothelial cells the phosphorylation of eNOS by protein kinase C is known to inhibit the activity and NO production by the enzyme.[74] Finally, there are indications that nitrate tolerance is associated with an upregulation of cyclic GMP degrading phosphodiesterases.[75,76] Taken together, nitrate tolerance is associated with an array of effects that decrease the bioavailability of NO either released from exogenous NO donors or generated from eNOS in response to physiological stimuli. Furthermore, the increased superoxide production and/or the formation of peroxynitrite will induce vascular injury and raise the expression of proinflammatory genes, thereby promoting intimal hyperplasia. The organic nitrate pentaerythrityl tetranitrate is less liable to the development of tolerance than nitroglycerin, and treatment with vitamin C or other antioxidants appears to protect against nitrate-induced superoxide radical formation and tolerance.[77] Another approach to reduce the development of tolerance is to combine a NO-releasing nitrate ester and a thiol-containing moiety, such as cysteine, in a single molecule. N-nitrotopivaloyl-S-(N'-acetylalanyl)-cysteine ethyl ester (SPM-5185) represents an example of this class of organic nitrates.[78,79]

Spontaneous NO donors

In contrast to organic nitrates these agents directly release NO. The inorganic salt sodium nitroprusside (SNP) contains a nitrosyl group and five cyanide anions liganded to iron. SNP releases NO in a non-linear fashion independent of pH. It should be noted that the relatively small amounts of NO released from SNP are not sufficient to account for its marked guanylate cyclase-activating and vasodilator potency.[61,62]

The diazeniumdiolate or NONOate (N(O)NO) class are organic compounds in which NO is covalently linked to diethylamine (DEA), diethylenetriamine (DETA) or spermine.[61–63] The sydnonimines are a class of heterocyclic NO donors. The best-studied compound is 3-morpholinosydnonimine (linsidomine, SIN-1), which arises from hepatic cleavage of the prodrug molsidomine. Linsidomine requires hydrolytic ring opening to form the nitrosamine SIN-1A, a hydroxyl-driven process that is strongly pH-dependent. This compound then requires molecular oxygen for the stoichiometrical release of NO and superoxide anion at physiological pH.[61,62] Other heterocyclic compounds are the furoxan class that require thiols to form *S*-nitrosothiols as the precursors of NO liberation. Finally, *S*-nitrosothiols of NO are naturally occurring donor molecules that spontaneously release NO. They are less liable to develop tolerance or to induce oxidative stress. *S*-nitroso-*N*-acetylpenicillamine (SNAP), *S*-nitroso-glutathione, and *S*-nitroso-albumin constitute examples of this class of compounds.[21,61–63]

Bifunctional NO donors

A new classes of drugs combines two activities, cyclooxygenase inhibition and NO release, in a single molecule, such as the nitroaspirins and *S*-nitroso nonsteroidal antiinflammatory drugs (*S*-nitroso NSAIDs). The objective is to oppose the gastrointestinal toxicity associated with the long-term use of cyclooxygenase 1 inhibitors by means of the cytoprotective properties of a low dose of NO. The nitroaspirins are nitrate ester derivatives of acetylsalicylic acid (aspirin) and require biotransformation to release NO. A prototype of this class is 2-acetoxybenzoate 2-(2-nitroxy-methyl)-phenyl ester (NCX-4215).[63,80,81] *S*-nitroso-diclofenac and flurbiprofen nitroxybutyl ester (HCT 1026) are examples of NSAIDs that spontaneously release NO.[63,82]

SYSTEMIC TREATMENT WITH NO DONORS AND INTIMAL HYPERPLASIA

In the rat denudation model, systemic nitroglycerin treatment decreased the early medial smooth muscle cell (SMC) proliferation, but was without effect on the intimal thickness after 3 weeks.[83] This may be due to the development of tolerance associated with this class of nitrovasodilators. Conversely, oral treatment with the cysteine-containing nitrate SPM-5185,[78] the spontaneous NO donor FK-409,[84] or chronic inhalation of NO,[85] reduced intimal thickening in the denuded rat carotid artery. In

contrast, oral treatment with molsidomine, a prodrug of the NO donor linsidomine, was without effect in this rat model.[24]

Similar results were obtained when intimal thickening was induced by perivascular collars in rabbits. Oral treatment of rabbits with the tolerance-resistant NO donors SPM-5185,[79] or FK-409,[86] reduced the collar-induced intimal thickening. In contrast, only a tendency towards inhibition was observed upon oral treatment with molsidomine.[79] It is not clear whether the difference between the drugs was related to the dose, or different characteristics of the NO donors (i.e. the presence of sulf-hydryl groups in SPM-5185 or the release of superoxide anion from linsidomine). In accordance with the findings in the rat and rabbit models, treatment with linsidomine did not influence intimal thickening following porcine carotid angioplasty, despite a significant inhibition of early platelet adhesion, mural thrombosis, neutrophil adhesion and medial SMC proliferation.[87–89]

In keeping with the lack of effects of molsidomine in animal models, the intravenous treatment of patients with stable angina with linsidomine during the PTCA procedure, followed by oral administration of molsidomine did not reduce late lumen loss or the rate of clinical restenosis.[90] However, the NO donor led to a modest improvement in long-term lumen patency. This beneficial effect was due to a better immediate result, which is in keeping with the attenuated postangioplasty vasoconstriction seen in carotid arteries of linsidomine-treated pigs.[89]

Recently, the effect of bifunctional NO donors has been reported. The NO-releasing derivative of flurbiprofen (HCT 1026) has been shown to reduce neointima formation in the rat carotid artery denudation model.[82] The reduction of intimal hyperplasia at day 14 was not seen with equimolar doses of flurbiprofen and was well correlated with an increase in plasma nitrite/nitrate levels. In the same model, oral treatment with nitroaspirin (NCX-4016) for 7 days before and 21 days after carotid artery denudation attenuated neointima formation in adult (6 months) and old (24 months) rats. The effect was associated with reduced vascular SMC proliferation and increased plasma nitrite and nitrate levels.[80] The inhibitory effect was not seen with an equimolar dose of acetylsalicylic acid (aspirin). The NO-releasing aspirin derivative NCX-4016 also attenuated the intimal thickening evoked by denudation injury of the carotid artery of hypercholesterolemic low density lipoprotein receptor-deficient mice receiving a cholesterol-rich diet.[81] NCX-4016 was effective both in therapeutic or preventive protocols. In the latter protocol the suppression of the intimal thickening by NCX-4016 amounted to 53%, whereas 32% reduction was seen upon treatment with an equimolar dose of aspirin. The anti-restenosis effect was associated with reduced SMC proliferation and macrophage deposition at the site of injury.[81]

LOCAL TREATMENT WITH NO DONORS

A single local treatment of the denuded rabbit femoral artery with S-nitroso albumin inhibited platelet deposition and intimal proliferation.[91] Local treatment with spermine-NONOate released from the collar suppressed intimal thickening as well.[92]

NO-releasing cross-linked poly-(ethylenimine) polymers containing diazeniumdiolate (NONOate) moieties have been shown to inhibit the in vitro proliferation of vascular SMCs and to display antiplatelet activity when coated on a normally thrombogenic graft situated in the circulation of baboons.[93] In vivo, polymeric-based perivascular delivery of spermine-NONOate inhibits intimal thickening after balloon denudation arterial injury in the rat. This is associated with suppression of NF-κB (nuclear factor kappa B) activation and elevation of the vascular cyclic GMP at the site of injury.[94] The effect of tantalum stents coated with polycaprolactone impregnated with DETA-NONOate as a slow release precursor of NO has been studied in pig coronary arteries.[95] Quantitative coronary angiography demonstrated a similar, severe decrease of the minimum lumen diameter for polymer-coated

stents with or without the slow release precursor of NO. Profuse neointima formation and inflammatory cell infiltration occurred in both types of polymer-coated stents. Therefore, the profuse and overwhelming stimulatory effects of the polymer in the coated stents or a lack of efficacy of NO might explain the disappointing result with this NO eluting stent.[95]

The effect of another NO eluting stent was recently studied in a porcine coronary artery stent injury model.[96] Sodium nitroprusside (SNP), the inorganic salt that releases NO via a nonenzymic mechanism, was incorporated into polyurethane polymers on to metallic stents and two types of stents with thin and thick barrier coatings were characterized. The SNP-coated stents led to an increase in local coronary artery cyclic GMP levels for up to 14 days, pointing to sustained delivery of SNP to the tissue. The neointimal area at 28 days was not influenced, however, by NO eluted from either stents of thin or thick barriers, and even showed a statistically non-significant tendency to increase. In this respect it should be noted that SNP cannot be regarded as an ideal NO donor since it affects additional regulatory systems unrelated to the generation of NO.[61,62] SNP may release cyanide and the relatively small amounts of NO released from SNP in vitro are not sufficient to account for its marked guanylate cyclase-activating and dilatory potency.

SYSTEMIC TREATMENT WITH L-ARGININE

Oral L-arginine supplementation suppressed intimal hyperplasia after balloon denudation of the rat carotid artery.[97–100] Similarly, neointima formation after balloon denudation and stent deployment in rat carotid arteries was 46% less upon systemic L-arginine treatment for two weeks. The beneficial effects of L-arginine on neointima formation with or without stenting occurred via NOS-dependent mechanisms since they were reversed by simultaneous administration of N^G-nitro L-arginine methyl ester.[97,101] The NOS involved is presumably iNOS,[43–45] since endothelial cells and eNOS activity do not recover in this model. The favorable effect of L-arginine in this rat model is associated with inhibition of smooth muscle cell (SMC) proliferation in the vessel wall and is not explained by increased vascular SMC apoptosis.[98]

The SMCs in the media are more sensitive to the antiproliferative effect of NO than those in the intima.[46]

Balloon angioplasty of lesion-free or atherosclerotic rabbit arteries creates more extensive injury of the media than gentle denudation.[8,102] It invokes thrombus formation and incorporation,[102] different phases of remodeling,[103–105] and the induction of iNOS in non-endothelial vascular cells,[9] predominantly in macrophages present in the adventitia and in organizing thrombi.[49] Systemic L-arginine supplementation has been shown to oppose the intimal hyperplasia after balloon angioplasty of naive arteries of normocholesterolemic rabbits,[8] and of atherosclerotic arteries in heritable hyperlipidemic rabbits.[106] Furthermore, this treatment inhibits monocyte tissue factor expression,[107] and the secondary intimal hyperplasia evoked by angioplasty in the iliac artery containing a primary lesion produced by balloon denudation 6 weeks earlier in combination with hypercholesterolemia.[108] However, in the latter experiment the compensatory vessel enlargement, seen in the control group at 4 weeks after angioplasty, did not occur in the L-arginine group. As a result, there was no significant lumen gain in the L-arginine group,[108] in contrast to local perivascular L-arginine delivery.[104] The discrepancy between both reports could be due to the time of evaluation (see below), the presence of pre-existing lesions, or the hypercholesterolemia.

LOCAL TREATMENT WITH L-ARGININE

Balloon angioplasty in normal rabbit carotid arteries evoked a complex process of remodeling.[104] Constrictive remodeling prevails in the first two weeks following angioplasty, while compensatory enlargement occurs thereafter. The remodeling had a greater impact on the lumen stenosis than the intimal thickening. Continuous subcutaneous infusion of L-arginine in the ventral neck area led to a significant inhibition of the constrictive remodeling during the first two weeks.[104] In combination with the reduced intimal hyperplasia this created a much greater vascular lumen in the arginine-treated animals when compared to the control group. Since the levels of circulating plasma L-arginine were not elevated by the treatment, these data may suggest that substrate delivery to iNOS that comes to expression in the adventitia following balloon angioplasty opposed the wound healing contraction by the myofibroblasts in the adventitia.

The effect of local intravascular application of L-arginine (800 mg, 5 ml) with a drug delivery balloon at the site of balloon angioplasty was studied in the iliac artery of cholesterol-fed rabbits.[109] Using radiolabeled L-arginine it was found that most of the L-arginine reached the systemic circulation since less than 1% of the total dose was associated with the target segment. Yet, the radioactivity at one day after application was modestly elevated (25%) above the radioactivity of contralateral vehicle-treated vessels.[109] Despite the low efficiency of the arginine delivery the output of iNOS metabolites was raised during the first week in L-arginine-treated segments and less monocyte binding to the intimal surface was seen 2–3 weeks following L-arginine application.[109] The local L-arginine delivery did not restore the endothelial dysfunction.[110] However, 2 weeks after the delivery of L-arginine the intima/media ratio was 38% less in segments treated with L-arginine compared with control segments, and the inhibition became even more apparent (64% reduction) 4 weeks after L-arginine delivery.[110] The efficacy of local L-arginine application to inhibit intimal hyperplasia is remarkable in view of the low efficiency of the intravascular instillation. It could indicate that interference with very early events after angioplasty is sufficient to exert protracted inhibitory effects on intimal hyperplasia.

In a pilot study of 50 patients receiving a single Palmaz-Schatz stent the effect of local delivery of L-arginine (600 mg) via the Dispatch catheter after stent deployment was studied.[111] At 6 month follow-up the neointimal volume in the L-arginine group ($n = 25$) was slightly less than in the group ($n = 25$) receiving 6 ml saline (25 vs 39 mm³). Similarly, the percentage neointimal volume was reduced in patients receiving L-arginine ($17 \pm 13\%$ vs $27 \pm 21\%$). Although the inhibition was rather modest, the results suggest that this approach may potentially suppress in-stent restenosis.[111]

NITRIC OXIDE-RELATED GENE THERAPY

In vivo eNOS gene transfer to the denuded rat carotid artery provided further evidence for the beneficial effects of nitric oxide (NO) on smooth muscle cell (SMC) accumulation in the intima. Transfection of the eNOS gene in the media not only restored the calcium-dependent NO production and concomitant relaxations of the denuded artery, it also inhibited neointima formation at day 14 after balloon injury by 70%.[112,113] Similarly, when rat SMCs transfected with the human eNOS gene were seeded on to the luminal surface of the balloon-denuded rat carotid artery, 37% inhibition of the neointimal hyperplasia was seen and oral administration of the NOS inhibitor nitro-L-arginine reversed the change.[114] In a further study it was shown that percutaneous eNOS gene transfer significantly reduced luminal narrowing, most likely through a combined inhibition of neointima formation and an effect on vessel remodeling leading to marked arterial dilatation after balloon angioplasty in pig coronary arteries.[115] Furthermore, eNOS gene transfer in rat aortic SMCs decreased MMP-2 and MMP-9 activities and increased the secretion of tissue inhibitor of metalloproteinase-2 (TIMP-2). Therefore, NO may favor the inhibition of SMC migration because of inhibition of extracellular matrix degradation.[116]

These experiments provide direct evidence that NO derived from eNOS is an endogenous inhibitor of vascular lesion formation in vivo. Furthermore, these experiments suggest the possibility of eNOS transfection, which has been successful in the human saphenous vein,[117] as a potential therapeutic approach to maintain patency after PTCA or in vein grafts.

Gene transfer of iNOS has also been reported to suppress injury-induced myointimal hyperplasia of isolated porcine arteries in vitro but NO biosynthesis and the antiproliferative effect required the exogenous supply of tetrahydrobiopterin.[118] Short-term but sustained increases in NO formation achieved with iNOS gene transfer at the time of vascular injury reduced intimal hyperplasia evoked by denudation of rat carotid or porcine iliac arteries.[119] Instillation of adenovirus expressing the murine iNOS gene in the rat carotid artery after stent deployment also led to a 30% reduction of the neointima formation after two weeks in comparison to arteries transfected with an adenovirus containing no transgene.[101] However, iNOS gene transfer did not lead to regression of pre-established intimal lesions.[119]

Several effects of NO are mediated by cyclic GMP and other approaches addressed the feasibility and effects of raising guanylate cyclase activity. Local expression of C-type natriuretic peptide to stimulate the particulate guanylate cyclase markedly suppressed neointima formation in a denudation model.[120] The combined adenoviral gene transfer of the α_1 and β_1 subunits of rat soluble guanylate cyclase (sGC) to the rat carotid artery after balloon denudation did not influence neointima formation two weeks after the injury in comparison to uninfected arteries or arteries infected with adenovirus not expressing a transgene.[24] However, the mean intima/media ratio was less when rats coinfected with α_1 and β_1 sGC subunits were treated with molsidomine (5 mg/kg bd). By contrast, molsidomine treatment did not affect neointima formation in non-infected rats or rats infected with adenovirus without transgene.[24] The balloon injury led to a loss of both the basal cyclic GMP levels and the response to application of exogenous NO. The coinfection with the α_1 and β_1 subunits of sGC did not restore the basal in vivo cyclic GMP levels of the medial SMCs, but led to a partial recovery of the response to the administration of molsidomine.[24] Therefore, gene transfer of the α_1 and β_1 subunits of sGC raised the responsiveness to exogenous NO, thereby enhancing the antimigratory and antiproliferative effects of NO donors on vascular SMCs.

DISCUSSION

Over recent years systemic NO-based interventions with S-nitrosothiols, the spontaneous donor FK-409 and the cysteine-containing nitrate SPM, have shown beneficial effects at intimal hyperplasia following various forms of injury to arteries of laboratory animals without inducing significant side effects. Administration of nitroglycerin or molsidomine was, however, without effect in the same animal models and systemic treatment with molsidomine failed to reduce late lumen loss following PTCA in patients with stable angina. An increased release of superoxide anion radicals could form an explanation for the disappointing results with the latter drugs. Nitroglycerin induces tolerance and this is associated with an increased production of superoxide radicals by endothelial cells and vascular SMCs. Superoxide anion is also stoichiometrically released from linsidomine, the active principle of molsidomine, together with NO. In this respect it would be interesting to investigate whether supplementary administration of antioxidant vitamins, which have been shown to oppose tolerance development,[66,77] could be used as a pharmaceutical adjunct to reduce oxidant stress during treatment with molsidomine or organic nitrates.

The extent to which the positive body of experimental data with the other classes of NO donors can be translated into the clinic remains to be determined. Most studies reporting benefit from NO donor treatment were conducted in normal, atherosclerosis-free arteries, in which intimal hyperplasia was evoked by creating a modest vascular injury by gentle endothelial denudation or placement of a flexible perivascular collar. These models may mimic the adaptive intimal cushions that normally develop during adolescence in certain human conduit arteries at atherosclerosis-prone sites, rather than the intimal thickening evoked by the vascular trauma of balloon angioplasty or stent placement. Few studies have documented

benefit from systemic NO donor treatment following a much more extensive vascular injury created by the repeated inflation of a slightly oversized angioplasty balloon or stent placement. Those models could be more relevant to PTCA interventions in the clinic since complex vascular remodeling processes, incorporation of mural thrombin inflammatory reactions as well as intimal hyperplasia are seen, whereas the gentle models mainly mimic the last aspect. Finally, in addition to species differences with regard to the mediators involved in processes of restenosis, or the pharmacokinetic and dose levels of the drugs, the presence or absence of advanced atherosclerotic plaques could also determine the outcome with a particular drug. This is illustrated by the observation that systemic administration of molsidomine showed little effect on intimal hyperplasia evoked by perivascular collar placement in normocholesterolemic rabbits,[79] whereas the same dose has been shown to strongly promote atherosclerotic plaque development in hypercholesterolemic animals.[121] Since the plaque burden of human coronary arteries is mostly not concentric, this could imply that beneficial effects of NO-releasing drugs on relatively normal sectors of the vessel wall are offset by the opposite effects on sectors that are more severely affected by atherosclerosis. In animal models a clear relationship between inhibition of SMC mitosis and neointima formation is lacking. SMC mitosis was influenced less than intimal thickening after eNOS gene transfer in denuded rat arteries,[112] or after NO donor treatment of rabbit collared arteries.[79] This suggests that NO exerts its major effect on SMC migration,[22,23] which is a crucial event in intimal thickening. Whether inhibition of migration is of importance to human atherosclerosis or restenosis remains to be determined, as atherosclerosis develops in an existing intima and migration of SMCs from media to intima is not considered a major determinant in atherogenesis.[4]

Few reports have documented benefit from local treatment with NO-releasing drugs on intimal hyperplasia, in contrast to the evidence presented for suppression of neointima formation upon systemic treatment. One possible explanation for this discrepancy could be the delicate balance between the anti-restenosis and pro-restenosis properties of NO. Low fluxes of NO are considered to suppress restenosis and stimulate compensatory vessel enlargement. However, the opposite is presumably true for high concentrations of NO, especially when generated in an environment where the vascular injury created by balloon angioplasty or stent placement, or the presence of an advanced atherosclerotic plaque, leads to an increased production of reactive oxygen species. Therefore, difficulties with the selection of the appropriate dose for local application, or the kinetics of the NO released from a stent platform, may counterbalance the advantage of reduced systemic side effects upon local drug delivery.

These detrimental effects were not reported when L-arginine was applied locally, or when gene transfer was used to raise the local expression and activity of iNOS, eNOS, or particulate or soluble guanylate cyclase following balloon angioplasty or stent deployment. The benefit from L-arginine may be several fold. By providing the substrate to the NOS isoforms, L-arginine may oppose the uncoupling of these enzymes that results in superoxide radical formation.[122] Furthermore, as well as raising NO biosynthesis, L-arginine has superoxide scavenging properties,[123] and arginase isoforms metabolize L-arginine to produce ornithine for the synthesis of proline, which is required for collagen synthesis and wound healing.[124] Finally, arginine is a potent stimulus for the secretion of insulin, and it has been suggested that the systemic vasomotor and antiplatelet effects of L-arginine upon systemic administration to humans are to a substantial part mediated by the release of endogenous insulin.[125]

The extent to which the positive experimental data with NOS gene transfer or local L-arginine application can be translated into the clinic remains to be determined. At present, systemic NO supplementation represents a potentially promising approach to help control restenosis, either alone or as a pharmaceutical adjunct to other local or systemic pharmacological interventions or stent deployment.

SUMMARY

The expression and impact of different isoforms of nitric oxide synthase (NOS) has been studied in animal models of adaptive intimal thickening (neointima formation) evoked by modest vascular injury (balloon denudation of rat or rabbit arteries, or positioning of a flexible, soft collar around the rabbit carotid artery), in models of remodeling, thrombus formation, and intimal hyperplasia evoked by more extensive vascular injury (repeated inflation of an oversized angioplasty balloon, or perivascular placement of rigid collars around murine arteries) and in models of in-stent restenosis. Collectively, the studies suggest that modest fluxes of nitric oxide (NO) generated from eNOS suppress intimal hyperplasia and stimulate chronic compensatory dilatation of the artery. The impact of iNOS, which is already expressed in advanced human plaques, and is induced in non-affected segments by mechanical insults, is more complex. Anti-restenosis effects of iNOS have been documented in models employing modest vascular injury, while stimulation of intimal hyperplasia may prevail when the vascular injury becomes more extensive. Systemic treatment with some classes of NO donors and the NOS substrate L-arginine has demonstrated potential benefits in animal models of neointima formation evoked by modest injury, restenosis after balloon angioplasty or in-stent restenosis. Studies with classical organic nitrates failed to document anti-restenosis effects. This class of NO donors requires intracellular biotransformation to release NO and is liable to the development of tolerance. Tolerance is associated with increased oxidative stress in vascular cells and this may counteract anti-restenosis properties of NO. Likewise, systemic treatment with molsidomine failed to suppress neointima formation or restenosis after angioplasty in most studies. Linsidomine, the active principle of molsidomine, spontaneously releases superoxide anion together with each molecule of NO that may inactivate NO and counterbalance its anti-restenosis properties. Donor molecules showing potential benefit either release NO spontaneously (e.g. NONOates, *S*-nitrosothiols) or are organic nitrates that are resistant to the development of tolerance. High concentrations of NO stimulate vascular injury, inflammation, and neointima formation, especially when superoxide anion is generated at the intervention site. This may explain why few studies could report benefit from local NO delivery or NO-releasing stents. In contrast local treatment with L-arginine or local gene transfer of eNOS, iNOS or particulate or soluble guanylate cyclase have demonstrated potential benefits in most animal models. Some of these interventions hold promise for ultimate pharmacotherapy of restenosis.

ACKNOWLEDGMENTS

The authors wish to thank Liliane Van den Eynde for secretarial help. This work was supported by the Fund for Scientific Research-Flanders (Belgium), grant No G.0427.02.

REFERENCES

1. Bauters C, Meurice T, Hamon M, et al. Mechanisms and prevention of restenosis: from experimental models to clinical practice. Cardiovasc Res 1996; 31:835–46.
2. Topol EJ, Serruys PW. Frontiers in interventional cardiology. Circulation 1998; 98:1802–20.
3. Bult H. Restenosis: a challenge for pharmacology. Trends Pharmacol Sci. 2000; 21:274–9.
4. Jackson CL. Animal models of restenosis. Trends Cardiovasc Med 1994; 4:122–30.
5. Schwartz RS, Topol EJ, Serruys PW, et al. Artery size, neointima, and remodeling: time for some standards. J Am Coll Cardiol 1998; 32:2087–94.
6. Weidinger FF, McLenachan JM, Cybulsky MI, et al. Hypercholesterolemia enhances macrophage recruitment and dysfunction of regenerated endothelium after balloon injury of the rabbit iliac artery. Circulation 1991; 84:755–67.
7. Weidinger FF, McLenachan JM, Cybulsky MI, et al. Persistent dysfunction of regenerated endothelium after balloon angioplasty of rabbit iliac artery. Circulation 1990; 81:1667–79.
8. Tarry WC, Makhoul RG. L-arginine improves endothelium-dependent vasorelaxation and reduces intimal hyperplasia after balloon angioplasty. Arterioscler Thromb 1994; 14:938–43.
9. Bosmans JM, Bult H, Vrints CJ, et al. Balloon angioplasty and induction of non-endothelial nitric oxide synthase in rabbit carotid arteries. Eur J Pharmacol 1996; 310:163–74.
10. Myers PR, Webel R, Thondapu V, et al. Restenosis is associated with decreased coronary artery nitric oxide synthase. Int J Cardiol 1996; 55:183–91.
11. Bult H. Nitric oxide and atherosclerosis: possible implications for therapy. Mol Med Today 1996; 2:510–18.
12. Matthys KE, Bult H. Nitric oxide function in atherosclerosis. Mediators Inflamm 1997; 6:3–21.
13. Rinaldo JE, Clark M, Parinello J, Shepherd VL. Nitric oxide inactivates xanthine dehydrogenase and xanthine oxidase in interferon-gamma-stimulated macrophages. Am J Respir Cell Mol Biol 1994; 11:625–30.
14. Clancy RM, Leszczynska-Piziak J, Abramson SB. Nitric oxide, an endothelial cell relaxation factor, inhibits neutrophil superoxide anion production via a direct action on the NADPH oxidase. J Clin Invest 1992; 90:1116–21.
15. Fukahori M, Ichimori K, Ishida H, et al. Nitric oxide reversibly suppresses xanthine oxidase activity. Free Radic Res 1994; 21:203–12.
16. De Caterina R, Libby P, Peng HB, et al. Nitric oxide decreases cytokine-induced endothelial activation. Nitric oxide selectively reduces endothelial expression of adhesion molecules and proinflammatory cytokines. J Clin Invest 1995; 96:60–8.
17. Spiecker M, Peng H-B, Liao JK. Inhibition of endothelial vascular cell adhesion molecule-1 expression by nitric oxide involves the induction and nuclear translocation of IκBα. J Biol Chem 1997; 272:30969–74.
18. Zeiher AM, Fisslthaler B, Schray-Utz B, Busse R. Nitric oxide modulates the expression of monocyte chemoattractant protein 1 in cultured human endothelial cells. Circ Res 1995; 76:980–6.
19. Bath PMW, Hassall DG, Gladwin A-M, et al. Nitric oxide and prostacyclin: divergence of inhibitory effects on monocyte chemotaxis and

adhesion to endothelium in vitro. Arterioscler Thromb 1991; 11:254–60.

20. Tsao PS, Lewis NP, Alpert S, Cooke JP. Exposure to shear stress alters endothelial adhesiveness. Role of nitric oxide. Circulation 1995; 92:3513–19.

21. Loscalzo J. Nitric oxide insufficiency, platelet activation, and arterial thrombosis. Circ Res 2001; 88:756–62.

22. Dubey RK, Jackson EK, Lüscher TF. Nitric oxide inhibits angiotensin II-induced migration of rat aortic smooth muscle cell. J Clin Invest 1995; 96:141–9.

23. Sarkar R, Meinberg EG, Stanley JC, Gordon D, Webb RC. Nitric oxide reversibly inhibits the migration of cultured vascular smooth muscle cells. Circ Res 1996; 78:225–30.

24. Sinnaeve P, Chiche JD, Nong Z, et al. Soluble guanylate cyclase alpha(1) and beta(1) gene transfer increases NO responsiveness and reduces neointima formation after balloon injury in rats via antiproliferative and antimigratory effects. Circ Res 2001; 88:103–9.

25. Gurjar MV, DeLeon J, Sharma RV, Bhalla RC. Mechanism of inhibition of matrix metalloproteinase-9 induction by NO in vascular smooth muscle cells. J Appl Physiol 2001; 91:1380–6.

26. Mooradian DL, Hutsell TC, Keefer LK. Nitric oxide (NO) donor molecules: effect of NO release rate on vascular smooth muscle cell proliferation in vitro. J Cardiovasc Pharmacol 1995; 25:674–8.

27. Assender JW, Southgate KM, Newby AC. Does nitric oxide inhibit smooth muscle proliferation? J Cardiovasc Pharmacol 1991; 17(suppl 3):S104–S107.

28. Cornwell TL, Arnold E, Boerth NJ, Lincoln TM. Inhibition of smooth muscle cell growth by nitric oxide and activation of cAMP-dependent protein kinase by cGMP. Am J Physiol 1994; 36:C1405–C1413.

29. Nakaki T, Nakayama M, Kato R. Inhibition by nitric oxide and nitric oxide-producing vasodilators of DNA synthesis in vascular smooth muscle cells. Eur J Pharmacol 1990; 189:347–53.

30. Garg UC, Hassid A. Nitric oxide-generating vasodilators and 8-bromo-cyclic guanosine monophosphate inhibit mitogenesis and prolif-

eration of cultured rat vascular smooth muscle cells. J Clin Invest 1989; 83:1774–7.

31. Fu Y, Blankenhorn EP. Nitric oxide-induced anti-mitogenic effects in high and low responder rat strains. J Immunol 1992; 148:2217–22.

32. Kawabe T, Isobe KI, Hasegawa Y, et al. Immunosuppressive activity induced by nitric oxide in culture supernatant of activated rat alveolar macrophages. Immunology 1992; 76:72–8.

33. Merryman PF, Clancy RM, He XY, Abramson SB. Modulation of human T-cell responses by nitric oxide and its derivative, S-nitrosoglutathione. Arthritis Rheum 1993; 36:1414–22.

34. Rudic RD, Shesely EG, Maeda N, et al. Direct evidence for the importance of endothelium-derived nitric oxide in vascular remodeling. J Clin Invest 1998; 101:731–6.

35. Moroi M, Zhang L, Yasuda T, et al. Interaction of genetic deficiency of endothelial nitric oxide, gender, and pregnancy in vascular response to injury in mice. J Clin Invest 1998; 101:1225–32.

36. Chyu KY, Dimayuga P, Zhu J, et al. Decreased neointimal thickening after arterial wall injury in inducible nitric oxide synthase knockout mice. Circ Res 1999; 85:1192–8.

37. Verbeuren TJ, Bonhomme E, Laubie M, Simonet S. Evidence for induction of non-endothelial NO-synthase in aortas of cholesterol-fed rabbits. J Cardiovasc Pharmacol 1993; 21:841–5.

38. Buttery LDK, Springall DR, Chester AH, et al. Inducible nitric oxide synthase is present within human atherosclerotic lesions and promotes the formation and activity of peroxynitrite. Lab Invest 1996; 75:77–85.

39. Esaki T, Hayashi T, Muto E, et al. Expression of inducible nitric oxide synthase in T lymphocytes and macrophages of cholesterol-fed rabbits. Atherosclerosis 1997; 128:39–46.

40. Luoma JS, Strålin P, Marklund SL, et al. Expression of extracellular SOD and iNOS in macrophages and smooth muscle cells in human and rabbit atherosclerotic lesions. Colocalization with epitopes characteristic of oxidized LDL and peroxynitrite-modified proteins. Arterioscler Thromb Vasc Biol 1998; 18:157–67.

41. Cromheeke KM, Kockx MM, De Meyer GRY, et al. Inducible nitric oxide synthase colocalizes

with signs of lipid oxidation/peroxidation in human atherosclerotic plaques. Cardiovasc Res 1999; 43:744–54.

42. Coers W, Timens W, Kempinga C, et al. Specificity of antibodies to nitric oxide synthase isoforms in human, guinea pig, rat, and mouse tissues. J Histochem Cytochem 1998; 46:1385–92.

43. Douglas SA, Vickery-Clark LM, Ohlstein EH. Functional evidence that balloon angioplasty results in transient nitric oxide synthase induction. Eur J Pharmacol 1994; 255:81–9.

44. Joly GA, Schini VB, Vanhoutte PM. Balloon injury and interleukin-1 β induce nitric oxide synthase activity in rat carotid arteries. Circ Res 1992; 71:331–8.

45. Hansson GK, Geng Y-J, Holm J, Hardhammar P, et al. Arterial smooth muscle cells express nitric oxide synthase in response to endothelial injury. J Exp Med 1994; 180:733–8.

46. Yan Z, Hansson GK. Overexpression of inducible nitric oxide synthase by neointimal smooth muscle cells. Circ Res 1998; 82:21–9.

47. De Meyer GRY, Bult H, Üstünes L, et al. Vasoconstrictor responses after neo-intima formation and endothelial denudation in the rabbit carotid artery. Br J Pharmacol 1994; 112:471–6.

48. De Meyer GRY, Kockx MM, Cromheeke KM, et al. Periadventitial inducible nitric oxide synthase expression and intimal thickening. Arterioscler Thromb Vasc Biol 2000; 20:1896–1902.

49. Bult H, Cromheeke KM, Bosmans JM, et al. Inducible NOS after experimental angioplasty and in human atherosclerosis. In Moncada S, Toda N, Maeda H, Higgs EA (eds), The Biology of Nitric Oxide. Part 6. Portland Press: London 1998:148.

50. Graham A, Hogg N, Kalyanaraman B, et al. Peroxynitrite modification of low-density lipoprotein leads to recognition by the macrophage scavenger receptor. FEBS Lett 1993; 330:181–5.

51. Beckman JS, Beckman TW, Chen J, et al. Apparent hydroxyl radical production by peroxynitrite: implications for endothelial injury from nitric oxide and superoxide. Proc Natl Acad Sci USA 1990; 87:1620–4.

52. Radi R, Beckman JS, Bush KM, Freeman BA. Peroxynitrite oxidation of sulfhydryls. The cytotoxic potential of superoxide and nitric oxide. J Biol Chem 1991; 266:4244–50.

53. Miles AM, Bohle DS, Glassbrenner PA, et al. Modulation of superoxide-dependent oxidation and hydroxylation reactions by nitric oxide. J Biol Chem 1996; 271:40–7.

54. Palmer RM, Bridge L, Foxwell NA, Moncada S. The role of nitric oxide in endothelial cell damage and its inhibition by glucocorticoids. Br J Pharmacol 1992; 105:11–12.

55. Shimizu S, Nomoto M, Naito S, et al. Simulation of nitric oxide synthase during oxidative endothelial cell injury. Biochem Pharmacol 1998; 55:77–83.

56. Fukuo K, Inoue T, Morimoto S, et al. Nitric oxide mediates cytotoxicity and basic fibroblast growth factor release in cultured vascular smooth muscle cells. J Clin Invest 1995; 95:669–76.

57. Szabo C, Zingarelli B, O'Connor M, Salzman AL. DNA strand breakage, activation of poly(ADP-ribose) synthetase, and cellular energy depletion are involved in the cytotoxicity in macrophages and smooth muscle cells exposed to peroxynitrite. Proc Natl Acad Sci USA 1996; 93:1753–8.

58. Gross SS, Wolin MS. Nitric oxide: pathophysiological mechanisms. Annu Rev Physiol 1995; 57:737–69.

59. Martinet W, Knaapen MWM, De Meyer GRY, et al. Oxidative DNA damage and repair in experimental atherosclerosis are reversed by dietary lipid lowering. Circ Res 2001; 88:733–9.

60. Schwarzacher SP, Tsao PS, Ward M, et al. Effects of stenting on adjacent vascular distensibility and neointima formation: role of nitric oxide. Vasc Med 2001; 6:139–44.

61. Feelisch M. The biochemical pathways of nitric oxide (NO) formation from nitrovasodilators: appropriate choice of exogenous NO donors and aspects of preparation and handling of aqueous NO solutions. J Cardiovasc Pharmacol 1991; 17:S25–S33.

62. Feelisch M. The use of nitric oxide donors in pharmacological studies. Naunyn Schmiedeberg's Arch Pharmacol 1998; 358:113–22.

63. Ignarro LJ, Napoli C, Loscalzo J. Nitric oxide donors and cardiovascular agents modulating the bioactivity of nitric oxide: an overview. Circ Res 2002; 90:21–8.

64. Chen Z, Zhang J, Stamler JS. Identification of the enzymatic mechanism of nitroglycerin bioactivation. Proc Natl Acad Sci USA 2002; 99:8306–11.

65. Parker JD, Parker JO. Nitrate therapy for stable angina pectoris. N Engl J Med 1998; 338:520–31.

66. Münzel T. Does nitroglycerin therapy hit the endothelium? J Am Coll Cardiol 2001; 38:1102–5.

67. Münzel T, Sayegh H, Freeman BA, et al. Evidence for enhanced vascular superoxide anion production in nitrate tolerance. J Clin Invest 1995; 95:187–94.

68. Sage PR, De la Lande IS, Stafford I, et al. Nitroglycerin tolerance in human vessels: evidence for impaired nitroglycerin bioconversion. Circulation 2000; 102:2810–15.

69. Laursen JB, Somers M, Kurz S, et al. Endothelial regulation of vasomotion in apoE-deficient mice: implications for interactions between peroxynitrite and tetrahydrobiopterin. Circulation 2001; 103:1282–8.

70. Abou-Mohamed G, Kaesemeyer WH, Caldwell RB, et al. Role of L-arginine in the vascular actions and development of tolerance to nitroglycerin. Br J Pharmacol 2000; 130:211–18.

71. Willis S, Allescher H-D, Weigert N, et al. Influence of the L-arginine-nitric oxide pathway on vasoactive intestinal polypeptide release and motility in the rat stomach in vitro. Eur J Pharmacol 1996; 315:59–64.

72. Soff GA, Cornwell TL, Cundiff DL, et al. Smooth muscle cell expression of type I cyclic GMP-dependent protein kinase is suppressed by continuous exposure to nitrovasodilators, theophylline, cyclic GMP, and cyclic AMP. J Clin Invest 1997; 100:2580–7.

73. Münzel T, Giaid A, Kurz S, et al. Evidence for a role of endothelin I and protein kinase C in nitroglycerin tolerance. Proc Natl Acad Sci USA 1995; 92:5244–8.

74. Fleming I, Fisslthaler B, Dimmeler S, et al. Phosphorylation of Thr(495) regulates Ca(2+)/calmodulin-dependent endothelial nitric oxide synthase activity. Circ Res 2001; 88:E68–E75.

75. Ahlner J, Andersson RGG, Torfgård K, Axelsson KL. Organic nitrate esters: clinical use and mechanisms of actions. Pharmacol Rev 1991; 43:351–423.

76. Kim D, Rybalkin SD, Pi X, et al. Upregulation of phosphodiesterase 1A1 expression is associated with the development of nitrate tolerance. Circulation 2001; 104:2338–43.

77. Dikalov S, Fink B, Skatchkov M, Bassenge E. Comparison of glyceryl trinitrate-induced with pentaerythrityl tetranitrate-induced in vivo formation of superoxide radicals: effect of vitamin C. Free Radic Biol Med 1999; 27:170–6.

78. Guo JP, Milhoan KA, Tuan RS, Lefer AM. Beneficial effect of SPM-5185, a cysteine-containing nitric oxide donor, in rat carotid artery intimal injury. Circ Res 1994; 75:77–84.

79. De Meyer GRY, Bult H, Üstünes L, et al. Effect of nitric oxide donors on neointima formation and vascular reactivity in the collared carotid artery of rabbits. J Cardiovasc Pharmacol 1995; 26:272–9.

80. Napoli C, Aldini G, Wallace JL, et al. Efficacy and age-related effects of nitric oxide-releasing aspirin on experimental restenosis. Proc Natl Acad Sci USA 2002; 99:1689–94.

81. Napoli C, Cirino G, del Soldato P, et al. Effects of nitric oxide-releasing aspirin versus aspirin on restenosis in hypercholesterolemic mice. Proc Natl Acad Sci USA 2001; 98:2860–4.

82. Maffia P, Ianaro A, Sorrentino R, et al. Beneficial effects of NO-releasing derivative of flurbiprofen (HCT-1026) in rat model of vascular injury and restenosis. Arterioscler Thromb Vasc Biol 2002; 22:263–7.

83. Wolf YG, Rasmussen LM, Sherman Y, et al. Nitroglycerin decreases medial smooth muscle cell proliferation after arterial balloon injury. J Vasc Surg 1995; 21:499–504.

84. Seki J, Nishio M, Kato Y, et al. FK409, a new nitric oxide donor, suppresses smooth muscle proliferation in the rat model of balloon angioplasty. Atherosclerosis 1995; 117:97–106.

85. Lee JS, Adrie C, Jacob HJ, et al. Chronic inhalation of nitric oxide inhibits neointimal formation after balloon-induced arterial injury. Circ Res 1996; 78:337–42.

86. Yasa M, Kerry Z, Yetik G, et al. Effects of treatment with FK409, a nitric oxide donor, on

collar-induced intimal thickening and vascular reactivity. Eur J Pharmacol 1999; 374:33–9.

87. Groves PH, Lewis MJ, Cheadle HA, Penny WJ. SIN-1 reduces platelet adhesion and platelet thrombus formation in a porcine model of balloon angioplasty. Circulation 1993; 87:590–7.

88. Groves PH, Banning AP, Penny WJ, et al. The effects of exogenous nitric oxide on smooth muscle cell proliferation following porcine carotid angioplasty. Cardiovasc Res 1995; 30:87–96.

89. Provost P, Tremblay J, Merhi Y. The antiadhesive and antithrombotic effects of the nitric oxide donor SIN-1 are combined with a decreased vasoconstriction in a porcine model of balloon angioplasty. Arterioscler Thromb Vasc Biol 1997; 17:1806–12.

90. Lablanche JM, Grollier G, Lusson JR, et al. Effect of the direct nitric oxide donors linsidomine and molsidomine on angiographic restenosis after coronary balloon angioplasty. The ACCORD Study. Angioplastic Coronaire Corvasal Diltiazem. Circulation 1997; 95:83–9.

91. Marks DS, Vita JA, Folts JD, et al. Inhibition of neointimal proliferation in rabbits after vascular injury by a single treatment with a protein adduct of nitric oxide. J Clin Invest 1995; 96:2630–8.

92. Yin ZL, Dusting GJ. A nitric oxide donor (spermine-NONOate) prevents the formation of neointima in rabbit carotid artery. Clin Exp Pharmacol Physiol 1997; 24:436–8.

93. Smith DJ, Chakravarthy D, Pulfer S, et al. Nitric oxide-releasing polymers containing the [N(O)NO]-group. J Med Chem 1996; 39:1148–56.

94. Kaul S, Cercek B, Rengstrom J, et al. Polymeric-based perivascular delivery of a nitric oxide donor inhibits intimal thickening after balloon denudation arterial injury: role of nuclear factor-kappaB. J Am Coll Cardiol 2000; 35:493–501.

95. Buergler JM, Tio FO, Schulz DG, et al. Use of nitric-oxide-eluting polymer-coated coronary stents for prevention of restenosis in pigs. Coron Artery Dis 2000; 11:351–7.

96. Yoon JH, Wu CJ, Homme J, et al. Local delivery of nitric oxide from an eluting stent to inhibit

neointimal thickening in a porcine coronary injury model. Yonsei Med J 2002; 43:242–51.

97. McNamara DB, Bedi B, Aurora H, et al. L-arginine inhibits balloon catheter-induced intimal hyperplasia. Biochem Biophys Res Commun 1993; 193:291–6.

98. Holm AM, Andersen CB, Haunso S, Hansen PR. Effects of L-arginine on vascular smooth muscle cell proliferation and apoptosis after balloon injury. Scand Cardiovasc J 2000; 34:28–32.

99. Taguchi J, Abe J, Okazaki H, et al. L-arginine inhibits neointimal formation following balloon injury. Life Sci 1993; 53:387–92.

100. Wu Z, Qian X, Cai D, et al. Long-term oral administration of L-arginine enhances endothelium-dependent vasorelaxation and inhibits neointimal thickening after endothelial denudation in rats. Chin Med J (Engl) 1996; 109:592–8.

101. Vermeersch P, Nong Z, Stabile E, et al. L-arginine administration reduces neointima formation after stent injury in rats by a nitric oxide-mediated mechanism. Arterioscler Thromb Vasc Biol 2001; 21:1604–9.

102. Bosmans JM, Kockx MM, Vrints CJ, et al. Fibrin(ogen) and von Willebrand factor deposition are associated with intimal thickening after ballon angioplasty of the rabbit carotid artery. Arterioscler Thromb Vasc Biol 1997; 17:634–45.

103. Kakuta T, Currier JW, Haudenschild CC, et al. Differences in compensatory vessel enlargement, not intimal formation, account for restenosis after angioplasty in the hypercholesterolemic rabbit model. Circulation 1994; 89:2809–15.

104. Bosmans JM, Vrints CJ, Kockx MM, et al. Continuous perivascular L-arginine delivery increases total vessel area and reduces neointimal thickening after experimental balloon dilatation. Arterioscler Thromb Vasc Biol 1999; 19:767–76.

105. Lafont A, Guzman LA, Whitlow PL, et al. Restenosis after experimental angioplasty. Intimal, medial, and adventitial changes associated with constrictive remodeling. Circ Res 1995; 76:996–1002.

106. Greenless C, Wadsworth RM, Martorana PA, Wainwright CL. The effects of L-arginine on

neointimal formation and vascular function following balloon injury in heritable hyperlipidaemic rabbits. Cardiovasc Res 1997; 35:351–9.

107. Corseaux D, Le Tourneau T, Six I, et al. Enhanced monocyte tissue factor response after experimental balloon angioplasty in hypercholesterolemic rabbit: inhibition with dietary L-arginine. Circulation 1998; 98:1776–82.

108. Le Tourneau T, Van Belle E, Corseaux D, et al. Role of nitric oxide in restenosis after experimental balloon angioplasty in the hypercholesterolemic rabbit: effects on neointimal hyperplasia and vascular remodeling. J Am Coll Cardiol 1999; 33:876–82.

109. Niebauer J, Schwarzacher SP, Hayase M, et al. Local L-arginine delivery after balloon angioplasty reduces monocyte binding and induces apoptosis. Circulation 1999; 100:1830–5.

110. Schwarzacher SP, Lim TT, Wang B, et al. Local intramural delivery of L-arginine enhances nitric oxide generation and inhibits lesion formation after balloon angioplasty. Circulation 1997; 95:1863–9.

111. Suzuki T, Hayase M, Hibi K, et al. Effect of local delivery of L-arginine on in-stent restenosis in humans. Am J Cardiol 2002; 89:363–7.

112. Von der Leyen HE, Gibbons GH, Morishita R, et al. Gene therapy inhibiting neointimal vascular lesion: in vivo transfer of endothelial cell nitric oxide synthase gene. Proc Natl Acad Sci USA 1995; 92:1137–41.

113. Janssens S, Flaherty D, Nong Z, et al. Human endothelial nitric oxide synthase gene transfer inhibits vascular smooth muscle cell proliferation and neointima formation after balloon injury in rats. Circulation 1998; 97:1274–81.

114. Chen L, Daum G, Forough R, et al. Overexpression of human endothelial nitric oxide synthase in rat vascular smooth muscle cells and in balloon-injured carotid artery. Circ Res 1998; 82:862–70.

115. Varenne O, Pislaru S, Gillijns H, et al. Local adenovirus-mediated transfer of human endothelial nitric oxide synthase reduces luminal narrowing after coronary angioplasty in pigs. Circulation 1998; 98:919–26.

116. Gurjar MV, Sharma RV, Bhalla RC. eNOS gene transfer inhibits smooth muscle cell migration and MMP-2 and MMP-9 activity. Arterioscler Thromb Vasc Biol 1999; 19:2871–7.

117. Cable DG, O'Brien T, Schaff HV, Pompili VJ. Recombinant endothelial nitric oxide synthase-transduced human saphenous veins: gene therapy to augment nitric oxide production in bypass conduits. Circulation 1997; 96:II–8.

118. Tzeng E, Shears LL, Robbins PD, et al. Vascular gene transfer of the human inducible nitric oxide synthase: characterization of activity and effects on myointimal hyperplasia. Mol Med Today 1996; 2:211–25.

119. Shears LL, Kibbe MR, Murdock AD, et al. Efficient inhibition of intimal hyperplasia by adenovirus-mediated inducible nitric oxide synthase gene transfer to rats and pigs in vivo. J Am Coll Surg 1998; 187:295–306.

120. Ueno H, Haruno A, Morisaki N, et al. Local expression of C-type natriuretic peptide markedly suppresses neointimal formation in rat injured arteries through an autocrine/paracrine loop. Circulation 1997; 96:2272–9.

121. Bult H, De Meyer GRY, Herman AG. Influence of chronic treatment with a nitric oxide donor on fatty streak development and reactivity of the rabbit aorta. Br J Pharmacol 1995; 114:1371–82.

122. Vasquez-Vivar J, Kalyanaraman B, Martasek P, et al. Superoxide generation by endothelial nitric oxide synthase: the influence of cofactors. Proc Natl Acad Sci USA 1998; 95:9220–5.

123. Wascher TC, Posch K, Wallner S, et al. Vascular effects of L-arginine: anything beyond a substrate for the NO-synthase? Biochem Biophys Res Commun 1997; 234:35–8.

124. Wu G, Morris SM, Jr. Arginine metabolism: nitric oxide and beyond. Biochem J 1998; 336:1–17.

125. Giugliano D, Marfella R, Verrazzo G, et al. The vascular effects of L-Arginine in humans. The role of endogenous insulin. J Clin Invest 1997; 99:433–8.

23

Vitamin E and its multiple properties: anti, pro, and non-oxidative activities

XianShun Liu and Ivan De Scheerder

INTRODUCTION

The term 'vitamin E' was introduced by Evans and Bishop in 1922 to describe an essential nutrient for reproduction in rats.[1] Vitamin E exists as at least eight naturally occurring compounds, including α-, β-, δ-, and γ-tocopherol and α-, β-, δ-, and γ-tocotrienol[2] and among these compounds, α-tocopherol has the greatest biological activity. In the 1960s vitamin E was associated with antioxidant function.[3] This antioxidant property has aroused the interest of many groups to study its ability to prevent chronic diseases, especially those believed to have an oxidative stress component, such as cardiovascular diseases, atherosclerosis, and cancer. Vitamin E was proposed as an effective treatment for heart disease in the 1940s,[4] which has since been confirmed by several epidemiologic studies and clinical trials.

However, recent interventional clinical trials demonstrated conflicting results of this benefi-cial effect. The equivocal outcomes of these studies cast additional doubt and confusion on the effectiveness of α-tocopherol supplementation in preventing cardiovascular disease (see below).

As well as antioxidant properties, prooxidant properties of vitamin E have also been observed.

In the 1990s, non-oxidant properties of vitamin E were proposed.[5] Many reports have subsequently confirmed the involvement of protein kinase C (PKC) in the effect of α-tocopherol in different cell types, such as monocytes, macrophages, neutrophils, fibro-blasts, and mesangial cells.[6–9] Vitamin E enrichment has been shown to inhibit the proliferation of smooth muscle cells, inhibit proinflammatory activity of monocytes, inhibit platelet adhesion and aggregation, inhibit the expression and function of adhesion molecules, attenuate the synthesis of leukotrienes, and potentiate the release of prostacyclin through upregulating the expression of cytosolic phospholipase A_2 and cyclooxygenase. These functions are not related to the antioxidant action of vitamin E.

VITAMIN E AND CORONARY HEART DISEASE

Vitamin E was first proposed as an effective treatment to heart disease more than 50 years ago,[4] and further gained considerable support from recent epidemiologic studies and clinical trials.[10,11] A prospective study revealed that large doses of vitamin E supplements (>100 IU/d) are associated with a significantly decreased risk of coronary heart disease.[10] A similar reduction in risk was observed in the Health Professionals' Follow-up Study.[11] Vitamin E consumption, in a population of postmenopausal women, was confirmed to be inversely associated with the risk of death from CHD.[12] Result from a clinical intervention trial (CHAOS) showed that vitamin E therapy significantly reduced the recurrence of heart attacks.[13] Another study demonstrated regression of existing atherosclerosis in patients who had coronary bypass surgery and who had an intake of over 100 IU/d of vitamin E.[14] However, results from prospective studies are equivocal. Steiner et al.[16] showed that patients who received α-tocopherol and aspirin had a significant reduction in transient ischemic attacks and ischemic strokes compared with those who took aspirin alone. The ATBC and HOPE studies showed no distinct benefit of having vitamin E supplementation.[15,17] The CHAOS and GISSI studies (four-way analyses) demonstrated that α-tocopherol supplementation was respectively associated with significant reduction in non-fatal myocardial infarction and cardiovascular deaths.[13,18] Despite one recent finding (SPACE) of a decrease in myocardial infarction in patients with endstage renal disease,[19] the conclusion from recent studies is that α-tocopherol is ineffective in decreasing coronary artery disease.[20–22]

In summary, although α-tocopherol is the most abundant lipid-soluble antioxidant in low density lipoprotein (LDL), controlled prospective clinical trials using vitamin E supplements have generated conflicting results. Overall, the treatment of high risk cardiovascular patients with daily vitamin E had no effect on cardiovascular outcomes. The reasons for these disappointing results are probably complex. A common criticism is that vitamin E may be more effective in primary rather than secondary interventions. Moreover, it is obvious that age, disease, gender, smoking habit, and diet may have strongly affected the outcomes of different trials on the efficacy of vitamin E.

ANTIOXIDANT ACTIVITY

Vitamin E is the major hydrophobic chain-breaking antioxidant that prevents the propagation of free radical reactions in the lipid components of membranes, vacuoles, and plasma lipoproteins.[23–26] The antioxidant properties of vitamin E are well known and documented.[27] In particular, prevention by α-tocopherol of low density lipoproteins (LDL) oxidation has been studied.[28] LDL is a key carrier of vitamin E in the bloodstream. It is estimated that for individuals who are not receiving any supplement, the average LDL particle contains 7 molecules of α-tocopherol and 0.5 molecule of α-tocopherol. Esterbauer et al.[29] reported that α-tocopherol-depleted LDL is able to undergo rapid lipid peroxidation, whereas LDL isolated from α-tocopherol-supplemented subjects exhibits increased resistance to ex vivo copper-induced oxidation.[30] Evidence so far demonstrates that both cell-mediated and metal-dependent oxidation of LDL can be suppressed by vitamin E supplementation. Enrichment of LDL with vitamin E was reported to protect LDL against ex vivo oxidative modification.[31–33] Conversely, enrichment of endothelial cells with vitamin E significantly attenuated their ability to oxidize LDL.[34] Similarly, in survivors of myocardial infarction, vitamin E content in LDL was inversely related to the severity of the coronary stenosis score as determined by angiograms.[35]

Taken together, vitamin E exerts a protective effect against free radical damage. These studies clearly demonstrate that as the vitamin E content in LDL or endothelial cells is increased, there is an overall protection against LDL oxidation.

PRO-OXIDANT ACTIVITY

In contrast to all the described antioxidant properties of vitamin E, it has been shown that lipid peroxidation of LDL is faster in the presence α-tocopherol, and is substantially accelerated by enrichment of the vitamin in LDL, either in vitro or in vivo.[36,37] Various investigators have reported that the resistance of LDL to oxidation does not correlate with its vitamin E content,[38,39] and that ubiquinol-10, not α-tocopherol, forms the first line of defense against oxidation in human LDL.[40] In particular, α-tocopherol can act as a pro-oxidant in LDL via α-tocopheroxyl radical-mediated formation of lipid radicals.[41] The presence of co-antioxidants, such as ascorbate (vitamin C),[42] and ubiquinol-10 in the vascular environment can convert α-tocopherol from a pro-oxidant into an antioxidant.[41] Pro-oxidative functions of α-tocopherol have been demonstrated in LDL isolated from healthy volunteers,[36] and a patient with a defect in the α-TTP gene.[43] However, the importance of pro-oxidation reactions of α-tocopherol in vivo appears to be questionable under physiological conditions.

In summary, vitamin E, like every redox-active compound, may exert anti- and pro-oxidative effects depending on the reaction partners present. The importance of a pro-oxidant role of vitamin E in vivo has yet to be demonstrated.

NON-OXIDATIVE PROPERTIES

In 1991, the first discovery of non-antioxidant action of α-tocopherol was represented by the inhibition of PKC activity and the related inhibition of vascular smooth muscle cell proliferation.[44] Many reports have subsequently confirmed the involvement of PKC in the effect of α-tocopherol on different cell types, including monocytes, macrophages, neutrophils, fibroblasts, and mesangial cells.[6–9,45] α-Tocopherol, but not β-tocopherol, was found to inhibit thrombin-induced PKC activation and endothelin secretion in endothelial cells.[46] These results show that alpha-tocopherol inhibits O^{-2} production by human adherent monocytes by impairing the assembly of the NADPH-oxidase and suggest that the inhibition of phosphorylation and translocation of the cytosolic factor p47(phox) results from a decrease in PKC activity.[47] Moreover, α-tocopherol has the important biological effect of inhibiting the release of the proinflammatory cytokine, IL-1β, via inhibition of the 5-lipoxygenase pathway.[48] It is becoming clear that α-tocopherol has activities that are unrelated to the LDL oxidation.

EFFECT ON SMOOTH MUSCLE CELLS (SMC): INHIBITION OF SMC PROLIFERATION

Smooth muscle cells found in the media form the bulk of normal arterial cellularity. Many stimuli can induce the migration of SMC from the media to the intima where cell proliferation can occur. The rate of SMC proliferation in lesions is an important determinant of lesion stability in patients, who exhibit excess cardiovascular events. Considerable in vitro data indicate that α-tocopherol inhibits the proliferation of SMC.[5] Using the A7r5 smooth muscle cell line, Boscoboinik and colleagues demonstrated that physiological concentrations of α-tocopherol (50 μM) inhibited [³H]-thymidine incorporation in response to serum, platelet-derived growth factor-BB, and endothelin.[5,44] Inhibition of cell proliferation in the A7r5 cells was associated with a reduction in PKC activity, suggesting that α-tocopherol inhibits smooth muscle cell proliferation principally as a consequence of PKC inhibition.[5] Inhibition of PKC by α-tocopherol in vascular SMC occurs at concentrations of α-tocopherol close to those measured in healthy adults.[49] A comparison of other tocopherol isomers showed that the effect of α-tocopherol was not related to its antioxidant property.[50] Another study showed that cellular proliferation was stimulated by either LDL or malondialdehyde-modified LDL.[51] Calphostin C, a specific PKC inhibitor, also inhibits SMC proliferation, which supports the notion that α-tocopherol acts through the inhibition of PKC stimulation.[52] However, it should be noted that the data on vitamin E inhibition of SMC proliferation is based almost completely on in vitro data, and experience in vivo has, therefore, so far been mixed.[53,54]

In short, the results presented above suggest that vitamin E may inhibit the proliferation of smooth muscle cells.

EFFECTS ON ENDOTHELIUM: PRESERVATION OF ENDOTHELIAL FUNCTION

The vascular endothelium is composed of a monolayer of endothelial cells. Although it functions as a barrier for nutrient transport, the endothelium is now regarded as an active and dynamic tissue involved in maintaining homeostasis in both healthy and diseased states. It is involved in pathophysiologic processes, such as inflammation, thrombosis formation, control of vasomotor tone, and cancer cell metastasis. Vitamin E was first recognized to potentially release prostaglandin I_2 (PGI_2) in rabbit aorta.[55,56] In ischemic-reperfused rat hearts, the release of PGI_2 by coronary vasculatures was inversely related to the levels of vitamin E in the diet.[57] When human endothelial cells in culture were enriched with different concentrations of vitamin E, PGI_2 synthesis was stimulated in a dose-dependent manner, suggesting that both cytosolic phospholipase A_2 ($cPLA_2$) and cyclooxygenase are upregulated.[58] In disease states, such as in diabetes, megadoses of vitamin E treatment were able to restore the diminished PGI_2 production.[59] Vitamin E enrichment can normalize the impaired PGI_2 production resulting from exposure of endothelial cells to oxidized LDL.[60] The mechanism by which vitamin E exerts its effect was recently identified as a higher expression of $cPLA_2$ and cyclooxygenase enzymes in endothelial cells and other cell types.[61,62] Therefore, the cardioprotective function of vitamin E is due in part to its augmentation of PGI_2 release.

Endothelium-derived nitric oxide (eNOS) is a pivotal molecule in the regulation of vascular tone and homeostasis.[63] eNOS not only stimulates vascular smooth muscle cell relaxation and vasodilation, it also exerts a number of potent antiatherogenic effects, including inhibition of smooth muscle cell proliferation, platelet aggregation, and leukocyte–endothelial cell interactions.[63] Animal studies have provided consistent evidence for a beneficial effect of α-tocopherol on vasodilation, as well as insight into underlying mechanisms. Supplementation of cholesterol-fed rabbits with α-tocopherol increased both the resistance of LDL to oxidation and agonist-induced relaxation of thoracic aortas, whereas supplementation with β-carotene had no effect on LDL oxidizability yet did enhance agonist-induced vasodilation.[64] These results suggest that α-tocopherol acts by increasing vascular antioxidant status rather than LDL antioxidant status. In addition, Keaney et al. proposed that α-tocopherol acts in the vascular wall by inhibiting PKC activation by oxidized LDL, hence inhibiting PKC-mediated phosphorylation of endothelial cell muscarinic receptors and enhancing agonist-induced NOS activation.[65]

A number of clinical studies have shown that α-tocopherol increases endothelium-dependent vasodilation in individuals with coronary risk factors.[66–70] Two of these studies also showed a reduction in markers of lipid oxidation.[66,67] Taken together, vitamin E enrichment can normalize the impaired PGI_2 production resulting from exposure of endothelial cells to oxidized LDL. The studies indicate that α-tocopherol may improve eNOS levels via the inhibition of PKC activity. However, in humans there are insufficient data to conclude that long-term treatment with α-tocopherol alone is beneficial.

EFFECT OF CYTOKINE RELEASE

Macrophages secrete several proinflammatory, proatherogenic cytokines, such as interleukin IL-1β and tumor necrosis factor (TNF-α).[71–73] IL-1β has been shown to augment monocyte–endothelial cell adhesion, increase procoagulant activity, promote cholesterol esterification in macrophages and stimulate smooth muscle cell proliferation.[74] TNF-α is a multifunctional cytokine that exerts pleiotropic biological actions. It activates endothelial cells, stimulates angiogenesis, and induces smooth muscle cell proliferation. Akeson et al.[75] showed in vitro that incubation of the human acute monocyte leukemia cell line (THP-1) cells with α-tocopherol significantly inhibits phorbol myristate acetate (PMA)-induced IL-1β secretion. Earlier, Cannon et al.[71] showed that α-tocopherol supplementation (800 IU/d) prevented the increase in IL-1β release from lipopolysaccharide (LPS)-activated mononuclear cells after exercise. α-Tocopherol has the important biological effect of inhibiting the release of the proinflammatory cytokine, IL-1β, via inhibition of the 5-lipoxygenase pathway.[48] The leukotrienes are potent chemotactic factors and mediators of inflammation derived from the 5-lipoxygenase pathway. Dietary vitamin E was shown to inhibit the synthesis of 5-hydroxy-eicosatetraenoic acid (5-HETE) and leukotriene B$_4$ (LTB$_4$) in a dose-dependent manner in rat peritoneal neutrophils.[76] This suppressive effect was demonstrated in humans given vitamin E supplementation from which urinary excretion of leukotriene E$_4$ (LTE$_4$) was monitored.[77,78]

α-Tocopherol has antiinflammatory properties at high doses. Irrespective of the mechanism, the antiinflammatory action of vitamin E could slow down the development of atherosclerosis.

EFFECT ON MONOCYTES: INHIBITION OF MONOCYTE REACTIVE OXYGEN SPECIES (ROS)

Monocytes, when appropriately stimulated, can produce many biologically active mediators that can influence virtually all aspects of atherogenesis. Monocytes have been shown to induce peroxidation of lipids, such as in LDL, by the generation of ROS, including superoxide anion, hydrogen peroxide, hydroxyl radical, peroxynitrite, myeloperoxidase, and hypochlorous acid. Cathcart et al.[79,80] showed that in vitro incubation of monocytes with butylated hydroxytoluene (BHT), vitamin E significantly reduced oxidation of LDL and formation of cytotoxic LDL. Recent data showed that LPS-activated monocytes from type 2 diabetic subjects with and without macrovascular disease released increasedlevels of superoxide anion compared with matched controls.[81] α-Tocopherol supplementation (1200 IU/d) signi-ficantly decreased superoxide anion release in control as well as diabetic monocytes to the same degree. Van Tits et al. showed that supplementation with RRR-AT (600 IU/d) significantly inhibited superoxide production by polymorphonuclear leukocytes (PMN) activated with phorbol ester, but not oxidized LDL or opsonized zymosan.[82] In addition, α-tocopherol inhibits superoxide production by monocytes by impairing the assembly of NADPH oxidase, the enzyme responsible for generating the respiratory burst.[47] This study also suggests that inhibition of PKC activity is not directly due to the antioxidant capacity of α-tocopherol, but requires α-tocopherol integration into the cell membrane where it can interact directly with PKC and NADPH oxidase.[47] Although one study found no change in PKC activity in endothelial cells treated with α-tocopherol, despite decreased E-selectin expression,[83] other studies showed decreased PKC activity paralleled by decreased ROS production in leukocytes treated with α-tocopherol.[6,84]

In summary, with regard to monocytes, α-tocopherol supplementation has been demonstrated to decrease the release of ROS. The mechanism of inhibition of superoxide and lipid oxidation by monocyte by α-tocopherol appear to be via inhibition of PKC.

EFFECT ON MACROPHAGES

Several studies have addressed the effect of α-tocopherol on foam cell formation. Van der Schroeff et al. reported that low doses of α-tocopherol failed to suppress accumulation of cholesteryl ester in J774 cells, which was induced by acetylated LDL.[85] However, Suzukawa et al. reported that enrichment of J774 cells with α-tocopherol inhibited cholesteryl ester formation in J774 cells.[86] Asmits et al. reported that enrichment of P338D macrophages with α-tocopherol decreased the ratio of cholesteryl ester to free cholesterol after incubation with fetal bovine serum but not with modified LDL. Shige et al.[87] subsequently showed that pretreatment of J774 macrophages with concentrations of α-tocopherol >50 μM significantly reduced the uptake of modified LDL and suppressed acyl-cholesterol-acyl-transferase activity, resulting in reduced cholesterol esterification in these macrophages.[88] Recently, α-tocopherol was demonstrated to downregulate SR-A activity and mRNA expression in rabbit and human monocyte-derived macrophages in vitro.[89] Ricciarelli et al. recently reported that α-tocopherol, but not β-tocopherol, reduced CD36 expression in a cultured human aortic smooth muscle cell line by downregulating CD36 mRNA and protein expression.[90] They also showed that α-tocopherol decreased CD36 activity in HL (human leukemia)-60 cells. Devaraj et al. recently showed that in human monocyte-derived macrophages.[91] α-Tocopherol enrichment (>50 μM) results in decreased CD36 expression by flow cytometry and decreased SR activity as assessed by (Dil)-labeled LDL uptake. It appears that this effect of α-tocopherol is not mediated via PKC because specific PKC inhibitors did not affect it in any way. Whereas inhibition of SR-A expression by α-tocopherol is at the level of mRNA. CD36 inhibition by α-tocopherol is a post-transcriptional effect. Baoutina et al. showed in vitro that α-tocopherol did not affect the rate of LDL oxidation or the amount of superoxide released from mouse peritoneal and human macrophages.[92] As previously reviewed, however, data showed that high doses of α-tocopherol significantly reduced further oxidation of LDL by J774 macrophages.[89,90] Although the limited studies to date suggest that α-tocopherol significantly decreases macrophage function relevant to atherogenesis, this area clearly needs further exploration.

INHIBITION OF MONOCYTE–ENDOTHELIAL CELL ADHESION

The recruitment of inflammatory cells into the vascular wall is an important component of vascular inflammation. The regulation of this process can occur at either the level of the endothelium and/or the leukocyte. The exact mechanism by which monocyte–endothelial cell adhesion occurs in vivo remains to be elucidated. Recent work has identified the specific adhesion molecules on endothelial cells and monocytes. These adhesion molecules include E-selectin, intercellular adhesion molecule-1 (ICAM-1), and vascular cell adhesion molecule-1 (VCAM-1) on endothelial cells and members of the β_2 integrin family, CD11a, CD11b, CD11c/18, and the β_1 integrin, VLA-4 (CD49d/29) on monocytes. On leukocytes, the CD11a and CD11b integrins as well as L-selectin have been implicated. In human atheroma, VCAM-1 and ICAM-1 are expressed on endothelial cells and to a smaller extent, on smooth muscle cells and macrophages.

Endothelial cells loaded with α-tocopherol demonstrate a reduction in agonist-induced monocyte adhesion.[83] In particular, the endothelial cell α-tocopherol content regulates the surface expression of E-selectin in response to IL-1β, thereby reducing monocyte adhesion to endothelial cells.[83] Cell culture studies have shown that pretreatment of endothelial cells with α-tocopherol inhibits cytokine or oxidized LDL-induced expression of ICAM-1, VCAM-1, or E-selectin and decreases adhesion of monocytes to these cells.[93–96] Cominacini et al. found that both LDL-associated and cellular α-tocopherol are able to inhibit upregulation of ICAM-1 and VCAM-1 by endothelial cells exposed to oxidized LDL.[94] α-Tocopherol also decreased stimulus-induced expression of β_1 and β_2 integrins on leukocytes and adhesion of these cells to cultured endothelial cells.[6,85,96] Ex vivo studies in humans have shown an inverse correlation between serum α-tocopherol levels and β_1 integrin expression on monocytes,[84] as well as decreased ex vivo monocyte–endothelial cell adhesion,[6] after supplementation with α-tocopherol. Another study, however, showed no effect on monocyte adhesiveness after supplementation of hypercholesterolemic patients with α-tocopherol.[97]

Despite convincing evidence that α-tocopherol decreases cell–cell adhesion in vitro and ex vivo, evidence is completely lacking in vivo.[98–100] For instance, α-tocopherol supplementation in hamsters had no effect on leukocyte–endothelial cell interactions induced by cigarette smoke,[98] or oxidized LDL.[99] More studies are needed to determine whether α-tocopherol exerts a consistent inhibitory effect on in vivo leukocyte–endothelial cell interactions and to further elucidate the underlying mechanisms.

EFFECT ON PLATELET FUNCTION: INHIBITION OF PLATELET ADHESION AND AGGREGATION

The trigger for cardiovascular disease is typically thrombus formation within the vessel lumen,[101] often precipitated by the adhesion and aggregation of platelets to a ruptured atherosclerotic plaque.[102] Plasma levels of platelet-derived thromboxane and prostaglandin metabolites are increased in patients with acute coronary syndromes.[103] Vitamin E has been shown to inhibit ex vivo platelet aggregation and the platelet release reaction.[104,105] The mechanism underlying this effect was shown to be mediated by the inhibition of platelet protein kinase C (PKC) activation.[8] However, the oxidized products of tocopherol (tocopherol quinone and tocopherol hydroquinone) were also reported to have the same inhibitory effect on platelets at a similar concentration, suggesting that the tocopherol effect is not necessarily due to its antioxidant property.[106] The inhibiting activity of different isoforms of α-tocopherol on platelet aggregation is restricted to the RRR-α-tocopherol.

In summary, PKC inhibition is accepted as a common denominator of cellular events regulated by α-tocopherol: cell proliferation, cell adhesion, enhancement of immune response, free radical production, and gene expression. The expression of several genes such as CD36,[90] SR class A,[89] collagenase, and ICAM-1,[107] appears to be regulated by α-tocopherol in a PKC-independent way. On the other hand, a few observations, such as PP2A,[50] and diacylglycerol kinase activation,[108] 5-lipoxygenase,[109] and cyclooxygenase inhibition,[110] still miss a mechanistic explanation.

SUMMARY

Vitamin E functions as a chain-breaking antioxidant evidenced by decreased LDL oxidative susceptibility and F2-isoprostanes. LDL oxidation is prevented by α-tocopherol either by diminishing radical production in macrophages or by scavenging the produced radicals.

Beyond the antioxidant and pro-oxidant properties of vitamin E, it has additional biologic effects that are related to its non-antioxidant properties. Vitamin E inhibits smooth muscle cell proliferation and migration, prevents endothelial function and limits platelet adhesion and aggregation. Vitamin E supplementation has shown its antiinflammatory effects on monocytes by decreasing the release of ROS, lipid oxidation, release of cytokines, such as IL-1β and TNF-α and by decreasing adhesion of monocytes to human endothelium. This mechanism appears to be via inhibition of PKC. However, clinical studies are still controversial concerning its effectiveness and require clarification. Recommendation on the uses and dosages of vitamin E and population selection can be provided by prospective intervention studies. Although biochemical, cellular, and molecular biology studies and ideas about vitamin E have increased dramatically, many molecular phenomena are still far from being fully elucidated. Further studies on the molecular events at the basis of α-tocopherol gene regulation are needed.

REFERENCES

1. Evans HM, Bishop BKS. Fetal resorption. Science (Washington, DC) 1922; 55:650.
2. Weiser H, Vecchi M, Schlachter M. Stereoisomers of -tocopheryl acetate: IV. USP units and α-tocopherol equivalents of all-rac-, 2-ambo- and RRR-tocopherol evaluated by simultaneous determination of resorption-gestation, myopathy and liver storage capacity in rats. Int J Vitam Nutr Res 1986; 56:45–56.
3. Tappel AL. Vitamin E as the biological lipid antioxidant. Vitam Horm 1962; 20:493–510.
4. Vogelsang A, Shute EV. Effect of vitamin E in coronary heart disease. Nature (Lond.) 1946; 157:772.
5. Boscoboinik D, Szewczyk A, Azzi A. α-Tocopherol (vitamin E) regulates vascular smooth muscle cell proliferation and protein kinase C activity. Arch Biochem Biophys 1991; 286:264–9.
6. Devaraj S, Li D, Jialal I. The effects of alpha tocopherol supplementation on monocyte function, decreased lipid oxidation, interleukin

1 beta secretion, and monocyte adhesion to endothelium. J Clin Invest 1996; 98:756–63.

7. Devaraj S, Adams-Huet B, Fuller CJ, Jialal I. Dose-response comparison of RRR-alpha-tocopherol and all-racemic alpha-tocopherol on LDL oxidation. Arterioscler Thromb Vasc Biol 1997; 17:2273–9.

8. Freedman JE, Farhat JH, Loscalzo J, Keaney JF Jr. Alpha-tocopherol inhibits aggregation of human platelets by a protein kinase C-dependent mechanism. Circulation 1996; 94:2434–40.

9. Tada H, Ishii H, Isogai S. Protective effect of D-alpha-tocopherol on the function of human mesangial cells exposed to high glucose concentrations. Metabolism 1997; 46:779–84.

10. Rimm EB, Stampfer MJ, Ascherio A, et al. Vitamin E consumption and the risk of coronary heart disease in men. N Engl J Med 1993; 328:1450–6.

11. Stampfer MJ, Hennekens CH, Manson JE, et al. Vitamin E consumption and the risk of coronary heart disease in women. N Engl J Med 1993; 328:1444–9.

12. Kushi LH, Folsom AR, Prineas RJ, et al. Dietary antioxidant and death from coronary heart disease in postmenopausal women. N Engl J Med 1996; 334:1156–62.

13. Stephens NG, Parsons A Schofield PM, et al. Randomised controlled trial of vitamin E in patients with coronary disease: Cambridge heart antioxidant study (CHAOS). Lancet 1996; 347:781–6.

14. Hodis HN, Mack WJ, LaBree L, et al. Serial coronary angiographic evidence that antioxidant vitamin intake reduces progression of coronary artery atherosclerosis. JAMA 1995; 21:1849–54.

15. Pryor WA. Vitamin E and heart disease. Free Radic Biol Med 2000; 28:141–64.

16. Steiner M, Glantz M, Lekos A. Vitamin E plus aspirin compared to aspirin alone in patients with TIA. Am J Clin Nutr 1995; 62:1381–4.

17. Jialal I, Devaraj S. HOPE trial. N Engl J Med 2000; 342:191.

18. Jialal I, Devaraj S, Huet BA, Traber MG. GISSI-Prevenzione Trial. Lancet 2000; 354:9189.

19. Boaz M, Smetana S, Weinstein T, et al. Secondary prevention with antioxidants of cardiovascular disease in endstage renal disease (SPACE): randomised placebo-controlled trial. Lancet 2000; 356:1213–18.

20. Gruppo Italiano per lo Studio della Sopravvivenza nell'Infarto miocardico. Dietary supplementation with n-3 polyunsaturated fatty acids and vitamin E after myocardial infarction: results of the GISSI-Prevenzione trial. Lancet 1999; 354:447–55.

21. Yusuf S, Dagenais G, Pogue J, et al. Vitamin E supplementation and cardiovascular events in high-risk patients. The Heart Outcomes Prevention Evaluation Study Investigators. N Engl J Med 2000; 342:154–60.

22. Lonn EM, Yusuf S, Dzavik V, et al. Effects of Ramipril and Vitamin E on Atherosclerosis: the Study to Evaluate Carotid Ultrasound Changes in Patients Treated With Ramipril and Vitamin E (SECURE). Circulation 2001; 103:919–25.

23. Burton GW, Joyce A, Ingold KU. Is vitamin E the only lipid-soluble, chain-breaking antioxidant in human blood plasma and erythrocyte membranes? Arch Biochem Biophys 1983; 221:281–90.

24. Ingold KU, Webb AC, Witter D, et al. Vitamin E remains the major lipid-soluble, chain-breaking antioxidant in human plasma even in individuals suffering severe vitamin E deficiency. Arch Biochem Biophys 1987; 259:224–25.

25. Packer L. Vitamin E is nature's master antioxidant. Sci Am Sci Med 1994; 1:54–63.

26. Kamal-Eldin A, Appelqvist LA. The chemistry and antioxidant properties of tocopherols and tocotrienols. Lipids 1996; 31:671–701.

27. Packer L, Weber SU, Rimbach G. Molecular aspects of alpha-tocotrienol antioxidant action and cell signalling. J Nutr 2001; 131:369S–373S.

28. Esterbauer H, Schmidt R, Hayn M. Relationships among oxidation of low-density lipoprotein, antioxidant protection, and atherosclerosis. Adv Pharmacol 1997; 38:425–56.

29. Esterbauer H, Jurgens G, Quehenberger O, Koller E. Autoxidation of human low density lipoprotein: loss of polyunsaturated fatty acids and vitamin E and generation of aldehydes. J Lipid Res 1987; 28:495–509.

30. Dieber-Rotheneder M, Puhl H, Waeg G, et al. Effect of oral supplementation with D-α-toco-

pherol on the vitamin E content of human low density lipoproteins and resistance to oxidation. J Lipid Res 1991; 32:1325–32.

31. Dieber-Rotheneder M, Puhl H, Waeg G, et al. Effect of oral supplementation with D-alpha-tocopherol on the vitamin E content of human LDL and resistance to oxidation. J Lipid Res 1991; 32:1325–32.

32. Jialal I, Fuller CJ, Huet BA. The effect of alpha-tocopherol supplementation on LDL oxidation. A dose-response study. Arterioscler Thromb Vasc Biol 1995; 15:190–8.

33. Reaven PD, Khouw A, Beltz WF, et al. Effects of dietary antioxidant combinations in humans: protection of LDL by vitamin E but not by beta-carotene. Arterioscler Thromb 1993; 13:590–600.

34. Steinbrecher UP, Parthasarathy S, Leake DS, et al. Modification of low density lipoprotein by endothelial cells involves lipid peroxidation and degradation of low density lipoprotein phospholipids. Proc Natl Acad Sci USA 1984; 81:3883–7.

35. Regnstrom J, Nilsson J, Strom K, et al. Inverse relationship between the concentration of LDL vitamin E and severity of coronary artery disease. Am J Clin Nutr 1996; 63:377–85.

36. Bowry VW, Ingold KU, Stocker R. Vitamin E in human low-density lipoprotein. When and how this antioxidant becomes a pro-oxidant. Biochem J 1992; 288:341–4.

37. Upston JM, Terentis AC, Stocker R. Tocopherol-mediated peroxidation of lipoproteins: implications for vitamin E as a potential antiatherogenic supplement. FASEB J 1999; 13:977–94.

38. Dieber-Rotheneder M, Puhl H, Waeg G, et al. Effect of oral supplementation with D-α-tocopherol on the vitamin E content of human low density lipoproteins and resistance to oxidation. J Lipid Res 1991; 32:1325–32.

39. Neuzil J, Thomas SR, Stocker R. Requirement for, promotion, or inhibition by alpha-tocopherol of radical-induced initiation of plasma lipoprotein lipid peroxidation. Free Radic Biol Med 1997; 22:57–71.

40. Stocker R, Bowry VW, Frei B. Ubiquinol-10 protects human low density lipoprotein more efficiently against lipid peroxidation than does alpha-tocopherol. Proc Natl Acad Sci USA 1991; 88:1646–50.

41. Bowry VW, Stocker R. Tocopherol-mediated peroxidation: the prooxidant effect of vitamin E on the radical-initiated oxidation of human low-density lipoprotein. J Am Chem Soc 1993; 115:6029–44.

42. Suarna C, Dean RT, May J, Stocker R. Human atherosclerotic plaque contains both oxidised lipids and relatively large amounts of alpha-tocopherol and ascorbate. Arterioscler Thromb Vasc Biol 1995; 15:1616–24.

43. Kontush A, Finckh B, Karten B, et al. Antioxidant and prooxidant activity of alpha-tocopherol in human plasma and low density lipoprotein. J Lipid Res 1996; 37:1436–48.

44. Boscoboinik D, Szewczyk A, Hensey C, Azzi A. Inhibition of cell proliferation by alpha-tocopherol. Role of protein kinase C. J Biol Chem 1991; 266:6188–94.

45. Tasinato A, Boscoboinik D, Bartoli GM, et al. D-alpha-Tocopherol inhibition of vascular smooth muscle cell proliferation occurs at physiological concentrations, correlates with protein kinase C inhibition, and is independent of its antioxidant properties. Proc Natl Acad Sci USA 1995; 92:12190–4.

46. Martin-Nizard F, Boullier A, Fruchart JC, Duriez P. Alpha-tocopherol but not beta-tocopherol inhibits thrombin-induced PKC activation and endothelin secretion in endothelial cells. J Cardiovasc Risk 1998; 5:339–45.

47. Cachia O, Benna JE, Pedruzzi E, et al. Alpha-tocopherol inhibits the respiratory burst in human monocytes. Attenuation of p47(phox) membrane translocation and phosphorylation. J Biol Chem 1998; 273:32801–5.

48. Devaraj S, Jialal I. Alpha-tocopherol decreases interleukin-1 beta release from activated human monocytes by inhibition of 5-lipoxygenase. Arterioscler Thromb Vasc Biol 1999; 19:1125–33.

49. Gey F. The antioxidant hypothesis of cardiovascular disease: epidemiology and mechanisms. Biochem Soc Trans 1990; 18(6):1041–5.

50. Ricciarelli R, Tasinato A, Clement S, et al. Alpha-tocopherol specifically inactivates cellular protein kinase C alpha by changing its phosphorylation state. Biochem J 1998; 334:243–9.

51. Ozer NK, Palozza P, Boscoboinik D, Azzi A. D-Alpha-tocopherol inhibits low density

lipoprotein induced proliferation and protein kinase C activity in vascular smooth muscle cells. FEBS Lett 1993; 322:307–10.

52. Tasinato A, Boscoboinik D, Bartoli GM, et al. D-alpha-tocopherol inhibition of vascular smooth muscle cell proliferation occurs at physiological concentrations, correlates with protein kinase C inhibition, and is independent of its antioxidant properties. Proc Natl Acad Sci USA 1995; 92:12190–4.

53. Sirikci O, Ozer NK, Azzi A. Dietary cholesterol-induced changes of protein kinase C and the effect of vitamin E in rabbit aortic smooth muscle cells. Atherosclerosis 1996; 126:253–63.

54. Ozer NK, Sirikci O, Tahal S, et al. Effect of vitamin E and probucol on dietary cholesterol-induced atherosclerosis in rabbits. Free Rad Biol Med 1998; 24:226–33.

55. Chan AC, Leith MK. Decreased prostacyclin synthesis in vitamin E-deficient rabbit aorta. Am J Clin Nutr 1981; 34:2341–7.

56. Szczeklik A, Gryglewski RJ, Domagala B, et al. Dietary supplementation with vitamin E in hyperlipoproteinemias: effects on plasma lipid peroxides, antioxidant activity, prostacyclin generation and platelet aggregability. Thromb Haemost 1985; 30:425–30.

57. Pyke DD, Chan AC. Effects of vitamin E on prostacyclin release and lipid composition of the ischemic rat heart. Arch Biochem Biophys 1990; 277:429–33.

58. Tran K, Chan AC. RRR-α-tocopherol potentiates prostacyclin release in human endothelial cells. Evidence for structural specificity of the tocopherol molecule. Biochim Biophys Acta 1990; 1043:189–97.

59. Gilbert VA, Zebrowski EJ, Chan AC. Differential effects of megavitamin E on prostacyclin and thromboxane synthesis in streptozotocin-induced diabetic rats. Horm Metab Res 1983; 15:320–5.

60. Thorin E, Hamilton CA, Dominiczak MH, Reid JL. Chronic exposure of cultured bovine endothelial cells to oxidized LDL abolishes prostacyclin release. Arterioscler Thromb 1994; 14:453–9.

61. Chan AC, Wagner M, Kennedy C, et al. Vitamin E up-regulates phospholipase A_2, arachidonic acid release and cyclooxygenase in endothelial cells. Aktuel Ernahr-Med 1998; 23:1–8.

62. Tran K, Wong KT, Lee E, et al. Vitamin E potentiates arachidonic acid release and phospholipase A_2 activity in rat heart myoblastic cells. Biochem J 1996; 319:385–91.

63. Furchgott RF. The discovery of endothelium-derived relaxing factor and its importance in the identification of nitric oxide. JAMA 1996; 276:1186–8.

64. Keaney JF, Gaziano JM, Xu A et al. Dietary antioxidants preserve endothelium-dependent vessel relaxation in cholesterol-fed rabbits. Proc Natl Acad Sci USA 1993; 90:11880–4.

65. Keaney JF, Guo Y, Cunningham D, et al. Vascular incorporation of alpha-tocopherol prevents endothelial dysfunction due to oxidized LDL by inhibiting protein kinase C stimulation. J Clin Invest 1996; 98:386–94.

66. Keaney JF, Gaziano JM, Xu A, et al. Low-dose α-tocopherol improves and high-dose β-tocopherol worsens endothelial vasodilator function in cholesterol-fed rabbits. J Clin Invest 1994; 93:844–51.

67. Motoyama T, Kawano H, Kugiyama K, et al. Vitamin E administration improves impairment of endothelium-dependent vasodilation in patients with coronary spastic angina. J Am Coll Cardiol 1998; 32:1672–9.

68. Heitzer T, Yla Herttuala S, Wild E, et al. Effect of vitamin E on endothelial vasodilator function in patients with hypercholesterolemia, chronic smoking or both. J Am Coll Cardiol 1999; 33:499–505.

69. Neunteufl T, Kostner K, Katzenschlager R, et al. Additional benefit of vitamin E supplementation to simvastatin therapy on vasoreactivity of the brachial artery of hypercholesterolemic men. J Am Coll Cardiol 1998; 32:711–16.

70. Green D, O'Driscoll G, Rankin JM, et al. Beneficial effect of vitamin E administration on nitric oxide function in subjects with hypercholesterolaemia. Clin Sci Lond 1998; 95:361–7.

71. Cannon JG, Meydani SN, Fielding RA. The acute phase response in exercise. Associations between vitamin E, cytokines and muscle proteolysis. Am J Physiol 1991; 260:R1235–R1240.

72. Libby P, Hansson G. Involvement of the human immune system in human atherogenesis:

current knowledge and unanswered questions. Lab Investig 1991; 64:5–15.

73. Raines E, Ross R. Multiple growth factors are associated with lesions of atherosclerosis: specificity or redundancy? Bioessays 1996; 18:271–82.

74. Devaraj S, Jialal I. Oxidized LDL and atherosclerosis. Int J Clin Lab Res 1996; 26:178–84.

75. Akeson AL, Woods CW, Mosher LB, et al. Inhibition of IL-1β expression in THP-1 cells by probucol and tocopherol. Atherosclerosis 1991; 86:261–70.

76. Chan AC, Tran K, Pyke DD, Powell WS. Effects of dietary vitamin E on the biosynthesis of 5-lipooxygenase products by rat polymorphonuclear leukocytes. Biochim Biophys Acta 1989; 1005:265–9.

77. Denzlinger C, Kless T, Sagebiel-Kohler S, et al. Modulation of the endogenous leukotriene production by fish oil and vitamin E. J Lipid Mediat Cell Signal 1995; 11:119–32.

78. Kohlschutter A, Mayatepek E, Finckh B, Hubner C. Effect of plasma alpha-tocopherol on leuktriene E$_4$ excretion in genetic vitamin E deficiency. J Inherit Metab Dis 1997; 20:581–6.

79. Cathcart MK, Morel DW, Chisolm GM. Monocytes and neutrophils oxidize LDL making it cytotoxic. J Leukoc Biol 1985; 38:341–50.

80. Cathcart MK, McNally AK, Morel DW, Chisolm GM. Superoxide anion participation in human monocyte-mediated oxidation of LDL and conversion of LDL to a cytotoxin. J Immunol 1989; 142:1963–9.

81. Devaraj S, Jialal I. LDL post-secretory modification, monocyte function and circulating adhesion molecules in type 2 diabetic patients: effect of AT supplementation. Circulation 2000; 102:191–6.

82. van Tits LJ, Demacker PN, deGraaf J, et al. AT supplementation decreases production of superoxide and cytokines by leukocytes ex vivo in both normolipidemic and hypertriglyceridemic individuals. Am J Clin Nutr 2000; 71:458–64.

83. Faruqi R, de la Motte C, DiCorleto PE. alpha-Tocopherol inhibits agonist-induced monocytic cell adhesion to cultured human endothelial cells. J Clin Invest 1994; 94:592–600.

84. Yoshida N, Yoshikawa T, Manabe H, et al. Vitamin E protects against polymorphonuclear leukocyte-dependent adhesion to endothelial cells. J Leukoc Biol 1999; 65:757–63.

85. van der Schroeff JG, Havekes L, Weerheim AM, et al. Suppression of cholesteryl ester accumulation in cultured human monocyte-derived macrophages by lipoxygenase inhibitors. Biochem Biophys Res Commun 1985; 127(1):366–72.

86. Suzukawa M, Abbey M, Clifton P, Nestel PJ. Effects of supplementing with vitamin E on the uptake of low density lipoprotein and the stimulation of cholesteryl ester formation in macrophages. Atherosclerosis 1994; 110(1):77–86.

87. Asmis R, Llorente VC, Gey KF. Prevention of cholesteryl ester accumulation in P388D1 macrophage-like cells by increased cellular vitamin E depends on species of extracellular cholesterol. Conventional heterologous non-human cell cultures are poor models of human atherosclerotic foam cell formation. Eur J Biochem 1995; 233(1):171–8.

88. Shige H, Ishikawa T, Suzukawa M, et al. Vitamin E reduces cholesterol esterification and uptake of acetylated low density lipoprotein in macrophages. Lipids 1998; 33(12):1169–75.

89. Teupser D, Thiery J, Seidel D. Alpha-tocopherol down-regulates scavenger receptor activity in macrophages. Atherosclerosis 1999; 144(1):109–15.

90. Ricciarelli R, Zingg JM, Azzi A. Vitamin E reduces the uptake of oxidized LDL by inhibiting CD36 scavenger receptor expression in cultured aortic smooth muscle cells. Circulation 2000; 102:82–7.

91. Devaraj S, Hugou I, Jialal I. Alpha-tocopherol decreases CD36 expression in human monocyte-derived macrophages. J Lipid Res 2001; 42(4):521–7.

92. Neuzil J, Baoutina A. Alpha-tocopherol in atherogenesis: do we know its real role? Cardiovasc Drugs Ther 1998; 12(5):421–3.

93. Yoshikawa T, Yoshida N, Manabe H, et al. Alpha-tocopherol protects against expression of adhesion molecules on neutrophils and endothelial cells. Biofactors 1998; 7:15–19.

94. Cominacini L, Garbin U, Pasini AF, et al. Antioxidants inhibit the expression of intercellular cell adhesion molecule-1 and vascular cell adhesion molecule-1 induced by oxidized LDL on human umbilical vein endothelial cells. Free Radic Biol Med 1997; 22:117–27.

95. Martin A, Foxall T, Blumberg JB, Meydani M. Vitamin E inhibits low-density lipoprotein-induced adhesion of monocytes to human aortic endothelial cells in vitro. Arterioscler Thromb Vasc Biol 1997; 17:429–36.

96. Islam KN, Devaraj S, Jialal I. alpha-Tocopherol enrichment of monocytes decreases agonist-induced adhesion to human endothelial cells. Circulation 1998; 98:2255–61.

97. Williams JC, Forster LA, Tull SP, et al. Dietary vitamin E supplementation inhibits thrombin-induced platelet aggregation, but not monocyte adhesiveness, in patients with hypercholesterolaemia. Int J Exp Pathol 1997; 78:259–66.

98. Lehr HA, Frei B, Olofsson AM, et al. Protection from oxidized LDL-induced leukocyte adhesion to microvascular and macrovascular endothelium in vivo by vitamin C but not by vitamin E. Circulation 1995; 91:1525–32.

99. Lehr H, Frei B, Arfors K. Vitamin C prevents cigarette smoke-induced leukocyte aggregation and adhesion to endothelium in vivo. Proc Natl Acad Sci USA 1994; 91:7688–92.

100. Koh KK, Blum A, Hathaway L, et al. Vascular effects of estrogen and vitamin E therapies in postmenopausal women. Circulation 1999; 100:1851–7.

101. DeWood MA, Spores J, Notske R, et al. Prevalence of total coronary occlusion during the early hours of transmural myocardial infarction. N Engl J Med 1980; 303:897–902.

102. Davies MJ, Thomas AC. Plaque fissuring: the cause of acute myocardial infarction, sudden ischemic death, and crescendo angina. Br Heart J 1985; 53:363–73.

103. Fitzgerald DJ, Roy L, Catella F, FitzGerald GA. Platelet activation in unstable coronary disease. N Engl J Med 1986; 315:983–9.

104. Higashi O, Kikuchi Y. Effects of vitamin E on the aggregation and lipid peroxidation of platelets exposed to hydrogen peroxide. Tohoku J Exp Med 1974; 112:271–8.

105. Steiner M, Anastasi J. Vitamin E: an inhibitor of the platelet release reaction. J Clin Invest 1976; 57:732–7.

106. Mower R, Steiner M. Synthetic byproducts of tocopherol oxidation as inhibitors of platelet function. Prostaglandins 1982; 24:137–47.

107. Wu D, Koga T, Martin KR, Meydani M. Effect of vitamin E on human aortic endothelial cell production of chemokines and adhesion to monocytes. Atherosclerosis 1999; 147:297–307.

108. Lee IK, Koya D, Ishi H, et al. D-alpha-tocopherol prevents the hyperglycemia induced activation of diacylglycerol (DAG)-protein kinase C (PKC) pathway in vascular smooth muscle cell by an increase of DAG kinase activity. Diabetes Res Clin Pract 1999; 45:183–90.

109. Jialal I, Devaraj S, Kaul N. The effect of alpha-tocopherol on monocyte proatherogenic activity. J Nutr 2001; 131:389S–394S.

110. Wu DY, Hayek MG, Meydani SN. Vitamin E and macrophage cyclooxygenase regulation in the aged. J Nutr 2001; 131:382S–388S.

24

The dexamethasone eluting stent

Zhongmin Zhou, Kai Wang, and A Michael Lincoff

STENT PHOTOGRAPH

See Figure 24.1.

TECHNICAL DESCRIPTION

- A 125 μm diameter tantalum wire configured into a 16 mm long balloon expandable coil stent (Wiktor, Medtronic) and coated with a monolithic matrix of poly-L-lactic acid (PLLA) and dexamethasone base (Upjohn).
- Two different forms of the biodegradable PLLA polymer were evaluated: a low molecular weight polymer of ~80 kDa and a high molecular weight polymer of ~321 kDa.
- The ratio of dexamethasone to PLLA in the coating was 2:1, with ~0.8 mg of dexamethasone and ~0.4 mg of PLLA per stent.

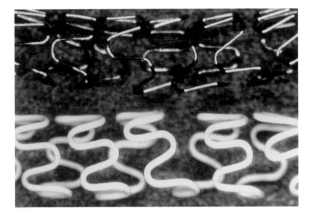

Fig. 24.1 *Top*: Uncoated control Wiktor tantalum coil wire stent. *Bottom*: eluting stent coated with high molecular weight poly-L-lactic acid and dexamethasone.

Dexamethasone elution in vitro: Figure 24.2.
Dexamethasone elution in vivo: Figure 24.3,
Figure 24.4.
Animal Studies: Table 24.1.

Biocompatibility: Figure 24.5.
Most relevant animal studies: Table 24.2.
Recent developments: Table 24.3.

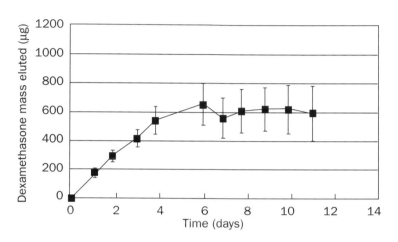

a

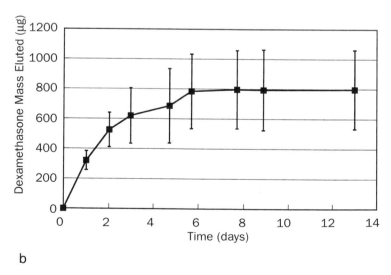

b

Fig. 24.2 Cumulative (mean ± SD) in vitro dexamethasone elution from poly-L-lactic acid (PLLA)-dexamethasone-coated stents over a 12 day period in pigs. Stents coated with low and high molecular weight PLLA polymer showed a similar elution curve, which was an initial rapid elution for the first 2 days, followed by a period of gradual slow elution. More than 50% of dexamethasone elution occurred within the first 2–3 days, with a leveling off of the elution curves after 6 to 7 days. (a) Low molecular weight PLLA (3 stents). (b) High molecular weight PLLA (5 stents).

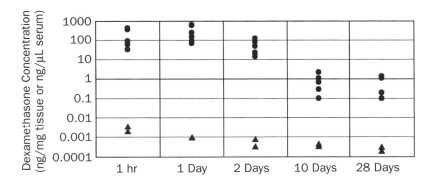

Fig. 24.3 Semilogarithmic plot of dexamethasone concentrations in stented arterial tissue (ng/mg wet tissue weight, ●) and serum (ng/µL serum, ▲) at 5 time points after implantation of three high molecular weight poly-L-lactic acid, dexamethasone stents in coronary arteries of ten pigs. At each time point, 2 serum samples and 6 stented vascular tissue samples were obtained from 2 pigs. For comparison, plasma concentrations of dexamethasone 1 h after intravenous administration of a 1 mg dose in humans range from 0.01 to 0.1 ng/µg. This demonstrates the feasibility of local delivery in an eluting stent coated with dexamethasone within high molecular weight PLLA to provide a drug residence time within the injured arterial tissue (≥28 days) that would be relevant for the clinical prevention of restenosis.

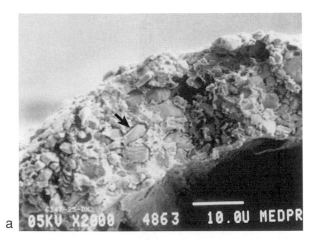

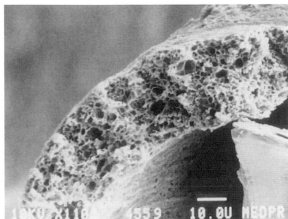

Fig. 24.4 Electron micrographs of high molecular weight poly-L-lactic acid-dexamethasone stent coatings before (a, ×2000) and 28 days after implantation (b, ×1100) in porcine coronary arteries. Dexamethasone crystals visible before elution (*arrow*) are no longer present after 28 days, although polymer matrix appears largely intact.

Table 24.1   Animal studies of the dexamethasone eluting stent in the porcine coronary injury model

Stent coating	Biocompatibility	Efficacy on restenosis
Low molecular weight PLLA	Unequivocal inflammatory reaction within the vascular wall. Normal architecture was variably destroyed	Not tested
High molecular weight PLLA	No evidence of inflammation	No significant change in the neointimal hyperplastic response to injury

PLLA, poly-L-lactic acid.

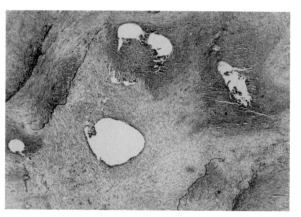
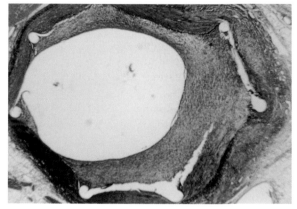

a   b

Fig. 24.5   Photomicrographs of porcine arterial cross-sections at 28 day sacrifice after injury with low (a) and high molecular weight poly-L-lactic acid (PLLA) control stents (b). (Hematoxylin and eosin stain: ×8.)

Table 24.2   Most relevant animal studies of the dexamethasone eluting stent

Year	Animal model	Delivery modality	Efficacy on restenosis	Source
1994	Rat carotid artery injury model	Periadventitial polymer matrices	Positive	Villa et al.[1]
1994	Porcine carotid artery injury model	Periadventitial polymer	Negative	Muller et al.[2]
1998	Canine femoral artery injury model	Coated metal stent	Positive	Strecker et al.[3]

Table 24.3   Recent human studies of the dexamethasone eluting stent

Year	Number of patients	Delivery modality	Efficacy on restenosis	Source
2003	71	Eluting stent	Positive, restenosis rate 13.3%	Liu et al.[4]
2004	30	Eluting stent	Negative, restenosis rate 31%	Hoffmann et al.[5]

REFERENCES

1. Villa AE, Guzman LA, Chen W, et al. Local delivery of dexamethasone for prevention of neointimal proliferation in a rat model of balloon angioplasty. J Clin Invest 1994; 93:1243–9.
2. Muller DWM, Golomb G, Gordon D, Levy RJ. Site-specific dexamethasone delivery for the prevention of neointimal thickening after vascular stent implantation. Coron Artery Dis 1994; 5:435–42.
3. Strecker EP, Gabelmann A, Boos I, et al. Effect on intimal hyperplasia of dexamethasone released from coated metal stents compared with non-coated stents in canine femoral arteries. Cardiovasc Intervent Radiol 1998; 21:487–96.
4. Liu X, Huang Y, Hanet C, et al. Study of anti-restenosis with the BiodivYsion dexamethasone-eluting stent (STRIDE): a first-in-human multicenter pilot trial. Catheter Cardiovasc Interv 2003; 60:172–8.
5. Hoffmann R, Langenberg R, Radke P, et al. Evaluation of a high-dose dexamethasone-eluting stent. Am J Cardiol 2004; 94:193–5.

25

Antiinflammatory approaches to restenosis

Ivan De Scheerder and Yanming Huang

Introduction • The inflammatory response to angioplasty and stenting • Neointimal formation
• Inflammatory markers • Therapeutic intervention • Conclusion

INTRODUCTION

Restenosis remains a major limitation of coronary angioplasty. A complex pathophysiological process, restenosis is thought to be the result of an exaggerated healing response induced by vascular injury subsequent to balloon predilatation, stent implantation and high pressure postimplantation balloon dilatation. The metallic prosthesis itself can provoke an immunological response with associated chronic inflammatory reaction. This chapter reviews the potential role of inflammation induced by stent implantation in the pathogenesis of restenosis. The effect of modulation of inflammation to prevent restenosis is evaluated.

THE INFLAMMATORY RESPONSE TO ANGIOPLASTY AND STENTING

The basic inflammatory cascade is shown in Table 25.1.

Thrombogenic surface

Inflammation is an initial and obligatory consequence of an angioplasty procedure. Angioplasty causes vascular injury, resulting in exposure of a thrombogenic surface. Circulat-

Table 25.1 Cells involved in the basic inflammatory cascade	
Inflammatory response	*Inflammatory cascade*
Aspecific	Polymorphonuclear cells→ neutrophils → eosinophils
Specific	Lymphocytes→plasmocytes→ monocytes → macrophages
Chronic	Macrophages→activated lymphocytes → giant cells

ing inflammatory cells adhere to the site of injury and migrate into the thrombus. Neutrophils, lymphocytes, and monocytes have been observed within the mural thrombus 1–5 days following angioplasty in an atherosclerotic rabbit model.[1] Scanning electron microscopy has demonstrated the presence of leukocytes and macrophages adherent to the luminal surface of stented arteries in other animal models.[2,3] Rogers et al. investigated the effects of placing endovascular metal stents in rabbit iliac arteries and observed peak monocyte adherence stimulated by early focal thrombus

3 days after stenting, with maximal intimal cell proliferation seen at 7 days.[4]

Vascular over-stretching

Over-stretching of the coronary vessel during angioplasty may also induce an inflammatory response by allowing inflammatory cell infiltration into the adventitial vessel wall. Kumar et al. observed inflammatory leukocyte recruitment around the lumen and in the adventitia after 3 days in a mouse carotid ligation model;[5] by day 7, inflammatory cells were found in the developing neointima, media, and adventitia.

Immune response to the stent

Stent deployment can cause a foreign body reaction. Karas et al. found reactive inflammatory infiltrates surrounding the stent wires at 4 weeks' follow-up in a porcine model of coronary artery injury.[6] In addition, multinucleated giant cells were found adjacent to the stent wires. Kornowski et al. reported that an inflammatory reaction at the arterial wall was frequently seen 1 month after stent implantation in pig coronary arteries.[7] Histiocytes, lymphocytes, neutrophils, and granuloma formation were also observed to be involved in the most severe inflammatory forms.

Clinical studies

Clinical studies have shown that an inflammatory reaction is common in neointimal hyperplasia. Using directional atherectomy, Kearney et al. retrieved tissue specimens from the peripheral arteries of 10 patients with in-stent restenosis and found that each specimen demonstrated inflammatory cell infiltration.[8] Komatsu et al. investigated 11 stented coronary arteries from 11 patients post mortem and observed thrombus formation with early formation of neointima composed of abundant macrophages at the stent site 9 and 12 days after stenting.[9] From 64 days onwards, the neointima still contained macrophages, but was composed predominately of α-actin positive smooth muscle cells (SMCs).

Recently, a large series of pathologic studies in stented humans has been reported.[10] Histologic analysis was performed on 55 stents in 35 coronary vessels (mean duration of stent placement: 39 days). Results showed acute inflammatory cells (neutrophils) surrounding the stent struts in 48 out of 61 arterial sections. Chronic inflammatory cells (lymphocytes and macrophages) surrounding the stent struts were also frequently observed at all time points.

Variability in the inflammatory response to angioplasty and stenting

The degree of the inflammatory response after angioplasty and stenting is related to both the local lesion characteristics and the extent of vessel injury. Atherosclerosis is considered to be a chronic inflammatory disease in which ongoing inflammation contributes to plaque formation and rupture.[11] Hence, prior to angioplasty, foci of inflammatory infiltrates may exist in atherosclerotic coronary lesions. Macrophage-rich areas are more frequently observed in coronary plaque tissue from patients with unstable angina than from patients with stable angina.[12] In addition, a marked inflammatory reaction is regularly observed within saphenous vein graft lesions. During angioplasty, deep vessel injury can increase the inflammatory response. Compared to balloon angioplasty, stent implantation induces deeper arterial injury resulting in greater macrophage accumulation in the neointima.[13] Inflammation is more pronounced at a more deeply lacerated arterial site, and a significant correlation between the degree of vascular injury and the inflammatory score (graded from 0–3) has been reported.[7]

The inflammatory response after stent deployment is also related to the material, design and surface of the stent (inflammation can be present around stent filaments with minimal arterial injury):

- Tanigawa et al. observed that copper stents elicit a more severe inflammatory response than stainless steel stents.[14]

- Changing the stent shape from a corrugated ring to a slotted tube has been shown to reduce the number of monocytes that adhere to the luminal surface of stented arteries.[15]
- Edelman et al. observed an increased inflammatory response to gold-coated stents in porcine coronary arteries.[16] However, results showed that modifying the coating surface by thermal processing could reduce inflammation to the level of uncoated stents. Results from studies with biological polymer coatings, such as fibrin and phosphoryl-choline (PC), have shown no increase in foreign body tissue reaction compared to uncoated stents.[3,17] However, most synthetic polymer coatings and polymeric stents are associated with an increased inflammatory response.[18]

NEOINTIMAL FORMATION

Inflammatory cells play a major role in the regulation of vascular repair and neointimal formation following angioplasty. A severe inflammatory response is associated with increased neointimal hyperplasia. The number of monocytes adhering to the luminal surface of stented arteries correlated linearly with the degree of neointimal hyperplasia in rabbit iliac arteries.[15] Polymer-coated stents have been demonstrated to induce an exaggerated inflammatory response with exuberant neointimal reaction.[18] The histiolymphocytic and fibromuscular reaction to polymer-coated metallic stents was found to correlate significantly with the luminal stenotic area in a porcine coronary artery model.[19] Furthermore, multiple regression analysis has shown that the extent of the inflammatory reaction is significantly correlated, both independently and in combination with the degree of arterial injury, with the amount of neointimal formation.[7]

Which inflammatory cell types are involved?

Leukocytes, monocytes, and macrophages all participate in the process of neointimal formation. The predominant inflammatory cell type present is dependent on the degree of vascular injury and the length of time that has elapsed since angioplasty. Leukocytes are recruited as a precursor to intimal thickening.[20] Rabbit iliac arteries with balloon denudation have been used to investigate inflammatory cell roles; results showed that macrophages were absent in these arteries and that neutrophil infiltration occurring early after endothelial denudation was positively related to medial SMC proliferation (inhibition of neutrophil infiltration was associated with inhibition of SMC proliferation).[21] Stent implantation was shown to increase the amount of neointimal formation in comparison with balloon angioplasty; this was related to more macrophages in the neointima after stent implantation.[13] Furthermore, it has been shown that the number of macrophages in arteries healing after coronary intervention is correlated with the amount of tissue growth.[22] Rogers et al. observed that heparin administration reduced monocyte adhesion as well as infiltration within the neointima after rabbit iliac stent implantation; this effect was correlated with suppression of neointimal hyperplasia and intimal cell proliferation.[4]

Released chemotactic/growth factors

The mechanisms of inflammatory cell involvement in restenosis are not fully understood – neointimal hyperplasia, thrombus organization, SMC migration and proliferation, and negative artery remodeling are all thought to play a part. The release of chemotactic and growth factors from inflammatory cells after arterial injury can promote SMC migration and proliferation. Macrophages produce a family of extracellular matrix metalloproteinases (MMPs). Inhibition of these MMPs after balloon injury could dramatically reduce the number of SMCs migrating into the intima.[26-28] Platelet-derived growth factor (PDGF) – secreted from activated platelets, macrophages and SMCs – can regulate the movement of SMCs from the media to the intima and is involved in the process of neointimal formation. Macrophages in neointimal lesions have been shown to express PDGF-A and -B mRNAs, PDGF-B protein and PDGF-B receptor proteins.[9] Furthermore, platelets that adhere to monocytes and leukocytes via P-selectin may migrate into the vessel wall with migratory inflammatory cells. Platelets at the vessel wall may further influence SMC migration and proliferation.[5]

Role of the adventitia in neointimal formation

The adventitia also plays an important role in neointimal formation and arterial remodeling after coronary angioplasty. Scott et al. observed that proliferating adventitial cells may migrate into the neointima after balloon over-stretched injury of porcine coronary arteries.[29] In another study, over-stretching the artery by high pressure stent deployment resulted in a severe perivasculitis, which was positively related to increased neointimal hyperplasia.[30] Using a rat balloon-injury model, Hayashi et al. found that accumulation of leukocytes in the injured vessel wall was frequently higher in the adventitia than in the neointima and media. Suppression of the adventitial inflammatory response could reduce adventitial fibrosis and vessel shrinking.[31] These studies suggest that the inflammatory response is also responsible for the adventitial constrictive response.

INFLAMMATORY MARKERS

Clinical studies have indicated that inflammatory markers in patients undergoing coronary angioplasty could predict the rate of restenosis and late complications. In patients with unstable angina, the number of macrophages in primary coronary plaque tissue from patients with restenosis was found to be significantly higher than that in tissue from patients without restenosis, and macrophage content was an independent predictor of restenosis.[22] Pietersma et al. observed that, at the time of intervention, the presence of activated blood monocytes was associated with late lumen loss after coronary angioplasty.[23] Inoue et al. observed that an increase in serum levels of circulating adhesion molecules, such as soluble intercellular adhesion molecule-1 (sICAM-1), sP-selectin and sL-selectin, after coronary angioplasty correlated

with the late loss index.[24] C-reactive protein (CRP) is a circulating marker of inflammation for vascular risk prediction: elevated CRP levels may reflect a prolonged inflammatory reaction and are also related to restenosis after angioplasty.[25]

THERAPEUTIC INTERVENTION

The inflammatory reaction in restenosis relates to neointimal formation and arterial remodeling. Therefore, inhibition of the inflammatory response after angioplasty may have some beneficial effects on restenosis. Inhibition of the adhesion, infiltration, and function of inflammatory cells has been investigated in various animal models.

There is emerging evidence for the utility of local drug delivery using coated or drug eluting stents. Although early polymer coatings were associated with development of an inflammatory response, newer coatings have improved biocompatibility.

P-selectin

P-selectin is stored in the α-granules of platelets and the Weibel-Palade bodies of endothelial cells.[32] P-selectin, which binds to circulating monocytes and leukocytes, plays a crucial role in the early inflammatory response. Using P-selectin-deficient mice, Kumar et al. found that inflammatory cells were completely absent from the neointima, media and adventitia.[5] Furthermore, neointimal formation of P-selectin knockout mice was reduced by 76% in the carotid ligation model.[5] Recently, Manka et al. reported that apolipoprotein E-deficient mice with targeted disruption of the P-selectin gene exhibited dramatically decreased monocyte infiltration into the arterial wall and significantly decreased neointimal formation in a carotid artery injury model.[33] In a rat balloon-injury model, anti-P-selectin monoclonal antibodies (MAbs) significantly inhibited leukocyte infiltration into the neointima, media, and adventitia – inhibition of both neointimal formation and vascular shrinkage was observed.[30]

Mac-1

Mac-1 (CD11b/CD18, $\alpha_M\beta_2$), a leukocyte integrin, promotes adhesion and transmigration of leukocytes and monocytes at sites of vascular injury. Upregulation of Mac-1 in patients is associated with increased restenosis.[34,35] Mac-1 deficient mice show decreased leukocyte accumulation with coincident reduction of neointimal thickening after angioplasty. M1/70, a CD11b blocking MAb, was shown to inhibit neutrophil infiltration and medial SMC proliferation in an artery balloon denudation model.[21] Furthermore, after balloon angioplasty and stent implantation in rabbit iliac arteries, M1/70 showed a reduction in both leukocyte recruitment and neointimal hyperplasia.[36]

Interleukin-10

Interleukin-10 (IL-10), an antiinflammatory cytokine, is a potent monocyte deactivator. In carotid arteries of hypercholesterolemic rabbits, recombinant human IL-10 (rhuIL-10) inhibited the activation of circulating monocytic cells after balloon angioplasty or stent implantation.[37] In addition, macrophage infiltration and proliferation in the intima and media were dramatically reduced, as was neointimal hyperplasia, after both balloon angioplasty and stent implantation.

Corticosteroids

Corticosteroids have a broad range of antiinflammatory, antirheumatic, and immunosuppressive activities.[38] Three randomized clinical trials of corticosteroids following percutaneous intervention have been reported. Single intravenous administration of methylprednisolone (MP),[39,40] or two intramuscular MP injections followed by oral prednisone administration for 7 days,[41] failed to demonstrate a positive effect on restenosis. As continuous systemic administration of hydrocortisone reduced neointimal hyperplasia in a rabbit arterial injury model,[42] it is possible that the treatment parameters – as opposed to the drug – in the investigations mentioned above could have contributed to the lack of efficacy.

To avoid systemic side effects, local corticosteroid delivery has been proposed. Periadventitial delivery of various doses of dexamethasone (DXM) has been evaluated. DXM-loaded silicone polymers implanted around rat balloon-injured carotid arteries significantly suppressed intimal proliferation.[43] However, this effect has not been found after stent implantation in porcine carotid arteries.[44] Intramural drug delivery at the site of arterial intervention negates the need for transadventitial delivery, therefore avoiding any additional injury. By using a perforated balloon, Valero et al. found that hydrocortisone-loaded polylactic-co-glycolide acid microspheres could significantly reduce intimal hyperplasia compared to unloaded microspheres.[45]

Stent-based drug delivery

Stent-mediated local drug delivery should theoretically provide sufficiently high drug concentrations at the target site to suppress inflammation without systemic side effects, hence allowing prolonged drug release. This approach has been evaluated in a number of different studies.

1. A tantalum wire stent, coated with DXM and impregnated with either low or high molecular weight poly-L-lactic acid (PLLA), achieved high and sustained DXM concentrations in the porcine arterial wall.[46] The tissue concentration of DXM was 3000-fold higher than that in blood at 28 days. However, DXM did not reduce neointimal hyperplasia.
2. Strecker stents coated with pure polylactide (dl-PLA), or a polylactide-co-polymer (PLA-Co-TMC) containing DXM, were evaluated in a canine femoral artery model. In vitro studies showed that 20% of the DXM was released within the first 24 hours and continuous elution was obtained for 40 days. DXM-loaded stents caused significantly less neointimal hyperplasia than uncoated stents.[47]

The discordance between the effects on neointimal hyperplasia in these two studies may be explained by the 10-fold higher drug concentrations used in the latter study, and the different animal models.

3. Wiktor stents coated with polyorganophosphazene impregnated with MP effectively inhibit the foreign body response induced by the polymer coating.[48]

To optimize local MP delivery, different coating methods have been studied to achieve high local drug concentrations and prolonged drug release.

4. Fluorinated polymethacrylate PFM-P75 dip-coated, spray-coated, and spray-coated combined with a barrier-coating metallic stents loaded with 5%, 10%, and 100% (g/g) MP, respectively, have been assessed in a porcine coronary artery model.[49] Approximately 10–15 mg and 20–25 mg of MP were loaded on 5% and 10% PFM-P75 dip-coated stents, respectively. By spray-coating, almost 100-fold more drug could be incorporated. The total amount of MP encrusted in a single spray-coated stent loaded with 9%, 33%, and 50% MP was calculated to be 100–150 mg, 400–450 mg and 700–1000 mg, respectively. Spray-coating therefore offers the possibility to achieve much higher local drug concentrations. The limitation of spray-coating is that the coating surface becomes irregular which leads to faster drug release, especially when high drug concentrations are used. Within 48 hours, approximately 20%, 50%, and 80% of the MP was released from 9%, 33%, and 50% MP-loaded stents, respectively. Adding a barrier coating could decrease the surface irregularities of MP-loaded PFM-P75 spray-coated stents. Furthermore, a barrier coating dramatically reduced MP release from a spray-coated 50% MP-loaded stent from 80% to 13% in the first 48 hours. In vivo studies in a porcine coronary model showed that MP-loaded stents could significantly inhibit the inflammatory response and neointimal hyperplasia. Barrier coating could further increase the biological effects of the active drug allowing use of a lower dose.

5. Phosphorylcholine (PC) is a highly hydrophilic component of the cell membrane and affords a biocompatible coating for stents, such that PC-coated stents do not elicit an antiinflammatory reaction in animal models. PC-coated stents have resulted in a low incidence of target vessel revascularization and angiographic restenosis in several clinical trials.[50,51] Furthermore, they have proven to be thromboresistant in in vitro and in vivo studies.[52,53] However, no reduction in neointimal thickness with PC-coated stents has been observed in animal studies.[2,54]

De Scheerder et al. used Bio*divY*sio stents with a PC drug delivery (DD) coating in a porcine coronary model to study the effects of local corticosteroid delivery on inflammation and neointimal hyperplasia.[19,48] The experiments were designed as acute and chronic studies with 5 day and 4 week follow-up, respectively. The results of the chronic study are presented in Table 25.2.

In the acute study, stents loaded with high dose MP, low dose DXM (LDD), high dose DXM (HDD), and bare DD stents (DD) were implanted in eight pigs. Stents loaded with low dose DXM (LDD), formulated DXM (FD) and bare DD stents (DD) were chosen for the chronic study in 15 pigs.

As the PC coating was thin (~1 mm), the quantity of DXM and MP loaded into each stent was limited. Adding drops of DXM or MP solution further increased the amount of DXM from 95 mg to 265 mg and MP from 34.3 mg to 269 mg. Drug release from the PC-coated stent appears to be dependent on the hydrophilic characteristics of the compound. Highly water soluble DXM phosphate (FD) exhibited fast release: approximately 95% of the DXM was released in 25 min, and the total amount of drug was released within 2 h. Release of LDD and high dose MP was slower than release of FD. Within 15 min, the total amount of MP was released.

Compared to other studies,[47,48] release of LDD was fast and nearly all of the DXM was released within 20 h (see Figure 25.1). The ratio of the larger size pores of the PC polymer to the molecular weight of DXM and MP may be responsible for these release characteristics.

Table 25.2 Quantitative coronary angiography at 4 weeks follow-up

	N	Pre-stenting (mm)	Balloon-size (mm)	Post-stenting (mm)	Oversizing (%)	Recoil (%)	Diameter at 4 weeks follow-up (mm)	Late loss (mm)
DD	10	2.80±0.24	3.23±0.13	3.18±0.17	16.00±10.45	1.50±4.65	2.58±0.63	0.60±0.66
FD	9	2.53±0.30	3.15±0.16	3.09±0.13	25.78±12.99	2.22±5.43	2.38±0.41	0.71±0.37
LDD	10	2.76±0.17	3.27±0.15	3.18±0.13	18.6±8.14	2.40±5.19	2.66±0.57	0.52±0.54

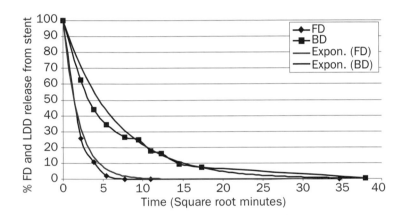

Fig. 25.1 Release of dexamethasone (FD and LDD) from Bio*divYsio* DD stents.

At 5 day follow-up, neointimal hyperplasia in the MP and HDD groups was significantly decreased compared to the control group. The inflammatory response to PC-coated stents implanted in porcine coronary arteries was minimal: leukocytes, macrophages, and macrophage giant cells were scarce in the neointima (see Table 25.3). A few inflammatory cells were present in the thrombotic meshwork and adjacent to the stent filaments in the neointima and the medial layers (see Figure 25.2). A few cases showed inflammatory cell infiltration into the adventitia (see Figure 25.3).

The inflammatory response was still low at 4 week follow-up, but higher than at the 5 day time point (see Table 25.3). It has been reported that the inflammatory response to metallic stents peaks between 3 and 7 days.[55] The different inflammatory response pattern of DD stents may be caused by the PC coating. However, in a long-term follow-up study (up to 12 weeks), no aggressive inflammation was observed.[2]

Local delivery of MP and HDD could further decrease the inflammatory response at 5 days. The inflammatory score of the MP group was significantly lower than that of the control group. The early inflammatory reaction after angioplasty may potently promote neointimal formation; therefore, inhibition of inflammation at an early stage with MP and HDD may affect late neointimal formation.

Neointimal hyperplasia and area stenosis of the MP and HDD groups were significantly decreased compared to the control group. Neointimal tissue early after stent implantation mainly consists of platelets, fibrin meshwork with trapped erythrocytes and some proliferating SMCs. Steroids have been shown to inhibit the formation of

Table 25.3 Histopathologic finding at 5 days and 4 weeks follow-up

	n	Injury	Thrombus	Inflammatory response
5 days				
DD	12	0.56±0.27	0.74±0.22	0.73±0.22
LDD	12	0.53±0.28	0.77±0.19	0.73±0.29
HDD	12	0.40±0.23	0.54±0.23*	0.57±0.20
MP	12	0.42±0.18	0.50±0.22*	0.51±0.25*
4 weeks				
DD	30	0.74±0.33	0.04±0.06	1.30±0.35
FD	27	0.71±0.42	0.03±0.06	1.26±0.49
LDD	30	0.63±0.40	0.04±0.06	1.30±0.52

*$p<0.05$ compared to the DD group

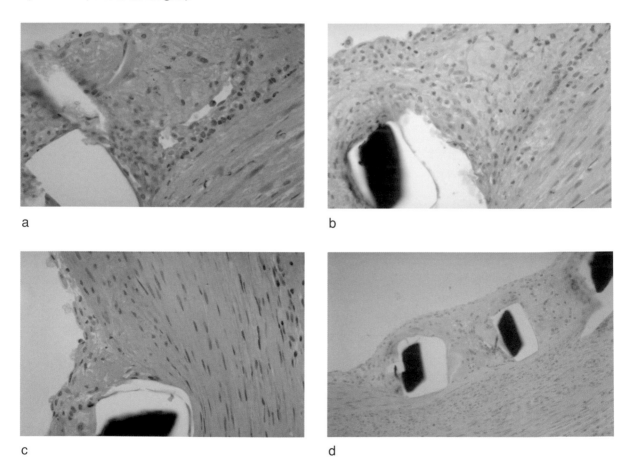

a   b

c   d

Fig. 25.2 Photomicrograph of a vessel segment stented with (a) a bare DD stent; (b) a LDD stent; (c) a HDD stent; (d) a MP stent at 5 days follow-up. A few inflammatory cells were present around the stent filaments and in the neointima in (a), which was comparable to (b). The histolymphocytic reaction surrounding the stent filaments in (c) and (d) were reduced by the local HDD and MP release. (Hematoxylin and eosin stain, magnification (a)–(c), ×400; (d) ×200.)

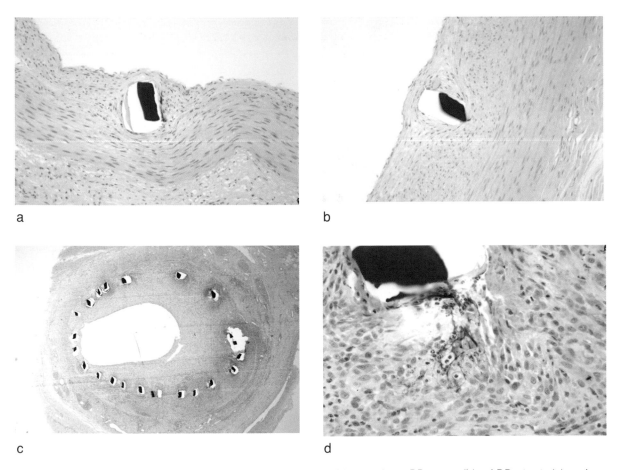

a b

c d

Fig. 25.3 Photomicrograph of a vessel segment stented with (a) a bare DD stent; (b) a LDD stent; (c) and (d) a bare DD stent at 4 weeks follow-up. The inflammatory response in (a) and (b) was low and comparable. (c) and (d) show another case of a DD stent with a more pronounced histolymphocytic reaction surrounding the stent filaments, the media and the adventitia. The narrowed lumen was surrounded by fibromuscular tissue. (Hematoxylin and eosin stain, magnification (a) and (b) ×200; (c) ×25; (d) ×400.)

platelet activating factor and may exert an antiplatelet effect.[56] The occurrence of thrombus surrounding the stent filaments in the MP and HDD groups was lower than in the control group. The effects of MP and HDD in reducing neointimal formation at 5 days are probably related to the reduction in inflammatory response and thrombus formation. In contrast, LDD was ineffective in reducing the inflammatory response and neointimal hyperplasia. Although the lumen area of the LDD group was significantly larger than that of the control group at 5 days (see Table 25.4), this effect was not observed at 4 week follow-up. This may be explained by the low DXM concentration on LDD-loaded stents.

FD was unable to suppress the inflammatory response and reduce neointimal formation: neointimal hyperplasia and area stenosis of the FD group were even higher than in the control group. This may be caused by the smaller artery size and the slightly higher over-sizing during stent

Table 25.4   Morphometric analysis of stented vessel segments at 5 days and 4 weeks follow-up

	n	Lumen area (mm²)	IEL area (mm²)	EEL area (mm²)	Neointimal hyperplasia (mm²)	Area stenosis (%)
5 days						
DD	12	7.94±0.49	8.74±0.44	10.44±0.39	0.80±0.16	9±2
LDD	12	8.94±0.53***	9.71±0.59***	11.65±0.97***	0.77±0.16	8±1
HDD	12	9.02±0.49***	9.70±0.49***	11.47±0.69***	0.68±0.12*	7±1**
MP	12	8.35±0.68	8.89±0.73	10.26±0.78	0.54±0.16**	6±2***
4 weeks						
DD	30	5.78±1.58	7.85±0.58	9.79±0.65	2.07±1.39	27±19
FD	27	4.95±1.79	7.26±0.70	9.18±0.77	2.31±1.50	33±22
LDD	30	6.05±1.57	8.11±1.06	10.19±1.31	2.06±1.21	26±15

*$p \leq 0.05$, **$p \leq 0.01$, ***$p \leq 0.001$ compared to the DD group

implantation. The fast drug release and low drug concentration may have contributed further to the less favorable effects.

The clinical efficacy of DXM loaded onto the Bio*divYsio* drug delivery stent is being investigated in the STRIDE study.

Other agents

Local drug delivery of ibuprofen and colchicine has also been investigated. Ibuprofen, a non-steroidal antiinflammatory agent that modulates the cyclooxygenase pathway of prostaglandin synthesis, failed to demonstrate a positive effect on neointimal hyperplasia in a porcine coronary model.[49] Colchicine, a drug with both anti-inflammatory and antiproliferative properties, also failed to demonstrate a favorable effect in reducing neointimal hyperplasia.[57]

Antioxidants, cholesterol-lowering agents, avoidance of aggressive balloon dilation and improvements in stent coatings all have the potential to modulate the inflammatory process and affect restenosis.

CONCLUSION

There is abundant scientific evidence that inflammatory cells surrounding the stent filaments after stent implantation play an important role in the induction of in-stent restenosis. These cells, when activated, can secrete a variety of mitogens that play a crucial role in smooth muscle cell dedifferentiation, migration, and proliferation. Interference with this inflammatory process is an attractive target for the prevention of in-stent restenosis.

REFERENCES

1. Wilensky RL, March KL, Gradus-Pizlo I, et al. Vascular injury, repair, and restenosis after percutaneous transluminal angioplasty in the atherosclerotic rabbit. Circulation 1995; 92(10):2995–3005.
2. Rodgers GP, Minor ST, Robinson K, et al. Adjuvant therapy for intracoronary stents. Investigations in atherosclerotic swine. Circulation 1990; 82(2):560–9.
3. Whelan DM, van der Giessen WJ, Krabbendam SC, et al. Biocompatibility of phosphorylcholine coated stents in normal porcine coronary arteries. Heart 2000; 83(3):338–34.
4. Rogers C, Welt FG, Karnovsky MJ, et al. Monocyte recruitment and neointimal hyperplasia in rabbits. Coupled inhibitory effects of heparin. Arterioscler Thromb Vasc Biol 1996; 16(10):1312–8.

5. Kumar A, Hoover JL, Simmons CA, et al. Remodeling and neointimal formation in the carotid artery of normal and P-selectin-deficient mice. Circulation 1997; 96(12):4333–42.

6. Karas SP, Gravanis MB, Santoian EC, et al. Coronary intimal proliferation after balloon injury and stenting in swine: an animal model of restenosis. J Am Coll Cardiol 1992; 20:467–74.

7. Kornowski R, Hong MK, Tio FO, et al. In-stent restenosis: contributions of inflammatory responses and arterial injury to neointimal hyperplasia. J Am Coll Cardiol 1998; 31(1):224–30.

8. Kearney M, Pieczek A, Haley L, et al. Histopathology of in-stent restenosis in patients with peripheral artery disease. Circulation 1997; 95(8):1998–2002.

9. Komatsu R, Ueda M, Naruko T, et al. Neointimal tissue response at sites of coronary stenting in humans: macroscopic, histological, and immunohistochemical analyses. Circulation 1998; 98(3):224–33.

10. Farb A, Sangiorgi G, Carter AJ, et al. Pathology of acute and chronic coronary stenting in humans. Circulation 1999; 99(1):44–52.

11. Alexander RW. Inflammation and coronary artery disease. N Engl J Med 1994; 331:468–9.

12. Moreno PR, Falk E, Palacios IF, et al. Macrophage infiltration in acute coronary syndromes. Implications for plaque rupture. Circulation 1994; 90(2):775–8.

13. Kollum M, Kaiser S, Kinscherf R, et al. Apoptosis after stent implantation compared with balloon angioplasty in rabbits. Role of macrophages. Arterioscler Thromb Vasc Biol 1997; 17(11):2383–8.

14. Tanigawa N, Sawada S, Kobayashi M. Reaction of the aortic wall to six metallic stent materials. Acad Radiol 1995; 2(5):379–84.

15. Rogers C, Edelman ER. Endovascular stent design dictates experimental restenosis and thrombosis. Circulation 1995; 91(12):2995–3001.

16. Edelman ER, Seifert P, Groothuis A, et al. Gold-Coated NIR Stents in Porcine Coronary Arteries. Circulation 2001; 103(3):429–34.

17. McKenna CJ, Camrud AR, Sangiorgi G, et al. Fibrin-film stenting in a porcine coronary injury model: efficacy and safety compared with uncoated stents. J Am Coll Cardiol 1998; 31(6):1434–8.

18. van der Giessen WJ, Lincoff AM, Schwartz RS, et al. Marked inflammatory sequelae to implantation of biodegradable and nonbiodegradable polymers in porcine coronary arteries. Circulation 1996; 94(7):1690–7.

19. De Scheerder IK, Wilczek KL, Verbeken EV, et al. Biocompatibility of polymer-coated oversized metallic stents implanted in normal porcine coronary arteries. Atherosclerosis 1995; 114(1):105–14.

20. Simon DI, Dhen Z, Seifert P, et al. Decreased neointimal formation in Mac-1(-/-) mice reveals a role for inflammation in vascular repair after angioplasty. J Clin Invest 2000; 105(3):293–300.

21. Welt FG, Edelman ER, Simon DI, et al. Neutrophil, not macrophage, infiltration precedes neointimal thickening in balloon-injured arteries. Arterioscler Thromb Vasc Biol 2000; 20(12):2553–8.

22. Moreno PR, Bernardi VH, Lopez-Cuellar J, et al. Macrophage infiltration predicts restenosis after coronary intervention in patients with unstable angina. Circulation 1996; 94(12):3098–102.

23. Pietersma A, Kofflard M, de Wit LE, et al. Late lumen loss after coronary angioplasty is associated with the activation status of circulating phagocytes before treatment. Circulation 1995; 91(5):1320–5.

24. Inoue T, Hoshi K, Yaguchi I, et al. Serum levels of circulating adhesion molecules after coronary angioplasty. Cardiology 1999; 91(4):236–42.

25. Gottsauner-Wolf M, Zasmeta G, Hornykewycz S, et al. Plasma levels of C-reactive protein after coronary stent implantation. Eur Heart J 2000; 21(14):1152–8.

26. Bendeck MP, Zempo N, Clowes AW, et al. Smooth muscle cell migration and matrix metalloproteinase expression after arterial injury in the rat. Circ Res 1994; 75:539–45 .

27. Michelle P, Colleen I, Reidy MA. Inhibition of matrix metalloproteinase activity inhibits smooth muscle cell migration but not neointimal thickening after arterial injury. Circ Res 1996; 78:38–43.

28. Zempo N, Koyama N, Kenagy RD, et al. Regulation of vascular smooth muscle cell migration and proliferation in vitro and in injured rat arteries by a synthetic matrix metalloproteinase inhibitor. Arterioscler Thromb Vasc Biol 1996;16:28–33.

29. Scott NA, Cipolla GD, Ross CE, et al. Identification of a potential role for the adventitia in vascular lesion formation after balloon overstretch injury of porcine coronary arteries. Circulation 1996; 93(12):2178–87.

30. De Scheerder I, Szilard M, Huang Y, et al. Evaluation of the effect of oversizing on vascular injury, thrombogenicity and neointimal hyperplasia using the Magic Wallstent™ in a porcine coronary model (abstract). J Am Coll Cardiol 2000; 35(2):70A.

31. Hayashi S, Watanabe N, Nakazawa K, et al. Roles of P-selectin in inflammation, neointimal formation, and vascular remodeling in balloon-injured rat carotid arteries. Circulation 2000; 102(14):1710–7.

32. McEver RP, Beckstead JH, Moore KL, et al. GMP-140, a platelet alpha-granule membrane protein, is also synthesized by vascular endothelial cells and is localized in Weibel-Palade bodies. J Clin Invest. 1989; 84:92–9.

33. Manka D, Collins RG, Ley K, et al. Absence of P-selectin, but not intercellular adhesion molecule-1, attenuates neointimal growth after arterial injury in apolipoprotein E-deficient mice. Circulation 2001; 103(7):1000–5.

34. Inoue T, Sakai Y, Morooka S, et al. Expression of polymorphonuclear leukocyte adhesion molecules and its clinical significance in patients treated with percutaneous transluminal coronary angioplasty. J Am Coll Cardiol 1996; 28(5):1127–33.

35. Mickelson, JK, Lakkis NM, Villarreal-Levy G, et al. Leukocyte activation with platelet adhesion after coronary angioplasty: a mechanism for recurrent disease? J Am Coll Cardiol 1996; 28:345–53.

36. Rogers C, Edelman ER, Simon DI. A mAb to the beta2-leukocyte integrin Mac-1 (CD11b/CD18) reduces intimal thickening after angioplasty or stent implantation in rabbits. Proc Natl Acad Sci USA 1998; 95(17):10134–9.

37. Feldman LJ, Aguirre L, Ziol M, et al. Interleukin-10 inhibits intimal hyperplasia after angioplasty or stent implantation in hypercholesterolemic rabbits. Circulation 2000; 101(8):908–16.

38. Fauci AS, Dale DC, Balow JE. Glucocorticosteroid therapy: mechanism of action and clinical consideration. Ann Intern Med 1976; 84:304–15.

39. Stone GW, Rutherford BD, McConahay DR, et al. A randomized trial of corticosteroids for the prevention of restenosis in 102 patients undergoing repeat coronary angioplasty. Cathet Cardiovasc Diagn 1989; 18:227–31.

40. Pepine CJ, Hirshfeld JW, MacDonald RG, et al, for the M-HEART Group. A controlled trial of corticosteroids to prevent restenosis after coronary angioplasty. Circulation 1990; 81:1753–61.

41. Lee CW, Chae JK, Lim HY, et al. Prospective randomized trial of corticosteroids for the prevention of restenosis after intracoronary stent implantation. Am Heart J 1999; 138:60–3.

42. Berk BC, Gordon JB, Alexander RW. Pharmacologic roles of heparin and glucocorticoids to prevent restenosis after coronary angioplasty. J Am Coll Cardiol 1991; 17(6 Suppl B):111B–117B.

43. Villa AE, Guzman LA, Chen W, et al. Local delivery of dexamethasone for prevention of neointimal proliferation in a rat model of balloon angioplasty. J Clin Invest 1994; 93(3):1243–9.

44. Muller DW, Golomb G, Gordon D, et al. Site-specific dexamethasone delivery for the prevention of neointimal thickening after vascular stent implantation. Coron Artery Dis 1994; 5(5):435–42.

45. Valero F, Hamon M, Fournier C, et al. Intramural injection of biodegradable microspheres as a local drug-delivery system to inhibit neointimal thickening in a rabbit model of balloon angioplasty. J Cardiovasc Pharmacol 1998; 31(4):513–9.

46. Lincoff AM, Furst JG, Ellis SG, et al. Sustained local delivery of dexamethasone by a novel intravascular eluting stent to prevent restenosis in the porcine coronary injury model. J Am Coll Cardiol 1997; 29(4):808–16.

47. Strecker EP, Gabelmann A, Boos I, et al. Effect on intimal hyperplasia of dexamethasone released from coated metal stents compared with non-coated stents in canine femoral arteries. Cardiovasc Intervent Radiol 1998; 21(6):487–96.

48. De Scheerder I, Wang K, Wilczek K, et al. Local methylprednisolone inhibition of foreign body

response to coated intracoronary stents. Coron Artery Dis 1996; 7(2):161–6.

49. De Scheerder I, Huang Y, Schacht E. New concepts for drug eluting stents. 6th local drug delivery meeting and cardiovascular course on radiation and molecular strategies. 27–29 January 2000, Geneva, Switzerland.

50. Galli M, Bartorelli A, Bedogni F, et al. Italian BiodivYsio open registry (BiodivYsio PC-coated stent): study of clinical outcomes of the implant of a PC-coated coronary stent. J Invasive Cardiol 2000; 12(9):452–8.

51. Zheng H, Barragan P, Corcos T, et al. Clinical Experience With a New Biocompatible Phosphorylcholine-Coated Coronary Stent. J Invasive Cardiol 1999; 11(10):608–14.

52. Campbell EJ, O'Byrne V, Stratford PW, et al. Biocompatible surfaces using methacryloylphosphorylcholine laurylmethacrylate copolymer. ASAIO J 1994; 40(3):M853–7.

53. Veil KR, Chronos NAF, Palmer SJ, et al. Phosphorylcholine: a biocompatible coating for coronary angioplasty devices (abstract). Circulation 1995; 685.

54. Kuiper KK, Robinson KA, Chronos NA, et al. Phosphorylcholine-coated metallic stents in rabbit iliac and porcine coronary arteries. Scand Cardiovasc J 1998; 32(5):261–8.

55. Edelman ER, Rogers C. Pathobiologic responses to stenting. Am J Cardiol 1998; 81(7A):4E–6E.

56. Parente L, Fitzgerald MF, Flower RJ, et al. The effect of glucocorticoids on lyso-PAF formation in vitro and in vivo. Agents Actions 1986; 17(3–4):312–3.

57. Eccleston D, Lincoff AM, Furst J. Administration of colchicine using a novel prolonged delivery stent produces a marked local biological effect within the porcine coronary artery (abstract). Circulation 1995; 92:I–87.

26

The role of matrix metalloproteinase inhibitors after arterial injury

Amit Segev, Marion J Sierevogel, Gerard Pasterkamp, and Bradley H Strauss

Introduction • **MMPs are upregulated after arterial injury**
• **The effect of MMPs on arterial remodeling**
• **Differences in MMP expression between BA and stent implantation**
• **MMPs in collagen turnover and cell migration** • **MMP inhibition as a strategy to prevent restenosis**
• **A clinical trial with MMP inhibitor coated stents** • **Conclusion**

INTRODUCTION

Coronary artery disease (CAD) is the leading cause of mortality and morbidity among adults in the western world. The last ten years have witnessed tremendous growth in percutaneous coronary interventions, with more than one million procedures performed worldwide. Nowadays, in most centers, stents are used in more than 80% of procedures, as they provide both a more reliable immediate result and improved restenosis rates compared to regular balloon angioplasty (BA). Nevertheless, in-stent restenosis persists as a significant limitation of this procedure, which is particularly resistant to reintervention.

The initial effect of arterial balloon injury is denudation of the smooth endothelial layer. Then, the process of restenosis consists of three phases.[1] (1) Thrombotic phase, which consists of platelet adhesion and aggregation and activation of coagulation cascade. This phase is mediated by tissue factor and several platelet–endothelial cell adhesion molecules and is targeted quite satisfactorily by the use of anticoagulants and platelet aggregation inhibitors, such as glycoprotein IIb/IIIa inhibitors; (2) The proliferative phase, which consists of medial smooth muscle cell (SMC) and fibroblast proliferation and migration towards the arterial lumen with the formation of neointima. This phase is stimulated by several growth factors, mainly platelet-derived growth factor (PDGF), and fibroblast growth factor (FGF); (3) The final phase, which consists of synthesis and accumulation of extracellular matrix (ECM) contributes to intimal formation and arterial remodeling. The synthesis and accumulation of ECM is stimulated by several growth factors and cytokines including transforming growth factor-β (TGF-β), endothelin,[2] and others. Matrix metalloproteinases (MMPs) play a key role in ECM degradation, which is required for arterial remodeling and cell migration into the intima and matrix remodeling after arterial injury.[3–4]

MMPs ARE UPREGULATED AFTER ARTERIAL INJURY

It was initially demonstrated that MMPs are important mediators of atherosclerotic plaque rupture and vulnerability as they degrade the fibrous cap layer, thereby exposing lipid core antigens to coagulation proteins in the bloodstream leading to in situ thrombosis and clinical acute coronary syndromes.[5]

In relation to restenosis, extracellular matrix (ECM) formation is a key aspect of the initial lesion that forms after balloon angioplasty (BA), ultimately contributing to approximately 90% of the volume of the lesion.[6] The major ECM proteins are collagen, elastin, glycoproteins (such as fibronectin, tenascin, osteopontin), laminin, and proteoglycans. Matrix metalloproteinases (MMPs) are a group of zinc- and calcium-dependent enzymes that degrade these ECM components. They produce chemotactic peptides, release mediators from the cell surface, and may activate latent enzymes that modify the ECM. They are broadly classified into three groups: collagenases, gelatinases, and stromelysins. The main sources of MMPs are smooth muscle cells (SMCs), endothelial cells and monocytes/macrophages. Cytokines such as TNF-α and interleukins, secreted by macrophages, induce the synthesis of MMPs. Previous work from our group has highlighted the role of collagen turnover in the arterial response to BA injury and the importance of MMP expression as a mediator of the ECM response.[7,8] We showed in the rabbit that MMP-2 activity was maximal at 1 week after balloon injury and remained detectable at 4 and 12 weeks. There was no evidence of gelatinase (MMP-9) activity in either balloon-injured or control non-dilated arteries at any time points.[8] On the other hand, Bendeck et al. in the rat model,[4] and Feldman et al. in the rabbit model,[9] showed that early MMP-9 expression was rapidly induced after arterial balloon injury followed by an increase in MMP-2 expression. In the rabbit, 1 day after injury, MMP-9 mRNA levels increased dramatically, remained stable until day 30 and then decreased. MMP-2 mRNA levels decreased

slightly 1 day after injury and then increased significantly over time with a peak at 30 days. In a human study, MMP-2 levels after BA have also been observed to be significantly increased in coronary sinus blood specimens.[10] Maximal MMP-9 expression coincides with cell migration into the neointima and preceded the positive geometrical remodeling of arteries, suggesting a potential role.[4] Thus, the relationship between increased MMP expression and subsequent arterial repair in the restenosis process has been well established in experimental arterial injury models.

THE EFFECT OF MMPs ON ARTERIAL REMODELING

Arterial remodeling is a major determinant of cardiovascular disease. Both expansive remodeling (e.g. enlargement) and constrictive remodeling (e.g. shrinkage) are observed in arterial occlusive diseases. Different triggers for geometrical arterial remodeling have been reported: de novo atherosclerosis, changes in arterial flow and subsequently shear stress, transplant vasculopathy, and the focus of our review – after arterial injury.[11] Constrictive remodeling is a major contributing factor to restenosis after angioplasty in humans. Longitudinal evaluation of restenosis after arterial injury with intravascular ultrasound (IVUS) imaging at several time points has shown that inward remodeling occurs predominantly between 1 and 6 months after the procedure, thus distinguishing it from early elastic recoil.[12] Since degradation of the ECM scaffold enables reshaping of tissue, participation of MMPs has become the object of intense recent interest in relation to physiological and pathological vascular remodeling.

In both expansive and constrictive remodeling, activation of MMP-2 and MMP-9 is enhanced and probably regulated at a post-transcriptional level. This enhanced MMP activity is an essential feature in the flow-induced remodeling response since enlargement of the arterial wall is limited by MMP inhibitors. Godin et al.[13] showed in a murine model of slow flow arterial remodeling, that MMP-9 induction is associated with the formation of intimal hyperplasia without the need of frank mechanical injury. They also showed that a significant increase in MMP-9 expression preceded the positive geometrical remodeling of arteries, suggesting a potential role for this matrix-degrading enzyme. Although outward remodeling is initially beneficial by preserving the lumen, recent evidence suggests it may ultimately increase the propensity for plaque destabilization and rupture,[14] and may be a trigger for SMC proliferation and migration.[15] Two studies of increased flow have reported that broad-spectrum MMP inhibitors prevented arterial enlargement induced by creation of arteriovenous fistulae.[16,17]

DIFFERENCES IN MMP EXPRESSION BETWEEN BA AND STENT IMPLANTATION

Although stents reduce restenosis rates by improving immediate luminal gain, in-stent restenosis remains a major clinical problem with limited interventional solutions. The biologic response to stent implantation differs from plain old balloon angioplasty (BA), particularly with respect to an enhanced inflammatory response and increased intimal hyperplasia formation. Studies have indicated that the neointima and collagen accumulation after stent implantation are in fact more then 2-fold greater than after BA, but an initially larger lumen in stenting more than compensates for this increased neointima. Two studies have shown there are also differences in MMP expression between balloon angioplasty and stent implantation.[9,18] Hypercholesterolemic rabbits underwent stent implantation and BA in the right and left iliac arteries, respectively. The expression of MMPs and their inhibitors (TIMPs) was assessed at various time points in the injured arteries. MMP-9 expression was rapidly induced after injury (1 day), whereas the increase in MMP-2 expression was delayed (7–30 days). At all time points (up to 60 days) MMP-9 activity and MMP-9 mRNA levels were significantly higher after stent implantation

than after BA. Although MMP-2 mRNA levels were upregulated in stent and BA treated arteries, MMP-2 activity was slightly higher in the stent implantation group up to 60 days after injury. No differences in TIMP expression were observed between stented and balloon-injured arteries. Furthermore, early inflammatory cell recruitment was more marked after stent implantation. The authors proposed a mechanism, which may explain the differential expression/activation patterns of MMPs in stented versus balloon-injured arteries. They suggest that proinflammatory cytokines (e.g. interleukin-1), are key contributors to in-stent intimal hyperplasia and may be responsible, at least in part, for the induction of MMP expression in stented arteries.[19,20] Galis et al. have previously demonstrated that gelatinolytic activity and expression of MMP-9 cosegregated with macrophage-derived foam cells in aortic lesions, further suggesting the role of inflammation in upregulating MMP expression.[21] Moreover, endothelial cells, through the release of soluble factors and through direct contact with monocyte cells, may regulate metalloproteinase synthesis by monocytes.[22] We also showed that at 1 week after injury, overall gelatinase activity was increased more than 2-fold in stented arteries, with both MMP-2 and MMP-9 activity.[18] Stented arteries also had increases in both intimal DNA content (1.5-fold) and absolute cell proliferation (4-fold).

MMPs IN COLLAGEN TURNOVER AND CELL MIGRATION

As mentioned before, medial SMC and fibroblast migration towards the injured endothelial surface is a crucial step in neointimal formation. This phase of migration is mediated by several growth factors and cytokines. In vivo, vascular SMCs (VSMCs) are surrounded by and embedded in a variety of ECM proteins that must be traversed during migration. One of the principal barriers to cell movement in the intact vessel is the basement membrane (BM) that surrounds each VSMC and separates the VSMC-containing medial cell layer from the endothelium. Because SMCs are surrounded by an encaging ECM, they can only migrate into the injured endovascular area by degrading this matrix. Pauly et al. showed that cultured VSMCs could migrate across a BM barrier and that this ability was dependent on the phenotypic state of the cell.[23] VSMCs maintained in a proliferative state readily migrated across a BM towards a chemoattractant. By use of a number of MMP inhibitors, the migration of proliferating VSMCs across the BM barrier was inhibited by over 80%. They demonstrated that type IV collagenase (MMP-2) was the principal MMP expressed and secreted by these cells. Antisera capable of selectively neutralizing MMP-2 activity also inhibited VSMC migration. Bendeck et al. characterized MMP expression in the rat carotid artery after injury.[4] Production of an 88 kD gelatinase was induced after BA, and proteinase (MMP-2 and MMP-9) production continued during the period of migration of SMCs from the media to the intima. Administration of MMP inhibitor resulted in a 97% reduction in the number of SMCs migrating into the intima. This group reported two years later that the administration of GM6001, an MMP inhibitor, resulted again in 97% decrease in the number of SMCs that migrated into the intima by 4 days after injury. However, neither intimal nor medial SMC replication rates were decreased by GM6001 treatment, supporting the hypothesis that the decrease in lesion size was due to inhibition of MMP-mediated migration and not inhibition of replication.[24] More recently, Shi et al. examined regional differences in cell outgrowth and the synthesis of MMPs and TIMP in different layers of porcine coronary arteries.[25] Coronary media demonstrated slower cell outgrowth than coronary adventitia. These observations were paralleled by the predominant expression of TIMP in the media, whereas higher MMP-2 and MMP-9 activities were released from the adventitia.

Two recent studies have also shown that MMP inhibitors can block collagen accumulation in the vessel wall in both neointimal in stented arteries,[18] and in the adventitia of balloon-injured arteries.[26] MMP inhibitor-treated animals showed less constrictive remodeling accompanied by less collagen content. It may seem paradoxical that an agent that inhibits matrix-degrading enzymes resulted in decreased collagen content. There are several potential reasons. Collagen degradation products have some detrimental effects that contribute to restenosis. These degradation products are chemotactic for inflammatory cells and fibroblasts that are intricately involved in neointimal formation.[27,28] Collagen degradation also enhances SMC migration, probably by exposing cryptic RGD sequences, which allow bind to α_v-β_3 integrin receptors that promote migration.[29] In contrast, intact (i.e. non-degraded) fibrillar type I collagen inhibits SMC proliferation by regulating cell cycle events, including cyclin E-associated kinase and cyclin-dependent kinase-2 phosphorylation.[30] Thus, MMPs, by virtue of blocking the formation of collagen degradation products, can have favorable effects on vessel repair. MMPs also appear to be involved in the process of collagen synthesis. This can be explained by in vitro studies showing that MMP inhibition, either by a non-specific MMPI, batimastat, or by antisense oligonucleotides directed against MMP-3 mRNA, can prevent phenotypic modulation and activation of vascular SMCs.[31,32] In vitro studies by our group have shown that MMP inhibition can block collagen synthesis in vitro.[18] Finally, MMP inhibitors may also block the activation of proinflammatory cytokines, such as endothelin,[33,34] and TNF-α.[35]

MMP INHIBITION AS A STRATEGY TO PREVENT RESTENOSIS

The role of natural MMP inhibitor (TIMP) in neointimal formation has been verified by Lijnen et al. who showed that more intimal formation occurred after injury in the TIMP knockout mouse.[36] TIMP deficiency resulted in higher intima/media ratio and higher intimal cells. Zymography of arterial extracts revealed a higher active MMP-2 level at 1 to 3 weeks after injury in TIMP knockout arteries, whereas active MMP-9 was only detected in TIMP knockout arteries 1 week after the injury.

However, in the rat carotid injury model, MMP inhibition resulted in significant inhibition of SMCs migration but not intimal formation due to a catch up phenomenon.[24] It has also been demonstrated that marimastat, an orally active specific MMP inhibitor, inhibits neointimal thickening in a model of human vein graft stenosis,[37] and in a model of human arterial intimal thickening.[38] This inhibition was paralleled by a significant reduction in the levels of MMP-2 and MMP-9 in the tissues. In vitro study showed that dexamethasone progressively inhibits VSMC migration in a dose-dependent fashion and via inhibition of MMP-2 secretion.[39]

In a study done on atherosclerotic iliac arteries of micropigs, batimastat, a non-specific MMP inhibitor, was administered after BA.[40] Angiographic and echocardiographic late lumen loss in the batimastat group were significantly reduced as compared to the vehicle group. Late media-bounded area loss, which was used as a measure of remodeling after BA, was significantly less in the treatment group. However, there were no differences in neointimal formation among the two groups. This observation was supported in a previously mentioned study.[24] Sierevogel et al. examined the effect of the oral MMP inhibitor, marimastat, on arterial remodeling (assessed by IVUS) after balloon dilation in pigs.[41] In the marimastat group, a significant reduction (53%) of late lumen loss was observed that was fully explained by impaired constrictive remodeling. In the marimastat group, the prevalence of constrictive remodeling was reduced (38% vs 75% in the control group) in favor of not only neutral but also expansive remodeling (21% and 42% vs 4% and 21% in the control group, respectively). In contrast to the control group, acute luminal gain in the marimastat group did not correlate with late vessel area loss.

As suggested previously by Feldman et al., stenting results in more pronounced inflammatory response and consequently increased expression of MMPs as compared to BA alone.[9] Cherr et al. studied the effects of RO113-2908, a broad-spectrum MMP inhibitor, on the response to iliac artery angioplasty and stenting in atherosclerotic cynomolgus monkeys.[42] They demonstrated that inhibition of MMP activity reduced angiogenesis but failed to prevent constrictive remodeling or intimal hyperplasia after BA and stenting.

We recently examined the effects of GM6001, a non-specific MMP inhibitor, on collagen synthesis in cultured SMCs and on collagen accumulation in the vessel wall after stenting.[18] In a double-injury rabbit model, adjacent iliac arteries received BA or stenting. Rabbits were treated for 1 week post procedure with either GM6001 or placebo. Compared to placebo, GM6001 significantly inhibited intimal hyperplasia and intimal collagen content, and it increased lumen area stented arteries without effects on proliferation rates (Figure 26.1). This study, as well as others in the past, strengthens the observation that MMP inhibition results in significant reduction of intimal collagen accumulation and cell migration with no effect on cell proliferation. The most novel and important finding of our study was that although no effects on cell proliferation were demonstrated, neointimal hyperplasia was significantly inhibited.

Several explanations may postulate the differences between our recent study and the negative study by Cherr and coworkers.[42] First, RO113-2908 has significantly less potency in inhibiting MMP-1 than GM6001; second, a potential factor that should be considered is the differences in animal models as Cherr et al. used a high cholesterol diet model with extremely high LDL levels. Moreover, Gobeil et al. recently showed that a Bio*divYsio* stent coated with an MMP inhibitor reduces neointimal hyperplasia in porcine coronary artery restenosis model.[43] (See Table 26.1.)

A CLINICAL TRIAL WITH MMP INHIBITOR COATED STENTS

Biocompatibles initiated human coronary trials with batimastat-coated stents in the summer of 2001. Although results of the Brilliant study have not been presented or published, these trials have been stopped, presumably due to lack of efficacy according to press releases. This

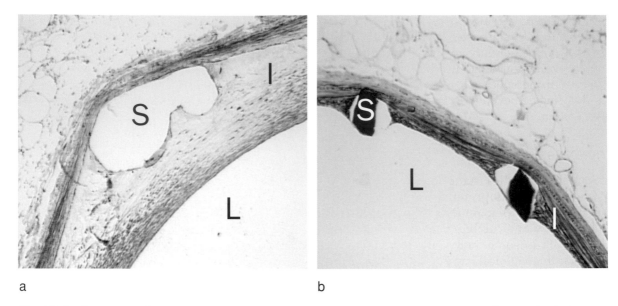

a b

Fig. 26.1 Representative photomicrograph of elastic trichrome-stained cross-sections of stented arteries showing increased intimal hyperplasia in (a) a placebo-treated artery, compared to (b) a GM6001 treated animal (×10 objective). I, intima; L, lumen; S, stent strut. (Reprinted with permission from the J Am Coll Cardiol 2002;**39**:1852–8.[18] © 2002 with permission from American College of Cardiology Foundation.)

Table 26.1   Studies on the effect of matrix metalloproteinase (MMP) inhibition after arterial injury

Study	Animal model	Experimental design/Type of inhibitor	Effect on neointimal formation	Other effects
Bendeck et al.[24]	Rats	BA/GM6001	No effect	97% ↓ in cell migration
Lijnen et al.[36]	Mice	BA/TIMP–/– vs +/+	72% ↓	45% ↓ in cell migration MMP-2 ↑ in TIMP –/–
Porter et al.[37]	Humen tissue	Human vein graft/marimastat	Significant inhibition: dose-dependent	Significant ↓ of tissue levels of MMP-2 and MMP-9
De Smet et al.[38]	Yucatán micropigs	BA/batimastat	24% ↓	Late lumen loss ↓ by ≈60%
Sierevogel et al.[41]	Pigs	BA/marimastat	No effect	Late lumen loss ↓ by 53%
Cherr et al.[42]	Monkeys	BA vs stenting/RO113-2908	No effects in stents or BA	No effect on lumen loss ↓ angiogenesis
Li et al.[18]	Rabbits	BA + stenting/GM6001	30% ↓ in stents No effect in BA	Lumen area ↑ by 14%

BA, balloon angioplasty; TIMP, tissue inhibitor of matrix metalloproteinase.

appears to be a major setback for the use of MMP inhibitors on stents, although at the present time there are inadequate data available. Several issues will need to be considered, including the specific MMP inhibitor studied and dosing achieved with this stent drug delivery system.

CONCLUSION

Preclinical studies have indicated efficacy of matrix metalloproteinases inhibitors for favorably affecting remodeling after balloon angioplasty and inhibition of in-stent intimal hyerplasia in some animal models. Although initial human clinical coronary stent trials with batimastat have been completed and further trials are on hold, no data have yet been presented on the results of these trials. Therefore, the future of this therapeutic approach to prevent in-stent restenosis is uncertain.

REFERENCES

1. Faxon DP, Coats W, Currier J. Remodeling of the coronary artery after vascular injury. Prog Cardiovasc Dis 1997; 40:129–40.
2. Barolet AW, Babaei S, Robinson R, et al. Administration of exogenous endothelin-1 following vascular balloon injury: early and late effects on intimal hyperplasia. Cardiovasc Res 2001; 52:468–76.
3. Dollery CM, McEwan JR, Henney AM. Matrix metalloproteinases and cardiovascular disease. Circ Res 1995; 77:863–8.
4. Bendeck MP, Zempo N, Clowes AW, et al. Smooth muscle cells migration and matrix metalloproteinases expression after arterial injury in the rat. Circ Res 1994; 75:539–45.
5. Galis ZS, Sukova GK, Lark MW, Libby P. Increased expression of matrix metalloproteinases and matrix degrading activity in vulnerable regions of human atherosclerotic plaques. J Clin Invest 1994; 94:2493–503.
6. Schwartz RS, Holmes DR, Topol EJ. The restenosis paradigm revisited: an alternative proposal for cellular mechanisms. J Am Coll Cardiol 1992; 20:1284–93.
7. Strauss BH, Chisolm R, Keeley FW, et al. Extracellular matrix remodeling after balloon angioplasty injury in a rabbit model of restenosis. Circ Res 1994; 75:650–8.
8. Strauss BH, Robinson R, Batchelor WB, et al. In vivo collagen turnover following experimental balloon angioplasty injury and the role of matrix metalloproteinases. Circ Res 1996; 79:541–50.
9. Feldman LJ, Mazighi M, Scheuble A, et al. Differential expression of matrix metalloproteinases after stent implantation and balloon angioplasty in the hypercholesterolemic rabbit. Circulation 2001; 103:3117–22.
10. Hojo Y, Ikeda U, Katsuki T, et al. Matrix metalloproteinases expression in the coronary circulation induced by coronary angioplasty. Atherosclerosis 2002; 161:185–92.
11. Ward MR, Pasterkamp G, Yeung AC, Borst C. Arterial remodeling. Mechanisms and clinical implications. Circulation 2000; 102:1186–91.
12. Kimura T, Kaburagi S, Tamura T, et al. Remodeling of human coronary arteries undergoing coronary angioplasty or atherectomy. Circulation 1997; 96:475–83.
13. Godin D, Ivan E, Johnson C, et al. Remodeling of carotid artery is associated with increased expression of matrix metalloproteinases in mouse blood flow cessation model. Circulation 2000; 102:2861–6.
14. Vink A, Schoneveld AH, Richard W, et al. Plaque burden, arterial remodeling and plaque vulnerability: determined by systemic factors? J Am Coll Cardiol 2001; 38:718–23.
15. Galis ZS, Khatri JJ. Matrix metalloproteinases in vascular remodeling and atherogenesis. The good, the bad, and the ugly. Circ Res 2002; 90:251–62.
16. Abbruzzese TA, Guzman RJ, Martin RL, et al. Matrix metalloproteinase inhibition limits arterial enlargement in a rodent arteriovenous fistula model. Surgery 1998; 124:328–35.
17. Karwowski JK, Markezich A, Whitson J, et al. Dose-dependent limitation of arterial enlargement by the matrix metalloproteinase inhibitor RS-113456. J Surg Res 1999; 87:122–9.
18. Li C, Cantor WJ, Nili N, et al. Arterial repair after stenting and the effects of GM6001, a matrix metalloproteinase inhibitor. J Am Coll Cardiol 2002; 39:1852–8.
19. Feldman LJ, Aguirre L, Ziol M, et al. Interleukin-10 inhibits intimal hyperplasia after

angioplasty or stent implantation in hyper-cholesterolemic rabbits. Circulation 2000; 101:908–16.

20. Nagase H, Woessner JF Jr. Matrix metalloproteinases. J Biol Chem 1999; 274:21491–4.

21. Galis ZS, Asanuma K, Godin D, Meng Z. N-acetyl-cysteine decreases the matrix-degrading capacity of macrophage-derived foam cells. New targets for antioxidant therapy. Circulation 1998; 97:2445–53.

22. Amorino GP, Hoover RL. Interactions of monocytic cells with human endothelial cells stimulate monocytic metalloproteinases production. Am J Pathol 1998; 152:199–207.

23. Pauly RR, Passaniti A, Bilato C, et al. Migration of cultured vascular smooth muscle cells through a basement membrane barrier requires type IV collagenase activity and is inhibited by cellular differentiation. Circ Res 1994; 75:41–54.

24. Bendeck MP, Irvin C, Reidy MA. Inhibition of matrix metalloproteinase activity inhibits smooth muscle cell migration but not neointimal thickening after arterial injury. Circ Res 1996; 78:38–43.

25. Shi Y, Patel S, Niculescu R, et al. Role of matrix metalloproteinases in the regulation of coronary cell migration. Arterioscler Thromb Vasc Biol 1999; 19:1150–5.

26. Sierevogel M, Velema E, van der Meer F, et al. Matrix metalloproteinase inhibition reduces adventitial thickening and collagen accumulation following balloon dilation. Cardiovasc Res 2002; 55:864.

27. Malone JD, Richards M, Jeffrey JJ. Recruitment of peripheral mononuclear cells by mammalian collagenase digests type I collagen. Matrix 1991; 11:289–95.

28. Albini A, Adelmann-Grill BC. Collagenolytic cleavage products of collagen type I as chemoattractants for human dermal fibroblasts. Eur J Cell Biol 1985; 36:104–7.

29. Stringa E, Knauper V, Murphy G, Gavrilovic J. Collagen degradation and platelet-derived growth factor stimulate the migration of vascular smooth muscle cells. J Cell Sci 2000; 113:2055–64.

30. Koyama H, Raines EW, Bornfeldt KE, et al. Fibrillar collagen inhibits arterial smooth muscle proliferation through regulation of Cdk2. Cell 1996; 87:1069–78.

31. Lövdahl C, Thyberg J, Hultgardh-Nilsson A. The synthetic metalloproteinase inhibitor batamistat suppresses injury-induced phosphorylation of MAP kinase ERK1/ERK2 and phenotypic modification of arterial smooth muscle cells in vitro. J Vasc Res 2000; 37:345–54.

32. Lövdahl C, Thyberg J, Cercek B, et al. Oligonucleotides to stromelysin mRNA inhibit injury-induced proliferation of arterial smooth muscle. Histol Histopathol 1999; 14:1101–12.

33. Fernandez-Patron C, Stewart KG, Zhang Y, et al. Vascular matrix metalloproteinase-2-dependent cleavage of calcitonin gene-related peptide promotes vasoconstriction. Circ Res 2000; 87:670–6.

34. Levy DE, Tang PC, Sweet K, et al. A hydroxamic acid matrix metalloproteinases inhibitor blocks the activity of endothelin converting enzyme in anesthetized rats. Med Chem Res 1994; 4:547–53.

35. McGeehan GM, Becherer JD, Bast RC Jr, et al. Regulation of tumour necrosis factor-alpha processing by a metalloproteinase inhibitor. Nature 1994; 370:558–61.

36. Lijnen HR, Soloway P, Collen D. Tissue inhibitor of matrix metalloproteinases-1 impairs arterial neointima formation after vascular injury in mice. Circ Res 1999; 85:1186–91.

37. Porter KE, Loftus IM, Peterson M, et al. Marimastat inhibits neointimal thickening in a model of human vein graft stenosis. Br J Surg 1998; 85:1373–7.

38. Peterson M, Porter KE, Loftus IM, et al. Marimastat inhibits neointimal thickening in a model of human arterial intimal hyperplasia. Eur J Vasc Endovasc Surg 2000; 19:461–7.

39. Pross C, Farooq MM, Angle N, et al. Dexamethasone inhibits vascular smooth muscle cell migration via modulation of matrix metalloproteinase activity. J Surg Res 2002; 102:57–62.

40. de Smet BJGL, de Kleijn D, Hanemaaijer R, et al. Metalloproteinase inhibition reduces constrictive arterial remodeling after balloon angioplasty. A study in the atherosclerotic Yucatán micropig. Circulation 2000; 101:2962–7.

41. Sierevogel MJ, Pasterkamp G, Velema E, et al. Oral matrix metalloproteinase inhibition and arterial remodeling after balloon dilation: an intravascular ultrasound study in the pig. Circulation 2001; 103:302–7.

42. Cherr GS, Motew SJ, Travis JA, et al. Metalloproteinase inhibition and the response to angioplasty and stenting in atherosclerotic primates. Arterioscler Thromb Vasc Biol 2002; 22:161–6.

43. Gobeil F, Laflamme M, Bouchard M, et al. BiodivYsio stent coated with metalloproteinase inhibitor reduces neointimal hyperplasia in a porcine coronary artery restenosis model. Circulation 2001; 104:1848 (abstract).

27

Methotrexate: a potential drug for stent-mediated local drug delivery: antiinflammatory and antiproliferative characteristics

Xianshun Liu and Ivan De Scheerder

Introduction • Cellular effects of methotrexate (MTX) • Immunosuppressive effect • Antiinflammatory effect • Antiproliferative effect • Summary

INTRODUCTION

Methotrexate (MTX) is a folate antagonist, first developed for the treatment of malignancies,[1] and subsequently used in non-neoplastic diseases as an antiinflammatory and/or immunosuppressive drug. Biochemical pharmacologic studies of MTX in tumor cell lines have shown that MTX, like physiological folates, is converted to polyglutamate forms that are not readily transported across the cell membrane.[2–4] Those polyglutamated derivatives not only inhibit dihydrofolate reductase (DHFR), the major MTX target, but also have markedly increased affinity for certain folate-dependent enzymes, such as thymidylate synthase (TS), 5-amino-imidazol-4-carboxamide ribonucleotide transformylase, and the triple complex of enzymes that interconvert various forms of reduced folate.[4,5] Low dose MTX is currently the most commonly used treatment for rheumatoid arthritis,[6,7] and other chronic inflammatory disorders. MTX is also effective in the prophylaxis of acute graft-versus-host disease either alone or in association with cyclosporin A and/or prednisone,[8–10] or FK506.[11] MTX has also been used as an adjunct therapy for persistent mild cardiac allograft rejection.[12] Most pharmacologic studies have addressed the use of MTX in cancer chemotherapy, where doses could be escalated up to 30 g/m^2 by administration of the antidote leucovorin (folinic acid, citrovorum factor). In autoimmune diseases and allografts, however, MTX dosage is usually given in a range of 7–15 mg per week, given orally or by intramuscular injections.

CELLULAR EFFECTS OF METHOTREXATE (MTX)

Methotrexate is a folate analog with an amino group (NH_2), a methyl group (CH_2), and a fully oxidized pteridine ring, rendering the molecule inactive as cofactor.[13] Once administered, MTX is delivered to cells in the same way as the parenteral folates; 3–12% is hydroxylated in the liver and circulates as 7-OH-MTX.[14] Extracellular MTX is brought into the cell by the folate receptors (FRα, FRβ). Thereafter, a portion of intracellular MTX and 7-OH-MTX is metabolized to polyglutamates (MTX-glu) in the same manner as naturally occurring folates.[15] MTX-glu represent long lived derivatives, which in rats may be detected in the skin for as long as two weeks after a single dose of the drug.[16] MTX binds dihydrofolate reductase (DHFR) with high affinity. MTX-glu binds DHFR and has fairly high affinity for enzymes that require folate cofactors, including thymidylate synthetase (TS) and 5-aminoimidazole-4-carboxamide ribonucleotide (AICAR) transformylase. The inhibition of TS, induced by MTX, interferes with DNA synthesis in actively dividing cells, and the increase of AICAR enzyme system, which plays a key part in the purine metabolism of the cell, leads to enhanced release of adenosine into the blood.[17–19] In fact, a number of antiinflammatory effects exerted by MTX seem to be related to the extracellular adenosine increase and its interaction with specific cell surface receptors, with subsequent inhibition such as interleukin-8 (IL-8) production by peripheral blood mononulcear cells (PBMC), IL-6 secretion by human monocytes, leucotriene B4 synthesis in neutrophils, and decreased synovial collagenase gene expression.[20,21]

IMMUNOSUPPRESSIVE EFFECT

Methotrexate typically blocks tetrahydrofolate dependent steps in cell metabolism. Because tetrahydrofolate and polyglutamyl derivatives of tetrahydrofolate are involved in purine biosynthesis several consequences can appear that result in adenosine overproduction. In purine biosynthesis, two steps are tetrahydrofolate-dependent. There is a preponderance of MTX-mediated inhibition of the second enzyme AICAR formyl transferase in comparison with the first enzyme GAR formyl transferase.[18,22] Thus, there will be a relative increase of AICAR. AICAR itself inhibits important steps of degradation of adenosine-5'-phosphate (AMP) and adenosine by the AMP deaminase and the adenosine deaminase (ADA), respectively. Inhibition of degradation of these two intracellular compounds leads to increased intracellular and extracellular AMP and adenosine.[18] At the surface of different types of immune competent cells, the ecto-5'-nucleotidase (CD73) converts AMP to adenosine.[23,24] This surface enzyme can be regulated by several immune mediators, such as interleukin-4 (IL-4) and interferon-γ (IFN-γ), which decrease the activity of the ecto-5'-nucleotidase on PBMC.[25,26] On the other hand, it has been reported that IL-1 and tumor necrosis factor (TNF) increase activity of this enzyme.[27] Thus, the local microenvironment determines the activity of this enzyme. Extracellular adenosine can bind to the seven transmembrane-spanning adenosine surface receptor types, A1, A2a, A2b, A3, which have been found on many different cell types.[28] The rank order of the affinity of adenosine binding to these receptor subtypes is A1>A2a>A2b.[29] The adenosine A1 receptor is coupled to a $G\alpha_{10}$ protein and the A2a and A2b receptors are coupled to $G\alpha_s$. Ligation of A1 receptors decreases intracellular cyclic AMP (cAMP), whereas binding of adenosine to A2 receptors increases intracellular cAMP. If the pathways through the two different receptor subtypes A1 or A2a/b were functionally intact one would expect a preponderance of the A1 pathway owing to the higher affinity of adenosine to the A1 receptor subtype. This would lead to a decrease of cAMP. Low dose MTX exerts its antiinflammatory effect, however, by inducing extracellular adenosine, which acts predominantly through A2a receptors.[28,30,31] Thus, it seems as if A1 receptor signaling is switched off. Similar effects have been described in a proinflammatory situation where the pathway through the two receptors is shifted to $G\alpha_s$ yielding an increase of cAMP.[32] Furthermore, it has been shown that cytokines can upregulate the A2 receptor subtype, which may be another mechanism to shift the pathway to $G\alpha_s$ rather than $G\alpha_{10}$.[33,34] It has

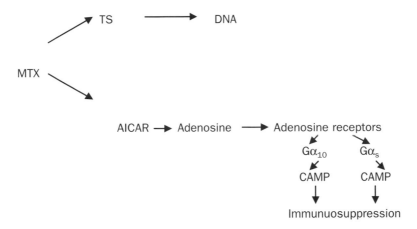

Fig. 27.1 Immunosuppressive action of methotrexate (MTX).

been repeatedly shown that an increase of cAMP leads to immunosuppression by inhibition of phagocytosis, inhibition of secretion of TNF, IFN-γ, IL-2, IL-12, HLA expression, and many others.[35–40] For adenosine via A2 receptor binding it has been specifically shown that this substance inhibits lymphocyte proliferation and production of TNF, IL-8, and IL-12[41,42] On the other hand, adenosine via A2 receptor binding increases secretion of IL-6 and IL-10.[43,44] Binding of adenosine to A3 receptors leads to inhibition of secretion of TNF, IL-12, and IFN-γ.[45,46] In conclusion, binding of adenosine to A2 and A3 receptors results in a favorable situation which is probably one of the important antiinflammatory mechanisms of MTX action (Figure 27.1).

ANTIINFLAMMATORY EFFECT

In considering IL-1 and TNF-α, which are cytokines with a central role in the inflammatory process and which are mainly produced by monocytes/macrophages at the level of rheumatoid arthritis (RA) synovial tissue, early studies suggested that MTX inhibits IL-1 production in vivo and ex vivo.[47] It has been suggested that MTX interferes directly with the binding of IL-1 receptor and thereby inhibits

the cellular responses to IL-1.[48] Alternatively, MTX, through adenosine increase and binding to A3 receptors, might promote the IL-1 receptor antagonist (Il-1ra) transcription and presumably its production. Recent studies seem to confirm this possibility, because it has been shown that MTX treatment generates a less inflammatory type of circulating monocyte in patients with RA treated with low doses, by inhibiting IL-1 and IL-8 secretion and, in parallel, by inducing the IL1-ra.[49,50]

A more recent study seems to confirm the possible IL-lra mediated antiinflammatory effects of MTX, at least on monocytes, because a significant increase of IL-lra was found with the low dose treatment of human cultured monocytic THP-1 cells.[51] The effects were clearly dose-dependent and gradually decreased with the lowest concentration at 24 h, while the presence of a steady state (at 48, 72, and 96 h) also indicated time-dependent effects. Interestingly, the high dose of MTX was found to cause a significant IL-lra decrease on cultured THP-1 cells compared with untreated control cells; this decrease was probably due to cell damage (apoptosis).[51] Monocytes produce greater amounts of IL-1 than IL-lra, whereas macrophages produce mainly IL-lra in in vitro cultures.[52] Recent results confirm these data, because IL-lra basal production was found to be significantly higher from untreated synovial RA macrophages than from untreated monocytic THP-1 cells.[51]

It has been also shown that adenosine inhibits TNF-α expression in a monocytic cell line and that monocytes release adenosine after treatment with MTX.[45,53] In addition, recent investigations showed both a late upregulation of the soluble TNF-α receptor (sTNFR p75) synthesis by PBMC after 24 h of MTX treatment and the MTX induced increased sTNFR p75 from cultured monoblastic leukemia cells, suggesting a further antiinflammatory mechanism through inhibition of TNF-α effects.[50] The short term antiinflammatory effects of MTX may include the inhibition of IL-6 secretion by cultured human monocytes and, in the course of RA treatment, a decreased production of IL-6, which might correlate with improvement of biological parameters of diseased activity.

In conclusion, MTX treatment in RA seems to reduce the production of proinflammatory monocytic/marcrophagic cytokines (IL-1, IL-6, and TNF-α), to increase gene expression of antiinflammatory Th2 cytokines (IL-4 and IL-10), and to decrease gene expression of proinflammatory Th1 cytokines (IL-2 and IFN-γ), with resulting antiinflammatory effects.

ANTIPROLIFERATIVE EFFECT

Several studies have recently shown that low dose MTX may well induce antiproliferative effects on immune cells owing to inhibition of dihydrofolate reductase and folate-dependent transmethylations as apoptosis-independent mechanisms. A recent study showed that patients with RA, treated with MTX, expressed low concentrations of circulation purines and pyrimidines, with consequent reduced availability for DNA and RNA synthesis and cell proliferation.[54] A recent paper confirmed that low concentrations of MTX inhibited in vitro thymidylate synthase activity in human peripheral blood mononuclear cells (PBMC).[55] It is difficult to relate observed changes in purine and pyrimidine levels directly to the pharmacokinetics of MTX because MTX clear-

ance from blood is rapid. Therefore, metabolic effects of MTX could be attributed predominantly to its polyglutamated derivatives that are formed and accumulated inside the cells. MTX polyglutamate derivatives may interfere with purine and pyrimidine metabolism and explain long-term antiproliferative effects in RA after low dose treatment with MTX once a week.[56] Recent data suggested that the disruption of the cell cycle caused by high dose MTX treatment may be the initial step of the apoptotic sequence of dying cells and may explain the antiproliferative effects of the drug.[57] The involvement of the APO-1/Fas (CD95) receptor/ligand system in MTX-induced apoptosis has been recently identified in leukemia cells, with a peak of apoptosis between 24 h and 48 h.[58] In addition, MTX was found to inhibit markedly the spontaneous proliferation of U937 monoblastic leukemia cells in vitro and induce the rapid expression of the apoptosis receptor CD95 also in presence of 1,25-OH-cholecalciferol.[59] Results of another recent investigation are in agreement with these latter studies and seem to suggest that intermediate MTX concentrations (50 μg/ml), as obtained in serum after low dose treatment, can induce both a significant cell growth inhibition and apoptosis, at least in monocytic immature cells (THP-1 cell line).[51] For cell proliferation, the lowest in vitro MTX concentrations (from 5 ng/mL to 500 ng/mL) were confirmed to be ineffective.[54] In that study, no significant effects on synovial macrophage proliferation were obtained with an MTX concentration of 50 μg/ml.[51]

The explanation for the lack of modulatory in vitro potency of MTX on synovial macrophage growth and apoptosis, as already found for cyclosporin A, may be that MTX affects only immature differentiating monocytes and not differentiated cells (i.e. tissue infiltrating monocytes and resident macrophages, respectively).[60,61] Therefore, these findings suggest that MTX might inhibit recruitment of immature and inflammatory monocytes into inflammatory sites and could reduce the survival of these cells in the inflamed synovial tissue.[51] A recent paper investigated whether other immunosuppressive properties of low dose MTX treatment were related to apoptosis.[62] The study showed that activated T cells from human peripheral blood underwent MTX induced apoptosis, which was completely abrogated by addition of folinic acid. Apoptosis of activated T-cells did not require interaction between CD95 (APO-1/Fas) and its ligand, and adenosine release accounted for only a small part of this MTX activity. Finally, in vitro activation of peripheral blood taken from patients with RA after MTX injection resulted in apoptosis.

Antiproliferative effect on endothelial and smooth muscle cells

In-stent restenosis, mainly caused by an abundant neointimal hyperplasia, remains the major limitation of coronary stent implantation. Mural thrombi, inflammatory response, smooth muscle cell (SMC) dedifferentiation, migration and proliferation, also extracellular matrix formation all participate to the pathogenesis of neointimal hyperplasia. Many investigators have reported that various chemotherapeutic agents inhibit SMC proliferation, and use of these compounds may result in decreased restenosis.[63,64] Such chemotherapeutic agents seem ideally suited for site-specific polymer-based delivery, given that toxic side

effects may limit systemic therapy. However, three reports showed a lack of efficacy for methotrexate in preventing restenosis. Muller et al. reported no effect of methotrexate in inhibiting neointimal proliferation after balloon injury to pig carotid arteries when MTX was delivered at the time of angioplasty by a perfusion catheter.[65] Murphy et al., in their study, which was also performed in a porcine model, showed that MTX (1.25 mg 5 days/week orally or 20 mg/week intramuscularly) given throughout a 28 day study period, failed to inhibit neointimal thickening in coronary arteries after implantation of oversized metallic stents.[66] Cox et al. report in an oversized stent porcine model showed that this model induced a significant proliferation response but the use of stents coated with methotrexate or a combination of the methotrexate and heparin resulted in no significant reduction in SMC proliferation when compared with arteries stented with uncoated tantalum coil stent.[67] However, we recently showed that stent-based delivery of 150 µg MTX using a SAE coating (Figure 27.2 shows the MTX release of the coating) reduces neointimal hyperplasia (1.13 ± 0.38 vs 1.92 ± 1.44 mm^2) compared with control in a porcine coronary stent model (unpublished data).

A few data are available in the literature with regard to the effect of MTX on endothelial and

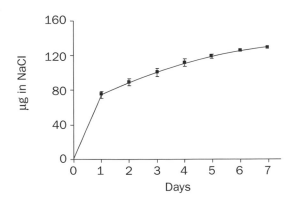

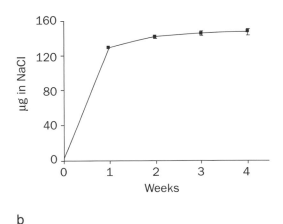

a

b

Fig. 27.2 In vitro accumulation of methotrexate released from three 3.0–18 mm biocompatible polymer coated coronary stents in 1 ml NaCl at 37°C. (a) Release over 1 week, (b) release over 4 weeks.

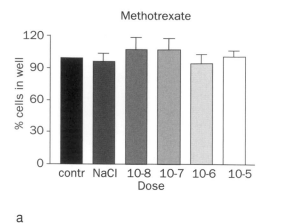

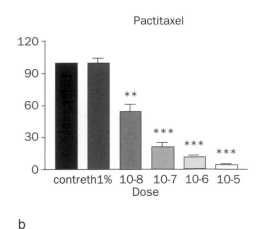

a

b

Fig. 27.3 Smooth muscle cell (SMC) proliferation assay. SMCs were incubated for 7 days with (a) methotrexate and (b) paclitaxel. ** $p<0.01$, *** $p<0.0005$ by one-way ANOVA.

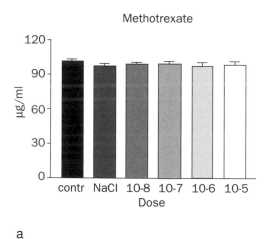

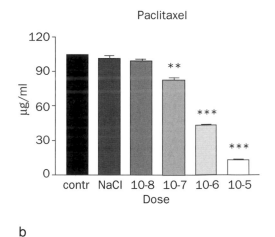

a

b

Fig. 27.4 Smooth muscle cell (SMC) total protein synthesis assay. SMCs were incubated for 7 days with (a) methotrexate and (b) paclitaxel. ** $p<0.005$, *** $p<0.0001$ by one-way ANOVA.

smooth muscle cell proliferation. Hirata et al. reported inhibition of vascular endothelial cell proliferation in vitro with concentrations of MTX as low as 5×10^{-9} M, and MTX inhibits endothelial cell proliferation in cell culture to a significantly greater degree than it inhibits fibroblast cell proliferation.[68] We recently showed no effect of vascular SMC proliferation in vitro with concentrations of MTX with a range of 10^{-8}–10^{-5} M in a rabbit aorta SMC proliferation assay. After 7 days of incubation with methotrexate, no reduction of the total number of SMCs was seen (10^{-8} M: 108 ± 24; 10^{-7} M: 107 ± 23; 10^{-6} M: 94 ± 18; 10^{-5} M: 100 ± 14; all data are a percentage of control cells in well; $n = 4$) (Figure 27.3). BrdU-labeling showed similar results. In addition, total protein synthesis was not diminished by methotrexate (control: 102.0 ± 2.6 vs 10^{-8} M: 99.3 ± 2.9; 10^{-7} M: 99.3 ± 4.0; 10^{-6} M: 97.0 ± 6.0; 10^{-5} M: 98.3 ± 7.5; all data are μg/mL; $n = 3$) (Figure 27.4). However, the remaining SMCs after methotrexate incubation showed excellent survival with 100% neutral red staining at all concentrations. This was in contrast with the paclitaxel incubated SMCs.

SUMMARY

Methotrexate has both antiproliferative and antiinflammatory effects in a dose-dependent manner. Knowledge about the basic mechanisms of action of MTX is not fully understood. The direct inhibitory effects on proliferation and the induction of apoptosis in cells were involved in the immune/inflammatory reaction. High dose MTX seems to induce cell cycle perturbations by metabolic effects and subsequently, as a consequence of the disruption of the cell cycle, inhibits a drug-specific apoptotic sequence. However, the mechanism of action of low dose MTX might be more antiinflammatory than immunosuppressive. Low dose MTX seems to exert antiinflammatory effects by inhibiting monocytic lymphocytic proinflammatory cytokines.

In-stent restenosis is the main limitation of coronary stent implantation. Methotrexate, with its antiinflammatory and antiproliferative characteristics may be a potential drug for stent-mediated local drug delivery. Nevertheless, methotrexate failed to inhibit restenosis in most animal models. Whether methotrexate truly fails to inhibit restenosis or whether polymer improvements to deliver greater quantities of the drug would decrease neointimal proliferation remains uncertain and requires further study.

REFERENCES

1. Farber S, Toch R, Manning Sears E, Pinkel D. Advances in Chemotherapy of Cancer in Man. In Haddow A, Greenstein J-P (eds), Advances in cancer research. Academic Press: New York 1956:2–73.

2. Jolivet J, Schilsky RL, Bailey BD, et al. Synthesis, retention, and biological activity of methotrexate polyglutamates in cultured human breast cancer cells. J Clin Invest 1982; 70:351–60.

3. Jolivet J, Chabner BA. Intracellular pharmacokinetics of methotrexate polyglutamates in human breast cancer cells. J Clin Invest 1983; 72:773–8.

4. Chabner PA, Allegra CJ, Curt GA, et al. Polyglutamation of methotrexate. Is methotrexate a prodrug? J Clin Invest 1985; 76:907–12.

5. Allegra CJ, Drake JC, Jolivet J, et al. Inhibition of phosphoribosyl-aminoimidazole-carboxamide tranformylase by methotrexate and dihydrofolic acid polyglutamates. Proc Natl Acad Sci USA 1985; 82:4881–5.

6. Weinblatt ME, Coblyn JS, Fox DA, et al. Efficacy of low-dose methotrexate in rheumatoid arthritis. N Engl J Med 1985; 312:818–22.

7. Williams HJ, Wilkens RF, Samuelson CO, et al. Comparison of low-dose oral pulse methotrexate and placebo in the treatment of rheumatoid arthritis: a controlled clinical trial. Arthritis Rheum 1985; 28:721–30.

8. Storb R, Deeg HJ, Whitehead J, et al. Methotrexate and cyclosporine compared with cyclosporine alone for prophylaxis of acute graft-versus-host disease after marrow transplantation for leukemia. N Engl J Med 1986; 314:729–35.

9. Nash RA, Pepe MS, Storb R, et al. Acute graft-versus-host disease: analysis of risk factors after allogeneic marrow transplantation and prophylaxis with cyclosporine and methotrexate. Blood 1992; 80:1838–45.

10. Chao NJ, Schmidt GM, Niland JC, et al. Cyclosporine, methotrexate, and prednisone compared with cyclosporine and prednisone for prophylaxis of acute graft-versus-host disease. N Engl J Med 1993; 329:1225–30.

11. Nash RA, Pineiro LA, Storb R, et al. FK506 combination with methotrexate for the prevention of graft-versus-host disease after marrow transplantation from matched unrelated donors. Blood 1996; 88:3634–41.

12. Olsen SL, O'Connel JB, Bristow MR, Renlund DG. Methotrexate as an adjunct in the treatment of persistent mild cardiac allograft rejection. Transplantation 1990; 50:773–5.

13. Seeger DR, Cosalich DDB, Smith JM, Hultquist ME. Analogs of pteroylglutamic acid: II. 4-aminoderivatives. J Am Chem Soc 1949; 71:1297–301.

14. Sonneveld P, Schultz FW, Nooter K, Hahlen K. Pharmacokinetics of methotrexate and 7-hydroxy-methotrexate in plasma and bone marrow of children receiving low-dose oral methotrexate. Cancer Chemother Pharmacol 1986; 18:111–16.

15. Baugh CM, Crumdieck Cl, Nair MG. Poly-gammaglutamyl metabolites of methotrexate. Biochem Biophys Res Commun 1973; 52:27–32.

16. Zimmerman CL, Franz TJ, Slattery IT. Pharmacokinetics of the polygammaglutamyl metabolites of methotrexate in skin and other

tissues of rats and hairless mice? J Pharmacol Exp Ther 1984; 231:242–7.

17. Cronstein BN, Eberle MA, Gruber HE, Levin RI. Methotrexate inhibits neutrophil function by stimulating adenosine release from connective tissue cells. Proc Natl Acad Sci USA 1991; 88:2441–5.

18. Baggott JE, Morgan SL, Ha TS et al. Antifolates in rheumatoid arthritis: a hypothetical mechanism of action. Clin Exp Rheumatol 1993; 11(suppl 8):101–5.

19. Gruber HE, Hoffer ME, McAllister DR, et al. Increased adenosine concentration in blood from ischemic myocardium by AICA riboside: effects on flow, granulocytes and injury. Circulation 1989; 80:1400–11.

20. Cronstein BN, Naime D, Ostad E. The antiinflammatory mechanism of methotrexate. Increased adenosine release at inflamed sites diminishes leukocyte accumulation in an in vivo model of inflammation. J Clin Invest 1993; 92:2675–82.

21. Bouma MG, Stad RK, van der Wildenberg FAJM, Buurman WA. Differential regulatory effects of adenosine on cytokine release by activated human monocytes. J Immunol 1994; 153:4159–68.

22. Allegra CJ, Drake JC, Jolivet J, Chabner BQ. Inhibition of phosphoribosylaminoimidazole-carbosamide transformylase by methotrexate and dihydrofolic acid polyglutamates. Proc Natl Acad Sci USA 1985; 82:4881–5.

23. Lazidins J, Karnoysky ML. Effect of phosphate esters, nucleotides and nucleosides on 5'-nucleotidase of cultured mouse macrophages. J Cell Physiol 1978; 96:115–22.

24. Edwards NL, Magilavy DB, Cassidy JT, Fox IH. Lymphocyte ecto-5' nucleotidase deficiency in agammaglobulinemia. Science 1978; 201:628–30.

25. Christensen LD, Andersen V, Nygaard P, Bendtzen K. Effects of immunomodulators on ecto-5'-nucleotidase activity on blood mononuclear cells in vitro. Scand J Immunol 1992; 35:407–13.

26. Armstrong MA, Shah S, Hawkins SA, Bell AL, Roberts SD. Reduction of monocyte 5'-nucleotidase activity by gamma-interferon in multiple sclerosis and autoimmune diseases. Ann Neurol 1988; 24:12–16.

27. Savic V, Stefanovic V, Ardaillou N, Ardaillou R. Induction of ecto-5'-nucleotide of rat cultured mesangial cells by interleukin-1 beta and tumour necrosis factor-alpha. Immunology 1990; 70:321–6.

28. Cronstein BN. The machanism of action of methotrexate. Rheum Dis Clin North Am 1997; 23:739–55.

29. Mazzom MR, Martin C, Bucacchini A. Regulation of agonist binding to A2A adenosine receptors effects of guanine nucleotides (GDP[s]) and GTP[s] and Mg2+. Biochem Biophys Acta 1993; 1220:76–80.

30. Morabito L, Montesinos M, Schreibman DM, et al. Methotrexate and sulfasalazine promote adenosine release by a mechanism that requires ecto-5'-nucleotidase-mediated conversion of adeninin nucleotides. J Clin Invest 1998; 101:295–300.

31. Montesinos MC, Chen JF, Desai A, et al. Adenosine acting at A2a receptors mediates the antiinflammatory effects of low-dose weekly methotrexate therapy. Arthritis Rheum 2000; 43:S354 (abstract).

32. Straub RH, Mannel DN. How the immune system puts the brain to sleep. Nature Med 1999; 5:877–9.

33. Xaus J, Mirabet M, Lloberas J, et al. IFN-gamma up-regulates the A2B adenosine receptor expression in macrophages: a mechanism of macrophage deactivation. J Immunol 1999; 162:3607–14.

34. Khoa ND, Montesinos MC, Cronstein BN. Inflammatory cytokines regulate expression of adenosine receptors in human monocytic THP-1 cells and human microvascular endothelial cells. Arthritis Rheum 2000; 43:S86 (abstract).

35. Figueiredo F, Uhing RJ, Okonogi K, et al. Activation of the cAMP cascade inhibits an early event involved in murine macrophage Ia expression. J Biol Chem 1990; 265:12317–23.

36. Renz H, Gong JH, Schmidt A, et al. Release of tumor necrosis factor-alpha from macrophages. Exhancement and suppression are dose-dependently regulated by prostaglandin E2 and cyclic nucleotides. J Immunol 1998; 141:2388–93.

37. Snijdewint FG, Kalinski P, Wierenga EA, et al. Prostaglandin E2 differentially modulates

cytokine secretion profiles of human T helper lymphocytes. J Immunol 1993; 150:5321–9.

38. Novogrodsky A, Patya M, Rubin AL, Stensel KH. Agents that increase cellular cAMP inhibit production of interleukin-2, but not its activity. Biochem Biophys Res Commun 1983; 114:93–9.

39. van der Pouw Kraan TC, Boeije LC, Smeenk RJ, et al. Prostaglandin-E2 is a potent inhibitor of human interleukin 12 production. J Exp Med 1995; 181:775–9.

40. Rossi AG, McCutcheon JC, Roy N, et al. Regulation of macrophage phagocytosis of apoptotic cells by cAMP. J Immunol 1998; 160:3562–8.

41. Kishiba M, Kojima H, Huang S, et al. Memory of extracellular adenosine A2A purinergic receptor-mediated signaling in murine T cells. J Biol Chem 1997; 272:25881–9.

42. Link AA, Kino T, Worth JA, et al. Ligand-activation of the adenosine A2a receptors inhibits IL-12 production by human monocytes. J Immunol 2000; 164:436–42.

43. Ritchie PK, Spangelo BL, Krzymowski DK, et al. Adenosine increases interleukin 6 release and decreases tumour necrosis factor release from rat adrenal zona glomerulosa cells, ovarian cells, anterior pituitary cells, and peritoneal macrophages. Cytokine 1997; 9:187–98.

44. Hasko G, Szabo C, Nemeth ZH, et al. Adenosine receptor agonists differentially regulate IL-10, TNF-alpha, and nitric oxide production in RAW 264.7 macrophages and in endotoxemic mice. J Immunol 1996; 157:4634–40.

45. Sajjadi FG, Takabayashi K, Foster AC, et al. Inhibition of TNF-alpha expression by adenosine: role of A3 adenosine receptors. J Immunol 1996; 156:3435–42.

46. Hasko G, Nemeth ZH, Vizi ES, et al. An agonist of adenosine A3 receptors decreases interleukin-12 and interferon-gamma production and prevents lethality in endotoxemic mice. Eur J Pharmacol 1998; 358:261–8.

47. Connolly KM, Stecher VJ, Danis E, et al. Alteration of interleukin-1 production and the acute phase response following medication of adjuvant arthritic rats with cyclosporin A or methotrexate. Int J Immunopharmacol 1988; 10:717–28.

48. Brody M, Bohm I, Barer R. Mechanism of action of methotrexate: experimental evidence that methotrexate blocks the binding of interleukin-1 beta to the interleukin-1 receptor on target cells. Eur J Chem Clin Biochem 1993; 31:667–74.

49. Seitz M, Loetscher B, Dewald B. Methotrexate action in rheumatoid arthritis: stimulation of cytokine inhibitor and inhibition of chemokine production by peripheral blood mononuclear cells. Br J Rheumatol 1995; 34:602–9.

50. Seitz M, Loetscher B, Dewald B. Interleukin-1 receptors antagonist, soluble tumor necrosis factor receptors, IL-1 and IL-8 markers of remission in rheumatoid arthritis during treatment with methotrexate. J Rheumatol 1996; 23:1512–16.

51. Cutolo M, Bisso A, Sulli A, et al. Antiproliferative and antiinflammatory effects of methotrexate on cultured differentiating myeloid monocytic cells (THP-1) but not on synovial macrophages from rheumatoid arthritis patients. J Rheumatol 2000; 27:2551–7.

52. Janson RW, Hance KR, Arend WP. Production of IL-1 receptor antagonist by human in vitro-derived marcrophages. Effect of lipopolysaccharide and granulocyte-macrophage colony stimulating factor. J Immunol 1991; 147:4218–23.

53. Merrill JT, Shen C, Scheibman D. Adenosine A1 receptor promotion of multinucleated giant cell formation by human monocytes: a mechanism for methotrexate-induced nodulosis in rheumatoid arthritis. Arthritis Rheum 1997; 40:1308–15.

54. Smolenska Z, Kaznowska Z, Zarowny D, et al. Effect of methotrexate on blood purine and pyrimidine levels in patients with rheumatoid arthritis. Rheumatology 1999; 38:997–1002.

55. Hornung N, Stengaard-Pedersen K, Ehrnrooth E, et al. The effects of low-dose methotrexate on thymidylate synthase activity in human peripheral blood mononuclear cells. Clin Exp Rheumatol 2000; 18:691–8.

56. Allegra CJ, Chabner BA, Drake JC. Enhanced inhibition of thymidylate synthase by methotrexate polyglutamates. J Biol Chem 1985; 260:9720–8.

57. Huschtascha LI, Martier WA, Andersson Ross CE, Tattersall MHN. Characteristics of cancer cell death after exposure to cytotoxic drugs in vitro. Br J Cancer 1996; 73:54–60.

58. Friesen C, Herr I, Krammer PH, Bebatin KM. Involvement of the CD95 (APO-1/Fas) receptor/

ligand system in drug-induced apoptosis in leukemia cells. Nature Med 1996; 2:574–6.

59. Seitz M, Zwicker M, Loetscher P. Effects of methotrexate on differentiation of monocytes and production of cytokine inhibitors by monocytes. Arthritis Rheum 1998; 41:2032–8.

60. Seitz M, Loetscher P, Dewald B, et al. In vitro modulation of cytokine, cytokine inhibitor, and prostaglandin E release from blood mononuclear cells and synovial fibroblasts by antirheumatic drugs. J Rheumatol 1997; 24:1471–6.

61. Cutolo M, Barone A, Accardo S, et al. Effects of cyclosporin A on apoptosis in human cultured monocytic THP-1 cells and synovial macrophages. Clin Exp Rheumatol 1998; 16:417–22.

62. Genestier L, Paillot R, Fournel S, et al. Immunosuppressive properties of methotrexate: apoptosis and clonal deletion of activated peripheral T cells. J Clin Invest 1998; 102(2):322–8.

63. Barath P, Arakawa K, Cao J, et al. Low dose of antitumor agents prevents smooth muscle cell proliferation after endothelial injury. J Am Coll Cardiol 1989; 13:252A (abstract).

64. Jonasson L, Holm J, Hansson GK. Cyclosporin A inhibits smooth muscle proliferation in the vascular response to injury. Proc Natl Acad Sci USA 1988; 85:2303–6.

65. Muller DWM, Topol EJ, Abrams G, et al. Intramural methotrexate therapy for the prevention of neointimal thickening after balloon angioplasty. J Am Coll Cardiol 1992; 20:460–6.

66. Murphy JG, Schwartz RS, Edwards WD, et al. Methotrexate and azathioprine fail to inhibit procine coronary restenosis. Circulation 1990; 82(suppl):III-429 (abstract).

67. Cox DA, Anderson PG Roubin GS, et al. Effect of local delivery of heparin and methotrexate on neointimal proliferation in stented porcine coronary arteries. Coron Artery Dis 1992; 3:137–248.

68. Hirata S, Matsubara T, Saura R, et al. Inhibition of in vitro vascular endothelial cell proliferation and in vivo neovascularization by low dose methotrexate. Arthritis Rheum 1989; 32(9):1065–73.

28

Actin-skeleton inhibitors: potential candidates for local drug delivery in the prevention of in-stent restenosis?

Koen J Salu, Johan M Bosmans, Hidde Bult, and Chris J Vrints

Introduction • Structure, organization, and function of actin filaments • Two groups of actin-skeleton inhibitors • Restenosis and actin-skeleton inhibitors • Conclusions

INTRODUCTION

The use of intracoronary stents has become the first choice of therapy in interventional cardiology, representing 70–80% of all percutaneous coronary interventions in the United States and Europe.[1,2] Metallic coronary stents reduce the incidence of restenosis compared to balloon angioplasty by opposing elastic recoil and late remodeling of the vessel.[3,4] However, an excessive neointimal hyperplasia inside the stent still induces a restenosis frequency in up to 10–30% of the treated patients.[1] This 'in-stent' restenosis is a local, chronic response of the vessel wall to a foreign body, which involves a cascade of thrombotic, proliferative, and inflammatory phases.[5] Many different cell types: platelets, smooth muscle cells (SMCs), myofibroblasts, endothelial cells, and inflammatory cells, are recruited to play a pivotal role in this wound healing phenomenon, with the subsequent release of several growth factors which, on their turn, again stimulate the fibromuscular proliferative response of the vessel wall.

Systemic administration of several drugs acting on one component of this entire cascade: heparin, abciximab, angiotensin-converting enzyme (ACE)-inhibitors, hirudin, angiopeptin, tranilast, nitric oxide donors, etc. showed good potency in animal studies, but all failed in the clinic.[6,7] This was probably due to inefficient local drug concentrations and an inappropriate knowledge of the complex restenosis pathophysiology in humans at that time. Moreover, in view of the multitude of cellular processes evoked by the vascular injury and the redundancy of mediators within each cascade, it can be anticipated that drugs acting on a single target (e.g. ACE) are not capable to sufficiently suppress the cascade of events that lead to restenosis. This view is supported by the observation that local intracoronary radiation therapy (brachytherapy), a very local approach acting by inhibiting cell-signaling, protein biosynthesis as well as cell proliferation, showed initially very promising results, in contrast to the 'clean' and specific drugs studies so far.[8,9] However, at later follow-up serious adverse effects such as delayed intimal thickening, delayed endothelial regeneration, late total occlusions and exaggerated tissue proliferation at the edges of the stent (the so called 'candy wrapper'), are now emerging.[10–12] Therefore, the combination of a stent together with local application of a wide acting pharmacological agent on top of it, could become a potential alternative for the prevention of in-stent restenosis. Both sirolimus[13] and paclitaxel[14] inhibit a large series of cell functions, important in neointima formation, due to their mode of action. Sirolimus is a pleiotropic macrolide antibiotic which shows, besides immunosuppression, a remarkable inhibition of SMC proliferation and migration by blocking G_1–S transition.[15] Paclitaxel, on the other hand, is a widely used anticancer agent which increases the assembly of dysfunctional and extraordinarily stable microtubules, thereby also reducing various cell functions, such as proliferation, migration, and signal transduction.[16]

The actin skeleton of the cell is another component which is involved in several cell functions including cytokinesis, cell migration, DNA replication, and cell cycle progression. All these processes are involved in the in-stent restenosis pathophysiology. Therefore, actin-skeleton inhibitors could be potential candidates for the prevention of in-stent restenosis. The goals of this chapter are threefold: (1) to give a brief overview of actin molecules and their function in general cell physiology; (2) to discuss two groups of actin-skeleton inhibitors – cytochalasins and latrunculins; and (3) to review preliminary results of these actin-skeleton inhibitors in the prevention of in-stent restenosis.

STRUCTURE, ORGANIZATION, AND FUNCTION OF ACTIN FILAMENTS

The actin molecule is the most important protein of the cytoskeleton of most eukaryotic cells (comprising typically 5–10% of total protein). Mammals have six distinct actin genes: four expressed in muscular cell types and two in non-muscle cells. All of the actins, however, are very similar in amino acid sequence and have been highly conserved throughout the evolution of eukaryotes. Individual actin molecules are globular proteins of 375 amino acids (43 kDa, G-actin). Globular G-actin monomers consist of a small and a large domain, with each domain further subdivided into two subdomains (Figure 28.1).[17] The small domain contains the subdomain 1 [with both the amino- (–) and carboxy- (+) terminus of actin] and subdomain 2, and the large domain consists of the subdomains 3 and 4.[18] In between the small and the large domain is a cleft with high affinity binding sites for one adenosine 5'-triphosphate (ATP) molecule or divalent cations, such as as Ca^{2+} or Mg^{2+}.

Each globular G-actin has tight binding sites that mediate head-to-tail interaction with two other actin monomers, first slowly forming a small aggregate of two and then three monomers (called 'nucleation') (Figure 28.1).[19–22] Finally, further reversible addition of monomers at both ends of the molecule leads to the formation of actin filaments (filamentous F-actin, or microfilaments), with a positive ('barbed') end growing five to ten times faster than the negative ('pointed') end. The actin filaments are thin, flexible fibers approximately 7 nm in diameter and up to several micrometers in length. During the assembly, each actin monomer is rotated by 166 degrees in the filaments, which therefore have the appearance of a double-stranded helix. Because all the actin filaments are orientated in the same direction, actin filaments have a distinct polarity. As already mentioned, actin monomers also bind ATP, which is hydrolyzed to ADP following filament assembly. Although ATP is not required for polymerization, actin monomers to which ATP is bound polymerize more readily than those to which adenosine 5'-diphosphate (ADP) is bound. Moreover, ATP-actin dissociates less readily than ADP-actin, resulting in a different concentration of monomers needed at either end of the filament (called the 'treadmilling' phenomenon). Therefore, ATP binding and hydrolysis play a key role in regulating the assembly and dynamic behavior of actin filaments.

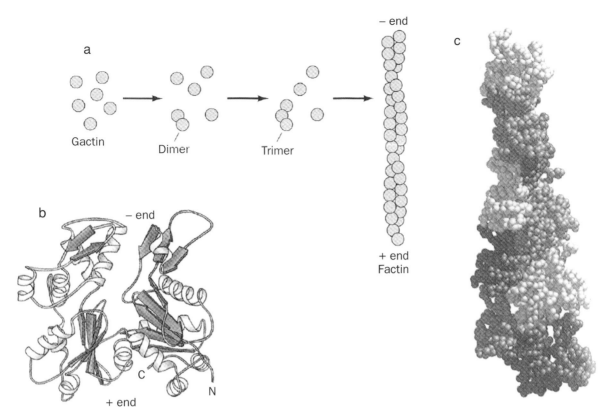

Fig. 28.1 Assembly and structure of actin filaments. (a) Actin monomers (G-actin) first form dimers and trimers, which then grow by the addition of monomers to both ends. (b) Structure of an actin monomer. (c) 3-D figure of an actin filament. (From Cooper G. M. *The Cell: A molecular approach*. Oxford University Press 1997.)

Because actin polymerization is reversible, filaments can depolymerize by the dissociation of actin subunits, predominantly at the negative end, allowing actin filaments to be broken down when necessary. Thus an apparent equilibrium exists between the actin monomers and filaments, which is dependent on the concentration of free actin monomers. This equilibrium resembles the critical concentration of free monomers when the rate of actin polymerization equals the rate of dissociation.[19] Also, the ionic strength of the environment influences the equilibrium between monomers and filaments, where the former are obtained in low salt buffers and the latter predominantly found in more physiological salt concentrations. Finally, temperature and divalent cation (Ca^{2+} and Mg^{2+}) concentrations play a pivotal role

here. However, the fact that, in vivo, the rate of polymerization is 100-fold greater than the steady state rate in vitro, indicates that the process is regulated by other factors than just free actin monomeric concentration. This regulation is performed by the so-called actin-binding proteins.[21] Within the cell, these proteins can act either by binding and sequestering actin monomers (as β-thymosin or profilin), thereby preventing their incorporation into filaments, or by binding or capping the ends of filaments and promoting (such as the Arp2/3 complex) or preventing as such further monomer addition (such as gelsolin or CapZ). Some of these proteins on their turn also promote the assembly (such as profilin) or disassembly (such as gelsolin or ADP/cofilin).[23] Sequestration of monomeric actin by these actin-binding proteins allows the cell to maintain a pool of unpolymerized actin, which is thus available to be incorporated into filaments when needed.

Within the cell, the actin filaments are organized into higher order structures, forming bundles or three-dimensional networks with the properties of semisolid gels. In bundles, the actin filaments are cross-linked into closely parallel arrays. In networks, the actin filaments are loosely cross-linked in three-dimensional orthogonal arrays. Actin filaments are particularly abundant beneath the plasma membrane, where they form a network that provides mechanical support. Actin filaments could also be organized into the so-called focal adhesion sites, which are discrete regions of the cell membrane that serve as attachment sites for large bundles of actin filaments ('stress fibers').[24] Thus, independent of its mechanical strength determining cell shape, the actin-skeleton forms a continuous, dynamic connection between nearly all cellular structures, and they present an enormous surface area on which proteins and other cytoplasmic components can dock.[25] The actin-skeleton allows, therefore, contact and movement of the cell surface, thereby enabling cells to contract (i.e. in muscular cells, in association with myosin), to migrate (i.e. invasion of tissues by white blood cells, the migration of fibroblasts during wound healing, phagocytosis by macrophages),[26–28] to engulf particles, and to divide (i.e. actin forms the contractile ring that divides the cell in two parts during cytokinesis following mitosis).[29,30] Besides these well known actions of the actin filaments, new cell functions were recently discovered wherein these filaments play a pivotal role. First, because the cytoskeleton is the only cellular structure directly linking the cell surface to the nucleus, a well organized cytoskeleton is of particular interest in growth factor-dependent cell cycle progression.[25,31,32] Second, the actin cytoskeleton on itself, acts as a checkpoint during cell division.[33] Third, they also are involved in mRNA regulation (i.e. localization and translational control). These are important for protein synthesis.[34–37] Many signal transduction pathways, involving several guanosine 5'-phosphate (GTP)-proteins, protein kinases, phosphoinositide kinases, and protein phosphatases, require an intact actin cytoskeleton.[25,32] Finally, some evidence was given that actin filaments are also required in the apoptosis process.[25,38–40] Therefore, in conclusion, the actin cytoskeleton is involved in fundamental processes associated with in-stent restenosis, as cell migration, cell proliferation, cell replication, protein synthesis, cell signaling, etc.[5] Inhibitors of the actin-skeleton could therefore mean potential candidates for the inhibition of in-stent restenosis.

TWO GROUPS OF ACTIN-SKELETON INHIBITORS

Cytochalasins

The cytochalasins are a group of small, naturally occurring, fungal metabolites derived from either *Helminthosporium dematioideum* (cytochalasin A and B) or *Metharrhizium anisopliae* (cytochalasin D). They bind (or 'cap') reversibly to the fast growing 'barbed' end of the F-actin filaments, thereby inhibiting both the association and the dissociation of G-actin monomers at that end. The stoichiometry of binding is about one cytochalasin molecule per actin filament.[41–43] In vitro experiments showed that the D-form (Figure 28.2) was the most active form, being 10 times more effective than the B-form, with a half maximal inhibition of actin elongation at the barbed end of 0.02 μM for cytochalasin D and 0.1 μM for cytochalasin B.[44,45] Moreover, cytochalasin D, in contrast to the other forms, is specific for actin, with a dissociation constant of only K_d = 2 nM. Other actin-related activities of cytochalasins include: (1) the rapid and loosely binding to actin monomers (with a higher K_d = 18 μM), forming a dimer and inducing a conformational change of the complex to a state that the cytochalasin is bound more tightly with a subsequent acceleration of the initial rate of actin assembly,[46–48] (2) cleavage of the actin filaments,[49–51] and (3) stimulation of the ATPase activity of F-actin.[52] Cytochalasins are also highly lipophilic, permeating cell membranes very rapidly.

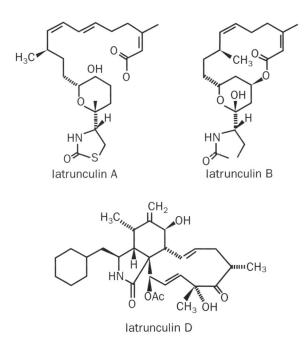

Fig. 28.2 Molecular formulas of the actin-skeleton inhibitors latrunculin A and B and cytochalasin D. (From Spector et al. Cell Motil Cytoskeleton 1989; 13:127–44.[98] © 1989 Reprinted with permission of Wiley-Liss, Inc. a subsidiary of John Wiley & Sons, Inc.)

The effects of cytochalasins on various cell functions have been extensively studied. The earliest effects of cytochalasins were reported by Carter.[53] He documented that in mouse fibroblasts, cytochalasin B induced the formation of ruffled cells and prevented cell growth by inhibiting the cytoplasmic cleavage at a concentration of only 0.5 µg/mL without interfering with nuclear division. Also, cell motility was inhibited at the same concentration. All these effects were reversible after removal of the compound. Later evidence that cytochalasins interfere with cell proliferation, showed that cytochalasin B inhibited the cytokinesis of epithelial cells by the formation of binucleated cells due to aberrant cleavage furrowing and inhibition of contractile ring microfilaments.[54] Later, Ornelles et al. demonstrated that cytochalasin D reversibly inhibited protein synthesis and released mRNA from the cytoskeletal framework in HeLa cells with a K_d of around 50% 1.4×10^{-5}M.[55] Cytochalasin D also inhibits

G_1–S phase cell cycle progression, DNA-, RNA, and protein synthesis in bovine epithelial and endothelial cells and in human dermal fibroblasts.[56–58] Moreover, transformed, malignant cell lines, having a large cell cycle turnover, are more sensitive to cytochalasin treatment than non-transformed cells.[59] Further, Rubtsova et al. showed that disruption of the actin filaments leads to the activation of the $p53$ molecule in rat fibroblasts treated with 1 µg/mL cytochalasin D. These cells underwent G_1–S cell cycle arrest or apoptosis.[60] Very high concentrations of cytochalasin D (100 µM) induce apoptosis in mouse 3C6 T-cells with a subsequent upregulation of the caspase-3 protease.[61] Also, in human airway and renal tubular epithelial cells and in porcine aortic endothelial cells, cytochalasin D induces apoptosis.[62–64] On the other hand, inhibition of actin filament assembly by 10 µM cytochalasin D prevented apoptosis in human B-cells.[65] Finally, cytochalasins also induce DNA fragmentation in various cell lines.[66]

Besides their effect on cell proliferation, DNA-, RNA-, protein synthesis, and apoptosis of various cell lines, cytochalasins also specifically influence certain cell lines which are of importance in the restenosis pathophysiology, such as inflammatory cells, platelets, and endothelial cells.

First, they inhibit the migration and phagocytosis of polymorphonuclear leukocytes and macrophages.[67–69] More recent reports suggest that, although cytochalasins do not inhibit macrophage adhesion, spreading or motility, they do inhibit macrophage fusion towards foreign body giant cells.[70] In a 1 µM concentration, cytochalasin D inhibits the migration of human neutrophils and induced a downregulation of the CD11b/CD18 integrin in these cells.[71] The transendothelial migration of monocytes is also inhibited by cytochalasin B.[72]

Second, the effects of cytochalasins on platelet function are diverse and partly contradictory. In thrombin-stimulated human platelets, 10^{-6} M cytochalasin D inhibited actin polymerization and also induces depolymerization of actin filaments formed during platelet shape change. However, no effects were seen on unstimulated platelets.[73–75] Also, no effect was seen of cytochalasin B on platelet [14C]-serotonin release.[76] On the other hand, Ruf et al. demonstrated that 0.1 μM cytochalasin D inhibited platelet degranulation and [3H]-serotonin release in unstimulated human platelets, whereas the opposite effects were seen in thromboxane-stimulated platelets (i.e. an enhanced degranulation and increased [3H]-serotonin release).[77] These data, later confirmed by Muallem et al., showed that actin filament disassembly is the final trigger for exocytosis in nonexcitable cells.[78] The degranulation of stimulated mast cells was also enhanced by cytochalasin D.[79] Also, the store-mediated Ca^{2+} entry, which plays a role in the activation of platelets and the secretion of granules, can be reduced to 50% by a long (40 min), but not a brief (1 min) exposure to cytochalasin D.[80] Finally, although cytochalasins D and E inhibit the fibrinogen redistribution and its binding to the $\alpha_{IIb}\beta_3$ receptor (glycoprotein IIb/IIIa) in activated platelets and thus inhibited platelet spreading in vitro, contradictory cytochalasin D also enhances the binding of fibrinogen to the $\alpha_{IIb}\beta_3$ receptor in unstimulated platelets.[81–83] Also the recruitment but not the activation of the $\alpha_{IIb}\beta_3$ receptor can be inhibited by cytochalasin D.[84] Although platelet aggregation could be inhibited by cytochalasin E in a dose-dependent manner, this effect was not shown by the B- or D-form.[76,82,84] Moreover, the platelet aggregation induced by von Willebrand factor (vWf) and high shear stress could even be enhanced by cytochalasin D.[85]

Third, vascular smooth muscle cell (SMC) migration is selectively and dose-dependently inhibited by cytochalasin D in a modified Boyden-chamber assay.[86] At a concentration of 10^{-7} M, this was already reduced by 20% and a complete inhibition was seen at 10^{-6} M cytochalasin D. Also, the outgrowth of α-SMC-actin positive cells in vitro was inhibited in the same manner.[86] Moreover, the expression of markers of cell differentiation can be altered by cytochalasin D in SMC.[87,88] Our group also demonstrated that SMC proliferation was dose-dependently reduced by cytochalasin D, estimated by both counting cells as using bromo-deoxyuridin-labeling (Salu et al., un-published data). Proliferation was almost completely (>80%) reduced at 10^{-6}M cytochalasin D (Figure 28.3). Also, stretch-induced extracellular signal-regulated kinases (ERKs) activation, known to play a role in cell growth in general and in the vascular remodeling process more specifically, is also inhibited by cytochalasin D.[89] The D-form also inhibits the activation of L-type Ca^{2+} channels, whereas the microtubule stabilizer paclitaxel (taxol) had no effect.[90] The inhibition due to cytochalasin incubation in vitro of Ca^{2+} regulation and signal transduction in SMCs was further shown by Tseng et al.[91] Finally, cytochalasins also depress the contraction and relaxation in rabbit and rat aortic rings.[86,92,93] A fourth and final group of important cell lines in the restenosis pathophysiology, are the endothelial cells (ECs). Only a few effects of cytochalasins on ECs are known: (1) the prostaglandin (E_2 and I_2) synthesis and release of human umbilical vein endothelial cells can be inhibited by the disruption of the actin-cytoskeleton;[94] and (2) cytochalasins also increase the number of fenestrae in rat liver sinusoidal endothelial cells.[95]

Latrunculins

The latrunculins are marine compounds isolated from the Red Sea sponge *Latrunculia magnifica*.[96] Two naturally occurring forms are known, the A- and B-forms (see Fig. 28.2). Latrunculins cause major but reversible alterations in the organization of the actin filaments, with the A-form being two to three times more potent than the B-form.[97] More importantly, effects on mouse neuroblastoma and fibroblasts showed that latrunculin A was even 10 to 20 times more potent than cytochalasin D, the most active cytochalasin.[97,98] Recently, new forms were synthesized (G-, H-, and I-forms), having even more drastic effects on the morphology and actin arrangement than the natural forms. The latrunculins form rapidly and specifically a 1:1 molar complex with the G-actin monomer, by mimicking the activity of monomer sequestering proteins (such as β-thymosin).[99] Thus, by sequestration of monomeric actin, the latrunculins remove the bound G-actin from the pool

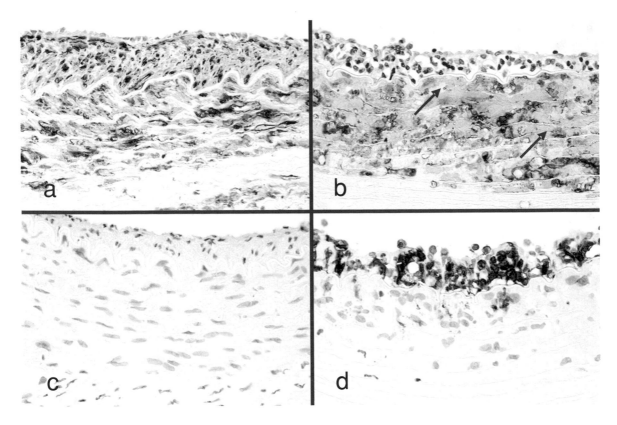

Fig. 28.3 Photomicrographs of control (saline; a, c) and cytochalasin D (10^{-4} M) treated rabbit carotid arteries in a collar model. (a) and (b), α-SMC-actin staining. Arrows indicate loose actin staining in the cytochalasin treated vessels. (c) and (d) CD-43 immunostaining. (From Bruijns RH, Bult H. Br J Pharmacol 2001; 134:473–83.[86])

of polymerizable actin, thereby inhibiting its polymerization and promoting the depolymerization of F-actin. For latrunculin A, which acts as a wedge that restricts the rotation of subdomains 2 and 4 of the G-actin monomer necessary for actin polymerization, a dissociation constant for the binding with G-actin of 0.2 μM was found.[100–102] In vitro effects of latrunculins include:

- The complete but reversible inhibition of cytokinesis, cell growth, DNA synthesis and cell motility in mouse and human fibroblasts and neuroblastoma cells.[57,98]
- Inhibition of phagocytosis by macrophages, as well as their fusion to giant cells, but not their adhesion, spreading or motility.[70,103]

- The inhibition of the transendothelial migration of monocytes.[72]
- The inhibition of egg fertilization in mice.[104]
- The inhibition of SMC differentiation.[87,88]
- A dose-dependent inhibition of SMC proliferation, with almost complete (>80%) inhibition at 10^{-6} M latrunculin A (Salu et al., unpublished data).
- The increased binding of fibrinogen to the $\alpha_{IIb}\beta_3$ receptor in human platelets.[83]
- The increase of vWf-induced platelet aggregation.[85]
- The increase of the number of fenestrae in rat liver sinusoidal endothelial cells.[95]
- The inhibition of the prostaglandin (E_2 and I_2) synthesis and release by human umbilical vein endothelial cells.[94]

Other actin-skeleton inhibitors

Recently, new naturally occurring antiactin drugs were discovered and isolated from several sponges.[99] The jasplakinolides were isolated from the Indo-Pacific sponge *Jaspis johnstoni*. They promote the polymerization of purified actin, stabilize actin filaments, and bind to F-actin with a K_d of 15 nM. They also cause a rapid nucleation of the actin polymerization and markedly lower the critical concentration of actin. They are very lipophilic and thus readily enter mammalian cells. Swinholide and misakinolide A were first isolated from the marine sponge *Theonella swinhoei*. Both bind to two actin monomers with high affinity (K_d around 50 nM), and prevent as such the actin subunits from participating in either actin filament nucleation or elongation reactions. Swinholide severs actin filaments and misakinolide caps the rapidly growing barbed ends of filaments. Mycalolides and aplyronines are marine macrolides isolated from several Pacific sponges. They inhibit actin polymerization by sequestration of actin monomers. They also induce rapid deploymerization of F-actin, suggesting that they may sever actin filaments. Halichondramide is another macrolide from the latter group, which exhibits barbed-end capping and F-actin severing activity. Finally, pectenotoxins are a family of macrolide toxins derived from the digestive glands of toxic shellfish. They sequester monomeric actin with a K_d of 20 nM, but do not possess severing or capping activity. All these compounds are still under investigation, but they all block cytokinesis, alter cell shape, and disrupt the organization of actin in a variety of cell types in a concentration- and time-dependent manner.[99] So also these drugs, could have potential benefit in the prevention of in-stent restenosis.

RESTENOSIS AND ACTIN-SKELETON INHIBITORS

The first studies of actin-skeleton inhibitors in the prevention of restenosis were done by Kunz et al. in the mid 1990s. During that time,

considerable interest was growing in the prevention of restenosis after balloon angioplasty, predominantly characterized by the late remodeling of the vessel wall.[105] They demonstrated that, using a microporous local drug delivery catheter, a single local application of 1 μg/mL cytochalasin B for 1.5–3 minutes immediately following balloon traumatization of pig femoral arteries, resulted in a sustained dilatation of these injured artery segments at 3 week follow-up.[106] Assessed by both angiographic and morphometrical analysis, an increase in luminal area of $140 \pm 27\%$ in cytochalasin B was seen compared to $20 \pm 17\%$ in control, untreated arteries. At 8 week follow-up, this significant increase in lumen was maintained. Proliferation of vascular SMCs, however, was not altered using this approach. The preliminary results in this peripheral pig model were later confirmed in porcine coronary arteries. Using the same catheter, the single local application of a low dose (0.1 μg/mL) or a high dose (1.5 μg/mL) cytochalasin B, resulted 3 weeks later in a lumen area of 55.8% (44.2% stenosis) in the saline control group, 92.1% (7.9% stenosis, $p<0.01$) in the low dose group, and 112.4% (12.4% dilatation, $p = 0.001$) in the high dose group. So application of the low dose resulted in the inhibition of restenosis and the high dose even resulted in an increase in luminal area, resulting in a chronic positive remodeling despite intimal proliferation.[107]

Based on these promising animal data, a small randomized, double blind, placebo-controlled, dose-finding clinical trial was started with 43 patients enrolled.[108] These patients were divided into two groups: 30 patients received cytochalasin B; and 13 received placebo (i.e. saline) using a microporous local drug delivery catheter. The treatment group was further stratified into four subgroups, respectively 0.1 μg/mL ($n = 8$), 0.5 μg/mL ($n = 8$), 1.5 μg/mL ($n = 8$), and 8.0 μg/ml ($n = 8$). The microporous balloon was inflated immediately after balloon angioplasty between 4 atm and 5 atm for 90 seconds. This inflation protocol delivered between 9 mL and 24 mL (at a flow rate of 6 to 18 mL/min) of the study drug to the treatment site, although in practice a wide variability in drug delivery rate was seen from patient to patient. Immediately after infusion, the mean lumen diameter (MLD) was significantly larger in the cytochalasin B group overall (1.86 ± 0.44 vs 1.49 ± 0.63 mm, $p = 0.03$). Only 17 patients underwent follow-up angiography at 4 or 6 week follow-up. They showed a paradoxical, although statistically non-significant (ns), trend towards less lumen gain (thus smaller improvement) in the treatment group compared towards the placebo group 0.09 ± 0.31 vs 0.42 ± 0.46, $p = $ ns. Yet, clinical restenosis, defined as >50% follow-up diameter stenosis, was 18% in the treatment group and 22% in the placebo group ($p = $ ns). The combined clinical study endpoint (death, non-fatal myocardial infarction, and/or repeat coronary revascularization) also showed a favorable trend towards less events in the treatment group (20%), as compared to the placebo group (38%) ($p = $ ns). The biochemical and electrocardiographic variables were not different among both groups. In their discussion, the authors explained the immediate larger MLD as a result of an additional biologic activity of the cytochalasins, namely its interference with platelet function.[81] Also the prevention of the postinjury vasospasm ('the acute recoil') by the inhibition of SMC contraction could have attributed to this beneficial effect.[86,93] The fact that at 4–6 week follow-up there was less gain in the MLD in the treatment group, was attributed to the fact that the drug-induced inhibition of remodeling not only involved blocking the short-term favorable but also the long-term unfavorable changes in MLD. In conclusion, this was not a rather convincing phase I study, with the consequence that no further studies were developed to prove that local cytochalasin delivery has its place in the prevention of restenosis. Probably the main reason for the failure lies in the fact that in using local drug delivery balloons only a very small fraction (<2.5%) of the drug is actually deposited within the arterial wall, with the remainder predominantly washed downstream into the systemic circulation.[109] Furthermore, the drug was not applied

in conjunction with a stent to inhibit acute recoil and late constrictive remodeling.

Bruijns and Bult used another approach for local delivery of cytochalasin D, namely, the perivascular infusion via a collar in the rabbit carotid artery.[86] Silicone collars were placed around rabbit carotid arteries, which were connected to subdermally placed osmotic mini-pumps containing cytochalasin D in various doses (10^{-8}–10^{-4} M). Collars were left in place for 14 days, and afterwards the arterial segments were removed and histologically and morphometrically analyzed. Although intimal hyperplasia was not inhibited after 14 days, the 10^{-5} M and 10^{-4} M doses caused an intima that was free of SMCs (see Figure 28.3). As cytochalasin D in their model had no effect on cell proliferation, they concluded that also in vivo, SMC migration was inhibited. Another finding was that the deeper layers of the media and the adventitia were free of leukocytes in the highest cytochalasin D treatment, suggesting paralysis of leukocytes infiltrating the vessel wall from the lumen. On the other hand, the fact that intimal hyperplasia was not reduced in this study, was explained as a consequence of the greater inflammatory response evoked by the drug eluting collar cuffs. Indeed, instead of containing SMCs, the intima of these vascular segments contained predominantly leukocytes (see Figure 28.3).

As this perivascular approach failed to prevent intimal hyperplasia, we evaluated an intramural delivery of cytochalasin D using a rigid stent platform in a porcine coronary in-stent restenosis model. Using the direct stent coating approach, we placed randomly 12 cytochalasin D-coated stents and 12 control (ethanol dipped only) stents in the right or left coronary artery.[110] Direct coating involved dipping the coronary stents in an ethanolic 1 mg/ml cytochalasin D solution for 1 minute, which were afterwards immediately air-dried. The dip-coating technique allows the drug to have immediate contact with the vessel wall, favoring rapid uptake by the arterial tissue, and does not have possible inflammatory responses as seen with the use of polymers.[111] Doing so, we applied 2 μg cytochalasin D on a stent, which was already after 2 hours completely eluted from the stent when placed in a physiological solution in vitro. Not withstanding this fast release in vitro, the quantitative angiographical analysis at 6 week follow-up showed a decreased late lumen loss in cytochalasin D-treated vessels (0.05 ± 0.04 vs 0.19 ± 0.05 mm, $p = 0.05$) compared to control segments. Morphometrical analysis of cross-sections of the stented coronary arteries also showed favorable results: a decreased intimal area (0.93 ± 0.09 vs 1.29 ± 0.14 mm^2, $p<0.05$), a decreased intimal thickness (200 ± 15 vs 264 ± 27 μm, $p<0.05$), a reduced percentage stenosis (14 ± 1 vs $21 \pm 3\%$, $p<0.005$), and a slightly larger luminal area (5.91 ± 0.24 vs 5.40 ± 28 mm^2, $p<0.05$) were seen in cytochalasin D-treated vessels compared to control segments (Figure 28.4). Moreover, histological analysis showed, as well as similar injury scores (1.48 ± 0.05 vs 1.53 ± 0.07, $p = 0.58$),[112] a favorable trend towards a smaller inflammatory response, as shown by the tendency to a reduced inflammation score in the cytochalasin D-coated stents (0.07 ± 0.03 vs 0.20 ± 0.09, $p = 0.12$).[113] No edge effects or thromboses were seen, and the stents were completely covered by endothelium. In conclusion, this study proved that local drug delivery of cytochalasins using a stent platform can be an interesting approach to inhibit restenosis. Further studies are, however, necessary to investigate optimized doses, toxicity and the pharmacokinetics of cytochalasins in the vascular wall. Also, longer follow-up studies and more controlled release forms, as polymers, should be evaluated in the future before clinical studies of cytochalasin coated stents can even be considered.

Using the same direct coating technique in the same model, we also evaluated whether latrunculin A could be used for the prevention of in-stent restenosis. Latrunculin A (1.5 μg) was applied to coronary stents, showing complete release after 4 hours incubation in physiological salt in vitro. At 6 week follow-up, quantitative angiographic analysis showed a reduced late lumen loss (-0.03 ± 0.20 vs 0.23 ± 0.029 mm, $p<0.05$) and percentage steno-

sis (15 ± 5 vs $30 \pm 14\%$, $p<0.005$) in latrunculin A-treated segments ($n = 11$) compared to control vessels ($n = 11$). However, morphometrical analysis showed similar intimal areas (1.50 ± 0.79 vs 1.60 ± 1.09 mm^2, $p = 0.68$) in both groups. The reasons for this discrepancy between quantitative coronary analysis (QCA) and morphometry are not clear. However, an increased injury score in the latrunculin A group (1.44 ± 0.46 vs 1.16 ± 0.28, $p<0.01$) was seen compared to control segments. This resulted in a reduced intima/injury value (1.0 ± 0.4 vs 1.3 ± 0.8 mm^2, $p = 0.08$) in the latrunculin A group. No edge effects or thromboses were seen, and vWf immunostaining showed complete re-endothelization at 6 weeks in both groups. Therefore, the applied dose, although showing the same inhibition of SMC proliferation in vitro and being, in the literature, 10–20 times as potent as cytochalasin D,[97,98] was insufficient for the inhibition of intimal hyperplasia in a porcine coronary in-stent restenosis model. Even larger injury scores were seen, suggesting that direct coating with latrunculin A could be deleterious for the vessel wall, even in low doses. Therefore, more controlled release forms, as polymers, need to be evaluated in larger animal studies and also toxicity and pharmacokinetics studies need to be performed in the future.

CONCLUSIONS

Actin-skeleton inhibitors have, due to their mode of action, a wide scale of effects on different cell types that are potentially useful for the inhibition of in-stent restenosis. In addition to suppressing smooth muscle cell (SMC) proliferation and migration, two important early pathophysiological phenomena in in-stent restenosis, they also exert interesting inhibitory effects on thrombocytes, inflammatory cells, and fibroblasts, which are all supposed to play a role in its pathophysiology. Porcine animal studies have shown promising effects, although further studies are absolutely necessary to prove that actin-skeleton inhibitors have their place in the prevention of in-stent restenosis. The future will tell whether they

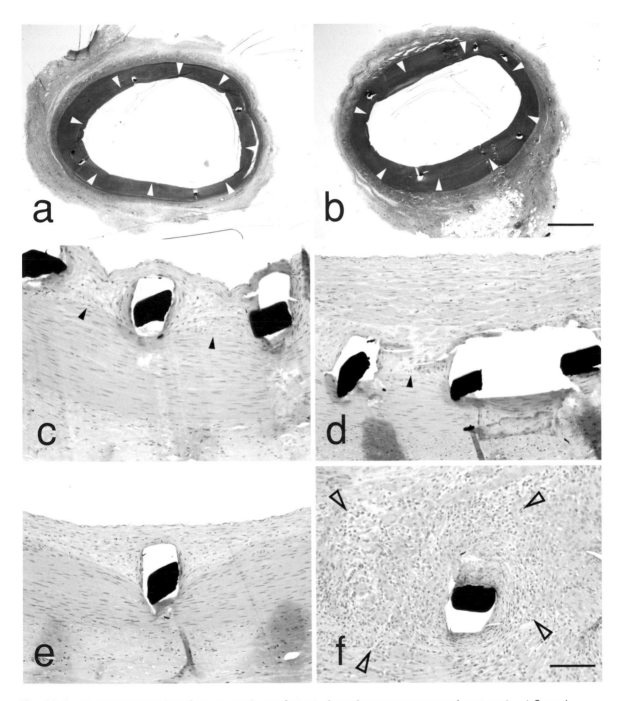

Fig. 28.4 Photomicrographs of cross-sections of stented porcine coronary vessel segments at 6 week follow-up. Cytochalasin D-treated vessels are in the right panels (a, d, f), the controls are in the left panels (a, c, e). (a), (b) Toluidin blue stain. (c–f) Hematoxylin-eosin stain. Bars in (a) and (b) represent 1 mm; in (c)–(f) 100 μm. White arrowheads: IEL, internal elastic lamina. Arrowheads: leukocytes.

may find a niche besides other drugs (i.e. sirolimus, paclitaxel), that currently dictate daily clinical work.

REFERENCES

1. Hoffmann R, Mintz GS. Coronary in-stent restenosis – predictors, treatment and prevention. Eur Heart J 2000; 21:1739–49.
2. Hofma SH, van Beusekom HM, Serruys PW, et al. Recent developments in coated stents. Curr Interv Cardiol Rep 2001; 3:28–36.
3. Serruys PW, de Jaegere P, Kiemeneij F, et al. A comparison of balloon-expandable-stent implantation with balloon angioplasty in patients with coronary artery disease. Benestent Study Group. N Engl J Med 1994; 331:489–95.
4. Fischman DL, Leon MB, Baim DS, et al. A randomized comparison of coronary-stent placement and balloon angioplasty in the treatment of coronary artery disease. Stent Restenosis Study Investigators. N Engl J Med 1994; 331:496–501.
5. Virmani R, Farb A. Pathology of in-stent restenosis. Curr Opin Lipidol 1999; 10:499–506.
6. Bult H. Restenosis: a challenge for pharmacology. Trends Pharmacol Sci 2000; 21:274–9.
7. Gruberg L, Waksman R, Satler LF, et al. Novel approaches for the prevention of restenosis. Expert Opin Investig Drugs 2000; 9:2555–78.
8. Teirstein PS, Massullo V, Jani S, et al. Catheter-based radiotherapy to inhibit restenosis after coronary stenting. N Engl J Med 1997; 336:1697–703.
9. Teirstein PS, Massullo V, Jani S, et al. Three-year clinical and angiographic follow-up after intracoronary radiation: results of a randomized clinical trial. Circulation 2000; 101:360–5.
10. Costa MA, Sabat M, van der Giessen WJ, et al. Late coronary occlusion after intracoronary brachytherapy. Circulation 1999; 100:789–92.
11. Albiero R, Nishida T, Adamian M, et al. Edge restenosis after implantation of high activity (32)P radioactive beta-emitting stents. Circulation 2000; 101:2454–7.
12. Verin V, Popowski Y, de Bruyne B, et al. Endoluminal beta-radiation therapy for the prevention of coronary restenosis after balloon angioplasty. N Engl J Med 2001; 344:243–9.

13. Sousa JE, Costa MA, Abizaid AC, et al. Sustained suppression of neointimal proliferation by sirolimus-eluting stents: one-year angiographic and intravascular ultrasound follow-up. Circulation 2001; 104:2007–11.
14. Honda Y, Grube E, de La Fuente LM, et al. Novel drug-delivery stent: intravascular ultrasound observations from the first human experience with the QP2-eluting polymer stent system. Circulation 2001; 104:380–3.
15. Gallo R, Padurean A, Jayaraman T, et al. Inhibition of intimal thickening after balloon angioplasty in porcine coronary arteries by targeting regulators of the cell cycle. Circulation 1999; 99:2164–70.
16. Rowinsky EK, Donehower RC. Paclitaxel (taxol). N Engl J Med 1995; 332:1004–14.
17. Bremer A, Aebi U. The structure of the F-actin filament and the actin molecule. Curr Opin Cell Biol 1992; 4:20–6.
18. Kabsch W, Vandekerckhove J. Structure and function of actin. Annu Rev Biophys Biomol Struct 1992; 21:49–76.
19. Korn ED. Actin polymerization and its regulation by proteins from nonmuscle cells. Physiol Rev 1982; 62:672–737.
20. Carlier MF. Control of actin dynamics. Curr Opin Cell Biol 1998; 10:45–51.
21. Cooper JA, Schafer DA. Control of actin assembly and disassembly at filament ends. Curr Opin Cell Biol 2000; 12:97–103.
22. Pantaloni D, Le Clainche C, Carlier MF. Mechanism of actin-based motility. Science 2001; 292:1502–6.
23. Theriot JA. Accelerating on a treadmill: ADF/cofilin promotes rapid actin filament turnover in the dynamic cytoskeleton. J Cell Biol 1997; 136:1165–8.
24. Small JV, Rottner K, Kaverina I. Functional design in the actin cytoskeleton. Curr Opin Cell Biol 1999; 11:54–60.
25. Janmey PA. The cytoskeleton and cell signaling: component localization and mechanical coupling. Physiol Rev 1998; 78:763–81.
26. Stossel TP. On the crawling of animal cells. Science 1993; 260:1086–94.
27. Lauffenburger DA, Horwitz AF. Cell migration: a physically integrated molecular process. Cell 1996; 84:359–69.

28. Mitchison TJ, Cramer LP. Actin-based cell motility and cell locomotion. Cell 1996; 84:371–9.
29. Wessells NK, Spooner BS, Ash JF, et al. Microfilaments in cellular and developmental processes. Science 1971; 171:135–43.
30. Fishkind DJ, Wang YL. New horizons for cytokinesis. Curr Opin Cell Biol 1995; 7:23–31.
31. Assoian RK, Zhu X. Cell anchorage and the cytoskeleton as partners in growth factor dependent cell cycle progression. Curr Opin Cell Biol 1997; 9:93–8.
32. Carpenter CL. Actin cytoskeleton and cell signaling. Crit Care Med 2000; 28:N94–N99.
33. Gachet Y, Tournier S, Millar JB, et al. A MAP kinase-dependent actin checkpoint ensures proper spindle orientation in fission yeast. Nature 2001; 412:352–5.
34. Mochitate K, Pawelek P, Grinnell F. Stress relaxation of contracted collagen gels: disruption of actin filament bundles, release of cell surface fibronectin, and down-regulation of DNA and protein synthesis. Exp Cell Res 1991; 193:198–207.
35. Sundell CL, Singer RH. Requirement of microfilaments in sorting of actin messenger RNA. Science 1991; 253:1275–7.
36. Hesketh J. Translation and the cytoskeleton: a mechanism for targeted protein synthesis. Mol Biol Rep 1994; 19:233–43.
37. Bassell G, Singer RH. mRNA and cytoskeletal filaments. Curr Opin Cell Biol 1997; 9:109–15.
38. Kayalar C, Ord T, Testa MP, et al. Cleavage of actin by interleukin 1 beta-converting enzyme to reverse DNase I inhibition. Proc Natl Acad Sci USA 1996; 93:2234–8.
39. Song Q, Wei T, Lees-Miller S, et al. Resistance of actin to cleavage during apoptosis. Proc Natl Acad Sci USA 1997; 94:157–62.
40. Brown SB, Bailey K, Savill J. Actin is cleaved during constitutive apoptosis. Biochem J 1997; 323(pt 1):233–7.
41. Cooper JA. Effects of cytochalasin and phalloidin on actin. J Cell Biol 1987; 105:1473–8.
42. Wodnicka M. Pierzchalska M, Bereiter-Hahn J, et al. Comparative study on effects of cytochalasins B and D on F-actin content in different cell lines and different culture conditions. Folia Histochem Cytobiol 1992; 30:107–11.
43. Ohmori H, Toyama S, Toyama S. Direct proof that the primary site of action of cytochalasin on cell motility processes is actin. J Cell Biol 1992; 116:933–41.
44. Yahara I, Harada F, Sekita S, et al. Correlation between effects of 24 different cytochalasins on cellular structures and cellular events and those on actin in vitro. J Cell Biol 1982; 92:69–78.
45. Sampath P, Pollard TD. Effects of cytochalasin, phalloidin, and pH on the elongation of actin filaments. Biochemistry 1991; 30:1973–80.
46. Goddette DW, Frieden C. The binding of cytochalasin D to monomeric actin. Biochem Biophys Res Commun 1985; 128:1087–92.
47. Goddette DW, Frieden C. The kinetics of cytochalasin D binding to monomeric actin. J Biol Chem 1986; 261:15970–3.
48. Goddette DW, Frieden C. Actin polymerization. The mechanism of action of cytochalasin D. J Biol Chem 1986; 261:15974–80.
49. Maruyama K, Hartwig JH, Stossel TP. Cytochalasin B and the structure of actin gels: II. Further evidence for the splitting of F-actin by cytochalasin B. Biochim Biophys Acta 1980; 626:494–500.
50. Schliwa M. Action of cytochalasin D on cytoskeletal networks. J Cell Biol 1982; 92:79–91.
51. Urbanik E, Ware BR. Actin filament capping and cleaving activity of cytochalasins B, D, E, and H. Arch Biochem Biophys 1989; 269:181–7.
52. Brenner SL, Korn ED. Stimulation of actin ATPase activity by cytochalasins provides evidence for a new species of monomeric actin. J Biol Chem 1981; 256:8663–70.
53. Carter SB. Effects of cytochalasins on mammalian cells. Nature 1967; 213:261–4.
54. Aubin JE, Osborn M, Weber K. Inhibition of cytokinesis and altered contractile ring morphology induced by cytochalasins in synchronized PtK2 cells. Exp Cell Res 1981; 136:63–79.
55. Ornelles DA, Fey EG, Penman S. Cytochalasin releases mRNA from the cytoskeletal framework and inhibits protein synthesis. Mol Cell Biol 1986; 6:1650–62.
56. Ingber DE, Prusty D, Sun Z, et al. Cell shape, cytoskeletal mechanics, and cell cycle control in angiogenesis. J Biomech 1995; 28:1471–84.

57. Iwig M, Czeslick E, Muller A, et al. Growth regulation by cell shape alteration and organization of the cytoskeleton. Eur J Cell Biol 1995; 67:145–57.

58. Böhmer RM, Scharf E, Assoian RK. Cytoskeletal integrity is required throughout the mitogen stimulation phase of the cell cycle and mediates the anchorage-dependent expression of cyclin D1. Mol Biol Cell 1996; 7:101–11.

59. Stournaras C, Stiakaki E, Koukouritaki SB, et al. Altered actin polymerization dynamics in various malignant cell types: evidence for differential sensitivity to cytochalasin B. Biochem Pharmacol 1996; 52:1339–46.

60. Rubtsova SN, Kondratov RV, Kopnin PB, et al. Disruption of actin microfilaments by cytochalasin D leads to activation of p53. FEBS Lett 1998; 430:353–7.

61. Suria H, Chau LA, Negrou E, et al. Cytoskeletal disruption induces T cell apoptosis by a caspase-3 mediated mechanism. Life Sci 1999; 65:2697–707.

62. DeMeester SL, Cobb JP, Hotchkiss RS, et al. Stress-induced fractal rearrangement of the endothelial cell cytoskeleton causes apoptosis. Surgery 1998; 124:362–71.

63. Anderson RJ, Ray CJ, Popoff MR. Evidence for Rho protein regulation of renal tubular epithelial cell function. Kidney Int 2000; 58:1996–2006.

64. White SR, Williams P, Wojcik KR, et al. Initiation of apoptosis by actin cytoskeletal derangement in human airway epithelial cells. Am J Respir Cell Mol Biol 2001; 24:282–94.

65. Melamed I, Gelfand EW. Microfilament assembly is involved in B-cell apoptosis. Cell Immunol 1999; 194:136–42.

66. Kolber MA, Broschat KO, Landa-Gonzalez B. Cytochalasin B induces cellular DNA fragmentation. FASEB J 1990; 4:3021–7.

67. Zigmond SH, Hirsch JG. Effects of cytochalasin B on polymorphonuclear leucocyte locomotion, phagocytosis and glycolysis. Exp Cell Res 1972; 73:383–93.

68. Klaus GG. Cytochalasin B. Dissociation of pinocytosis and phagocytosis by peritoneal macrophages. Exp Cell Res 1973; 79:73–8.

69. Newman SL, Mikus LK, Tucci MA. Differential requirements for cellular cytoskeleton in human macrophage complement rece. J Immunol 1991; 146:967–74.

70. DeFife KM, Jenney CR, Colton E, et al. Disruption of filamentous actin inhibits human macrophage fusion. FASEB J 1999; 13:823–32.

71. Anderson SI, Hotchin NA, Nash GB. Role of the cytoskeleton in rapid activation of CD11b/CD18 function and its subsequent downregulation in neutrophils. J Cell Sci 2000; 113:2737–45.

72. Kielbassa K, Schmitz C, Gerke V. Disruption of endothelial microfilaments selectively reduces the transendothelial migration of monocytes. Exp Cell Res 1998; 243:129–41.

73. Fox JE, Phillips DR. Inhibition of actin polymerization in blood platelets by cytochalasins. Nature 1981; 292:650–2.

74. Casella JF, Flanagan MD, Lin S. Cytochalasin D inhibits actin polymerization and induces depolymerization of actin filaments formed during platelet shape change. Nature 1981; 293:302–5.

75. Hartwig JH. Mechanisms of actin rearrangements mediating platelet activation. J Cell Biol 1992; 118:1421–42.

76. Kirkpatrick JP, McIntire LV, Moake JL, et al. Differential effects of cytochalasin B on platelet release, aggregation and contractility: evidence against a contractile mechanism for the release of platelet granular contents. Thromb Haemost 1979; 42:1483–9.

77. Ruf A, Patscheke H, Morgenstern E. Role of internalization in platelet activation induced by collagen fibers – differential effects of aspirin, cytochalasin D, and prostaglandin E1. Thromb Haemost 1991; 66:708–14.

78. Muallem S, Kwiatkowska K, Xu X, et al. Actin filament disassembly is a sufficient final trigger for exocytosis in nonexcitable cells. J Cell Biol 1995; 128:589–98.

79. Frigeri L, Apgar JR. The role of actin microfilaments in the down-regulation of the degranulation response in RBL-2H3 mast cells. J Immunol 1999; 162:2243–50.

80. Rosado JA, Sage SO. The actin cytoskeleton in store-mediated calcium entry. J Physiol 2000; 526(pt 2):221–9.

81. Olorundare OE, Simmons SR, Albrecht RM. Cytochalasin D and E: effects on fibrino-

gen receptor movement and cytoskeletal reorganization in fully spread, surface-activated platelets: a correlative light and electron microscopic investigation. Blood 1992; 79:99–109.

82. Fox JE, Shattil SJ, Kinlough-Rathbone RL, et al. The platelet cytoskeleton stabilizes the interaction between alphaIIbbeta3 and its ligand and induces selective movements of ligand-occupied integrin. J Biol Chem 1996; 271:7004–11.

83. Bennett JS, Zigmond S, Vilaire G, et al. The platelet cytoskeleton regulates the affinity of the integrin $\alpha(IIb)\beta(3)$ for fibrinogen. J Biol Chem 1999; 274:25301–7.

84. Addo JB, Bray PF, Grigoryev D, et al. Surface recruitment but not activation of integrin $\alpha_{IIb}\beta_3$ (GPIIb–IIIa) requires a functional actin cytoskeleton. Arterioscler Thromb Vasc Biol 1995; 15:1466–73.

85. Mistry N, Cranmer SL, Yuan Y, et al. Cytoskeletal regulation of the platelet glycoprotein Ib/V/IX-von Willebrand factor interaction. Blood 2000; 96:3480–9.

86. Bruijns RH, Bult H. Effects of local cytochalasin D delivery on smooth muscle cell migration and on collar-induced intimal hyperplasia in the rabbit carotid artery. Br J Pharmacol 2001; 134:473–83.

87. Sotiropoulos A, Gineitis D, Copeland J, et al. Signal-regulated activation of serum response factor is mediated by changes in actin dynamics. Cell 1999; 98:159–69.

88. Mack CP, Somlyo AV, Hautmann M, et al. Smooth muscle differentiation marker gene expression is regulated by RhoA-mediated actin polymerization. J Biol Chem 2001; 276:341–7.

89. Numaguchi K, Eguchi S, Yamakawa T, et al. Mechanotransduction of rat aortic vascular smooth muscle cells requires RhoA and intact actin filaments. Circ Res 1999; 85:5–11.

90. Nakamura M, Sunagawa M, Kosugi T, et al. Actin filament disruption inhibits L-type Ca(2+) channel current in cultured vascular smooth muscle cells. Am J Physiol Cell Physiol 2000; 279:C480–C487.

91. Tseng S, Kim R, Kim T, et al. F-actin disruption attenuates agonist-induced [Ca2+], myosin phosphorylation, and force in smooth muscle. Am J Physiol 1997; 272:C1960–C1967.

92. Dresel PE, Knickle L. Cytochalasin-B and phloretin depress contraction and relaxation of aortic smooth muscle. Eur J Pharmacol 1987; 144:153–7.

93. Saito SY, Hori M, Ozaki H, et al. Cytochalasin D inhibits smooth muscle contraction by directly inhibiting contractile apparatus. J Smooth Muscle Res 1996; 32:51–60.

94. Sawyer SJ, Norvell SM, Ponik SM, et al. Regulation of PGE(2) and PGI(2) release from human umbilical vein endothelial cells by actin cytoskeleton. Am J Physiol Cell Physiol 2001; 281:C1038–C1045.

95. Braet F, De Zanger R, Jans D, et al. Microfilament-disrupting agent latrunculin A induces an increased number of fenestrae in rat liver sinusoidal endothelial cells: comparison with cytochalasin B. Hepatology 1996; 24:627–35.

96. Kashman Y, Groweiss A, Shmueli U. Latrunculin, a new 2-thiazolidinone macrolide from the marine sponge *Latrunculia magnifica*. Tetrahedron Lett 1980; 21:3629–32.

97. Spector I, Shochet NR, Kashman Y, et al. Latrunculins: novel marine toxins that disrupt microfilament organization in cultured cells. Science 1983; 219:493–5.

98. Spector I, Shochet NR, Blasberger D, et al. Latrunculins – novel marine macrolides that disrupt microfilament organization and affect cell growth: I. Comparison with cytochalasin D. Cell Motil Cytoskeleton 1989; 13:127–44.

99. Spector I, Braet F, Shochet NR, et al. New anti-actin drugs in the study of the organization and function of the actin cytoskeleton. Microsc Res Tech 1999; 47:18–37.

100. Coué M, Brenner SL, Spector I, et al. Inhibition of actin polymerization by latrunculin A. FEBS Lett 1987; 213:316–18.

101. Yarmola EG, Somasundaram T, Boring TA, et al. Actin-latrunculin A structure and function. Differential modulation of actin-binding protein function by latrunculin A. J Biol Chem 2000; 275:28120–7.

102. Morton WM, Ayscough KR, McLaughlin PJ. Latrunculin alters the actin-monomer subunit interface to prevent polymerization. Nat Cell Biol 2000; 2:376–8.

103. de Oliveira CA, Mantovani B. Latrunculin A is a potent inhibitor of phagocytosis by macrophages. Life Sci 1988; 43:1825–30.

104. Schatten G, Schatten H, Spector I, et al. Latrunculin inhibits the microfilament-mediated processes during fertilization, cleavage and early development in sea urchins and mice. Exp Cell Res 1986; 166:191–208.

105. Mintz GS, Popma JJ, Pichard AD, et al. Arterial remodeling after coronary angioplasty: a serial intravascular ultrasound study. Circulation 1996; 94:35–43.

106. Kunz LL, Anderson PG, Schroff RW, et al. Sustained dilation and inhibition of restenosis in a pig femoral artery injury model. Circulation 1994; 90(suppl):I-297 (abstract).

107. Kunz LL, Tatalick LM, Anderson PG, et al. Efficacy of cytochalasin B in inhibiting coronary restenosis caused by chronic remodeling after balloon trauma in swine. J Am Coll Cardiol 1995; 25(suppl A):302A (abstract).

108. Lehmann KG, Popma JJ, Werner JA, et al. Vascular remodeling and the local delivery of cytochalasin B after coronary angioplasty in humans. J Am Coll Cardiol 2000; 35:583–91.

109. Camenzind E, Kutryk MJ, Serruys PW. Use of locally delivered conventional drug therapies. Semin Interv Cardiol 1996; 1:67–76.

110. Salu KJ, Yanming H, Bosmans JM, et al. Direct cytochalasin D stent coating inhibits neointimal formation in a porcine coronary model. Circulation 2001; 104:II-506 (abstract).

111. Heldman AW, Cheng L, Jenkins GM, et al. Paclitaxel stent coating inhibits neointimal hyperplasia at 4 weeks in a porcine model of coronary restenosis. Circulation 2001; 103:2289–95.

112. Schwartz RS, Huber KC, Murphy JG, et al. Restenosis and the proportional neointimal response to coronary artery injury: results in a porcine model. J Am Coll Cardiol 1992; 19:267–74.

113. Kornowski R, Hong MK, Tio FO, et al. In-stent restenosis: contributions of inflammatory responses and arterial injury to neointimal hyperplasia. J Am Coll Cardiol 1998; 31:224–30.

29

Local delivery of antisense oligomers to *c-myc* for the prevention of restenosis

Michael JB Kutryk and Patrick W Serruys

Introduction • **Proto-oncogenes** • **Antisense compounds** • **LR-3280 antisense to *c-myc*** • **Phosphorothioate morpholino oligomer antisense to *c-myc*** • **Conclusions**

INTRODUCTION

The focus of the treatment of restenosis over the last two decades has been through the application of pharmacologic active agents and mechanical approaches using a host of different devices. Unfortunately, with only a few exceptions, this frequent and costly complication of percutaneous revascularization techniques has proven refractory to all such therapies. Characteristic of the restenosis process is neointimal proliferation that involves the migration of vascular smooth muscle cells (SMCs) from the media and the adventitia and their intraluminal proliferation and vascular remodeling which potentially involves all three layers of the vessel wall. The inciting stimuli involved in restenosis include disruption of the endothelial barrier layer, mechanical factors which disrupt the medial smooth muscle layer and serve as stimuli for SMC proliferation and migration, and the contact of this disrupted layer with circulating blood factors and mitogens which serve as further stimuli to neointimal formation.

Vascular injury sets into motion a cascade of events that result in the final hyperplastic response shown by the neointima. Early in our understanding of the pathophysiologic processes involved in restenosis, attention was concentrated on factors that interact with SMCs through cell surface receptors. These include compounds like thrombin, platelet-derived growth factor (PDGF), angiotensin-II, interleukin-1, insulin growth factor-1 (IGF-1), basic fibroblast growth factor (bFGF), and a whole host of other mitogenic factors. Initial treatments for restenosis targeted these receptors with pharmacologic agents in an attempt to inhibit their effects. It soon became apparent, however, that none of these stimuli work through a unique pathway. Instead, through the process of signal transduction, these stimuli interact at an intracellular level through second messenger systems, which confers redundancy to the system. Ultimately, these second messenger systems converge on a final common pathway at the cellular DNA level.

PROTO-ONCOGENES

The proto-oncogenes are a family of genes, each of which encodes a protein that is implicated in signal transduction. Signals from a wide variety of sources including the interaction of growth factors with cell surface receptors, activation by trophic factors, such as insulin and cytokines, as well as the binding of adhesion molecules with their corresponding ligands, all converge on this common pathway. An important member of this pathway is the *c-myc* proto-oncogene. The product of the *c-myc* gene, the Myc protein, is in low abundance in adult tissues but its enhanced expression is an early event with peak expression at 2 to 4 hours after angioplasty.[1] Myc regulates the expression of other important proteins including cyclin D1 which initiates the progression of cells through the cell cycle, ICAM-cell adhesion is required for thrombus formation and matrix metalloproteinases are required for vascular wall remodeling. Induction and transcription of the proto-oncogene *c-myc* inexorably commits the cell to at least one round of DNA replication and cell division.

The life cycle of a normal cell can be considered in five different cell phases. G_0 (G = gap) is the quiescent state in which the cell is biologically active but is neither actively dividing nor replicating. Under appropriate stimuli the cell can enter the cell cycle at G_1, or interphase, in which biosynthetic activities of the cell prepare the cell to enter into the next phase of the cell cycle, the S phase. The S phase begins when DNA synthesis starts, and ends when the DNA content of the nucleus has doubled and the chromosomes have replicated. The S phase is followed by G_2, which ends when mitosis starts signaling the start of the M phase. Activation of the cell cycle is responsible both for normal physiological growth and cell division as well as for pathophysiological processes, such as restenosis.

A large number of genes are involved in the control of cell cycle progression in eukaryotic cells. They can be divided into early G_1 genes (such as *c-fos*, *c-myc*, etc.), late G_1 genes (*c-myb*, *Rb*, etc.), genes involved in G_1/S transition (*cdc/ckd* kinases, etc.), S phase genes involved in DNA synthesis (DNA polymerases, PCNA, etc.), genes involved in G_2/M transition (*cdc/ckd* kinases, etc.), and genes involved in mitosis (cytoskeletal proteins, mitosis specific kinases, etc.). In theory, suppression of any one of these genes will lead to interruption of cell cycle progression, a strategy that is being explored for the prevention of restenosis.

ANTISENSE COMPOUNDS

The nucleotide sequence of DNA or RNA that contains the information for the amino acid sequence of the protein is called the sense strand. In double-stranded DNA, the other nucleotide sequence is complementary to the sense strand and is termed the antisense strand. Antisense oligodeoxyribonucleotides (ODNs) are synthetic, relatively short single strands of deoxyribonucleic acid (DNA) with sequences that are complementary to their ribonucleic acid (RNA) targets. Binding of the antisense oligodeoxyribonucleotide to mRNA inhibits translation and the production of protein (Figure 29.1). The theoretical high affinity and sequence specificity of these relatively short sequences of DNA for their target messenger RNA has led to their use as a method of suppressing specific gene products in vitro and in vivo.

The major mechanisms of action of antisense compounds are through the sequence specific interaction with messenger RNA, although sequence specific and sequence non-specific effects for many of the antisense compounds have also been demonstrated (Figure 29.2). On binding to the target, the antisense compound sterically inhibits the interaction of ribosomes with the messenger RNA. Another mechanism of action, which may be as important as the steric inhibition of ribosome binding is a consequence of the DNA/RNA hybrid being more susceptible to degradation by intracellular RNAse than single stranded messenger RNA. The result is an increased clearance of target mRNA from the cell. In principle, any gene may be selected for antisense suppression; inhibition of certain genes will certainly be more biologically effective. Important factors in this regard include the abundance of the messenger RNA, the half-life of the protein product, and

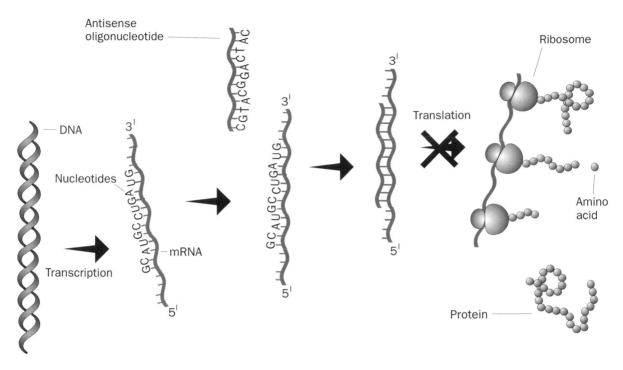

Fig. 29.1 One of the proposed mechanisms of action of antisense deoxyribonucleotides. Normal gene transcription of DNA into mRNA is followed by translation into protein. Antisense oligonucleotides to a complementary portion of the mRNA prevents translation by the steric inhibition of ribosome binding.

the existence of redundancy within the cell, such that other proteins are capable of performing similar functions to that which is targeted. Given these considerations, it is not surprising that most of the attention of antisense technology has been focused on the short-lived regulators of the final common pathway of mitogenic stimuli – the cell cycle. Inhibition of the production of several of the mediators of the cell cycle with antisense oligonucleotides has been shown to be effective for the prevention of restenosis in several different animal models of vascular injury (Table 29.1).

LR-3280 ANTISENSE TO *c-myc*

LR-3280 is a synthetic 15-mer phosphorothioate-modified oligodeoxyribonucleotide (ODN) directed against the 5'-translation-initiation region of the *c-myc* nuclear proto-oncogene with the sequence 5'-AACGTTGAGGGGCAT-3'. Phosphorothioate modification of the oligo-

deoxyribonucleic acid involves replacement of an oxygen atom of the phosphate group with a sulfur atom, which provides increased stability against nucleases (see Figure 29.3). LR-3280 has been reported to:

1. Decrease *c-myc* expression and inhibit growth of rat and human vascular smooth muscle cells (SMCs) in vitro, indicating an important role of *c-myc* activation in the process of SMC proliferation.[1,2] The effect on gene expression was not due to a cytotoxic action of the compound, and could not be prevented by an excess of the sense oligomer. Sense and mismatch oligomers did not inhibit the growth.
2. Inhibit type I and type III collagen secretion of SMCs.[3] The inhibition was sequence- and dose-specific.
3. Reduce neointimal formation when applied in a gel to the adventitial surface of the vessel wall in the rat artery injury model of intimal hyperplasia.[1]

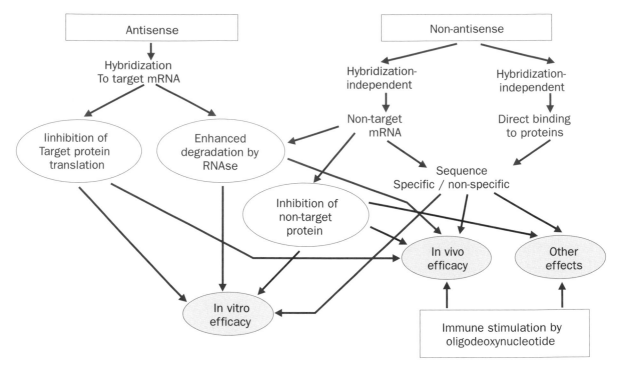

Fig. 29.2 Extra- and intracellular interactions of antisense oligonucleotides. Some of the effects of antisense compounds may be due to non-antisense specific events.

4. Reduce neointimal hyperplasia in a porcine saphenous vein–carotid artery interposition graft model when applied ex vivo.[4]
5. Reduce neointimal formation when intra-luminally delivered locally at the site of postangioplasty, over-stretched porcine coronary arteries.[5] The oligomers persisted at the site of delivery for more than 3 days, but were rapidly cleared from the plasma ($t_{1/2}$ = 12 minutes). A single transcatheter delivery of 1 mg of LR-3280 at the time of the acute injury resulted in a 70% decrease in neointimal area and a 20% increase in lumen area.

Clinical safety of LR-3280 was shown in a multicenter, randomized, controlled, open label, sequential escalating-dose safety study. The oligomer LR-3280 was administered through a guiding catheter directly into the same vessel as the target lesion in low risk patients approximately 15 minutes after balloon angioplasty at 5 centers in Buenos Aires. The study monitored clinical safety immediately post treatment, at 7 days, and at 1, 3, and 6 months. Overall safety was evaluated by clinical laboratory tests, adverse experiences, and clinical outcome. Patients were randomized either to control (no treatment) or LR-3280 treatment. The doses administered were 1 mg (n = 8), 2 mg (n = 8), 4 mg (n = 8), 8 mg (n = 8), and 16 mg (n = 12). In the 16 mg cohort, a few adverse experiences were reported. One patient experienced nausea and vomiting, while a second patient demonstrated a moderate drop in blood pressure immediately following injection of LR-3280, which persisted for 4 hours post treatment. Both of these events were considered 'possibly' related to the trial medication. Based on these experiences, the Safety Review Board (SRB) recommended that an additional six patients be treated with 16 mg. There were no adverse experiences reported in the subsequently treated six patients, however, the SRB felt that prudence should be exercised and the next dose be 24 mg

Table 29.1 In vivo antisense studies

Source	Experimental model	Gene	Delivery vehicle	% intimal suppression
Simons et al.[16]	Rat	c-myb	Pluronic gel	84%
Edelman et al.[17]	Rat	c-myb	Evac	80%
Azrin et al.[18]	Pig	c-myb	Hydrogel catheter	NR
Gunn et al.[19]	Pig	c-myb	None	65%
Bennet et al.[1]	Rat	c-myc	Pluronic gel	53%
Edelman et al.[17]	Rat	c-myc	Evac	90%
Shi et al.[9]	Pig	c-myc	None	70%
Mannion et al.[4]	Pig	c-myc	None	29%
Morishita et al.[20]	Rat	cdc-2/PCNA	Sendai virus/ liposome	68%
Abe et al.[21]	Rat	cdc-2	Pluronic gel	47%
Abe et al.[21]	Rat	cdk-2	Pluronic gel	55%
Morishita et al.[22]	Rat	cdk-2	HVJ	40%
Simons et al.[23]	Rat	PCNA	Pluronic gel	80%
Sirois et al.[24]	Rat	PDGF-β receptor	Evac	70%

HVJ, hemagglutinating virus of Japan; Evac, ethylenevinylacetate; PCNA, proliferating cell nuclear antigen; PDGF, platelet-derived growth factor; NR, not reported.
Modified from: Simons M. Endogenous expression modification: antisense approaches. In March KL (ed), *Gene Transfer in the Cardiovascular System. Experimental Approaches and Therapeutic Implications*. Kluwer: Boston 1997.

and not 32 mg as originally planned. Eight patients were treated with 24 mg, and one of these patients developed a significant skin rash. After reviewing all of the data, it was the conclusion of the investigators that up to 24 mg of LR-3280 was well tolerated despite the minor adverse reactions.

The results of the preclinical efficacy studies, and clinical safety trial supported the use of LR-3280 in a clinical efficacy trial. The ITALICS trial examined the safety and efficacy of LR-3280 for the inhibition of the development of restenosis when given by local delivery immediately after coronary stent implantation using the Transport™ local delivery catheter. A total of 85 patients were randomly assigned to receive either 10 mg of phosphorothioate

modified 15-mer ODN or saline vehicle by intracoronary local delivery after Wallstent™ coronary stent implantation. The primary endpoint was percentage neointimal volume obstruction measured by computerized analysis of ECG-gated intravascular ultrasound (IVUS) at 6 month follow-up. Secondary endpoints included clinical outcome and quantitative coronary angiography analysis. Analysis of follow-up IVUS data was performed on 77 patients. In-stent volume obstruction was similar between groups ($44 \pm 16\%$ and $46 \pm 14\%$, placebo vs ODN; $p = 0.57$; 95% CI, -1.13–0.85). Minimum luminal diameter increased from 0.84 ± 0.36 and 0.90 ± 0.45 ($p = 0.55$) to 2.70 ± 0.37 and 2.80 ± 0.37 ($p = 0.28$) after stent implantation, which decreased to 1.50 ± 0.61

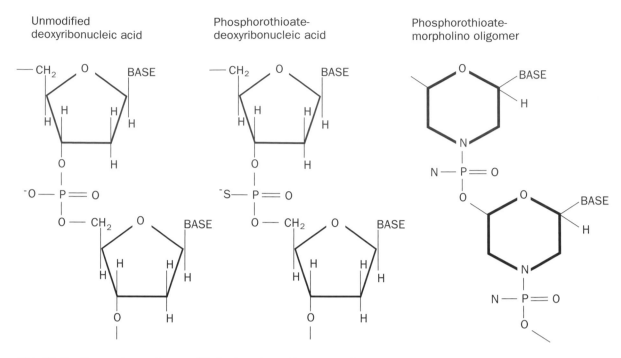

Fig. 29.3 Comparison of unmodified, phosphorothioate-modified and phosphorothioate morpholino oligomers. Phosphorothioate-modification involves substitution of one free oxygen atom of the phosphate by a sulfur atom, providing increased stability against nucleases. Phosphorothioate morpholino oligomers (PMOs) represent an unusual DNA chemistry with a 6-membered morpholino and an uncharged phosphodiester internucleoside linkage. The lack of internucleoside charge allows the PMO to avoid non-specific effects through binding of cellular and extracellular proteins.

and 1.50 ± 0.53 ($p = 0.98$) by 6 months yielding similar loss indices (placebo vs ODN respectively). There were no differences in angiographic restenosis rates (38.5% and 34.2%, $p = 0.81$; placebo vs ODN) or in clinical outcome. The investigators concluded that treatment with 10 mg of phosphorothioate modified ODN directed against *c-myc* did not reduce neointimal volume obstruction or the angiographic restenosis rate in this patient population.

Several reasons for the lack of effect of locally delivered LR-3280 for the prevention of restenosis have been proposed. First, the local concentration of antisense compound achieved may not have been high enough, or maintained long enough, to show a significant effect. Using the same antisense compound and a porous balloon delivery catheter, Shi et al. have shown that the efficiency of delivery is less than 1% in

a swine coronary model of vessel injury.[5] In diseased human vessels, the tissue retention of compound delivered via local intracoronary administration using a coil balloon has been shown to be between 1% and 8% of the initially administered dose.[6] It is possible that the choice of delivery catheters contributed to the apparent lack of effect of LR-3280 and it may be that the use of a delivery device that targets the media could have resulted in higher tissue concentrations of AS-ODNs. It is also possible that delivery into a diseased arterial wall is less efficient that delivery into an injured normal vessel in an animal model.

Second, paradoxically the concentration of LR-3280 may have been too high. It is well recognized that different mechanisms are responsible for the effects of AS-ODNs. In addition to RNA binding, non-antisense effects – both sequence specific (aptamer effect) and sequence independent – are also mediated by AS-ODNs.[7] These effects can be either beneficial or detrimental. It has been suggested that non-sequence specific effects predominate when phosphorothioate AS-ODNs are employed at concentrations higher than 5 μM.[8] It may be that the local concentrations achieved with the administration of 10 mg of compound exceeded 5 μM and detrimental side effects of the antisense compound may have masked any beneficial effects of specific binding to *c-myc* RNA.

Third, the single administration of AS-ODN employed in this trial may not have been effective. It is known that after acute vessel injury, *c-myc* expression shows a biphasic response, with early and late expression peaks.[9–11] The delivered antisense compound may have been effective in suppressing early c-Myc protein production, but washout and degradation may have resulted in tissue concentrations too low to suppress expression by the later peak. Very little is known about the expression of *c-myc* in stented vessels, in which there is protracted vessel injury to the metal scaffold. In this regard, the self-expanding nature of the stent chosen for use in this trial, with its persistent radial strain on the vessel wall, may have further confounded the results.[12]

Finally, it has been shown that the intraluminal delivery of saline using a local delivery device can exaggerate the intimal proliferative response.[13] It is possible that the use of a saline vehicle in the ITALICS trial aggravated the neoproliferative response and masked any beneficial effect of LR-3280.

PHOSPHOROTHIOATE MORPHOLINO OLIGOMER ANTISENSE TO *c-myc*

The development of an antisense compound that appears to overcome many of the pharmaceutical limitations inherent in other antisense approaches and the development of a local delivery device which allows for medial administration of compounds has led to renewed interest into an antisense approach for the prevention of restenosis following coronary interventions. Phosphorothioate morpholino oligomers (PMO) represent an unusual DNA chemistry with a six-membered morpholino and an uncharged phosphodiester internucleoside linkage (Figure 29.3). The lack of internucleoside charge allows the PMO to avoid non-specific effects through binding of cellular and extracellular proteins. The antisense mechanism of action appears to be limited to the PMO hybrid duplex with mRNA, which inhibits its translation.[15]

Preclinical in vitro assessment of antisense PMO to *c-myc* has been performed. Acute studies in pigs have shown that the degree of injury correlates with the expression of *c-myc*, and that after either balloon angioplasty or stent implantation *c-myc* expression was similar. Local delivery of antisense PMO to *c-myc* blocked expression of *c-myc* in a dose-dependent fashion. In vivo assessment of antisense PMO in a porcine model of restenosis has also been performed. Local delivery of 1 mg, 5 mg and 10 mg of antisense PMO in pig coronaries using an Infiltrator catheter has shown a significant reduction in intimal area at 5 mg and 10 mg. These observations provided critical dose justification and delivery validation for further clinical trials antisense PMO to prevent restenosis. A phase II, randomized, evaluator blinded, three arm study of the efficacy of antisense PMO (Resten-NG™, AVI BioPharma) for the prevention of restenosis has been initiated at New York's Lenox Hill Hospital. Resten-NG will be delivered into the coronary arteries of patients undergoing balloon angioplasty. The control group will be treated with the Infiltrator® intramural delivery catheter only and compared to groups treated with 3 mg and 10 mg of antisense PMO. A total of 120 patients will be studied in order to obtain 100 evaluable patients (33 per arm). Patients with both de novo and in-stent restenoses will be included. Angiographic endpoints will be assessed by quantitative coronary angiography and intravascular ultrasound. Clinical endpoints include an assessment of major adverse clinical events at 30 days and 6 months and revascularization rates at 6 months.

CONCLUSIONS

Despite the lack of efficacy of LR-3280 for the prevention of restenosis in clinical trials, promising animal data support the continued investigation of antisense to *c-myc*. With the introduction of newer antisense agents, such as phosphorothioate morpholino oligomers, and the availability of superior drug delivery devices, antisense against *c-myc* may prove clinically effective for the prevention of restenosis.

REFERENCES

1. Bennet MR, Anglin S, McEwan JR, et al. Inhibition of vascular smooth muscle cell proliferation in vitro and in vivo by *c-myc* antisense oligodeoxynucleotides. J Clin Invest 1994; 93:820–8.

2. Shi Y, Hutchinson HG, Hall DJ, Zalewski A. Downregulation of *c-myc* expression by antisense oligonucleotides inhibits proliferation of human smooth muscle cells. Circulation 1993; 88:1190–5.

3. Shi Y, Dodge GR, Hall DJ, et al. Inhibition of type I collagen synthesis in vascular smooth muscle cells by *c-myc* antisense oligomers. Circulation 1994; 90(suppl):I-514.

4. Mannion JD, Ormont ML, Magno MG, et al. Sustained reduction of neointima with *c-myc* antisense oligonucleotides in saphenous vein grafts. Ann Thorac Surg 1998; 66:1948–52.

5. Shi Y, Fard A, Galeo A, et al. Transcatheter delivery of *c-myc* antisense oligomers reduces neointimal formation in a porcine model of coronary artery balloon injury. Circulation 1994; 90:944–51.

6. Camenzind E, Bakker WH, Reijs A, et al. Site-specific intracoronary heparin delivery in man after balloon angioplasty: A radioisotopic assessment of regional pharmacokinetics. Circulation 1997; 96:154–65.

7. Bennett MR, Schwartz SM. Antisense therapy for angioplasty restenosis; some critical considerations. Circulation 1995; 92:1981–93.

8. Stein CA. Does antisense exist? Nature Medicine 1995; 1:119–21.

9. Shi Y, Hutchinson HG, Hall DJ, Zalewski A. Downregulation of *c-myc* expression by antisense oligonucleotides inhibits proliferation of human smooth muscle cells. Circulation 1993; 88:1190–5.

10. Kindy MS, Sonenshein GE. Regulation of oncogene expression in cultured aortic smooth muscle cells. J Biol Chem 1986; 261:12865–8.

11. Gadeau AP, Campan M, Desgranges C. Induction of cell cycle dependent genes during cell cycle progression of arterial smooth muscle cells in culture. J Cell Physiol 1991; 146:356–61.

12. von Birgelen C, Airiian SG, de Feyter PJ, et al. Coronary Wallstents show significant late, post-procedural expansion despite implantation with adjunct high pressure balloon inflations. Am J Cardiol 1998; 82:129–34.

13. Kim WH, Hong MK, Kornowski R, et al. Saline infusion via local drug delivery catheters is associated with increased neointimal hyperplasia in a porcine coronary in-stent restenosis model. Coron Artery Dis 1999; 10:629–32.

14. Morishita R, Gibbons GH, Ellison KE, et al. Single intraluminal delivery of antisense *cdc2* kinase and proliferating-cell nuclear antigen oligonucleotides results in chronic inhibition of neointimal hyperplasia. Proc Natl Acad Sci USA 1993; 90:8474–8.

15. Hudziak RM, Summerton J, Weller DD, Iversen PL. Antiproliferative effects of steric blocking phosphorodiamidate morpholino antisense agents directed against *c-myc*. Antisense Nucleic Acid Drug Dev 2000; 10:163–76.

16. Simons M, Edelman ER, DeKeyser JL, et al. Antisense *c-myb* oligonucleotides inhibit intimal arterial smooth muscle cell accumulation in vivo. Nature 1992; 359:67–70.

17. Edelman ER, Simons M, Sirois MG, Rosenberg RD. *c-Myc* in vasculo-proliferative disease. Circ Res 1995; 76:176–82.

18. Azrin MA, Mitchel JF, Pedersen C. Inhibition of smooth muscle cell proliferation in vivo following local delivery of antisense c-myb oligonucleotide during angioplasty. J Am Coll Cardiol 1994; 23 (suppl):396A (abstract).

19. Gunn J, Holt CM, Shepherd L, et al. Local delivery of *c-myb* antisense attenuates neointimal thickening in porcine model of coronary

angioplasty. J Am Coll Cardiol 1995; 25 (suppl):201A (abstract).

20. Morishita R, Gibbons GH, Ellison KE, et al. Single intraluminal delivery of antisense *cdc2* kinase and proliferating-cell nuclear antigen oligonucleotides results in chronic inhibition of neointimal hyperplasia. Proc Natl Acad Sci USA 1993; 90:8474–8.

21. Abe J, Zhou W, Taguchi J, et al. Suppression of neointimal smooth muscle cell accumulation in vivo by antisense *cdc-2* and *cdk-2* oligonucleotides in rat carotid artery. Biochem Biophys Res Comm 1994; 198:16–24.

22. Morishita R, Gibbons GH, Ellison KE, et al. Intimal hyperplasia after vascular injury is inhibited by antisense cdk-2 oligonucleotides. J Clin Invest 1994; 93:1458–64.

23. Simons M, Edelman ER, Rosenberg RD. Antisense PCNA oligonucleotides inhibit intimal hyperplasia in a rat carotid injury model. J Clin Invest 1994; 93:2351–6.

24. Sirois MG, Simons M, Edelman ER, Rosenberg RD. Platelet release of platelet derived growth factor is required for intimal hyperplasia in rat vascular injury model. Circulation 1994; 90(suppl I):1-511 (abstract).

30

Site-specific delivery of cytostatic agents

Martin Oberhoff, Christian Herdeg, and Karl R Karsch

Introduction • Doxorubicine, cytarabine, etoposide, vincristine • Methotrexate
• All-*trans*-retinoic acid • Colchicine and colchicine analogs • Paclitaxel • Conclusions

INTRODUCTION

The massive smooth muscle cell (SMC) proliferation after percutaneous interventions and especially after stent implantation resulted in the idea that antineoplastic agents might be a promising approach in the search for a solution to the complex problem of restenosis.

In the past, several cytostatic agents have been used preclinically and clinically to prevent restenosis which completely differ in their mode of action. All cytostatic agents have a dose-dependent toxicity which make a systemic therapy difficult and dangerous for the patient. (See Table 30.1.)

DOXORUBICINE, CYTARABINE, ETOPOSIDE, VINCRISTINE

Doxorubicine leads to DNA intercalation with subsequent DNA rupture and inhibition of topoisomerase II. Cytarabine inhibits the DNA polymerase α. Etoposide leads to a complex of topoisomerase II and DNA and subsequent DNA rupture. Vincristine inhibits the production of microtubules and the mitotic spindle.[1,2] All four are strong cytostatic substances and were so far investigated in vitro only and showed dose-dependent significant reduction of SMC growth.[3,4] In a recent study, tissue factor targeted acoustic nanoparticles incorporating doxorubicin inhibited SMC proliferation in a dose-related fashion. The specific binding of nanoparticles to smooth muscle cells was confirmed by nuclear magnetic resonance (NMR) fluorine spectroscopy.[5]

METHOTREXATE

Methotrexate is an inhibitor of the folic acid reductase and leads to an inhibition of purine synthesis. Muller et al. presented the first in vivo results delivering methotrexate to the carotid arteries of pigs. Methotrexate was delivered locally with a total dose of 25 mg using a perforated balloon catheter. The animals were sacrificed 30 days after intervention. They could demonstrate a >1000-fold greater wall concentration compared to the circulating blood. However, there was no significant difference between the methotrexate treated animals and the control. The authors suggested inadequate tissue concentration, non-uniform distribution within the arterial wall, inadequate duration of therapy, the detrimental effects of endothelial cell regeneration as possible explanations for the negative outcome.[6]

Table 30.1 Preclinical and clinical studies on cytostatic agents

Year	Research model	Delivery modality	Compound	Volume/ Conc	Results	Source
1992	Farm pigs	Wolinsky infusion balloon catheter	Methotrexate	4 mL; 25 mg	No effect on neointimal thickness	Muller et al.[6]
1992	Rabbits	Porous balloon catheter	Colchicine	1 mL; 0.1 and 10 μmol/L	No effect on neointimal thickness	Wilensky et al.[14]
1993	Human stenotic SMC	In vitro	Cytarabine Vincristine	0.005–500 μg/mL 0.0001–10 μg/mL	Inhibition of SMC proliferation	Voisard et al.[3]
1994	Bovine aortic SMC	In vitro	Microspheres + hydrophobic Colchicine analog	10–17% of weight	Inhibition of SMC proliferation	March et al.[5]
1995	Human stenotic SMC	In vitro	Colchicine Etoposide Doxorubicin	0.00004–4 pg/mL 0.002–200 μg/mL 0.0005–50 μg/mL	Inhibition of SMC proliferation	Voisard et al.[4]
1995	New Zealand white rabbits	Porous balloon catheter	Colchizine Hydrophobic Colchicine analog Microparticles + Colchicine	0.1–10 μmol/L 10 μmol/L ~10% of weight	No effect on neointima formation	Gradus-Pizlo et al.[16]
1997	Human SMC and EC	In vitro	Paclitaxel	0.1–10 μmol/L	Dose-dependent inhibition of SMC growth	Axel et al.[9]
1999	Domestic pigs	Double balloon catheter (before stent implantation)	Paclitaxel	10 mL; 10 μmol/L	No inhibition of neointima formation	Oberhoff et al.[22]

Table 30.1 *Continued*

Year	Research model	Delivery modality	Compound	Volume/ Conc	Results	Source
2000	New Zealand rabbits	Double balloon catheter	Paclitaxel	10 mL; 10 μmol/L	Inhibition of neointima formation, enlargement of vessel area	Herdeg et al.[21]
2000	Domestic pigs	Intrapericardial delivery	Paclitaxel	10–50 mg	Inhibition of neointima formation, enlargement of vessel area	Hou et al.[24]
2000	Domestic pigs	Double balloon catheter	Paclitaxel	10 mL; 10 μmol/L	Inhibition of neointima formation, enlargement of vessel area	Oberhoff et al.[23]

SMC, smooth muscle cell; EC, endothelial cell.

ALL-*trans*-RETINOIC ACID

All-*trans*-retinoic acid (atRA) is a naturally occurring metabolite of vitamin A. Mediated by nuclear receptors, retinoids are key elements in the regulation of cellular proliferation and differentiation on a genetic basis.[7,8] In vitro it could be demonstrated that atRA was able to inhibit human SMC proliferation and migration in mono- and coculture systems together with extracellular matrix (ECM) formation and matrix metalloprotein (MMP) production.[9] In vivo it was demonstrated that the local delivery of atRA (10 ml; 10 μmol/L) with the double balloon catheter resulted in a significant reduction of vessel area stenosis in the rabbit carotid artery.[10]

COLCHICINE AND COLCHICINE ANALOGS

Colchicine binds to tubulin, disrupting spindle formation and resulting in the metaphase arrest of cell division. Colchicine has been shown to inhibit chemotaxis,[11] and platelet aggregation.[12] Bauriedel et al. investigated the effect of colchicine on arterial smooth muscle cells cultivated from human plaque tissue excised from 22 coronary and peripheral lesions. In this study, colchicine caused a concentration-dependent inhibition of smooth muscle cell proliferation with a half-maximal inhibitory concentration (IC_{50}) of 5 nmol/L. Smooth muscle cell migratory activity was reduced by colchicine in a concentration-dependent manner (IC_{50}) of 5 nmol/L. Transmission electron microscopy revealed severe disorganization of cytoplasmic structures, especially of organelles.[13]

In rabbit femoral arteries the effect of 0.1 μmol/L and 10 μmol/L of colchicine delivered with a porous balloon catheter were investigated after induction of an atherosclerotic lesion. There was no difference in neointima area between the treatment and control groups. In addition, the authors observed a rapid decrease in colchicine wall concentration one day after delivery.[14]

In another study, a colchicine analog was incorporated into biodegradable microspheres composed of a lactic acid/glycolic acid copolymer. The drug release behavior and their effect on bovine aortic SMCs in culture were studied. Drug release was evaluated by spectrophotometric assay. Drug effects on DNA synthesis were measured by thymidine incorporation. The polymeric microspheres incorporated 10–17% of drug by weight. The microspheres were found to release the colchicine analog in buffered saline solution over more than several weeks. Drug-loaded particles inhibited DNA synthesis completely, with IC_{50} values ranging from 0.001 g% to 0.005 g% (wt/wt).[15] The same group investigated the delivery efficiency, intramural retention, and anti-restenotic efficacy of soluble colchicine and colchicine analog locally delivered into the arterial wall. In addition, they evaluated the effect after prolonged local release from biodegradable microparticles. Delivery efficiency was 0.01% and intramural retention <24 h. Neither soluble colchicine formulation reduced restenosis. Microparticles releasing the colchicine analog reduced restenosis compared with control and colchicine microparticles but not angioplasty alone. Delivery outside the artery was observed, and the long-term release of both colchicines resulted in toxicity to the adjacent musculature.[16]

PACLITAXEL

Paclitaxel is one of the most promising antimicrotubule agents under research. Paclitaxel causes the formation of numerous decentralized and disorganized microtubules and enhances the assembly of extraordinarily stable microtubules.[17,18] Sollott et al. could demonstrate that paclitaxel interferes with platelet-derived growth factor-stimulated rat SMC migration and with rat SMC proliferation at nanomolar levels in vitro. In vivo, systemic paclitaxel treatment prevented medial SMC proliferation and neointimal SMC accumulation in the rat carotid artery after balloon dilatation.[19]

Similar results have been reported by Axel et al. in the human cell culture model. Monocultures of human smooth muscle cells and cocultures with human arterial endothelial cells were investigated. Cell growth after 4, 8, and 14 days was determined in the absence and presence of platelet-derived growth factor, basic fibroblast growth factor, or thrombin. Nonstop paclitaxel exposure, as well as single-dose applications of paclitaxel for 24 h or even 20 min (0.1 to 10.0 μmol/L), caused a complete and prolonged inhibition of smooth muscle cell growth up to day 14, with an IC_{50} of 2.0 nmol/L. Mitogens or cocultures with stimulating human endothelial cells did not significantly attenuate paclitaxel-induced effects.[20] In a subsequent in vivo study the effect of local paclitaxel delivery was determined in the carotid arteries of rabbits after induction of an atherosclerotic plaque. The extent of stenosis in paclitaxel-treated animals was significantly reduced compared with the control animals. Marked vessel enlargement after local paclitaxel treatment compared with balloon-dilated control animals could be observed. Tubulin staining and electron microscopy revealed changes in microtubule assembly, which were limited to the intimal area. Vasocontractile function after paclitaxel treatment showed major impairment.[21]

Local delivery of paclitaxel (10 ml; 10 μmol/L) prior to stent implantation was investigated in pig coronary arteries using the double-balloon-perfusion-catheter. The animals were sacrificed 28 days after intervention. Neointimal thickness, neointimal area and lumen area showed no significant differences between the treatment and control groups.[22]

In contrast, local delivery of paclitaxel after balloon over-stretch injury in the pig coronary artery, using the double balloon perfusion catheter, demonstrated a significant inhibitory effect on neointima formation 28 days after intervention.[23]

In a recent study, catheter-based intrapericardial delivery of paclitaxel after over-stretch injury of porcine coronary arteries was investigated. Micellar paclitaxel was delivered intrapericardially with a low (10 mg) and high (50 mg) dose. The neointimal area, maximal intimal thickness, and adventitial thickness were significantly reduced in both treatment groups compared with the control group. The

vessel circumference of paclitaxel-treated vessels was significantly larger than the control circumference. However, the high dose treated animals showed significant damage of pericardial tissue.[24]

CONCLUSIONS

In addition to the fact that different cytostatic agents have been investigated, paclitaxel appears to be one of the most promising compounds for the treatment of restenosis after percutaneous interventions and stent implantation. However, further preclinical and ongoing clinical trials have to be awaited before we can decide on the clinical value of this method.

REFERENCES

1. Cheson BD. New antimetabolites in the treatment of human malignancies. Semin Oncol 1992; 19:695–706.
2. Chabner BA, Collins C (eds). Cancer Chemotherapy: Principles and Practice. Lippincott: Philadelphia, 1990.
3. Voisard R, Dartsch PC, Seitzer U, et al. The invitro effect of antineoplastic agents on proliferative activity and cytoskeletal components of plaque-derived smooth-muscle cells from human coronary arteries. Coron Artery Dis 1993; 4(10):935–42.
4. Voisard R, Seitzer U, Baur R, et al. A prescreening system for potential antiproliferative agents: implications for local treatment strategies of postangioplasty restenosis. Int J Cardiol 1995; 51(1):15–28.
5. Lanza GM, Abendschein DR, Hall CS, et al. Targeted delivery of doxorubicin to vascular smooth muscle cells using a novel, tissue factor-specific acoustic nanoparticle contrast agent. Circulation 2000; 102(suppl):II-561 (abstract).
6. Muller DW, Topol EJ, Abrams GD, et al. Intramural methotrexate therapy for the prevention of neointimal thickening after balloon angioplasty. J Am Coll Cardiol 1992; 20(2):460–6.
7. Favennec L, Cals MJ. The biological effects of retinoids on cell differentiation and

proliferation. J Clin Chem Clin Biochem 1988; 26(8):479–89.

8. Miano JM, Topouzis S, Majesky MW, Olson EN. Retinoid receptor expression and all-trans retinoic acid-mediated growth inhibition in vascular smooth muscle cells. Circulation 1996; 93(10):1886–95.

9. Axel DI, Dittmann J, Runge H, et al. All-trans retinoic acid inhibits human arterial smooth muscle cell proliferation, migration, differentiation, and matrix formation. Circulation 1999; 100(suppl):I-21 (abstract).

10. Herdeg C, Axel DI, Blattner A, et al. Assessment of the biological effects of retinoic acid in cell cultures in vitro and in vivo after local delivery in the rabbit carotid artery. J Am Coll Cardiol 1999; 33:268A (abstract).

11. Caner JE. Colchicine inhibition of chemotaxis. Arthritis Rheum 1965; 8(5):757–64.

12. Soppitt GD, Mitchell JR. The effect of colchicine on human platelet behaviour. J Atheroscler Res 1969; 10(2):247–52.

13. Bauriedel G, Heimerl J, Beinert T, et al. Colchicine antagonizes the activity of human smooth muscle cells cultivated from arteriosclerotic lesions after atherectomy. Coron Artery Dis 1994; 5(6):531–9.

14. Wilensky R, Gradus-Pizlo I, March K, et al. Efficacy of local intramural injection of colchicine in reducing restenosis following angioplasty in the atherosclerotic rabbit model. Circulation 1992; 86(suppl):I-52 (abstract).

15. March KL, Mohanraj S, Ho PP, et al. Biodegradable microspheres containing a colchicine analogue inhibit DNA synthesis in vascular smooth muscle cells. Circulation 1994; 89(5):1929–33.

16. Gradus-Pizlo I, Wilensky RL, March KL, et al. Local delivery of biodegradable microparticles containing colchicine or a colchicine analogue: effects on restenosis and implications for catheter-based drug delivery. J Am Coll Cardiol 1995; 26(6):1549–57.

17. Schiff PB, Fant J, Horwitz SB. Promotion of microtubule assembly in vitro by taxol. Nature 1979; 277(5698):665–7.

18. Jordan MA, Toso RJ, Thrower D, Wilson L. Mechanism of mitotic block and inhibition of cell proliferation by taxol at low concentrations. Proc Natl Acad Sci USA 1993; 90(20):9552–6.

19. Sollott SJ, Cheng L, Paully RR, et al. Taxol inhibits neointimal smooth muscle cell accumulation after angioplasty in the rat. J Clin Invest 1995; 95(4):1869–76.

20. Axel DI, Kunert W, Goggelmann C, et al. Paclitaxel inhibits arterial smooth muscle cell proliferation and migration in vitro and in vivo using local drug delivery. Circulation 1997; 96(2):636–45 (see comments).

21. Herdeg C, Oberhoff M, Baumbach A, et al. Local paclitaxel delivery for the prevention of restenosis: biological effects and efficacy in vivo. J Am Coll Cardiol 2000; 35(7):1969–76.

22. Oberhoff M, Cetin S, Al Ghobainy R, et al. Local delivery of paclitaxel before stent implantation using the perfusion double balloon in a porcine restenosis model. Circulation 1999; 100(suppl):I-306 (abstract).

23. Oberhoff M, Cetin S, Al Ghobainy R, et al. Intracoronary delivery of paclitaxel after experimental balloon angioplasty using the double balloon perfusion catheter. Circulation 2000; 102(suppl):II-564 (abstract).

24. Hou D, Rogers PI, Toleikis PM, et al. Intrapericardial paclitaxel delivery inhibits neointimal proliferation and promotes arterial enlargement after porcine coronary overstretch. Circulation 2000; 102(13):1575–81.

31

Catheter-based delivery of NOS gene

Stefan Janssens

Introduction • **Current gene transfer devices** • **NOS cardiovascular gene transfer** • **Is human restenosis a relevant target for intracoronary NOS gene transfer?** • **Conclusions**

INTRODUCTION

Nitric oxide is a structurally simple heterodiatomic molecule, synthesized from L-arginine by the catalytic reaction of a class of enzymes called nitric oxide synthases (NOS). NO is short-lived and its synthesis involves a complex array of biochemical interactions which, in turn, participate in a wide variety of physiological functions, including neurotransmission, cellular communication, inflammation, and regulation of vascular tone.[1] In the cardiovascular system, NO has an important role in basic homeostasis by way of mediating vasorelaxation and attenuating platelet and leukocyte activation. In addition, NO also mediates essential cellular functions in the vessel wall including smooth muscle migration, proliferation, and apoptosis, as well as endothelial cell growth.[2] NO interacts with several intracellular molecular targets, one of which is soluble guanylate cyclase (sGC), a heterodimer consisting of α and β subunits, linked by disulfide bonds. Binding of NO to the heme-Fe group in sGC stimulates conversion of guanosine 5'-triphosphate GTP to the intracellular second messenger cyclic GMP, which, in turn, mediates the vasorelaxation, regulation of apoptosis, migration, and proliferation of smooth muscle

cells by binding to a cyclic GMP-dependent protein kinase (Figure 31.1).

A common hallmark of patients with increased cardiovascular risk profiles, such as hyperlipidemia, hypertension, smoking, and diabetes, is the impaired endothelium-dependent vasorelaxation caused by reduced NO bioavailability.[3–6] Moreover, reduced NO production by the dysfunctional endothelium plays a pivotal role in the genesis of vascular lesions and atherothrombotic complications, and inhibition of the constitutive endothelial NOS enzyme causes accelerated atherosclerosis in experimental models.[7] Alternatively, NO also has antiatherogenic and antiinflammatory properties by inhibiting signaling pathways that promote endothelial–leukocyte interaction and oxidative stress.[8] Strategies aimed at increasing vascular NO bioavailability are therefore being considered to target a number of cardiovascular diseases, including coronary restenosis following angioplasty or stenting, unstable angina, and ischemia-reperfusion injury.

At present, two distinct NOS isoforms have been identified and characterized, the constitutive form present in endothelial cells, cardiomyocytes, and neurons and an inducible isoform expressed in a variety of inflammatory

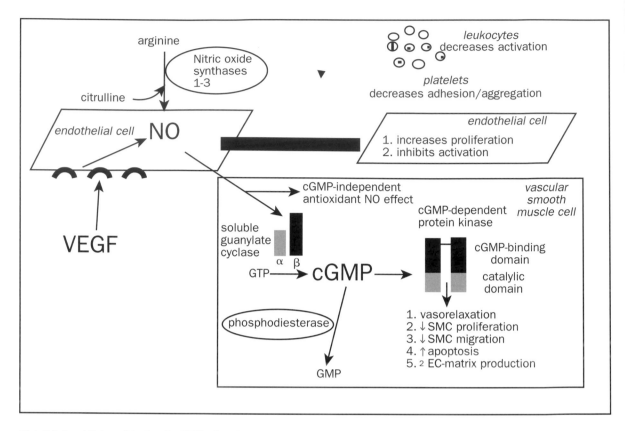

Fig. 31.1 Nitric oxide/cyclic GMP signal transduction. VEGF, vascular endothelial growth factor; SMC, smooth muscle cell; ECM, extracellular matrix.

cells, neuronal, and vascular cells upon stimulation with cytokines or infectious pathogens.[9,10] The genes encoding these different isoforms have been cloned and intensively studied in experimental cardiovascular gene targeting and gene transfer protocols. Whereas the constitutive low output enzymes are predominantly regulated at the post-translational level (see below), an important level of regulation for the inducible high output isoforms is their rate of transcription. At present, deficient local production of NO, shown to contribute to the pathophysiology of a variety of cardiovascular diseases, has spurred widespread interest in strategies to increase local NO production using either supplemental L-arginine,[11,12] pharmacologic NO-donors,[13] or NOS gene transfer technology.[14–17] These have recently resulted in the initiation of a phase 1 clinical gene transfer trial in patients with in-stent restenosis.

CURRENT GENE TRANSFER DEVICES

Most readily applicable strategies for intravascular or intracardiac gene transfer require percutaneous catheter-mediated local delivery of a safe and effective vector system. For site-specific intravascular gene transfer, existing catheter technology can be, in general, divided into various diffusion-type catheters (using passive diffusion at variable pressure) and delivery devices using some form of mechanical facilitation (intramural infusion). The effficiency of the respective pressure-driven and mechanical delivery devices has been studied in a variety of animal models using either (radio)isotopes, fluorescently labeled molecules or marker genes allowing at best a semiquantitative assessment of vector distribution and transfer efficacy. The double balloon catheter was the first device used for in vivo gene transfer but still required surgical isolation and direct visualization of the targeted artery, with ligation of side branches and prolonged occlusion times,[18] which all prohibit intracoronary application. However, these dwell techniques remain a promising approach to transduce and to modify the phenotype of segments from saphenous veins used as bypass grafts.[19] The first percutaneous intracoronary administration of a DNA–lipofectin complex was realized in dogs using a modified perfusion balloon catheter, but gene transfer efficiency in these uninjured arteries was limited to the endothelium and to the vasa vasorum of the adventitia.[20] Using first-generation adenoviral vectors, we have compared the intracoronary gene transfer profiles of different pressure-driven devices and of a mechanical intramural delivery device and found similar intracoronary gene transfer efficiency with both types of catheters. Most strikingly, the levels of transgene expression were highly variable between the animals with transduction rates ranging from 0.01 to 3 copies of the transgene per cell.[21] Interestingly, a positive correlation was observed between gene transfer efficiency and the degree of arterial injury for the pressure-driven diffusion catheters (Channeled® balloon, Crescendo®, and Infusasleeve® catheter), but not for the intramural Infiltrator® catheter.

Depending on the vector system used for gene transfer, biocompatibility issues of the delivery catheters may also profoundly affect transfer efficiency. This important restriction was evidenced by Marshall et al. who observed that commonly used catheter constituents including stainless steel, nitinol, and polycarbonate rapidly and effectively inactivate adenovirus vector infectivity.[22] Moreover, the parameters that influence adenovirus-mediated gene delivery to the injured vessel wall, were recently reviewed for different commercially available local delivery catheters.[23] It was found that viral particles are transported into the vessel wall in a manner consistent with diffusion rather than pressure-driven convection and that transduction levels of nearly 20% were achieved using low volumes of concentrated adenoviral vectors at low pressure.[23] Expression profiles thus obtained are comparable to those achieved after direct intramural injection of adenoviral vectors. This issue is likely to be particularly important when using less effective gene vector systems including naked DNA molecules complexed to cationic lipid formulations or oligonucleotides.

NOS CARDIOVASCULAR GENE TRANSFER

Gene transfer with constitutive and inducible NOS isoforms

The constitutive nitric oxide synthases (NOS3 or NOS1) differ significantly from the inducible isoforms (NOS2) both in the regulation of gene expression as well as in the biological activity of their translation product.[9] Constitutively expressed NOS are calcium- and calmodulin-dependent enzymes, and are regulated predominantly at the post-translational level. NOS activation occurs in an Akt-dependent phosphorylation reaction in response to agonist stimulation or increased shear stress. They in turn release low levels of NO shown to contribute to cellular communication and blood pressure regulation and to mediate, in part, the antiplatelet and antiinflammatory properties of the endothelium. The pivotal role of NOS3 in cardiovascular disease was clearly evidenced by the increased neointimal reaction to local arterial injury in mice with targeted deletion of the endothelial NOS gene,[24] and by decreased neointimal thickening following perivascular injury in inducible NOS knockout mice.[25]

Whereas low level, endothelium-derived NO production has a vasculoprotective effect, high output NO production following expression of the inducible NOS isoform is often associated with local inflammation and oxidant stress injury in atherosclerotic vessels.[26] Systemic and cardiac induction of inducible NOS during sepsis is thought to be responsible for the hypotension and cardiac depression characteristic of these pathological conditions.[27] For therapeutic purposes it is therefore important to carefully control the level of local NO production following gene transfer. This is all the more

Table 31.1 Vectors for cardiovascular gene transfer

	Efficiency	Integration	Stability	Safety issues
Viral vectors				
Retrovirus	Low	Yes	Months	Insertional mutagenesis
Adenovirus	High	No	Weeks	Inflammation, immunogenicity
AAV	Intermediate	Yes (chr 19)	Months	Variable integration
Nonviral vectors				
Cationic liposomes	Low	No	h, days	None
HVJ liposomes	Low	No	days	None
Naked DNA	Low	No	h, days	None

important in biomedical research because we have come to appreciate much better the intricate relationship between nitric oxide and apoptosis or programmed cell death, a key regulator in vascular homeostasis and in pathophysiological conditions including restenosis and depressed left ventricular function in various forms of cardiomyopathy and myocarditis. Recent experimental data suggest that physiologically relevant levels of NO are capable of suppressing apoptosis by inhibiting caspase activity via *S*-nitrosylation. In contrast, higher rates of NO production within a cell induce apoptosis probably via a cGMP-independent mechanism (i.e. by way of direct DNA damage) or through interaction with superoxide anions to form the potent oxidant peroxynitrite.

Vectors for vascular catheter-based NOS gene transfer

From the above, it should be stressed that for any given dose of NOS genes, the local production levels of NO in the vessel wall or in the heart will ultimately mediate the biological response in the host. In considering this equation one should not only remember the differences in the respective transgene products (constitutive vs inducible NO-synthesizing enzymes) but also consider the vast differences in efficacy of the delivery device and gene vector system. Over the years, vectors for cardiovascular gene transfer have been divided in viral and non-viral vectors, each with a specific safety, efficacy, and feasibility profile (Table 31.1).

For coronary NOS gene transfer to be successful, a sufficiently large number of vascular cells had to be transduced following catheter-mediated delivery. A major advantage of NOS gene transfer is the easy and rapid diffusion of the gaseous transgene product to surrounding cells, thereby significantly amplifying the biological response by way of this so-called paracrine 'bystander' effect. We have confirmed the beneficial effect of constitutive NOS3 gene transfer in both the balloon- and stent-injured coronary vessel wall of pigs. Intramural adenoviral delivery of 1.5×10^9 plaque-forming-units of the recombinant first-generation adenoviral vector at the site of injury was capable of efficiently transducing medial and adventitial cells and increasing cGMP production, an effect that resulted in a significant reduction in neointima formation after 28 days (Figure 31.2).[15] In NOS3-infected pigs, the neointimal area normalized to the fracture length of the internal elastic lamina, a measure of injury severity, was

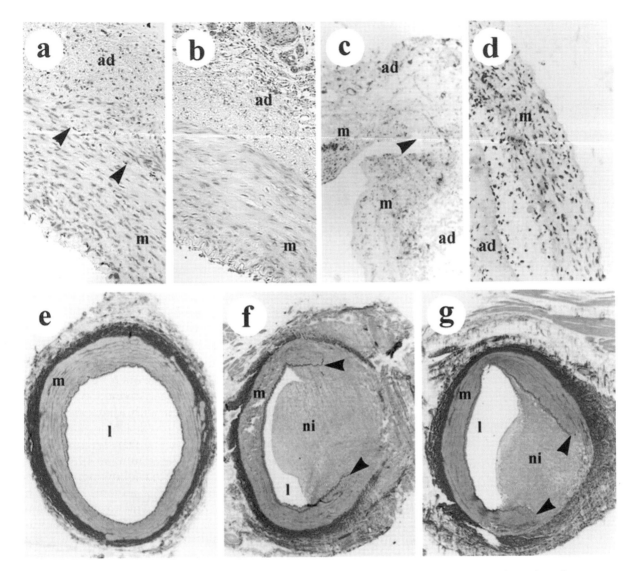

Fig. 31.2 (a)–(d) Distribution of transgene expression in the coronary arterial wall following adenovirus-mediated transfer of a construct carrying the *E. Coli LacZ* gene encoding a nuclear localizing variant of β-galactosidase (**a**) or no transgene, AdRR5 (**b**) (× 100). Marked β-galactosidase activity, as assessed by blue staining of nuclei of infected cells, was detected in medial (***m***) and adventitial (***ad***) cell layers of Adβ-gal infected (**a**) but not in control AdRR5-infected animals (**b**). Injured coronary arteries were infected with an adenoviral vector carrying the human NOS3 cDNA (**c**) or with a control virus AdRR5 (**d**) and were stained with a specific anti-NOS3 antiserum. Medial smooth muscle cells and adventitial cells of coronary arteries infected with AdNOS3 (**c**) but not with AdRR5 (**d**) showed diffuse NOS immunoreactivity. (e)–(g) Hart's-stained coronary arterial sections 28 days after angioplasty. In noninjured untransduced control LAD (**f**) no neointima is observed. After angioplasty and infection with AdRR5 (**g**), marked neointima formation (***ni***) results in 78% stenosis, while arteries infected with AdNOS3 (**h**) show significantly reduced neointimal area normalized to fracture length of the internal elastic membrane (arrow heads) and a larger residual lumen (***l***). (Reproduced from Varenne et al. Circulation 1998; 98:216–26 with permission from Lippincott Williams & Wilkins.)

significantly smaller (0.59 ± 0.14 vs 0.80 ± 0.19 mm, $p = 0.02$) and the maximal neointimal thickness was significantly thinner (0.70 ± 0.35 vs 0.32 ± 0.18 mm^2, $p = 0.007$) than in control adenovirus-infected animals. Although it was unlikely that the adenoviral vector per se modulated the vascular response, irrespective of the transgene, one can not exclude that adenoviral dose-related inflammatory cell infitration may in part impact on final outcome.

We have therefore also examined the effect of NOS3 gene transfer in a more severe stent-induced coronary injury model in pigs where extensive matrix modification, smooth muscle dedifferentiation and migration and inflammatory cell infiltration was observed in the absence of adenoviral administration. As was observed in balloon angioplastied pigs, NOS gene transfer in the stented area by way of the intramural Infiltrator catheter was associated with significant reduction of in-stent stenosis and more importantly with better preservation of the collagen matrix, with less smooth muscle cell dedifferentiation and with less inflammatory cell infiltration.

To reduce potential adenovirus-related toxicity and inflammation while at the same time retaining sufficiently high NO production, log-fold lower virus concentrations of the inducible NOS isoform have been administered intravascularly. In the rat carotid injury (100- to 1000-fold less virus administered) and porcine iliac injury (3- to 20-fold less virus administered) model, this approach was capable of reducing neointimal hyperplasia by 97% and 52%, respectively, without prohibitive side effects.[17] It has also been successfully applied in a porcine model of in-stent stenosis.[28]

IS HUMAN RESTENOSIS A RELEVANT TARGET FOR INTRACORONARY NOS GENE TRANSFER?

Although the field of vascular gene therapy has emerged as a viable approach during the last decade to target restenosis, one has to carefully consider the advantages and potential disadvantages of such an approach at the present time. As outlined above, one of the major hurdles to overcome is the suboptimal vector profile, especially with regard to the inflammatory side-effects and the immunogenicity of adenoviral vectors. We have investigated the prevalence of pre-existing antiadenoviral immunity in a random population of ischemic heart disease patients and found high levels of pre-existing neutralizing antibodies in >50% of patients. Because pre-existing immunity significantly reduces the efficacy of adenoviral regional myocardial gene transfer in pigs and is associated with increased toxicity, indiscriminate intracoronary injection of these vectors in patients is not indicated. In contrast, intramural delivery of small quantities of the vector in immunized pigs did not elicit these problems probably because of less exposure of foreign antigens to the immune system.[29] Whether the advantage of this delivery modality will translate into enhanced clinical benefit and safety, remains unknown. As scientists and physicians, we need to avoid raising premature public expectations for rapid and large-scale clinical applications. The primary goal in gene therapy with NOS and similarly active molecules should be to carefully dissect their respective contributions in the pathogenesis of restenosis and to foster intense cooperation between academia, industry, and regulatory agencies which will undoubtedly propel the development of new, improved gene vector systems.

CONCLUSIONS

There still remain significant gaps in our understanding of the molecular events that unfold in the hours and days after a percutaneous coronary intervention and that ultimately result in a restenotic lesion, refractory to conventional therapies. In principle, restored NOS gene function at the site of injury has the great potential of interfering with several key steps in the pathophysiology of this complication. It therefore provides a viable therapeutic option which needs to be tested in patients, because no single animal model in the end can predict the outcome in the atherosclerotic patient. In this respect, small-scale clinical trials are warranted, provided that the vector systems applied demonstrate a robust safety profile. There is justified hope that the recently started trial using liposome-mediated transfer of the inducible NOS2 isoform to target in-stent restenotic lesions will unravel some of these questions.

REFERENCES

1. Schmidt H, Walter U. NO at work. Cell 1994; 78:919–25.
2. Lloyd-Jones DM, Bloch KD. The vascular biology of nitric oxide and its role in atherogenesis. Annu Rev Med 1996; 47:365–75.
3. Stroes ES, Koomans HA, de Bruin TW, Rabelink TJ. Vascular function in the forearm of hypercholesterolaemic patients off and on lipid-lowering medication. Lancet 1995; 346:467–71.
4. Williams SB, Cusco JA, Roddy MA, et al. Impaired nitric oxide-mediated vasodilation in patients with non-insulin-dependent diabetes mellitus. J Am Coll Cardiol 1996; 27:567–74.
5. Panza JA, Garcia CE, Kilcoyne CM, et al. Impaired endothelium-dependent vasodilation in patients with essential hypertension. Evidence that nitric oxide abnormality is not localized to a single signal transduction pathway. Circulation 1995; 91:1732–8.
6. Heitzer T, Yla-Herttuala S, Luoma J, et al. Cigarette smoking potentiates endothelial dysfunction of forearm resistance vessels in patients with hypercholesterolemia. Role of oxidized LDL. Circulation 1996; 93:1346–53.
7. Cayatte AJ, Palacino JJ, Horten K, Cohen RA. Chronic inhibition of nitric oxide production accelerates neointima formation and impairs endothelial function in hypercholesterolemic rabbits. Arterioscler Thromb 1994; 14:753–9.
8. Qian H, Neplioueva V, Shetty GA, et al. Nitric oxide synthase gene therapy rapidly reduces adhesion molecule expression and inflammatory cell infiltration in carotid arteries of cholesterol-fed rabbits. Circulation 1999; 99:2979–82.
9. Nathan C, Xie QW. Nitric oxide synthases: roles, tolls, and controls. Cell 1994; 78:915–18.
10. Lowenstein CJ, Glatt CS, Bredt DS, Snyder SH. Cloned and expressed macrophage nitric oxide synthase contrasts with the brain enzyme. Proc Natl Acad Sci USA 1992; 89:6711–15.
11. Hamon M, Vallet B, Bauters C, et al. Long-term oral administration of L-arginine reduces intimal thickening and enhances neoendothelium-dependent acetylcholine-induced relaxation after arterial injury. Circulation 1994; 90:1357–62.
12. Wang BY, Candipan RC, Arjomandi M, et al. Arginine restores nitric oxide activity and inhibits monocyte accumulation after vascular injury in hypercholesterolemic rabbits. J Am Coll Cardiol 1996; 28:1573–9.
13. Seki J, Nishio M, Kato Y, et al. FK409, a new nitric-oxide donor, suppresses smooth muscle proliferation in the rat model of balloon angioplasty. Atherosclerosis 1995; 117:97–106.
14. VonDerLeyen H, Gibbons G, Morishita R, et al. Gene therapy inhibiting neointimal vascular lesion: In vivo transfer of endothelial cell nitric oxide synthase gene. Proc Natl Acad Sci USA 1995; 92:1137–41.
15. Varenne O, Pislaru S, Gillijns H, et al. Local adenovirus-mediated transfer of human endothelial nitric oxide synthase reduces luminal narrowing after coronary angioplasty in pigs. Circulation 1998; 98:919–26.
16. Janssens S, Flaherty D, Nong Z, et al. Human endothelial nitric oxide synthase gene transfer inhibits vascular smooth muscle cell proliferation and neointima formation after balloon injury in rats. Circulation 1998; 97:1274–81.
17. Shears LL, II, Kibbe MR, Murdock AD, et al. Efficient inhibition of intimal hyperplasia by adenovirus-mediated inducible nitric oxide synthase gene transfer to rats and pigs in vivo. J Am Coll Surg 1998; 187:295–306.
18. Nabel E, Plautz G, Nabel G. Site specific gene expression in vivo by direct gene transfer into the arterial wall. Science 1990; 249:1285–8.
19. Mann MJ, Whittemore AD, Donaldson MC, et al. Ex-vivo gene therapy of human vascular bypass grafts with E2F decoy: the PREVENT single-centre, randomised, controlled trial. Lancet 1999; 354:1493–8.
20. Chapman GD, Lim CS, Gammon RS, et al. Gene transfer into coronary arteries of intact animals with a percutaneous balloon catheter. Circ Res 1992; 71:27–33.
21. Varenne O, Gerard RD, Sinnaeve P, et al. Percutaneous adenoviral gene transfer into porcine coronary arteries: is catheter-based gene

delivery adapted to coronary circulation? Hum Gene Ther 1999; 10:1105–15.

22. Marshall DJ, Palasis M, Lepor J, Leiden JM. Biocompatibility of cardiovascular gene delivery catheters with adenovirus vectors: an important determinant of the efficiency of cardiovascular gene transfer. Mol Ther 2000; 1:423–8.

23. Palasis M, Luo Z, Barry JJ, Walsh K. Analysis of adenoviral transport mechanisms in the vessel wall and optimization of gene transfer using local delivery catheters. Hum Gene Ther 2000; 11:237–46.

24. Kawashima S, Yamashita T, Ozaki M, et al. Endothelial NO synthase overexpression inhibits lesion formation in mouse model of vascular remodeling. Arterioscler Thromb Vasc Biol 2001; 21:201–7.

25. Chyu KY, Dimayuga P, Zhu J, et al. Decreased neointimal thickening after arterial wall injury in inducible nitric oxide synthase knockout mice. Circ Res 1999; 85:1192–8.

26. Kockx MM, De Meyer GR, Buyssens N, et al. Cell composition, replication, and apoptosis in atherosclerotic plaques after 6 months of cholesterol withdrawal. Circ Res 1998; 83:378–87.

27. Balligand JL, Ungureanu-Longrois D, Simmons WW, et al. Cytokine-inducible nitric oxide synthase (iNOS) expression in cardiac myocytes. Characterization and regulation of iNOS expression and detection of iNOS activity in single cardiac myocytes in vitro. J Biol Chem 1994; 269:27580–8.

28. von der Leyen H, Muhs A, Schrader J. Inhibition of in-stent plaque formation by inducible nitric oxide synthase-lipoplex-mediated gene therapy in a pig femoral artery stent model. J Am Coll Cardiol 2000; 35:A280.

29. Szelid Z, Sinnaeve P, Vermeersch P, et al. Pre-existing anti-adenoviral immunity and regional myocardial gene transfer: Modulation by nitric oxide. Circulation 2000; 102:A38.

32

Carbon-coated stents: diamond-like stent coatings

Ivan De Scheerder, and Yanming Huang

Introduction • Materials and methods • Results • Discussion

INTRODUCTION

Randomized clinical trials have revealed a significant reduction in angiographic restenosis rate (>50% diameter stenosis) when adjunctive stenting was performed after conventional coronary angioplasty.[1,2] Completely in line with previous experimental observations,[3] this beneficial effect of stenting was not related to inhibition of the neointimal cellular proliferation following vascular injury but simply the mechanical result of over-stretching the treated vessel segment. In addition, the reduced restenosis rate was obtained using a stringent antithrombotic regimen leading to an excess in bleeding complications and prolonged hospitalization. Both these considerations are now boosting the search for stent coatings suited to deliver high local intramural concentrations of antiproliferative and antithrombotic agents as well.

In this regard, polymers are especially attractive since a large variety of vasoactive substances can easily be embedded in their network without firm chemical bindings. Consequently, they potentially can act as an intramural slow release formulation for vasoactive drugs. Different polymer stent coatings have shown not to be sufficiently biocompatible for clinical use. Either they resulted in an increased thrombogenicity or induced severe histolymphocytic inflammatory foreign body reaction resulting in severe vessel narrowing.[4–5]

New, more inert materials are becoming available and are now under preclinical testing as potential stent coating materials. Phosphorylcholine stent coatings have been shown to decrease the thrombogenicity of coronary stents but have not been shown to influence neointimal hyperplasia. Hydrogenated diamond-like carbon films (DLC, a-C:H), deposited using plasma-assisted or ion beam-assisted techniques, offer great potential as self-lubricating coatings in many tribological applications.[6] Additionally, studies on their biocompatibility have shown that DLC is an inert, impervious hydrocarbon with properties suitable for use in the biomedical field.[7] One particular class of modified DLC coatings is diamond-like nanocomposite coatings (DLN or Dylyn™), offering a promising solution for many industrial applications. In this study the biocompatibility of two diamond-like stent coatings are evaluated in a porcine coronary stent model.

MATERIALS AND METHODS

Stents

The Freedom Coronary Stent (Global Therapeutics, Broomfield, CO) consists of a preconditioned, non-ferromagnetic, highly polished stainless steel wire, which is mechanically twisted in a zig-zag shape forming a fishscale design. The particular design allows folding on any conventional balloon catheter, resulting in a low profile 6 Fr guiding catheter compatible stent delivery system. Percentage of shortening is limited (<5%) and the stent is available in a large variety of lengths from 12 mm up to 40 mm allowing customized stenting. These stents are available as bare stents or mounted stents. For this study stents of 16 mm were used.[8–9]

Preparation and coating of the stents

The coatings described in this study have been deposited using a plasma-assisted CVD process. A plasma is created from liquid siloxane precursors using electron emission from a heated filament combined with an RF or DC voltage on the substrate. The rotating sample holder has a diameter of 73 cm. Prior to deposition, all substrates are in situ cleaned using an Ar plasma etch.

Two coating types have been deposited. Coating 97070800 is a DLN coating, covered with a DLC (a-C:H) top layer, while 97070900 is a single DLN layer. Both coating types have a thickness of typically 2–3 μm.

Procedures

Domestic cross-bred pigs of both sexes weighing 25–30 kg were used. They were fed with a standard natural grain diet without lipid or cholesterol supplementation throughout the study. All animals were treated and cared for in accordance with the National Institute of Health Guide for the Care and Use of Laboratory Animals. The pigs were sedated with 1 mL/kg Azaperone (Stresnil®, Janssens Pharmaceutics, Beerse, Belgium) and anesthetized with intravascular ketamine (10 mg/kg) for induction and a mixture of ketamine

(Ketalar®, Parke-Davis NV, Warner Lambert, Belgium) (0.1 mg/kg/h) and Pacuronium (Pavulon®, Organon NV, Oss, Holland) (0.4 mg/kg/h) for maintenance intravenously, adequate anesthesia was determined by the loss of the limb withdrawal reflex. The pigs were intubated in 6 Fr tracheal tubes and ventilation (Mark 7A, Bird Cooperation, Palm Springs, CA) was started using a mixture of 20 vol% of pure oxygen and 80 vol% of room air. Ventilation was adjusted by frequent blood gas analysis in order to maintain a minimum PaO$_2$ of 100 mmHg and physiologic PaCO$_2$ and pH parameters. Throughout the procedure the electrocardiogram (ECG), blood pressure, and temperature were monitored continuously. An external carotid artery was surgically exposed and an 8 Fr intra-arterial sheath was introduced over a 0.035 inch guidewire.

Heparin (10 000–12 500 IU) and acetylsalicylic acid (250 mg) were administered intravenously as bolus. Right coronary arteries were visualized using an 8 Fr Judkins L 3.0 catheter and Hexabrix (Hexabrix® 320, France) was used as contrast agent. Either coated or non-coated stents were randomly implanted in two coronary arteries of 20 pigs so that each group contained 13 stents. The stents were mounted on a conventional 3.0 mm or 3.5 mm coronary angioplasty balloon catheter by hand crimping and then deployed in the selected artery segment using an inflation pressure of 8 atm for 30 seconds. Arterial angiography, after intra-arterial administration of nitroglycerine (0.25 mg), confirmed vessel patency in all animals. Finally, the carotid arteriotomy was repaired and the dermal layers were closed using standard techniques. No antiplatelet agents or additional anticoagulants were administered during follow-up.

Six weeks after implantation, control angiography of stented vessel was performed and subsequently pigs were sacrificed using an intravenous bolus of 20 ml over-saturated potassium chloride. At that time, their average weight was about 70 kg. For these follow-up studies, the instrumentation of the pigs and angiographic technique were identical to those used during the implantation procedure.

Measurements

Quantitative coronary angiography

Angiographic analysis of stented vessel segments was performed before, immediately after stenting, and at follow-up using the Polytron 1000® system as described previously by De Scheerder et al.[4,5] The Polytron 1000® system was previously validated in vitro and in vivo,[10] with a metal bar as a calibration device.[11] The diameters of the vessel segments were measured before, immediately after stent implantation, and at follow-up. The degree of oversizing was expressed as measured maximum balloon size (i.e. selected artery diameter divided by selected artery diameter). Recoil was expressed as measured maximum balloon size – minimal stent lumen diameter measured 15 minutes after stent implantation divided by measured maximum balloon size.

Histopathology and morphometry

After 6 weeks follow-up, the pigs were sacrificed and the stented coronary pressure fixed using a 10% formalin solution at 80 mmHg. Coronary segments were carefully dissected together with a 1 cm minimum vessel segment both proximal and distal to the stent. The segment was fixed in a 10% formalin solution. Tissue specimens were embedded in a cold-polymerizing resin (Technovit 7100, Heraeus Kulzer GmbH, Wehrheim, Germany). Sections, 5 microns thick, were cut with a Rotary heavy duty microtome HM 360 (Microm-Walldorf, Germany) equipped with a hard metal knife, and stained with hematoxylin-eosin, Masson's trichrome, elastic stain, and a phosphotungstic acid hematoxylin stain. Light microscopic examination was performed by an experienced pathologist who was blinded to the type of stent used. Injury of the arterial wall due to stent deployment was evaluated for every stent filament site, and graded as described by Schwartz et al.:[12]

0: internal elastic membrane intact, media compressed but not lacerated
1: internal elastic membrane lacerated, media visibly lacerated
2: external elastic membrane compressed but intact
3: large lacerations of the media extending through the external elastic membrane
4: stent filament residing in the adventitia.

Inflammatory reaction at every stent filament site was carefully examined searching for inflammatory cells, and scored as follows:

I: sparsely located histolymphocytes around the stent filament
II: more densely located histolymphocytes covering the stent filament, but no lymphogranuloma and/or giant cells formation found
III: diffusely located histolymphocytes, lymphogranuloma and/or giant cells, also involving the media.

Appearance of thrombus was evaluated for every stent filament on the phosphotungstic acid hematoxylin stained slide and graded as follows:

1: small thrombus adjacent to the stent filament
2: thrombus totally covering the stent filament
3: large thrombus resulting in an area stenosis of <50%
4: big thrombus resulting in an area stenosis ≥50%.

The mean score for every factor was calculated as:

$$\text{Mean score} = \text{Sum of score for each filament}/\text{Number of filaments present}$$

Finally, morphometric analysis of the coronary segments harvested was performed using a computerized morphometry program (Leitz CBA 8000). Measurements of lumen area, lumen inside the internal elastic lamina, and lumen inside the external elastic lamina were performed on the arterial sites, visually appreciated as being most proliferative. Furthermore, area stenosis and neointimal hyperplasia area were calculated.

Statistics

Arteriographic measurements before, immediately after, and 6 weeks after stent deployment were compared using paired t-tests. For comparison among different groups non-paired t-tests were used. Data are presented as mean value ± SD. A p-value < 0.05 was considered statistically significant.

RESULTS

All stent deployments were successful, routine control angiogram obtained 15 minutes after stent implantation showed that all stented vessel segments were patent. One pig died (two stents) after 48 hours. Post mortem examination showed patent stented vessels.

Quantitative coronary analysis

The results of angiographic measurements in the three groups are presented in Table 32.1. Baseline selected arteries, measured balloon diameter, and post-stenting diameter were similar in the three groups. Oversizing and recoil were also similar. At 6 weeks follow-up a somewhat larger minimal luminal stent diameter and a somewhat decreased late loss was found in the 97070900 group, however, these factors did not reach statistical significance.

Histopathology

Injury was similar in the three groups (control group: 0.84 ± 0.32, 97070900: 0.74 ± 0.48,

97070800: 1.02 ± 0.46). Inflammation surrounding the stent filaments was significantly more pronounced in the 97070800 group (1.98 ± 0.28 vs 1.09 ± 0.48 in the control bare stent group, $p = 0.000$, and 0.78 ± 0.54 in the 97070900 group, $p = 0.144$). Thrombus formation surrounding the stent filaments was significantly decreased in the coated stent groups compared to the control bare stent group (control bare: 0.14 ± 0.20, 97070800: 0.02 ± 0.04 ($p = 0.045$), 97070900: 0.00 ± 0.00 ($p = 0.024$)).

Morphometry (Table 32.2)

The largest lumen area at follow-up was found in the 97070900 group. However, there was no significant difference in the control group ($p = 0.074$), nor with the 97070800 group ($p = 0.254$). Both the internal elastic lamina (IEL) area and the external elastic lamina (EEL) area were similar in the three study groups. Neointimal hyperplasia was decreased in both coated-stent groups. However, the differences in the control group were not statistically significant. Area stenosis was lowest in the 97070900 group (41 ± 17 vs 54 ± 15% in the control group, $p = 0.06$).

DISCUSSION

It is known that coronary stents increase the arterial lumen size better than conventional

Table 32.1 Angiographic measurements of the stented vessel segments

	Control bare stent (n = 12)	97070900 (n = 12)	97070800 (n = 13)
Pre-stenting (mm)	2.52 ± 0.18	2.57 ± 0.22	2.41 ± 0.18
Balloon size (mm)	2.93 ± 0.16	2.96 ± 0.10	2.91 ± 0.15
Post-stenting (mm)	2.68 ± 0.16	2.71 ± 0.20	2.64 ± 0.14
Oversizing (%)	16 ± 6	16 ± 8	21 ± 7
Recoil (%)	8 ± 4	8 ± 4	9 ± 6
6 weeks follow-up (mm)	2.52 ± 0.29	2.65 ± 0.27	2.54 ± 0.37
Late loss (mm)	0.16 ± 0.28	0.06 ± 0.27	0.10 ± 0.34

Table 32.2 Morphometric analyis of stented vessel segments at 6 week follow-up

	Control (n = 12)	97070900 (n = 12)	97070800 (n = 13)
Lumen area (mm^2)	1.71 ± 0.66	2.31 ± 0.89	1.93 ± 0.73
IEL area (mm^2)	3.87 ± 1.39	3.84 ± 0.67	3.59 ± 0.54
EEL area (mm^2)	5.74 ± 2.06	5.15 ± 0.89	4.95 ± 0.66
Hyperplasia (mm^2)	2.16 ± 1.48	1.53 ± 0.54	1.66 ± 0.38
Area stenosis (%)	54 ± 15	41 ± 17	48 ± 16

IEL, internal elastic lamina; EEL, external elastic lamina.

balloon angioplasty, however, in-stent restenosis still remains the major limitation. Although the mechanisms underlying in-stent restenosis are not well understood, injury during balloon angioplasty and consequent stent implantation and a foreign body reaction induced by the implant are considered to be the major contributing factors for in-stent restenosis.[3,12,13] In order to increase the biocompatibility of coronary stents, metallic surface treatment using electrochemical polishing,[14] and surface coatings,[4] have been proposed. Heparin coatings,[15,16] and phosphorylcholine coatings[17] have shown a positive effect on thrombogenicity but studies evaluating the effect on neointimal hyperplasia have conflicting results.[15–17] Most polymer stent coatings result in an increased foreign body response causing a severe inflammatory response finally resulting in an increased neointimal hyperplasia and severe in-stent stenosis.[4,18–20] Therefore, the search for more inert stent coatings enabling also local drug delivery is actually very intense.

Hydrogenated diamond-like carbon films (DLC, a-C:H), deposited using plasma-assisted or ion beam-assisted techniques, offer great potential as self-lubricating coatings in many tribological applications.[6] Additionally, studies on their biocompatibility have shown that DLC is an inert, impervious hydrocarbon with properties suitable for use in the biomedical field.[7] However, the commercial introduction of DLC coatings is impeded by some intrinsic application difficulties, such as the high internal stress impeding adhesion, the low temperature stability, and the moisture sensitivity of the coefficient of friction.[21] One particular class of modified DLC coatings is diamond-like nanocomposite coatings (DLN or Dylyn™), offering a promising solution for many industrial applications. DLNs consist of two amorphous interpenetrating networks, a diamond-like (a-C:H) network and a glass-like (a-Si:O) network.[22] The internal residual stress, as determined by measuring the substrate curvature of thin Si wafers, is below 1 GPa, although a typical hardness, as measured by depth sensing indentation, between 12 GPa and 17 GPa is reached. The low friction and low wear properties of these coatings, combined with their good adhesion to steel, make them an excellent candidate for application (e.g. on cutting tools for paper or textiles, on biomedical prostheses, as release coatings for molds, on cold forming tools and sliding machine elements eliminating the need for lubrication). In this study, stainless steel coronary stents were coated with the two coating types. Coating 97070800 consists of a DLN coating, covered with a DLC top layer, while 97070900 consists of a single DLN layer. Quantitative coronary analysis did not show any significant difference in minimal luminal stent diameter or late lumen loss at follow-up. Histopathology revealed an increased inflammatory response to the 97070800 coating. Thrombus formation was decreased in both coated stent groups. Finally, morphometry showed the biggest lumen area in the 97070900 group caused by a decreased neointimal hyperplasia in this group. The results indicate that the DLN stent coatings behave as biocompatible stent coatings resulting in a decreased thrombogenicity and a decreased neointimal hyperplasia. Covering this coating with DLC resulted in an increased inflammatory reaction and no additional advantage compared to the single layer DLN coating.

REFERENCES

1. Serruys PW, De Jaegere P, Kiemeneij F, et al. for the Benestent Study Group. A comparison of balloon-expandable-stent implantation with balloon angioplasty in patients with coronary artery disease. New Engl J Med 1994; 331:489–95.

2. Fishman D, Leon M, Baim D, et al. A randomized comparison of coronary stent placement and balloon angioplasty in the treatment of coronary artery disease. New Engl J Med 1994; 331:496–501.

3. Karas SP, Gravanis MB, Santioian EC, et al. Coronary intimal proliferation after balloon injury and stenting in swine: an animal model of restenosis. J Am Coll Cardiol 1992; 20:467–74.

4. De Scheerder IK, Wilczek KL, Verbeken EV, et al. Biocompatibility of polymer-coated oversized metallic stents implanted in normal porcine coronary arteries. Atherosclerosis 1995; 114:105–14.

5. De Scheerder I, Wilzek K, Van Dorpe J, et al. Local angiopeptin delivery using coated stents reduces neointimal proliferation in overstretched porcine coronary arteries. J Invas Cardiol 1996; 8:215–22.

6. Holmberg K, Matthews A. Coatings tribology. Elsevier, Amsterdam 1994.

7. Evans AC, Franks J, Revell PJ. Surface and coatings technology. 1991; 47:662.

8. Wang K, Verbeken E, Mukherjee S, et al. Experimental evaluation of a new single wire stainless steel fishscale coronary stent (Freedom™). J Invasive Cardiol 1996; 8:357–62.

9. De Scheerder I, Wang K, Kerdsinchai P, et al. Clinical and angiographic experience with coronary stenting using the Freedom stent. J Invasive Cardiol 1996; 8:418–27.

10. Barth K, Eicker B, Bittner U, Marhoff P. The improvement of vessel quantification with image processing equipment for high resolution digital angiography. In Lemke HV (ed), Computer Assisted Radiology. Springer: Berlin 1989:220–5.

11. Desmet W, Willems JL, Vrolix M, et al. Intra- and interobserver variability of a fast on-line quantitative coronary angiographic system. Int J Cardiac Imaging 1993; 9:249–56.

12. Schwartz R, Huber K, Murphy J, et al. Restenosis and the proportional neointimal response to coronary artery injury: Results in a porcine model. J Am Coll Cardiol 1992; 19:267–74.

13. Schwartz RS, Murphy JG, Edwards WD, et al. Restenosis after balloon angioplasty: practical proliferative model in porcine coronary arteries. Circulation 1990; 82:2190–200.

14. De Scheerder I, Sohier J, Wang K, et al. Metallic surface treatment using electrochemical polishing decreases thrombogenicity and neointimal hyperplasia of coronary stents. J Interv Cardiol 2000; 13:179–85.

15. De Scheerder I, Wang K, Wilczek K, et al. Experimental study of thrombogenicity and foreign body reaction induced by heparin-coated coronary stents. Circulation 1997; 95:1549–53.

16. Härdhammar PA, Beusekom HMM, Emanuelsson HU, et al. Reduction in thrombotic events with heparin-coated Palmaz-Schatz stents in normal porcine coronary arteries. Circulation 1996; 93:423–30.

17. Chronos NAF, Robinson KA, Kelly AB, et al. Thromboresistant phosphorylcholine coating in porcine coronary arteries. Eur J Cardiol 1997; 18(suppl):153.

18. Schwartz RS, Murphy JG, Edwards WD, Holmes DR. Bioabsorbable, drug-eluting, intracoronary stents: design and future applications. In Sigwart U and Frank GI (eds), Coronary Stents. Springer: Heidelberg: 1992:135–54.

19. Lincoff AM, Schwartz RS, van der Giessen WJ, et al. Biodegradable polymers can evoke a unique inflammatory response when implanted in the coronary artery. Circulation 1992; 86 (suppl):I-800.

20. van Beusekom HM, van der Giessen WJ, van Ingen S, Slager CJ. Synthetic polymers as an alternative to metal in stents? In vivo and mechanical behaviour of polyethylene-terephtalate. Circulation 1992; 86(suppl):I-731.

21. Grill A. Review of the tribology of diamond-like carbon. Wear 1993; 168:143–53.

22. Dorfman VE. Diamond-like nanocomposites (DLN). Thin Solid Films 1992; 212:267–73.

33

Long-term biocompatibility evaluation of poly-bis-trifluorethoxyphosphazene (PTFEP): a novel biodegradable polymer stent coating in a porcine coronary stent model

Yanming Huang, Xiaoshun Liu, Lan Wang, Shengqiao Li, Eric Verbeken, and Ivan De Scheerder

Introduction • **Materials and methods** • **Results** • **Discussion**

INTRODUCTION

Metal coronary stents are widely used in clinical practice and can improve the immediate and long-term outcomes in some subset lesions as compared to percutaneous transluminal coronary angioplasty (PTCA) alone. However, foreign body reaction and deep arterial injury induced by stent deployment can increase the tissue response.[1,2] The rate of in-stent restenosis is still unacceptable, especially in complex lesions.[3–6] Intravascular ultrasound (IVUS) studies have demonstrated that in-stent neointimal formation is the main contributor to restenosis after stenting.[7,8] It has been reported that modification of the metal stent surface with polymer coatings can alter the response of both blood and the arterial wall to stent implantation.[9–14] Furthermore, polymer coat-

ings have been used as a matrix for stent-based local drug delivery. Drug eluting stents using rapamycin, paclitaxel, and dexamethasone have shown beneficial effects on in-stent restenosis in animal models and clinical studies.[15–18] The biocompatibility of the polymer coating is furthermore a crucial determinant of the performance of the drug eluting stent.

Poly-bis-trifluorethoxyphosphazene (PTFEP) is a biodegradable polymer, which has shown excellent blood compatibility in in vitro investigations. In this study, we used PTFEP dip-coated stents and assessed the biocompatibility in a porcine coronary stent model. The blood biocompatibility, wound healing, and neointimal formation at different time points up to 6 months were evaluated.

MATERIALS AND METHODS

Stent and stent coating

Balloon mounted stainless steel balloon expandable coronary stents (Coroflex stent, Germany), 16 mm long, were used for this study. The bare stents were dip-coated in PTFEP solution to achieve a homogenous coating (Figure 33.1).

The bare stents and polymer-coated stents were sterilized using ethylene oxide.

Stent implantation

Thirty five domestic cross-bred pigs of both sexes weighing 20–25 kg were used. They were fed with a standard natural grain diet without lipid or cholesterol supplementation throughout the study. All animals were treated and cared for in accordance with the Belgium National Institute of Health Guidelines for the care and use of laboratory animals.

Acute study

In this study control bare Coroflex stents ($n = 8$) and polymer coated Coroflex stents ($n = 9$) were randomly implanted in the coronary arteries of nine pigs. The pigs were sacrificed after 5 days to evaluate injury, acute inflammatory response, and thrombus formation.

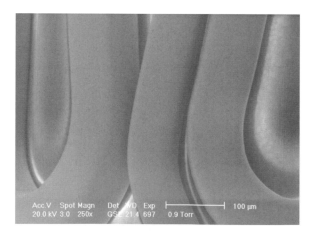

Fig. 33.1 Scanning electron micrograph (SEM) of PTFEP dip-coated stent wire (bar = 100 μm).

Chronic study

In this study bare Coroflex stents and polymer-coated Coroflex stents were implanted randomly in the coronary arteries of pigs. The 26 pigs were sacrificed after 6 weeks (bare $n = 9$, coated $n = 8$) and 6 months (bare $n = 13$, coated $n = 14$) to evaluate injury, peristrut inflammation, and neointimal hyperplasia. In addition, a further three bare and coated stents were evaluated at 3 months follow-up.

Stent implantation in the right coronary artery and left anterior descending coronary artery or left circumflex coronary artery was performed according to the method described by De Scheerder et al.[14,19] The guiding catheter was used as a reference to obtain a balloon-to-artery ratio 1.1–1.2:1. A stented segment with a balloon-to-artery ratio of more than 1.2:1 was excluded for quantitative coronary angiography and histomorphometric evaluation.

Five days, 6 weeks, and 6 months after implantation, control angiography of the stented vessels was performed to confirm the arterial patency after administration of 0.25 mg of nitroglycerin. The pigs were sacrificed using an intravenous bolus of 20 ml oversaturated potassium chloride. For these follow-up studies, the instrumentation of the pigs and angiographic technique were identical to those used during the implantation procedure.

Scanning electron microscopy (SEM)

Scanning electron microscopy was used to evaluate the presence of platelet adhesion, fibrin disposition, endothelium coverage, and maturity. Tissue segments for SEM were fixed in 2.5% glutaraldehyde and postfixed in osmium tetroxide, both kept at pH = 7.2 with phosphate buffer. Subsequently, they were dehydrated through a series of increasing concentrations of acetone, and finally, critical point dried with CO_2 and sputtered with gold. The specimens were examined in a Philips XL40 SEM.

Quantitative coronary angiography

Angiographic analysis of stented vessel segments was performed before stenting, immediately after, and at follow-up using the polytron 1000® system as described by De Scheerder et al.[14,19] The diameter of the vessel segments was measured before, immediately after stent implantation, and at follow-up. The degree of oversizing was expressed as measured maximum balloon size minus selected artery diameter divided by selected artery diameter. Recoil was expressed as measured maximum balloon size minus the minimal stent lumen diameter, measured 15 minutes after stent implantation divided by measured maximum balloon size.

Histopathology and morphometry

At different follow-up time points, the pigs were sacrificed and the stented coronary arteries pressure fixed using a 10% formalin solution at 80 mmHg. Coronary segments were carefully dissected together with a 1 cm vessel segment both proximal and distal to the stent. The segments were fixed in a 10% formalin solution. Each segment was cut into a proximal, middle, and distal stent segment for histomorphometric analysis. The region between the proximal and middle stent segment was harvested for SEM evaluation at 5 days and 6 weeks. Tissue specimens were embedded in a cold-polymerizing resin (Technovit 7100, Heraus Kulzer GmbH and Wehrheim, Germany). Sections, 5 μm thick, were cut with a rotary heavy duty microtome HM 360 (Microm, Walldorf, Germany) equipped with a hard metal knife and stained with hematoxylin-eosin, Masson's trichrome, elastic stain, and phosphotungstic acid hematoxylin stain. Light microscopic examination was performed by an experienced pathologist who was blinded to the type of stent used. Injury of the arterial wall due to stent deployment (and eventually inflammation induced by the polymer) was evaluated for each stent filament and graded as described by Schwartz et al.[20] Inflammatory reaction at each stent filament was carefully examined, searching for inflammatory cells, and scored as follows:

1. sparsely located histolymphocytes surrounding the stent filament;

2. more densely located histolymphocytes covering the stent filament, but no lymphogranuloma and/or giant cell formation found;
3. diffusely located histolymphocytes, lymphogranuloma and/or giant cells, also invading the media.

Appearance of thrombus was evaluated for every stent filament on the phosphotungstic acid hematoxylin stained slides and graded as follows:

1. small thrombus adjacent to the stent filament;
2. more pronounced, covering the stent filament;
3. large thrombus resulting in an area stenosis of <50%;
4. large thrombus resulting in an area stenosis ≥50%.

The mean score was calculated as the sum of scores for each filament/number of filaments present.

Morphometric analysis of the coronary segments harvested was performed using a computerized morphometry program (Leitz CBA 8000). The areas of, respectively, the arterial lumen, the area inside the internal elastic lamina (IEL), and the area inside the external elastic lamina (EEL) were measured. Furthermore, the area of the stenosis (1 – lumen area/ IEL area) and the area of neointimal hyperplasia (IEL area – lumen area) were calculated.

Statistics

Arteriographic measurements before, immediately after, and several time points after stent deployment were compared using a paired t-test. For comparison among different groups, a non-paired t-test is used. Data are presented as mean values ± SD. A p-value <0.05 is considered to be statistically significant.

RESULTS

The stents were easily maneuvered from the carotid artery access site to a predetermined position in the coronary arteries. All stents were easily and accurately deployed in all cases. All the pigs survived until sacrifice and no stent thrombosis occurred in either group. Three coated stents at 6 month follow-up were excluded from further analyses as the balloon-to-artery ratio was more than 1.2:1.

SEM evaluation of stented artery

The endothelialization of stent luminal surface was confirmed morphologically with SEM. At 5 days, the stent luminal surface was totally covered by endothelium at both the bare and the coated stents. Fibrous strands were detected on the luminal surface (Figure 33.2). Fibrin deposition and platelet adhesion of the coated stents were no different to the bare stents. At 6 weeks, the endothelial cells were oval and oriented along the direction of blood flow. No clear differentiation of endothelium coverage and endothelial immaturity, fibrin deposition, and platelet adhesion were observed between the bare and coated stents.

Quantitative coronary angiography (QCA)
(Table 33.1)

Angiographic measurements showed that selected arterial segments, balloon size, and post-stenting size of the two groups were similar in both the acute and the chronic studies (Table 33.1). The oversizing of the two groups was also comparable, although in the acute study the oversizing of the bare stent group was slightly higher than the coated stent group ($12.14 \pm 7.95\%$ vs $8.90 \pm 2.51\%$, $p = 0.263$).

The late loss of the bare stent group was somewhat lower (not significant) than the coated stent group at 6 weeks (0.52 ± 0.35 vs 0.62 ± 0.27 mm, $p = 0.524$). At 3 months, the late loss in the bare stent group was 0.62 ± 0.23 vs 0.55 ± 0.42 mm in the coated stent group. No difference of the late loss was observed at 6 months (0.86 ± 0.40 vs 0.86 ± 0.40 mm).

Histopathology (Table 33.2)

At 5 days, the inflammatory response of both coated and bare stents was low. A few inflammatory cells were seen adjacent to the stent struts. A thin thrombotic mesh covering the stent struts was observed (Figure 33.3). The inflammatory (1.11 ± 0.19 vs 1.08 ± 0.15, $p = 0.725$) and thrombus scores (0.92 ± 0.14 vs 0.87 ± 0.23, $p = 0.591$) of coated stents and bare stents were not significantly different. Compressed or lacerated internal elastic lamina were observed. Arterial injury caused by stent

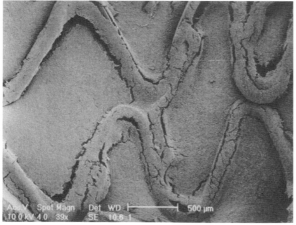
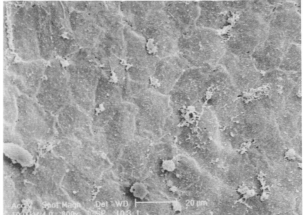

a   b

Fig. 33.2 Scanning electron micrograph (SEM) of a coated stent luminal surface at 5 days shows a complete re-endothelialized surface with macrophages rolling on the luminal surface (a) and (b), (bar = 500 μm and 20 μm, respectively). A few fibrin strands with erythrocytes and platelets are present on the luminal surface.

Table 33.1 Quantitative coronary angiography at 5 day, 6 week, and 6 month follow-up

Stent	n	Prestenting (mm)	Balloon size (mm)	Poststenting (mm)	Oversizing (%)	Recoil (%)	Late loss (mm)
5 days							
Bare	8	2.77 ± 0.23	3.11 ± 0.40	2.96 ± 0.35	12.14 ± 7.95	4.15 ± 1.37	0.41 ± 0.16
Coated	9	2.70 ± 0.43	2.94 ± 0.48	2.82 ± 0.49	8.90 ± 2.51	4.76 ± 2.52	0.42 ± 0.16
6 weeks							
Bare	9	2.71 ± 0.24	3.02 ± 0.42	2.92 ± 0.37	11.16 ± 10.36	2.99 ± 2.06	0.52 ± 0.35
Coated	8	2.83 ± 0.29	3.15 ± 0.42	3.07 ± 0.38	11.12 ± 5.01	2.49 ± 3.12	0.62 ± 0.27
6 months							
Bare	13	2.66 ± 0.26	3.04 ± 0.34	2.92 ± 0.34	12.00 ± 5.00	3.00 ± 4.00	0.86 ± 0.40
Coated	11	2.56 ± 0.22	2.81 ± 0.28	2.71 ± 0.26	10.00 ± 6.00	2.00 ± 3.00	0.86 ± 0.40

p-Values were not significant between the bare and the coated stent groups at all time points.

Table 33.2 Histomorphometric analysis of stented coronary segments at different time points

Stent	n	Lumen area (mm²)	Neointimal hyperplasia (mm²)	Area stenosis (%)	Inflammation score	Injury score
5 days						
Bare	8	6.35 ± 1.70	0.47 ± 0.11	7 ± 2	1.08 ± 0.15	0.24 ± 0.13
Coated	9	6.48 ± 1.92	0.51 ± 0.11	8 ± 3	1.11 ± 0.19	0.24 ± 0.20
6 weeks						
Bare	9	5.88 ± 1.80	1.30 ± 0.79	19 ± 12	1.22 ± 0.42	0.29 ± 0.22
Coated	8	5.27 ± 1.45	2.04 ± 1.24	27 ± 15	1.50 ± 0.54	0.50 ± 0.37
6 months						
Bare	13	5.77 ± 0.89	1.15 ± 0.40	17 ± 4	1.02 ± 0.03	0.22 ± 0.12
Coated	11	5.44 ± 1.41	1.37 ± 0.44	21 ± 7	1.05 ± 0.05	0.36 ± 0.31

p-Values were not significant between the bare and the coated stent groups at all time points.

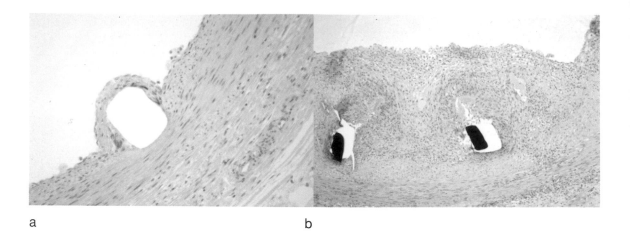

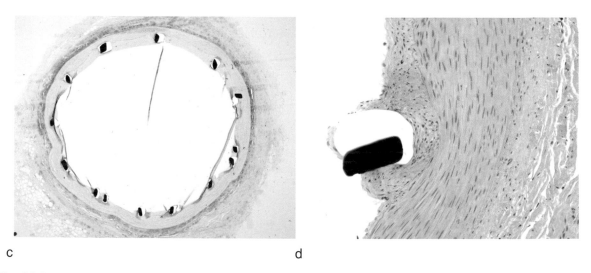

Fig. 33.3 Photomicrographs of vessel segments stented with coated stents. (a) At 5 days, the media is mildly compressed, occasional inflammatory cells infiltrated into the neointima or attached to the endothelium were found (hematoxylin-eosin stain, ×200). (b) At 6 weeks, increased inflammatory response with increased neointimal formation are observed at some stent struts (hematoxylin-eosin stain, ×200). (c, d) At 6 months, the internal elastic lamina is still compressed. The peristrut inflammation and neointimal hyperplasia is minimal (c, elastic stain ×25; d, hematoxylin-eosin stain, ×200).

deployment was low and identical for both groups.

At 6 weeks, the neointima of the bare stent group consisted of smooth muscle cells within an extracellular matrix. The medial and adventitial layers showed a normal appearance. The peristrut inflammatory response at that point was increased, but it was still low and not significantly different compared to the 5 day period (1.22 ± 0.42 vs 1.08 ± 0.15, $p = 0.387$). Inflammatory cells were present around the stent struts and in the neointima. The injury score at this time point was comparable to the 5 day point (0.29 ± 0.22 vs 0.24 ± 0.13, $p = 0.583$). The coated stents, however, showed a moderate peristrut inflammatory reaction (Figure 33.3). Inflammatory cells infiltrating into the medial layer and adventitia were observed at some stent struts. As compared to the bare control group, the inflammatory response (1.50 ± 0.37 vs 1.22 ± 0.42, $p = 0.248$) of the coated stent group was higher. The mean vessel injury induced by the individual stent struts of the coated stent group was also increased from 0.24 ± 0.20 at the 5 days point to 0.50 ± 0.37, which was higher than that of the bare group (0.50 ± 0.37 vs 0.29 ± 0.22, $p = 0.170$). Arterial media were lacerated at some stent struts. Both the coated and the bare stents however showed a heterogeneous response from pig to pig, which was more pronounced in the coated stent group. Some stented segments showed about no inflammation and very mild neointimal hyperplasia, compared to other segments showing quite distinct inflammation and clearly more pronounced neointimal hyperplasia. Furthermore, a severe inflammatory response could extend into the adventitia when deeper arterial injury was observed.

At 3 months, the peristrut inflammation (bare stents: 1.12 ± 0.14, coated stents: 1.17 ± 0.15) was minimal and similar in the bare and the coated stent groups. Occasional inflammatory cells were observed around the stent struts. A few stent struts showed a moderate inflammatory response.

At 6 months, the inflammatory response of bare and coated stent groups was consistently decreased. No significant differences of inflammatory response and arterial injury were observed between the bare and the coated stent groups. Furthermore, the arterial injury of coated stent group was less pronounced compared to the 6 weeks time point (Figure 33.3).

Morphometry (Table 33.2)

The vessel wall reaction was comparable between the coated stent and the bare stent group at 5 days. There was no significant difference in the neointimal hyperplasia (0.51 ± 0.11 vs 0.47 ± 0.11 mm^2) and area stenosis ($8 \pm 3\%$ vs $7 \pm 2\%$) between the coated and the bare stents. At 6 weeks, the lumen area of bare stents was larger than the coated stents, but without significant difference. The coated stent

group showed an increased neointimal hyperplasia (2.04 ± 1.24 vs 1.30 ± 0.79 mm^2, $p = 0.158$) and area stenosis ($27 \pm 15\%$ vs $19 \pm 12\%$, $p = 0.241$) compared to the bare stent group. Neointimal hyperplasia of the bare and the coated stents were variable, especially in the coated stent group. At 3 month (1.34 ± 0.19 vs 1.20 ± 0.28 mm^2) and 6 month (1.37 ± 0.44 vs 1.15 ± 0.40 mm^2, $p = 0.213$), the neointimal hyperplasia was decreased in both groups. No significant differences of neointimal hyperplasia and area stenosis were noted.

DISCUSSION

The present study demonstrates the long-term biocompatibility of PTFEP-coated stents in a porcine coronary stent model. No (sub)acute or late thrombus complications up to 6 months were present. Compared to the bare stents, no significant differences in neointimal formation and peri-strut inflammation were observed at all time points. The neointimal hyperplasia and area stenosis of coated stents at 6 months were only 1.37 ± 0.44 mm^2 and $21 \pm 7\%$, respectively. In contrast to previous synthetic polymer-coated stent studies,[14,21] PTFEP coating shows a good biocompatibility to both blood and coronary arterial tissue, and seems to be an excellent candidate for stent based local drug delivery.

Effect of the polymer coating on stent thrombogenicity

Stent deployment induces arterial wall injury, which initiates platelet activation and thrombus formation. The degree of arterial injury and the stent material itself determines this process. Activated platelets produce and release various cytokines and growth factors, such as platelet-derived growth factor (PDGF), which plays a role in the early inflammatory response after vascular injury and subsequently smooth muscle cell migration and proliferation. The substances and factors generated in the thrombi either directly or indirectly influence neointimal hyperplasia after stent implantation. Platelet depletion and prolonged thrombin inhibition have been shown to decrease the neointimal formation in different animal models.[22,23] Furthermore, in a canine femoral artery model, the neointima of stents with flow restriction resulted from replacement of stent thrombus.[24]

Polymer coating can alter the stent surface properties and influence thrombus formation after stent implantation. Polymers, such as polytetrafluoroethylene (PTFE) and polyethylene terephthalate (PET), have a lower thrombogenicity than stainless steel.[25] Altering the stent with a polymer coating showed significantly reduced thrombosis rates in coated stents compared to uncoated stents.[26] In vitro studies have found that the PTFEP-coated surface yielded the lowest platelet adhesion compared to other coated surfaces, including PTFE, PET, and silicone. Furthermore, in a perfusion model using human platelet-rich plasma, PTFEP-coated stents showed significantly less platelet adhesion than the non-coated stents. The activation of platelets and the mean glycoprotein IIb/IIIa receptor density on platelets were also significantly reduced (pers comm). In our study, both the bare and PTFEP-coated stents showed excellent blood biocompatibility. At 5 days, the thrombus score of coated stents was low and identical to the bare stents even though no antiplatelet drugs were administrated during follow-up. This non-thrombogenic coating may have potential benefits with respect to thrombotic outcomes after stent implantation. Furthermore, no late thrombotic complications were observed during follow-up.

Effect of the polymer coating on tissue responses

Biocompatible polymer coatings should not delay the wound healing process. The rate of re-endothelialization after stent implantation has been used as a parameter of arterial wound healing. The lack of complete endothelialization of endoluminal grafts is a major factor for the development of intimal hyperplasia and late graft failure.[27,28] Polymer coatings might influence the process of re-endothelialization on the stent surface. It has been found that the migration distance of endothelial cells on polydimethylsiloxane (PDMS) covered stainless steel was significantly reduced compared to bare stainless steel.[29] Polymer coatings can influence the binding of plasma proteins on the stent surface, which may consequently alter bindings of endothelial cells to the stent surface.[29] In animal studies, the process of endothelial regrowth after arterial denuding injury begins within the first 24 hours and is completed by 4 weeks.[30-32] Therefore, we observed the endothelial regrowth until 6 weeks follow-up. In our study, a complete endothelial cell recovery within fibrin strands was found on the stent luminal surface at 5 days. No clear difference was observed between the coated and the bare stents. The process of regenerated endothelium is faster than in other studies,[33,34] probably caused by less arterial injury and the stent itself. Furthermore, no differences in endothelium maturity, fibrin deposition, and platelet adhesion were observed between the bare and the coated stents at 6 weeks. The PTFEP coating did not delay endothelial regrowth.

In addition, stent coatings should not elicit excessive inflammatory, proliferative, or degenerative responses. Previous studies with biodegradable polymer coatings have shown an important vessel wall inflammatory reaction and an exuberant neointimal hyperplasia.[14,21] Furthermore, biocompatibility testing in vitro may lack accord with in vivo studies in coronary arteries.[21,35] With improvement of polymer technology and coating methods, more biocompatible polymer coatings have been reported. In a porcine coronary injury model, fibrin-film stents did not provoke neointimal hyperplasia at 28 day, 90 day, 3 month, and 6 month follow-up compared to bare stents.[36] Phosphorylcholine coating showed an excellent blood and tissue biocompatibility in porcine coronary arteries. No difference in inflammatory response and neointimal hyperplasia were noted between the coated and the bare metal stents at 5 days, 4 weeks, and 12 weeks.[34] By using a biodegradable elastomeric poly(esteramide) (co-PEA) coating, the inflammatory and injury scores of polymer-coated stents were also identical to bare stents. The neointimal hyperplasia of coated stents was even less than bare stents.[37] In our study, PTFEP-coated stents did not induce an increased peristrut inflammation at 5 days. The neointima of coated stents was identical to the bare stents. At 6 weeks, the coated stents showed an increased inflammatory response correlating to increased arterial injury and resulting in increased neointimal hyperplasia. However, compared to the bare stents, no significant differences were observed. The increased inflammatory reaction may relate to the increased injury score. Furthermore, heterogeneous responses of inflammation and neointimal hyperplasia from pig to pig were observed in both the coated and bare stents, which was more obvious in the coated stent group. At 3 and 6 months, the injury score and the inflammatory scores of coated stents were similar to the bare stents. Also, the neointimal hyperplasia and area stenosis of coated stents were comparable to the bare stents.

In conclusion, PTFEP stent coating is safe and does not delay regrowth of endothelial cells after stent implantation. Both the bare and the PTFEP-coated Coroflex stents showed long-term biocompatible performance in a porcine coronary stent model. Since no increased tissue response up to 6 months was observed, this PTFEP coating may serve as an excellent vehicle for local drug delivery.

REFERENCES

1. Karas SP, Gravanis MB, Santoian EC, et al. Coronary intimal proliferation after balloon injury and stenting in swine: an animal model of restenosis. J Am Coll Cardiol 1992; 20:467–74.
2. Edelman ER, Rogers C. Pathobiologic responses to stenting. Am J Cardiol 1998; 81:4E–6E.
3. Fischman DL, Leon MB, Baim DS, et al. A randomized comparison of coronary-stent placement and balloon angioplasty in the treatment of coronary artery disease. N Engl J Med 1994; 331(8):496–501.
4. Serruys PW, de Jaegere P, Kiemeneij F, et al. A comparison of balloon-expandable-stent implantation with balloon angioplasty in patients with coronary artery disease. N Engl J Med 1994; 331(8):489–95.
5. Abizaid A, Kornowski R, Mintz GS, et al. The influence of diabetes mellitus on acute and late clinical outcomes following coronary stent implantation. J Am Coll Cardiol 1998; 32(3):584–9.
6. Akiyama T, Moussa I, Reimers B, et al. Angiographic and clinical outcome following coronary stenting of small vessels: a comparison with coronary stenting of large vessels. J Am Coll Cardiol 1998; 32(6):1610–18.
7. Hoffmann R, Mintz GS, Dussaillant GR, et al. Patterns and mechanisms of in-stent restenosis. A serial intravascular ultrasound study. Circulation 1996; 94(6):1247–54.
8. Hoffmann R, Mintz GS, Haager PK, et al. Relation of stent design and stent surface material to subsequent in-stent intimal hyperplasia in coronary arteries determined by intravascular ultrasound. Am J Cardiol 2002; 89(12):1360–4.
9. Palmaz JC. Intravascular stents: tissue-stent interactions and design considerations. AJR 1993; 160:613–18.
10. Fontaine AB, Koelling K, Clay J, et al. Decreased platelet adherence of polymer-coated tantalum stents. JVIR 1994; 5:567–72.
11. Matsuhashi T, Miyachi H, Ishibashi T, et al. In vivo evaluation of a fluorine-acryl-styleneurethane-silicone antithrombogenic coating material copolymer for intravascular stents. Acad Radiol 1996; 3(7):581–8.
12. Malik N, Gunn J, Shepherd L, et al. Phosphorylcholine-coated stents in porcine coronary arteries: in vivo assessment of biocompatibility. J Invasive Cardiol 2001; 13(3):193–201.
13. Holmes DR, Camrud AR, Jorgenson MA, et al. Polymeric stenting in the porcine coronary artery model: differential outcome of exogenous fibrin sleeves versus polyurethane-coated stents. J Am Coll Cardiol 1994; 24(2):525–31.
14. De Scheerder IK, Wilczek KL, Verbeken EV, et al. Biocompatibility of polymer-coated oversized metallic stents implanted in normal porcine coronary arteries. Atherosclerosis 1995; 114(1):105–14.
15. Suzuki T, Kopia G, Hayashi S, et al. Stent-based delivery of sirolimus reduces neointimal formation in a porcine coronary model. Circulation

16. Sousa JE, Costa MA, Abizaid A, et al. Lack of neointimal proliferation after implantation of sirolimus-coated stents in human coronary arteries: A quantitative coronary angiography and three-dimensional intravascular ultrasound study. Circulation 2001; 103:192–5.

17. Heldman AW, Cheng L, Jenkins GM, et al. Paclitaxel stent coating inhibits neointimal hyperplasia at 4 weeks in a porcine model of coronary restenosis. Circulation 2001; 103(18):2289–95.

18. De Scheerder I, Huang Y. Anti-inflammatory approach to restenosis. In Rothman MT (ed), Restenosis: Multiple Strategies for Stent Drug Delivery. ReMedica: London 2001:13–31.

19. De Scheerder IK, Wang K, Kerdsinchai P, et al. The concept of the home-made coronary stent: experimental results and initial clinical experience. Cathet Cardiovasc Diagn 1996; 39:191–6.

20. Schwartz RS, Huber KC, Murphy JG, et al. Restenosis and the proportional neointimal response to coronary artery injury: results in a porcine model. J Am Coll Cardiol 1992; 19:267–74.

21. van der Giessen WJ, Lincoff AM, Schwartz RS, et al. Marked inflammatory sequelae to implantation of biodegradable and nonbiodegradable polymers in porcine coronary arteries. Circulation 1996; 94:1690–7.

22. Sirois MG, Simons M, Kuter DJ, et al. Rat arterial wall retains myointimal hyperplastic potential long after arterial injury. Circulation 1997; 96(4):1291–8.

23. Gallo R, Padurean A, Toschi V, et al. Prolonged thrombin inhibition reduces restenosis after balloon angioplasty in porcine coronary arteries. Circulation 1998; 97(6):581–8.

24. Richter GM, Palmaz JC, Noeldge G, Tio F. Blood flow and thrombus formation determine the development of stent neointima. J Long Term Eff Med Implants 2000; 10:69–77.

25. Palmaz JC. Review of polymeric graft materials for endovascular applications. JVIR 1998; 9:7–13.

26. Rogers C, Edelman ER. Endovascular stent design dictates experimental restenosis and thrombosis. Circulation 1995; 91(12):2995–3001.

27. Clowes AW, Gown AM, Hanson SR, Reidy MA. Mechanisms of arterial graft failure: 1. Role of cellular proliferation in early healing of PTFE prostheses. Am J Pathol 1985; 118:43–54.

28. van der Giessen WJ, Serruys PW, Visser WJ, et al. Endothelialization of intravascular stents. J Intervent Cardiol 1988; 1:109–20.

29. Palmaz JC. The 2001 Charles T. Dotter lecture: understanding vascular devices at the molecular level is the key to progress. J Vasc Interv Radiol 2001; 12(7):789–94.

30. Isner JM, Asahara T, Losordo DW, Vale P. Pro-endothelial cell approach to restenosis. In Rothman MT (ed), Restenosis: Multiple Strategies for Stent Drug Delivery. ReMedica: London 2001:55–81.

31. Van Belle E, Tio FO, Couffinhal T, et al. Stent endothelialization. Time course, impact of local catheter delivery, feasibility of recombinant protein administration, and response to cytokine expedition. Circulation 1997; 95(2):438–48.

32. Schatz RA, Palmaz JC, Tio FO, et al. Balloon-expandable intracoronary stents in the adult dog. Circulation 1987; 76:450–7.

33. Hårdhammar PA, van Beusekom HMM, Emanuelsson HU, et al. Reduction in thrombotic events with heparin-coated Palmaz-Schatz stents in normal porcine coronary arteries. Circulation 1996; 93:423–30.

34. Whelan DM, van der Giessen WJ, Krabbendam SC, et al. Biocompatibility of phosphorylcholine coated stents in normal porcine coronary arteries. Heart 2000; 83(3):338–45.

35. Huang Y, Wang L, Verweire I, et al. Optimization of local methylprednisolone delivery to inhibit inflammatory reaction and neointimal hyperplasia of coated coronary stents. J Invasive Cardiol 2002; 14(9):505–13.

36. McKenna CJ, Camrud AR, Sangiorgi G, et al. Fibrin-film stenting in a porcine coronary injury model: efficacy and safety compared with uncoated stents. J Am Coll Cardiol 1998; 31(6):1434–8.

37. Lee SH, Szinai I, Carpenter K, et al. In-vivo biocompatibility evaluation of stents coated with a new biodegradable elastomeric and functional polymer. Coron Artery Dis 2002; 13(4):237–41.

34

Biocompatibility evaluation of biosoluble stent coatings in a porcine coronary stent model

Shengqiao Li, Yanming Huang, Lan Wang, Eric Verbeken, and Ivan De Scheerder

Introduction • Materials and methods • Results • Conclusions

INTRODUCTION

Drug eluting stents comprise three components: stent backbone, stent/drug interface (coating), and the therapeutic agent. Currently, most commercially available drug eluting stents are coated with biostable polymer coatings containing the therapeutic agent. These synthetic polymers are fairly biocompatible, however, animal research has shown increased inflammation and neointimal response induced by these polymers. In this chapter, biosoluble oil-based stent coatings are evaluated in a porcine coronary model. These coatings are: (1) biosoluble biocompatible oils and (2) α-tocoferol. Mixtures of these components were either used in a single layer or used in multiple layers.

MATERIALS AND METHODS

Stent and stent coating

Balloon-mounted stainless steel balloon expandable coronary stents, 16 mm long, were used for these studies. The bare stents were sterile and dipped in a bicarbonate solution and air-dried, then dip-coated in the polymer coating solution. The coated stents were air-dried before implantation in porcine coronary arteries. The surface characteristics of the coated stents were examined by light and scanning electron microscopy (SEM).

Stent implantation

Domestic cross-bred pigs of both sexes, weighing 20–25 kg were used. They were fed with a standard natural grain diet without lipid or cholesterol supplementation. All the animals were treated and cared for in accordance with the Belgium National Institute of Health Guidelines for the care and use of laboratory animals.

Acute study

In this study control bare stents and polymer-coated stents (Biolog1, Biolog2, and Biolog3; five stents in each group) were randomly implanted in the coronary arteries of pigs. Pigs were sacrificed after 5 days to evaluate acute inflammatory response and thrombus formation.

Chronic study

In this study, control bare stents ($n = 16$) and polymer-coated stents (Biolog1, $n = 13$; Biolog2, $n = 16$; Biolog3, $n = 3$) were implanted randomly in the coronary arteries of pigs. (Biolog, NVGMS, Zulte, Belgium.) Pigs were sacrificed after 4 weeks to evaluate peristrut inflammation and neointimal hyperplasia.

Surgical procedures and stent implantation in the coronary arteries were performed according to the method described by De Scheerder et al.[1,2] The guiding catheter was used as a reference to obtain oversizing from 10% to 20%.

Tissue processing for histomorphometric analysis

At 5 day or 4 week follow-up, the pigs were sacrificed and the stented coronary arteries were perfused with a 10% formalin solution at 80 mmHg. Artery segments were carefully dissected together with a 1 cm vessel segment both proximal and distal to the stent. The segments were then fixed in a 10% formalin solution. Each segment was cut into a proximal, middle, and distal stent region for histomorphometric analysis. Tissue specimens were embedded in a cold-polymerizing resin (Technovit 7100, Heraus Kulzer GmbH, and Wehrheim, Germany). Sections, 5 μm thick, were cut with a rotary heavy duty microtome HM 360 (Microm, Walldorf, Germany) equipped with a hard metal knife, and stained with hematoxylin-eosin, Masson's trichrome, elastic stain, and a phosphotungstic acid hematoxylin stain. Light microscopic examination was performed blinded to the type of stent used. Injury of the arterial wall due to stent deployment was evaluated for each stent filament site and graded as described by Schwartz et al.[3] Inflammatory reaction at every stent filament site was carefully examined searching for inflammatory cells, and scored as followed:

1. sparsely located histiolymphocytic infiltrate around the stent filament;
2. more densely located histiolymphocytic infiltrate covering the stent filament, but no foreign body granuloma or giant cells;

3. diffusely located inflammatory cells and/or giant cells, also invading the media.

Appearance of thrombus was evaluated for every stent filament on the phosphotungstic acid hematoxylin stained slides and graded as follows:

1. small thrombus adjacent to the stent filament;
2. more pronounced, covering the stent filament;
3. large thrombus resulting in an area stenosis of <50%;
4. large thrombus resulting in an area stenosis >50%.

The mean score was calculated as the sum of scores for each filament/number of filaments present.

Morphometric analysis of the coronary segments harvested was performed on three slices (proximal, middle, and distal stent) by using a computerized morphometry program (Leitz CBA 8000). The areas of respectively the arterial lumen, the area inside the internal elastic lamina (IEL), and the area inside the external elastic lamina (EEL) were measured. Furthermore, the area stenosis (1 – lumen area/IEL area) and the area of neointimal hyperplasia (IEL area – lumen area) were calculated.

Statistics

For comparison among different groups, the non-paired t-test is used. Data are presented as mean value $\pm$ SD. A p-value ≤ 0.05 was considered to be statistically significant.

RESULTS

SEM images of the coated stents

The thickness of coating covering the stent filaments was 10 μm. The stent surface was smooth.

Histopathologic findings (Table 34.1)

At 5 day follow-up, both the bare and the polymer-coated stents induced an identical histopathologic response. The stent filaments

Table 34.1   Histomorphometric response to the coated stents at 4 week follow-up

Stent	n	Lumen area (mm²)	Neointimal hyperplasia (mm²)	Area stenosis (%)	Inflammation score	Injury score
Bare	48	5.17 ± 1.19	1.50 ± 0.76	23 ± 13	1.10 ± 0.29	0.28 ± 0.39
Biolog1	39	5.59 ± 1.39	1.25 ± 0.61	19 ± 10	1.02 ± 0.07	0.19 ± 0.19
Biolog2	48	4.19 ± 0.93***	1.60 ± 0.66	28 ± 12	1.00 ± 0.01*	0.31 ± 0.26
Biolog3	9	6.37 ± 0.97**	0.96 ± 0.20*	13 ± 3*	1.00 ± 0.00	0.21 ± 0.16

In comparison to bare stents: *$p<0.05$, **$p<0.01$, ***$p<0.001$.

showed a good alignment to the vascular wall. The internal elastic membrane was beneath the stent filaments and the media were compressed. Arterial injury induced by stent implantation was not significantly different among the groups. A thin fibrin layer covering the stent filaments was observed. A few inflammatory cells trapped within a thrombotic mesh covering the stent struts were observed. No significant differences in inflammatory and thrombus scores for Biolog1, Biolog3 coated stents and bare stents were observed (Figure 34.1).

At 4 week follow-up, histopathological examination revealed that the lumen surface of the polymer-coated stents and bare stents were completely covered with endothelial cells. A few inflammatory cells were found adjacent to the stent struts. A peristrut inflammation score

>2 was rare. The mean inflammation scores of all polymer-coated stents were lower than the bare stents, although only Biolog2-coated stents showed a significant decrease ($1.10 ± 0.29$ vs $1.00 ± 0.01$, $p<0.05$). Lacerated internal elastic lamina and media were observed. Compared to bare stents, the arterial injury scores of Biolog1-coated ($0.28 ± 0.39$ vs $0.19 ± 0.19$, $p>0.05$) and Biolog3-coated stents ($0.28 ± 0.39$ vs $0.21 ± 0.16$, $p>0.05$) were lower (Figure 34.2).

Morphometry

At 4 week follow-up, the neointima of all polymer-coated and bare stents was well organized and consisted of extracellular matrix and SMCs (Figure 34.3). The lumen area of bare stents was significantly larger than the Biolog2-

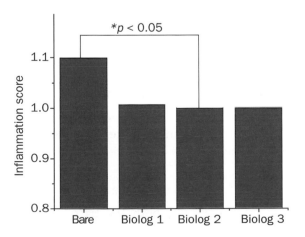

Fig. 34.1   Inflammation scores at 5 day follow-up.

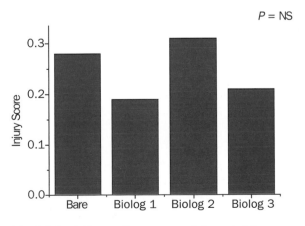

Fig. 34.2   Inflammation scores at 4 week follow-up.

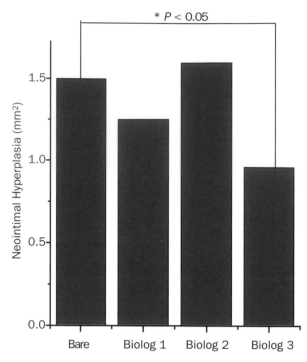

Fig. 34.3 Neointimal hyperplasia at 4 week follow-up.

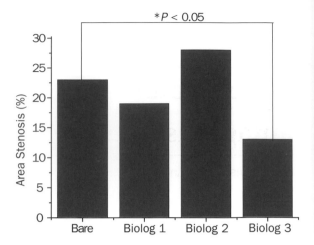

Fig. 34.4

coated stents (5.17 ± 1.19 vs 4.19 ± 0.93, p<0.001), but smaller than Biolog3 stents (5.17 ± 1.19 vs 6.37 ± 0.97, p<0.01). The neointimal hyperplasia of bare stents was comparable to Biolog2 stents, but higher than Biolog1 stents (1.50 ± 0.76 vs 1.25 ± 0.61, p>0.05) and Biolog3 (1.50 ± 0.76 vs 0.96 ± 0.20, p<0.05) (Figures 34.3 and 34.4).

CONCLUSIONS

All three coated and bare stents elicited a similar tissue response at 5 day follow-up. No additional inflammatory response and increased thrombus formation were observed with coated stents at that time point. At 4 week follow-up, all coated stents showed a mild inflammatory response. The inflammatory scores of coated stents were lower than the bare stents, especially

using the Biolog2 coating. Biolog1 and Biolog3 coated stents showed a decreased neointimal hyperplasia compared to the bare stents. The decreased lumen area of Biolog2-coated stents may be caused by smaller selected stented arteries as the neointimal hyperplasia of Biolog1-coated stents was comparable to bare stents.

In summary, all these coatings showed an excellent Biolog compatibility to vascular tissue and could therefore serve as a vehicle for local drug delivery. The best results were obtained with the Biolog3 combination.

REFERENCES

1. De Scheerder IK, Wilzek KL, Verbeken EV, et al. Biocompatibility of polymer-coated oversized metallic stents implanted in normal porcine coronary arteries. Atherosclerosis 1995; 114:105–14.
2. De Scheerder IK, Wang K, Kerdsinchai P, et al. The concept of the home-made coronary stent: experimental results and initial clinical experience. Cathet Cardiovac Diagn 1996; 39:191–6.
3. Schwartz RS, Huber KC, Murphy JC, et al. Restensosis and the proportional neotimal response to coronary artery injury: results in a porcine model. J Am Coll Cardiol 1992; 19:267–74.

35

Glycoprotein (GP) IIb/IIIa receptor antagonist eluting stents

Neil Swanson and Anthony Gershlick

Introduction • Abciximab (ReoPro) • Tirofiban • Conclusions

INTRODUCTION

The problem of acute stent thrombosis is rare with modern adjunctive therapy, such as clopidogrel, and with optimal, high pressure stent deployment. However, platelet-rich thrombi, which are the cause of stent thrombosis, create problems in 3.6% of patients with small vessels stented.[1] Patients with complex problems, such as bifurcation lesions, are also at a higher risk of thrombosis. In reported vascular brachytherapy trials, 9.1% of patients have suffered acute occlusion of the treated area, 40% of these with resultant myocardial infarction, for as long as 9 months post treatment.[2]

Activation of the GPIIb/IIIa receptor on platelets, with subsequent fibrinogen binding, represents the final common pathway of platelet activation and adhesion. Therefore, antagonists to this receptor including monoclonal antibodies may be expected to prevent platelet adhesion and thrombus formation.

ABCIXIMAB (ReoPro)

The antibody fragment GPIIb/IIIa inhibitor, abciximab (Figure 35.1), has been shown in clinical trials to substantially decrease composite endpoints after high risk percutaneous intervention. Abciximab, initially known as 'c7e3', was used in the EPIC trial in 'high risk' angioplasty.[3] Abciximab appears to reduce the immediate thrombotic complications of intervention.

Abciximab and restenosis

Furthermore, an apparent reduction in restenosis, as judged by the need for target vessel revascularization, was seen at six months.[3] This effect may be attributable to the binding of abciximab to a second glycoprotein, the integrin vitronectin, on smooth muscle cells (SMCs). This is because abciximab targets the RGD peptide sequence on the β-subunit of both integrins. Vitronectin facilitates the proliferation and migration of SMCs. Cell culture studies have shown that blockade of this integrin with abciximab inhibits SMC proliferation.[4] Further studies with abciximab have not shown any reduction in restenosis, so the clinical relevance of these interactions is unclear.

Research findings with abciximab eluting stents

Extensive evaluation of polymer-coated stents absorbed with either abciximab, AZ1 (the

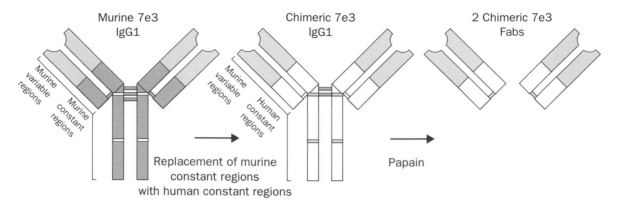

Fig. 35.1 Diagrammatic representation of the processing and final structure of c7e3 (abciximab). An initial murine immunoglobulin (IgG) antibody is formed to the GPIIb/IIIa receptor. This has the constant portions of the antibody replaced with human IgG chains. This chimeric antibody is cleaved to form Fab fragments. This is c7e3, or abciximab. (Diagram used with permission from Eli Lilly and Company Limited.)

Table 35.1   Studies using abciximab/c7E3 or the rabbit equivalent AZ1, bound to polymer coated stents

Year	Study	Results
1995	Combined AZ1/urokinase releasing stents[4]	In vitro abolition of platelet aggregation in response to ADP. This studied AZ1, the rabbit analog of abciximab
1996	In vivo reduction in AZ1-stent thrombosis[5]	>50% improvement in stent patency rates at 28 days in a rabbit iliac model of stenting. This again studied AZ1
1997	In vitro antithrombotic effect of abxicimab stents[6]	In vitro >90% reduction in platelet adhesion with c7e3 stents
1998	Efficacy after c7e3-stent sterilization[7]	Antiplatelet effect maintained after sterilization and storage over several months
1999	In vitro study of abxicimab absorption/elution kinetics[8]	Sustained release as shown in Figure 35.2

rabbit equivalent antibody) or AZ1 and urokinase together have been performed in our laboratory. The results of these studies are summarized in Table 35.1 and Figure 35.2.

TIROFIBAN (Figure 35.3)

Tirofiban (Aggrastat) is another GPIIb/IIIa receptor blocker. Clinical studies in unstable angina have suggested a beneficial effect, at least over short follow-up periods.[10] A non-peptide analog of tirofiban, L-703081, has been tested in a canine model. When bound to a polycaprolactone-coated stent, the drug showed a significant 56% reduction in platelet deposition 2 hours after stent deployment. In vitro, when perfused with buffered saline, 18% of the drug was released in

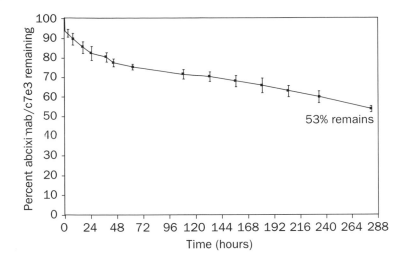

Fig. 35.2 Prolonged elution of abciximab (c7e3) from a polymer-coated stent. (Reproduced from Baron et al. Eur Heart J 1999; (suppl 18):503–P2902 by permission of Oxford University Press.)

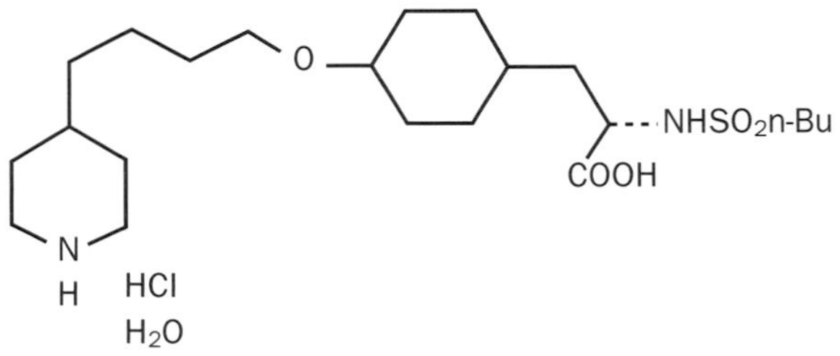

Fig. 35.3 Structure of tirofiban, a non-peptide GPIIb/IIIa blocker.

the first 2 hours, with >90% released by 90 hours.[11]

CONCLUSIONS

Neither tirofiban nor abciximab have been tested in a large-scale clinical trial of a drug-eluting stent.

The GRII stent was used briefly to deliver abciximab in a small group of patients without complication, but not in a controlled trial setting (G. Roubin, pers comm 1998). This stent has since been withdrawn from the market as the (drug-free) stent appeared to have a high restenosis rate.

The benefit of a GPIIb/IIIa antagonist eluting stent would most likely be in smaller stented vessels or after brachytherapy, where thrombosis is more of a risk or in diabetics, since use of abciximab in these patients leads to complication rates comparable to non-

diabetics.[12] These patient groups would be the subjects of a helpful controlled trial of GPIIb/IIIa antagonist eluting stents.

REFERENCES

1. Savage MP, Fischman DL, Rake R, et al. Efficacy of coronary stenting versus balloon angioplasty in small coronary arteries. Stent Restenosis Study (STRESS) Investigators. J Am Coll Cardiol 1998; 31(2):307–11.

2. Waksman, R. Total occlusion rates across VBT trials. 10th Endovascular Therapy Course, Paris, 25 May 1999 (conference presentation).

3. Anonymous. Use of a monoclonal antibody directed against the platelet glycoprotein IIb/IIIa receptor in high-risk coronary angioplasty. The EPIC Investigation. N Engl J Med 1994; 330(14):956–61.

4. Baron J, Moiseeva EP, de Bono D, et al. Inhibition of vascular smooth muscle cell adhesion and migration by c7e3 Fab (abciximab): a possible mechanism for influencing restenosis. Cardiovasc Res 2000; 48(3):464–72.

5. Aggarwal RK, Ireland DC, de Bono DP. Platelet-targeted urokinase: Preparation, characterisation and antithrombotic potential when bound to stent wire. Circulation 1995; 92(8):1437–1–302 (abstract).

6. Aggarwal RK, Ireland DC, Azrin MA, et al. Antithrombotic potential of polymer-coated stents eluting platelet glycoprotein IIb/IIIa receptor antibody. Circulation 1996; 94(12):3311–17.

7. Baron J, Ezekowitz MD, Azrin MA, et al. Polymer-coated stent wires eluting c7e3 Fab inhibit platelet aggregation in vitro. Am J Cardiol 1997; 9S:TCT–30 (abstract).

8. Baron JH, Aggarwal RK, Azrin MA. Development of c7e3 Fab (abciximab) eluting stents for local drug delivery: Effect of sterilization and storage. AHA 71st sessions 1998; 1:855–4487 (abstract).

9. Baron JH, Aggarwal RK, de Bono DP. Adsorption and elution of c7e3 Fab from polymer-coated stents in vitro. Eur Heart J 1999:(suppl 18); 503-P2902 (abstract).

10. Anonymous. Inhibition of the platelet glyco-protein IIb/IIIa receptor with tirofiban in unstable angina and non-Q-wave myocardial infarction. Platelet Receptor Inhibition in Ischemic Syndrome Management in Patients Limited by Unstable Signs and Symptoms (PRISM-PLUS) Study Investigators. N Engl J Med 1998; 338(21):1488–97.

11. Santos RM, Tanguay JF, Crowley JJ, et al. Local administration of L-703,081 using a composite polymeric stent reduces platelet deposition in canine coronary arteries. Am J Cardiol 1998; 82(5):673–5.

12. Bhatt DL, Marso SP, Lincoff AM, et al. Abciximab reduces mortality in diabetics following percutaneous coronary intervention. J Am Coll Cardiol 2000; 35(4):922–8.

36

Activated protein C eluting stents

Neil Swanson, Roger Foo, and Anthony Gershlick

Introduction • **Research findings with APC eluting stents** • Conclusions

INTRODUCTION

Stent thrombosis occurs rarely in the era of adjunctive therapies, such as clopidogrel or ticlopidine. However, in smaller vessels, thrombosis occurs in up to 3.6% of treated patients.[1] An antithrombotic stent will be of benefit especially in patients with lesions in smaller arteries. One attractive candidate for delivery using a drug-eluting stent would be activated protein C.

Activated protein C (APC) is an endogenous anticoagulant and inhibitor of thrombin generation. The inactive zymogen (protein C) is activated in vivo via a thrombin–thrombomodulin complex found on intact endothelial surfaces.

APC then cleaves and then deactivates Factors Va and VIIIa of the coagulation cascade. It also deactivates Xase and prothrombinase. Furthermore, APC has been shown in vivo to inhibit platelet activation.[2] APC has these effects without appreciable hemorrhagic side effects.[3] These many actions make APC an attractive means of inhibiting the processes that lead to stent thrombosis.

RESEARCH FINDINGS WITH APC ELUTING STENTS

Research using a polymer-coated stent has been carried out that suggests that this agent

Table 36.1 Studies using activated protein C (APC) bound to Cook, polymer (cellulose) coated stents

Year	Study	Results
1999	In vitro assays of APC coated-stents and thrombogenicity[4]	48% reduction in fibrin adhesion after 4 h immersion in plasma ($p < 0.001$)
2000	In vivo efficacy of APC stents in preventing stent occlusion[5]	0/14 stent occlusions of APC stents placed in rabbit iliac arteries after 2 h vs 9/15 in control group. 55% reduced platelet deposition ($p < 0.005$)

may well be of benefit clinically if delivered locally by a drug-eluting stent. The results of this research are summarized in Table 36.1.

CONCLUSIONS

Activated protein C is a key part of the natural coagulation system that inhibits thrombus formation. It has been demonstrated that APC can be absorbed into the structure of a polymer-coated stent, that it will elute from this polymer and produce antithrombotic effects and that this effect is retained when tested in an animal model. The animal model chosen is highly thrombogenic and a wide difference was seen between the control and APC stents in the proportion of vessels that occluded with thrombus.

An APC-coated stent may therefore become useful in patients where a high risk of stent thrombosis is anticipated. This would include stented small vessels, complex lesion, lesions where thrombus can be seen angiographically at the outset, and for patients who have had vascular brachytherapy in whom the phenomenon of 'late thrombosis' has been encountered.

APC stents are yet to be tested in humans, although work on a clinical trial is ongoing.

REFERENCES

1. Savage MP, Fischman DL, Rake R et al. Efficacy of coronary stenting versus balloon angioplasty in small coronary arteries. Stent Restenosis Study (STRESS) Investigators. J Am Coll Cardiol 1998; 31(2):307–11.

2. Gruber A, Griffin JH, Harker LA, Hanson SR. Inhibition of platelet-dependent thrombus formation by human activated protein C in a primate model. Blood 1989; 73(3):639–42.

3. Arnljots B, Dahlback B. Antithrombotic effects of activated protein C and protein S in a rabbit model of microarterial thrombosis. Arterioscler Thromb Vasc Biol 1995; 15(7):937–41.

4. Foo R, Hogrefe K, Baron JH. Activated protein C adsorbed on a stent reduces its thrombogenicity. Eur Heart J 1998 (suppl I):4488.

5. Foo R, Gershlick AH, Hogrefe K, et al. Inhibition of platelet thrombosis using an activated protein C loaded stent: in vitro and in vivo results. Throm Haemost 2000; 83(3):496–502.

37

Local methylprednisolone (MP) delivery using a Bio*divYsio* phosphorylcholine (PC)-coated drug delivery stent reduces inflammation and neointimal hyperplasia in a porcine coronary stent model

Yanming Huang, Xiaoshun Liu, Lan Wang, Eric Verbeken, Shengqiao Li, and Ivan De Scheerder

Introduction • Materials and methods • Measurements • Results • Discussion
• Conclusions • Acknowledgments

INTRODUCTION

Inflammatory response, induced by vessel injury and stent implantation, is considered to be an important contributing factor to in-stent neointimal hyperplasia. Stent-mediated local drug delivery has been proposed to provide high local drug concentrations at the target site to suppress neointimal hyperplasia and in-stent stenosis. A prolonged drug release without systemic side effects can be achieved. Most synthetic polymer coatings are, however, hampered by inducing an inflammatory reaction that may counteract the potential beneficial effects of pharmacologic agents.[1,2] Phosphorylcholine (PC) is a major component of the cell membrane. PC-coated devices have shown thromboresistance in in vitro and in vivo studies.[3,4] Furthermore, the PC coating can improve the biocompatibility of the stent surface and did not

elicit an inflammatory reaction in animal models, although no reduction of neointimal hyperplasia was observed.[5,6] Previous studies showed that local methylprednisolone (MP) delivery could significantly inhibit inflammation and neointimal hyperplasia, induced by polymer-coated stents.[7] This study aimed to assess whether local methylprednisolone delivery from a methylprednisolone-loaded PC-coated stent has a beneficial effect on the in-stent neointimal hyperplasia induced after implantation of an oversized PC-coated stent.

MATERIALS AND METHODS

Stent and drug-loaded stent

Balloon expandable stents coated with a 1 μm layer of phosphorylcholine (Bio*divYsio* DD stents, Biocompatibles, Farnham, UK) were used in this study. The stents are cut from 316 L stainless steel tubing and present a metallic strand mesh that can expand to a range of diameters from 3.0 mm to 4.0 mm. Each stent has a predeployment diameter of 1.6 mm with a length of 18 mm and is supplied premounted on a 3.5 mm (or 3.0 mm) × 20 mm balloon delivery system.

Methylprednisolone (MP) with different dose concentrations was loaded on to dose delivery (DD) stents by dipping the stent in a methylprednisolone solution.

Low dose methylprednisolone (LDMP): DD stents loaded by immersion of the stents into a 12 mg/ml MP solution for 5 minutes at room temperature. Solutions were prepared in ethanol (100%). The stents were removed from the MP solution and allowed to air dry for 5 minutes.

High dose methylprednisolone (HDMP): loading was increased on DD stents following LDMP loading by adding four 10 μL aliquots of drug solution on to the stents.

Using these methods a total dose of 34 ± 6 μg and 269 ± 47 μg of MP could be loaded, respectively.

In vitro drug release

To measure the release in vitro, a MP-loaded DD stent was incubated in a 5 ml phosphate buffer solution at 25°C. At regular time intervals, the medium was analyzed for the concentration of the drug by means of high performance liquid chromatography (HPLC).

Stent implantation

Domestic cross-bred pigs of both sexes, weighing 20–25 kg were used. They were fed with a standard natural grain diet without lipid or cholesterol supplementation throughout the study. All animals were treated and cared for in accordance with the Belgium National Institute of Health Guidelines for care and use of laboratory animals. Antiplatelet therapy with ticlopidine (250 mg/d) and aspirin (81 mg/d) were administered to each study animal beginning

3 days prior to the scheduled stent implantation. Ticlopidine therapy was discontinued on the postoperative day 5 and aspirin therapy was continued until the day of scheduled animal sacrifice.

Acute study

In this study, four stents loaded with high dose MP (HDMP) and four bare DD stents were randomly implanted in the right coronary artery of eight pigs. The pigs were sacrificed after 5 days to evaluate acute inflammatory response and thrombus formation.

Chronic study

In this study 12 stents loaded with high dose MP and 11 bare DD stents were implanted randomly in a coronary artery of 12 pigs. Pigs were sacrificed after 4 weeks to evaluate peri-strut inflammation and neointimal hyperplasia.

Stent implantation in the right coronary artery and left anterior descending was performed randomly according to the method described by De Scheerder et al.[2,7] Five days or 4 weeks after implantation, control angiography of the stented vessels was performed to confirm stent patency after administration of 0.25 mg of nitroglycerin. Pigs were sacrificed using an intravenous bolus of 20 ml oversaturated potassium chloride. For these follow-up studies, the instrumentation of the pigs and angiographic technique were identical to those used during the implantation procedure.

MEASUREMENTS
Quantitative coronary angiography (QCA)

Angiographic analysis of stented vessel segments was performed before stenting, immediately after, and at follow-up using the polytron 1000® system as described previously by De Scheerder et al.[2,7] The diameters of the vessel segments were measured before, immediately after stent implantation, and at follow-up. The degree of oversizing was expressed as measured maximum balloon size minus selected artery diameter divided by selected artery diameter.

Histopathologic evaluation

After 5 days or 4 weeks of follow-up, the pigs were sacrificed and the stented coronary artery was fixed using a 10% formalin solution at 80 mmHg. Coronary segments were carefully dissected together with a 1 cm minimal vessel segment, both proximal and distal to the stent. The segment was fixed in a 10% formalin solution. Each segment was cut into a proximal, middle, and distal stent segment for histomorphometric analysis. Tissue specimens were embedded in a cold-polymerizing resin (Technovit 7100, Heraus Kulzer GmbH, and Wehrheim, Germany). Sections, 5 μm thick, were cut with a rotary heavy duty microtome HM 360 (Microm, Walldorf, Germany) equipped with a hard metal knife and stained with hematoxylin-eosin, Masson's trichrome, elastic stain, and a phosphotungstic acid hematoxylin stain. Light microscopic examination was performed by an experienced pathologist who was blinded to the type of stent used. Injury of the arterial wall due to stent deployment was evaluated for each stent filament site and graded as described by Schwartz et al.[8] Inflammatory reaction at every stent filament site was carefully examined searching for inflammatory cells, and scored as described by De Scheerder et al.[7] Appearance of thrombus was evaluated for every stent filament on the phosphotungstic acid hematoxylin stained slides and graded as follows:

1. small thrombus adjacent to the stent filament;
2. more pronounced, covering the stent filament;
3. large thrombus resulting in an area stenosis of <50%;
4. large thrombus resulting in an area stenosis >50%.

Mean score = Sum of score for each filament/number of filaments present.

Morphometric analysis

Morphometric analysis of coronary stenting segment was performed on three slices (proximal, middle and distal region) using a com-puterized morphometry program (Leitz CBA 8000). Measurements of lumen area, lumen area inside the internal elastic lamina (IEL), and lumen inside the external elastic lamina (EEL) were performed. Furthermore, area stenosis and neointimal hyperplasia areas were calculated.

Statistics

Arteriographic measurements before, immediately after and 5 days or 4 weeks after stent deployments were compared using paired *t*-tests. For comparison among different groups, non-paired *t*-tests were used. Data are presented as mean value ± SD. A *p*-value <0.05 was considered to be statistically significant.

RESULTS

In vitro drug release

The high dose MP-loaded stents showed a slow progressive MP release: approximately 16% of MP loaded was released in the first 15 minutes. The low dose MP-loaded stents showed a burst release: within 15 minutes, the total amount of MP was released (Figure 37.1).

In vivo studies

All stent deployment procedures were successful. All pigs had arteriographically patent arteries immediately after stent implantation. All animals survived the follow-up period without stent-related complications. A HDMP stented segment with a balloon-to-artery ratio of more than 1.35:1 was excluded for further analysis.

Quantitative coronary angiography (QCA)

In the acute study, angiographic measurements showed that the selected arterial segments, post-stenting size and recoil ratio of the two groups were similar. The balloon-to-artery ratio was between 1.12 and 1.25 (mean value 1.18 ± 0.08). In the chronic study, the selected arterial segments of the two groups (HDMP 2.65 ± 0.19 vs DD 2.60 ± 0.16 mm, *p*>0.05) were

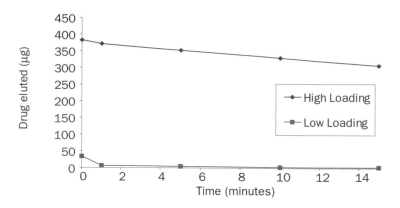

Fig. 37.1 Release of low and high doses of methylprednisolone (MP) from Bio*divYsio* dose delivery (DD) stents.

similar. No significant differences of post-stenting, oversizing (HDMP 21.93 ± 5.30 vs DD 22.59 ± 4.54%, $p>0.05$) and recoil ratio were found between the two groups.

Histopathology

At 5 day follow-up, the inflammatory response of non-MP-loaded DD stents was limited. A few inflammatory cells were present in the thrombotic meshwork adjacent to the stent filaments (Figure 37.2). The inflammatory score (0.51 ± 0.20 vs 0.73 ± 0.12, $p>0.05$) and thrombus score of HDMP-loaded DD stent group (0.50 ± 0.18 vs 0.74 ± 0.18, $p>0.05$) were lower than in the control group (Table 37.1).

At 4 week follow-up, the inflammatory response of DD stents was more pronounced than at 5 days, but it was still low (1.44 ± 0.28). Inflammatory cells were present around the stent struts, neointima, and medial layers. A few cases showed inflammatory cells infiltrating the adventitia (Figure 37.3). The injury score after 4 week follow-up was comparable to 5 day follow-up (Table 37.1). As compared to the DD control group, the inflammatory response of the HDMP group was lower, but without significant difference. The injury score of the control group was higher than in the HDMP group (0.52 ± 0.20 vs 0.35 ± 0.25, $p>0.05$).

Morphometry

At 5 day follow-up, the neointimal hyperplasia of the HDMP group was significantly decreased as compared to the control group

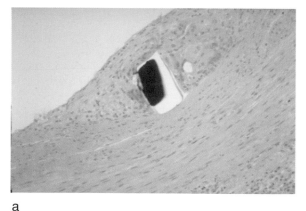

a

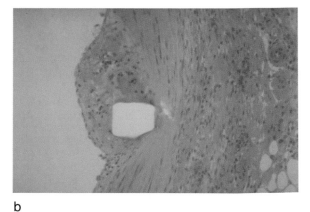

b

Fig. 37.2 Photomicrograph of vessel segments stented with (a) a bare DD stent, (b) a methylprednisolone (MP)-loaded stent at 5 day follow-up. (a) A few inflammatory cells are present around the stent filaments and in the neointima. (b) The histolymphocytic reaction surrounding the stent filaments is reduced (hematoxylin-eosin stain, ×200).

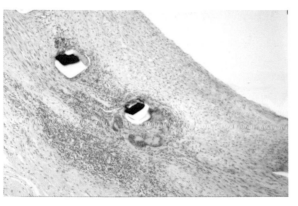

a

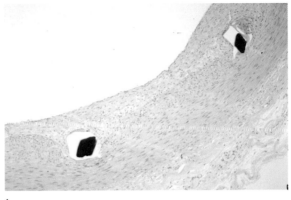

b

Fig. 37.3 Photomicrograph of vessel segments stented with (a) a bare drug delivery (DD) stent and (b) a HDMP-loaded stent at 4 week follow-up. The bare DD stent in this case shows a more pronounced histolymphocytic reaction surrounding the stent filaments, the media, and the adventitia. Giant cells are present. The locally released methylprednisolone (MP) can abolish the inflammatory reaction, limiting the neointimal hyperplasia. (Hematoxylin-eosin stain, ×100.)

Table 37.1 Morphometric analysis of stented vessel segments at 5 day and 4 week follow-up

Drug	n	Lumen area (mm²)	Neointimal hyperplasia (mm²)	Area stenosis (%)	Inflammation score	Injury score
5 days						
DD	4	7.94 ± 0.51	0.80 ± 0.10	9 ± 1	0.73 ± 0.12	0.56 ± 0.21
HDMP	4	8.20 ± 0.27	0.48 ± 0.10**	6 ± 1**	0.51 ± 0.20	0.42 ± 0.15
4 weeks						
DD	11	4.36 ± 1.59	2.42 ± 0.87	37 ± 16	1.44 ± 0.28	0.52 ± 0.20
HDMP	11	5.39 ± 1.75	1.62 ± 0.71*	25 ± 14	1.26 ± 0.31	0.35 ± 0.25

HDMP, high dose methylprednisolone. *$p < 0.05$, **$p < 0.01$ compared to the DD group.

$(0.48 \pm 0.10$ vs 0.80 ± 0.10 mm², $p<0.01$). At 4 weeks, the luminal area of the HDMP group was larger than the control group $(4.36 \pm 1.59$ vs 5.39 ± 1.75 mm², $p>0.05$). The neointimal hyperplasia $(2.42 \pm 0.87$ vs 1.62 ± 0.71 mm², $p<0.05$) of the HDMP group was significantly lower than in the control group.

DISCUSSION

Historically, coronary stenting was hampered by two major problems: (sub)acute stent throm-bosis and increased in-stent neointimal hyper-plasia resulting in in-stent restenosis. With the introduction of more optimal stent deployment and the use of more aggressive antiplatelet treatment, stent thrombosis was dramatically reduced. In-stent restenosis caused by neointi-mal hyperplasia is related to thrombus forma-tion, inflammation, and smooth muscle cell migration and proliferation. Phosphorylcholine (PC) coating of coronary stents has been intro-duced to improve stent biocompatibility of metal stents. Clinical trials with PC-coated stents have shown a low incidence of target vessel revasculation and angiographic restenosis but these incidences were not significantly lower compared to bare stainless steel stents.[9,10] The PC coating is, however, able to absorb drugs that can play a potential role in inhibiting the restenosis cascade.

This study demonstrates that a high dose methylprednisolone (MP) delivered using a PC-coated stent can suppress thrombus formation and inflammation at the early stage after stent implantation. At 4 week follow-up, implantation of high dose MP-loaded stents could furthermore decrease peristrut arterial injury and in-stent neointimal hyperplasia.

Phosphorylcholine (PC) coatings for local drug delivery

Polymer coatings have been used as a reservoir for local drug delivery. Drugs embedded into the polymer matrix can diffuse out of the matrix or be released during the degradation of the matrix. The use of synthetic polymers, however, is hampered by the potential inflammatory response induced by the polymer, resulting in increased neointimal hyperplasia. The PC coating mimics the outer cellular membrane and is well known to be biocompatible. In this study, the PC coating was loaded with MP. The loading was carried out by immersion of the stent in a MP solution. The solvent causes the polymer to swell and the drug is absorbed into the PC polymer matrix. As the PC coating is quite thin (1 μm), the amount of MP loaded on each stent is limited. Adding drops of the MP solution to the standard loading procedure could increase the amount of MP loaded from 34 μg to 269 μg. The drug release kinetics from the PC-coated stent appeared to be dependent on the total loading dose. The release of high dose MP was slower than the release of low dose MP. Comparing, however, studies using synthetic polymers,[7,11] the release of high dose MP was still rapid. The larger pore size of the PC polymer compared to the molecular volume of MP may be responsible for this release characteristic.

PC-coated MP eluting stent

Corticosteroids potently inhibit monocyte and macrophage function. The production and release of several soluble mediators of cell-mediated immunity, including macrophage aggregating factor and migration inhibitory factor is markedly diminished by steroids. In addition, in vitro studies found that corticosteroids could inhibit the proliferation of smooth muscle cells derived from human stenosing and restenosing plaques.[12,13]

Our study found that the inflammatory response of PC-coated DD stents was low at 5 day follow-up, even in this oversized injury model. A few inflammatory cells were present in the thrombotic meshwork adjacent to the stent wires. The inflammatory response was still low at 4 week follow-up, but higher than at 5 day follow-up. It has been reported that the inflammatory reaction of metallic stent implantation peaks between 3 and 7 days.[14] The different inflammatory response pattern of DD stents may be caused by the PC coating material. In a 12 week follow-up study, however, no aggressive inflammation was observed.[2] Local delivery of HDMP could further decrease the inflammatory response at 5 days. The inflammatory score of the HDMP group was lower than in the control group. Early inflammatory reaction after angioplasty may have a potent promoting effect on neointimal formation. Furthermore, the neointimal hyperplasia and area stenosis of the HDMP group at 5 days was significantly decreased compared to the control group. The thrombus score of the HDMP group was lower than in the control group. Neointimal hyperplasia early after stent implantation mainly consists of platelets, and a fibrin meshwork with trapped erythrocytes. It has been found that inflammation and thrombosis are correlated in vascular pathology. Antiinflammatory therapy may suppress thrombosis as a hypothesis recent has proposed.[15] Steroids have been shown to inhibit the formation of platelet activating factor and may exert an anti-platelet effect.[16] The early effect of MP in reducing neointimal formation at 5 days probably relates to the decreased inflammatory response and thrombus burden.

At 4 week follow-up, the inflammation and arterial injury of HDMP-loaded stents were lower than the bare DD stents. Vascular injury accompanying stent implantation is related to the balloon–artery ratio, stent geometry, and wound healing process. As the oversizing of the HDMP and DD control group was similar, the arterial injury caused by mechanical force during stent implantation is supposed to be identical. The lower vascular injury with MP-loaded stents may be related to the decreased inflammatory response and improvement of vascular repair.

Inflammatory response and arterial injury, both independently and in combination, are positively correlated with the amount of neo-intimal formation.[17] The consistently low inflammation and decreased arterial injury may both contribute to the reduction of neointimal hyperplasia with MP-loaded stents in the study.

CONCLUSIONS

Local vascular delivery of high doses of methyl-prednisolone from Bio*divYsio* dose delivery (DD) stents can decrease the inflammatory response and neointimal hyperplasia after oversized stent deployment in porcine coronary arteries.

ACKNOWLEDGMENTS

We wish to thank T Stassen and D De Coux for technical assistance. Ivan De Scheerder is holder of the Andreas Gruntzig Chair for Interventional Cardiology sponsored by Medtronic AVE.

REFERENCES

1. van der Giessen WJ, Lincoff AM, Schwartz RS, et al. Marked inflammatory sequelae to implantation of biodegradable and nonbiodegradable polymers in porcine coronary arteries. Circulation 1996; 94(7):1690–7.

2. De Scheerder IK, Wilczek KL, Verbeken EV, et al. Biocompatibility of polymer-coated over-sized metallic stents implanted in normal porcine coronary arteries. Atherosclerosis 1995; 114(1):105–14.

3. Campbell EJ, O'Byrne V, Stratford PW, et al. Biocompatible surfaces using methacryloyl-phosphorylcholine laurylmethacrylate co-polymer. ASAIO J 1994; 40(3):M853–7.

4. Veil KR, Chronos NAF, Palmer SJ, et al. Phosphorylcholine: a biocompatible coating for coronary angioplasty devices. Circulation 1995; 92:685. (abstract).

5. Whelan DM, van der Giessen WJ, Krabbendam SC, et al. Biocompatibility of phosphorylcholine coated stents in normal porcine coronary arteries. Heart 2000; 83(3):338–45.

6. Kuiper KK, Robinson KA, Chronos NA, et al. Phosphorylcholine-coated metallic stents in rabbit iliac and porcine coronary arteries. Scand Cardiovasc J 1998; 32(5):261–8.

7. De Scheerder I, Wang K, Wilczek KL, et al. Local methylprednisolone inhibition of foreign body response to coated intracoronary stents. Coron Artery Dis 1996; 7(2):161–6.

8. Schwartz RS, Huber KC, Murphy JG, et al. Restenosis and the proportional neointimal response to coronary artery injury: results in a porcine model. J Am Coll Cardiol 1992; 19(2):267–74.

9. Galli M, Bartorelli A, Bedogni F, et al. Italian BiodivYsio open registry (BiodivYsio PC-coated stent): study of clinical outcomes of the implant of a PC-coated coronary stent. J Invasive Cardiol 2000; 12(9):452–8.

10. Zheng H, Barragan P, Corcos T, et al. Clinical experience with a new biocompatible phospho-rylcholine-coated coronary stent. J Invasive Cardiol 1999; 11(10):608–14.

11. De Scheerder I, Huang Y, Schacht E. New concepts for drug eluting stents. 6th Local Drug Delivery Meeting and Cardiovascular Course on Radiation and Molecular Strategies, Geneva, Switzerland, 27–29 January 2000.

12. Fauci AS, Dale DC, Balow JE. Gluco-corticosteroid therapy: mechanism of action and clinical consideration. Ann Intern Med 1976; 84:304–15.

13. Voisard R, Seitzer U, Baur R, et al. Cortico-steroid agents inhibit proliferation of smooth

muscle cells from human atherosclerotic arteries in vitro. Int J Cardiol 1994; 43(3):257–67.

14. Edelman ER, Rogers C. Pathobiologic responses to stenting. Am J Cardiol 1998; 81(7A):4E–6E.

15. Libby P, Simon DI. Inflammation and thrombosis: The clot thickens. Circulation 2001; 103:1718–20.

16. Parente L, Fitzgerald MF, Flower RJ, et al. The effect of glucocorticoids on lyso-PAF formation in vitro and in vivo. Agents Actions 1986; 17(3–4):312–13.

17. Kornowski R, Hong MK, Tio FO, et al. In-stent restenosis: contributions of inflammatory responses and arterial injury to neointimal hyperplasia. J Am Coll Cardiol 1998; 31(1):224–30.

38

Methotrexate-loaded BOBSC-coated coronary stents reduce neointimal hyperplasia in a porcine coronary model

Yanming Huang, Koen Salu, Xiaoshun Liu, Shengqiao Li, Lan Wang, Eric Verbeken, Johan Bosmans, and Ivan De Scheerder

Introduction • **Materials and methods** • **Results** • **Discussion**

INTRODUCTION

In-stent restenosis, caused by neointimal formation, has been a vexing problem of coronary stenting intervention. Coronary stent implantation induces an important arterial injury at the stenting site, which initiates the cascade of in-stent restenosis. Although the molecular mechanism of in-stent restenosis is not completely understood, inflammatory response, smooth muscle cell dedifferentiation, migration and proliferation, and extracellular matrix formation within the intima have been known to play an important role in the development of neointimal hyperplasia.[1,2] Stent-based drug delivery results in a high drug concentration and sustained drug release at the stenting site with low systemic side effects. Local delivery with antiinflammatory and/or antiproliferative agents has been shown to reduce neointimal hyperplasia in animal models and clinical trials.[3-5] As the pathogenesis of in-stent restenosis is multifactorial and consists of elaboration of cytokines and growth factors, agents with both antiinflammatory and antiproliferative proper-

ties could have a potential advantage to suppress neointimal formation.

Methotrexate (MTX), as a folate analog, has been used in the treatment of rheumatoid arthritis, psoriasis, and graft-vs-host disease after transplantation.[6-9] It has also been used for the treatment of leukemia, choriocarcinoma, head and neck cancer, etc.[10,11] MTX has shown immunosuppressive effects by blocking the tetrahydrofolate-dependent steps of cell metabolism. It may also directly inhibit the secretion and production of cytokines from inflammatory cells. Furthermore, as a cytotoxic agent, MTX could inhibit proliferation of inflammatory cells and induce apoptosis.[12-14]

MTX, incorporated into a polymer matrix, however, has failed to decrease neointimal formation in a porcine coronary model.[15] In the present study, we used a biological polymer to deliver MTX to the injured coronary artery wall. The biocompatibility of the polymer, feasibility, safety, and efficacy of stent-based MTX delivery using this polymer were evaluated in a porcine coronary stenting model.

MATERIALS AND METHODS

Stent and stent coating

Stainless steel balloon expandable stents, 16 mm long, were used for these studies. The bare stents were dip-coated in a biological polymer (BOBSC, Global Medical Systems, Belgium) or in a 10 mg/mL MTX/BOBSC solution, resulting in a total load of 150 µg MTX/stent. The surface characteristics of the coated stents were examined by scanning electron microscopy (SEM).

The stents were sterilized with ethylene oxide before implantation in porcine coronary arteries.

In vitro methotrexate (MTX) release kinetics

To study the release of methotrexate in vitro, three MTX-loaded stents were placed in vials containing 1 mL 0.9% NaCl at 37°C and ultraviolet (UV) absorbance (Cary 4 E spectrophotometer, Varian Inc., CA, USA) was measured at 222 nm each day for the first 14 days and after 3 and 4 weeks to determine MTX release. After every time point, the stents were replaced in a new vial containing NaCl. One control polymer-only stent underwent the same procedure and the UV absorbance values were subtracted from the values of the drug eluting stents.

Impact of MTX on vascular smooth muscle cells (SMCs) in vitro

SMC proliferation assay

To determine the effect of MTX on SMC proliferation, SMCs were isolated from the rabbit aorta and passaged according to techniques described previously.[16] Cells were rinsed with fetal bovine serum (FBS, Gibco Ltd, Paisley, UK), trypsinized (Gibco Ltd, UK), counted with a Coulter counter, and seeded at a density of 5×10^4 cells/well on six-well plates (Corning, Cambridge, MA, USA), containing 2 mL Dulbecco's modified Eagle's medium (DMEM) (Gibco, UK), antibiotics (penicillin 100 U mL^{-1}, streptomycin 100 µg mL^{-1}, gentamycin 100 µg mL^{-1}, and polymixin B sulfate 100 U mL^{-1}), and 10% heat-inactivated FBS (Gibco Ltd, UK).

Methotrexate (0, 10^{-8}, 10^{-7}, 10^{-6}, and 10^{-5} M), dissolved in 20 µL ethanol (Merck, Darmstadt, Germany, final concentration 1%), was added every third day in combination with changes in medium. Also, a 1% ethanol solution was added to investigate any effect of ethanol on SMC proliferation. After 7 days incubation, final cell numbers were measured by cell counting (Coulter Counter) or by total protein determination by means of the BCA Protein Assay Kit (Pierce, Rockford, IL, USA). For the latter assay, 25 µl of each culture well was added to new microwell plate wells (Corning), and 200 µL of the BCA Working Reagent was added, and placed on a plate shaker for 30 seconds. After an incubation period at 37°C for 30 minutes, the plate was cooled and finally the UV absorbance was read at 562 nm (Titertek Multiskan®, MCC/340, Flow Laboratories NV, Brussels, Belgium). This was also done for the diluted BCA standards (i.e. dilution of 1 mL of the 2.0 mg/mL BSA stock standard) and for blank samples (i.e. 25 µL diluent only), so that a standard curve could be retracted, by which the several protein concentrations could be determined. To determine the potency of methotrexate on SMC proliferation, its effect was compared with that of paclitaxel, a potent antiproliferative agent of SMCs. Paclitaxel was used in the same concentrations (dissolved in 0.9% NaCl) and underwent the same procedure.

Effects on SMC viability

Finally, cell viability was measured using neutral red staining (Sigma). For this assay, 100 µL of the 0.1% stock solution of neutral red was added to the 1 mL media of each culture well. After 2 hours of incubation (37°C, CO_2), the wells were washed with PBS (137 mM NaCl, 2.68 mM KCl, 1.47 mM KH_2PO_4, and 6.46 mM $Na_2HPO_4 \cdot 2H_2O$; pH = 7.4; all from Merck-Belgolabo, Overijse, Belgium) and the neutral red was extracted again from the cells using NaH_2PO_4 0.05 M in 50% ethanol. Finally, the UV absorption was measured at 540 nm for the treated and the control wells, as also for a blank sample (i.e. pure extraction solution). The percentage viability is then defined as

100 × (abs treated − abs blank/abs control − abs blank), and the percentage cytotoxicity = 100 − % viability.

Stent implantation

Domestic cross-bred pigs of both sexes, weighing 20–25 kg were used. They were fed with a standard natural grain diet without lipid or cholesterol supplementation throughout the study. All animals were treated and cared for in accordance with the Belgium National Institute of Health Guide for the care and use of laboratory animals.

Surgical procedures and stent implantation in the coronary arteries were performed according to the method described by De Scheerder et al.[17,18]

Biocompatibility of the coated stents

To evaluate the biocompatibility of the BOBSC coating, 30 BOBSC-coated stents and bare stents were randomly deployed in the right and left coronary arteries of 15 pigs. Arterial segments were selected to obtain a 1.1:1 stent-to-artery ratio.

The pigs were sacrified after 5 days (10 stents) and 4 weeks (20 stents), respectively. Peristent inflammation, thrombus formation, arterial injury, and neointimal hyperplasia were evaluated.

MTX coated stents

Ten BOBSC-coated stents and 10 BOBSC-coated stents loaded with 150 μg MTX were randomly deployed in the coronary arteries of 10 pigs. Arterial segments were selected to obtain a 1.2:1 stent-to-artery ratio. Pigs were sacrificed after 4 weeks to evaluate the efficacy of local methotrexate delivery on neointimal hyperplasia.

Tissue processing and histomorphometric analysis

At 5 day or 4 week follow-up, the pigs were sacrificed and the stented coronary arteries were perfused with a 10% formalin solution at 80 mmHg. Artery segments were carefully dissected together with a minimum 1 cm vessel segment both proximal and distal to the stent. The segments were furthermore fixed in a 10% formalin solution. Each segment was cut into a proximal, middle, and distal stent segment for histomorphometric analysis. Tissue specimens were embedded in a cold-polymerizing resin (Technovit 7100, Heraus Kulzer GmbH, and Wehrheim, Germany). Sections, 5 μm thick, were cut with a rotary heavy duty microtome HM 360 (Microm, Walldorf, Germany) equipped with a hard metal knife, and stained with hematoxylin-eosin, Masson's trichrome, elastic stain, and a phosphotungstic acid hematoxylin stain. Light microscopic examination was performed by a technician blinded to the type of stent used. Injury of the arterial wall due to stent deployment was evaluated for each stent filament site and graded as described by Schwartz et al.[19] Inflammatory reaction at every stent filament site was carefully examined searching for inflammatory cells, and scored as follows:

1. sparsely located histiolymphocytic infiltrate around the stent filament;
2. more densely located histiolymphocytic infiltrate covering the stent filament, but no foreign body guanuloma or giant cells;
3. diffusely located inflammatory cells and/or giant cells, also invading the media.

The mean score was calculated as the sum of scores for each filament/number of filaments present.

Morphometric analysis of the coronary segments harvested was performed on three slices (proximal, middle, and distal stent region) by using a computerized morphometry program (Leitz CBA 8000). The areas of, respectively, the arterial lumen, the area inside the internal elastic lamina (IEL), and the area inside the external elastic lamina (EEL) were measured. Furthermore, the area stenosis (1 − lumen area/IEL area) and the area of neointimal hyperplasia (IEL area − lumen area) were calculated.

Statistics

In vitro data are presented as mean values ± SEM. Histomorphometric data are presented as mean values ± SD. The in vitro data (proliferation and viability assay) were evaluated by means of a one-way analysis of variance (ANOVA) and Dunnett's multiple comparison post-hoc test. For comparison of histomorphometric data among different groups, a non-paired t-test was used. A p-value <0.05 was considered to be statistically significant.

RESULTS

SEM images of the coated stents

The thickness of coating covering the stent filaments was 10 μm. The stent surface was

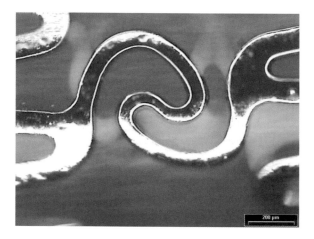

Fig. 38.1 Photograph of a BOBSC dip-coated stent wire.

smooth (Figure 38.1). Loaded MTX into the BOBSC did not influence the surface characteristic (Figure 38.2).

In vitro methotrexate release kinetics

The release curves showed that after 24 hours, 50% of the MTX was already released from the stent (Figure 38.3a). After the first 24 hours, the release was slower, showing an 87% release at 1 week. Finally, after 4 weeks of incubation in NaCl at 37°C, complete release was found (Figure 38.3b).

Effect of MTX on SMC proliferation and viability

After 7 days of incubation with MTX, no reduction of the total number of SMCs was seen (10^{-8}M: 108 ± 24; 10^{-7}M: 107 ± 23; 10^{-6}M: 94 ± 18; 10^{-5}M: 100 ± 14; all data are the percentage of control cells in wells; $n = 4$) as opposed to the dose-dependent reduction in SMC proliferation by paclitaxel (10^{-8}M: 55 ± 13, $p<0.05$; 10^{-7}M: 22 ± 7, $p<0.0005$; 10^{-6}M: 13 ± 3, $p<0.0001$; 10^{-5}M: 5 ± 2, $p<0.0001$; all data are a percentage of control cells in wells, $n = 4$) (Fig 38.4). Similar results were obtained by the total protein synthesis assay. MTX did not reduce SMC proliferation (control: 102.0 ± 2.6 vs 10^{-8}M: 99.3 ± 2.9; 10^{-7}MS: 99.3 ± 4.0; 10^{-6}M: 97.0 ± 6.0; 10^{-5}M:

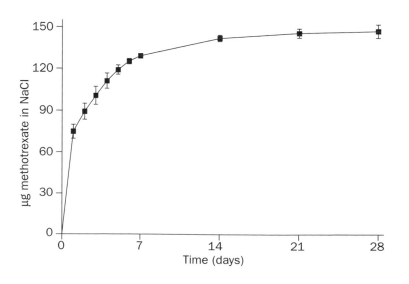

Fig. 38.2 In vitro accumulation of methotrexate released from three SAE coated coronary stents in 1 mL NaCl at 37°C.

a

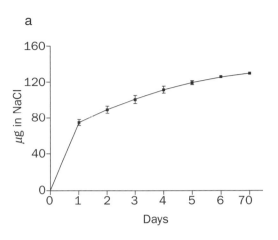

b

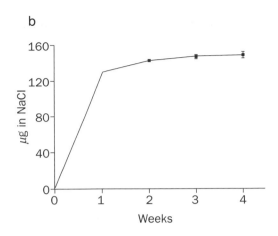

Fig. 38.3 The in vitro accumulation of methotrexate released from three BOBSC coated coronary stents in 1 mL NaCl at 37°C. (a) Release over 1 week and (b) release over 4 weeks.

98.3 ± 7.5; all data are μg/mL; $n = 3$) as opposed to the dose-dependent reduction by paclitaxel (control: 87.3 ± 1.2 vs 10^{-8} M: 82.7 ± 3.8; 10^{-7}M: 69.3 ± 2.5, $p<0.001$; 10^{-6}M: 36.3 ± 1.2, $p<0.0001$; 10^{-5}M: 10.7 ± 2.5, $p<0.0001$; all data are μg/mL; $n = 3$) (Figure 38.5). However, the remaining SMCs after methotrexate incubation showed excellent survival with 100% neutral red staining at all concentrations. This was in contrast with the paclitaxel-incubated SMCs, which showed a dose-dependent decrease in survival, with 93%, 84% 76%, and only 42% of the remaining cells that stained for neutral red at 10^{-8}M, 10^{-7}M, 10^{-6}M, and 10^{-5}M, respectively ($n = 3$).

In vivo biocompatibility of BOBSC-coated stents (Table 38.1)

At 5 day follow-up, both the bare and the BOBSC-coated stents induced an identical histopathological response. The stent filaments showed a good alignment to the vascular wall. The internal elastic membrane was beneath the stent filaments and most of them kept intact. The media were mildly compressed. Arterial injury induced by stent implantation was not significantly different between the two groups. A thin fibrin layer covering the stent filaments was observed. A few inflammatory cells trapped within a thrombotic mesh were observed. The vascular segment without stent filaments appeared normal. No significant differences in the inflammatory score and thrombus score of coated stents and bare stents were observed. At 4 week follow-up, the neointima of both coated and bare stents was well organized, and consisted of extracellular matrix with SMCs. A few inflammatory cells were adjacent to the stent struts. A peristrut inflammation score >2 was rare. The mean inflammation score (1.02 ± 0.08 vs 1.11 ± 0.30, $p>0.05$) and arterial injury score (0.21 ± 0.21 vs 0.28 ± 0.41, $p>0.05$) of the BOBSC-coated and the bare stents were not significantly different. The mean lumen area, neointimal hyperplasia (1.32 ± 0.66 vs 1.73 ± 0.93, $p>0.05$) and area stenosis (20 ± 11 vs 26 ± 16%, $p>0.05$) were similar in both groups.

In vivo effect of stent-based MTX delivery on neointimal formation (Table 38.2)

Histopathological examination found that both the lumen surfaces of the BOBSC-coated and MTX-loaded stents were completely covered with endothelial cells. With an increased stent-to-vessel ratio, a moderate to severe medial compression and stretching were observed.

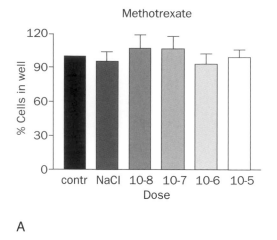

A

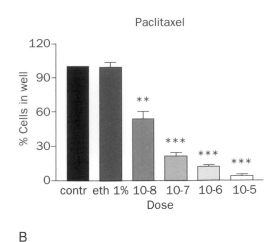

B

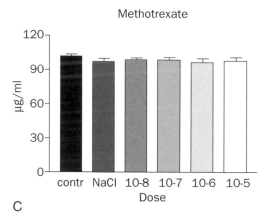

C

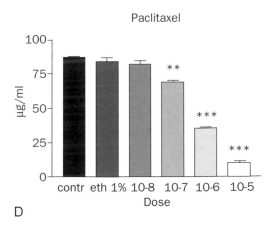

D

Fig. 38.4 (a,b) SMC proliferation by means of cell counting and (c,d) total protein assay. SMCs were incubated for 7 days with (a,c) methotrexate and (b,d) paclitaxel. ** $p<0.01$, *** $p<0.0005$ by one-way ANOVA.

Internal elastic lamina disruption and medial laceration by stent filaments were more frequently observed in the BOBSC-coated stent group. A few sections of BOBSC-coated stents showed a pronounced inflammatory response around some stent filaments, although the inflammatory response from the stent filaments through the media was rare. Compared to the BOBSC-coated stent group, MTX-loaded stents showed a significantly decreased inflammatory response (1.01 ± 0.06 vs 1.30 ± 0.62, $p<0.05$). Furthermore, the neointimal hyperplasia of MTX-loaded stents was limited and developed predominantly around the stent filaments. The neointimal hyperplasia (1.92 ± 1.44 vs 1.13 ± 0.38, $p<0.01$) as well as area stenosis (29 ± 23 vs $17 \pm 6\%$, $p<0.05$) of the BOBSC-coated stents was significantly higher compared to the MTX-loaded stents.

DISCUSSION

In the present study, metallic bare stents coated with a BOBSC biological coating did not provoke increased peristrut inflammatory response at 5 day and 4 week follow-up. The

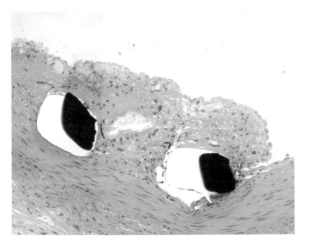

a

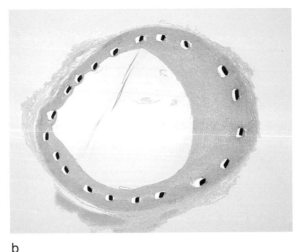

b

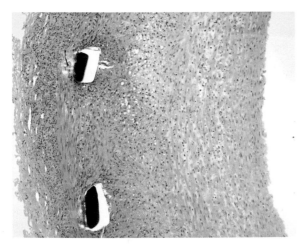

c

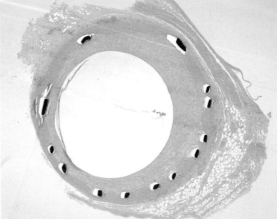

d

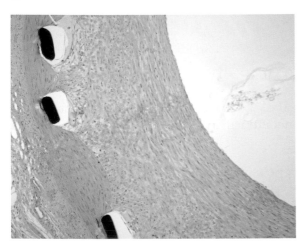

e

Fig. 38.5 (a) Photomicrograph of a coronary segment stented with a BOBSC-coated stent at 5 days. A few inflammatory cells are infiltrating into a thrombus mesh, with leukocytes rolling on the neointimal surface. (b,c) Coronary segment stented with a bare stent, (d–f) BOBSC-coated, or (g) loaded with methotrexate at 4 weeks. (b,c) An eccentric and well organized neointima is observed. Around some stent struts a moderate inflammatory response is present (d,e). With the increased stent/artery ratio, the media are compressed or even lacerated around some stent filaments. However, only occasional inflammatory cells are observed around the stent filaments. (f) In another case, increased peristrut inflammatory reaction and neointimal hyperplasia are noted. (g) Local released MTX significantly inhibits peristrut inflammation and neointimal hyperplasia (hematoxylin-eosin stain. (b) and (d); (c)–(f); (a) and (g): ×25, ×100, and ×200 respectively).

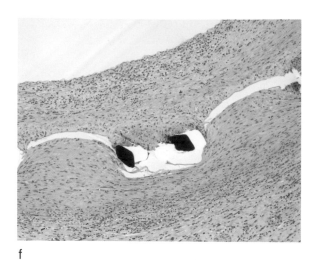

f

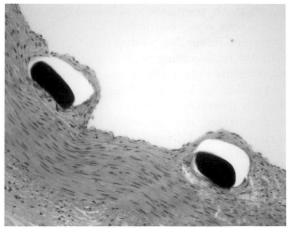

g

Fig. 38.5 *Continued*

Table 38.1   Histomorphometric response to BOBSC-coated stents at 4 week follow-up

Stent	n	Lumen area (mm²)	Neointimal hyperplasia (mm²)	Area stenosis (%)	Inflammation score	Injury score
Bare	30	5.21 ± 1.60	1.73 ± 0.93	26 ± 16	1.11 ± 0.30	0.28 ± 0.41
BOBSC-coated	30	5.65 ± 1.35	1.32 ± 0.66	20 ± 11	1.02 ± 0.08	0.21 ± 0.21

Compared to the bare control stents, no significant differences were observed.

Table 38.2   Histomorphometric analysis of MTX-loaded stents at 4 week follow-up

Stent	n	Lumen area (mm²)	Neointimal hyperplasia (mm²)	Area stenosis (%)	Inflammation score	Injury score
BOBSC-coated	30	4.96 ± 1.93	1.92 ± 1.44	29 ± 23	1.30 ± 0.62	0.43 ± 0.54
Methotrexate-loaded	30	5.80 ± 1.25*	1.13 ± 0.38**	17 ± 6**	1.01 ± 0.06*	0.23 ± 0.17

Compared to BOBSC-coated stents: *$p \leq 0.05$, **$p < 0.01$.

neointimal hyperplasia of BOBSC-coated stents at 4 weeks was even lower than bare stents implanted in similar conditions. Impregnation of the BOBSC coating with 150 μg MTX could significantly reduce the peristrut inflammation and neointimal hyperplasia in an overstretched porcine coronary stenting model. This study demonstrated the feasibility of stent-based methotrexate delivery to prevent in-stent restenosis.

Biocompatible coating: a crucial determinant for the success of drug eluting stents

Polymers have been used as a matrix to incorporate drugs for local delivery. With improving coating methods, ultrathin and homogenous stent coating surfaces could be obtained. Polymer coatings have shown a biocompatibility to blood in ex vivo and in vivo models.[20,21] A reduction of thrombotic events with heparin-coated stents has been reported in animal studies and clinical trials.[18,22] However, poor biocompatibility to coronary arterial tissue has been observed with some polymer coatings.[23] An important inflammatory response induced by the polymer coating resulting in an increased neointimal formation has also been reported.[23,24] The increased inflammation could counteract the efficacy of drug eluting stents. In the present study, a biological polymer was applied to a metallic stent surface to serve as a matrix for local drug delivery. At 5 days the BOBSC-coated stents showed an identical histopathologic response to bare non-coated stents. No significant difference in peristrut inflammation and thrombus formation was observed between the two stent groups. This low inflammatory response to BOBSC-coated stents was also observed at 4 week follow-up. The neointimal hyperplasia and area stenosis of BOBSC-coated stents were even lower than the bare stents. All these data suggest that the BOBSC coating is biocompatible to both blood and coronary arterial tissue. BOBSC-coated stents can therefore serve as a vehicle for local drug delivery.

Methotrexate eluting stents: anti-restenosis effects and postulated mechanisms

It has been found that inflammatory cells and proinflammatory cytokines play an important role in vascular healing. The number of monocytes adhering to the luminal surface of stented arteries correlated linearly with the degree of neointimal hyperplasia in rabbit iliac arteries.[25] Using transgenic mice, Rectenwald et al. demonstrated that tumor necrosis factor (TNF)-α and interleukin (IL)-1 directly participated in the pathogenesis of neointimal hyperplasia.[26] In addition, the antiinflammatory cytokine rhuIL-10 could reduce intimal hyperplasia after both balloon angioplasty and stent implantation in carotid arteries of hypercholesterolemic rabbits.[27]

Methotrexate possesses a variety of antiinflammatory effects. Extracellular MTX penetrates into cells by the reduced folate carrier protein and the folate receptors.[14,28] By inhibition of dihydrofolate reductase and other folate-dependent enzymes, methotrexate can interfere with DNA synthesis in dividing cells and enhance extracellular adenosine release. Extracellular adenosine, binding to its surface receptors, exerts its immunosuppression properties by inhibition of phagocytosis and production of proinflammatory cytokines, as TNF, IL-2, IL-12.[29,30] In addition, MTX can interfere directly with cellular response to IL-1 and increase the gene expression of antiinflammatory cytokines IL-4 and IL-10 from stimulated peripheral blood mononuclear cells (PBMC) of patients with rheumatoid arthritis.[12,31,32] Furthermore, methotrexate can induce apoptosis of activated T-cells and inhibit recruitment of inflammatory monocytes into inflammatory sites.[14,33]

These characteristics have led to some enthusiasm for using MTX to prevent neointimal formation after angioplasty. As oral (1.25 mg 5 days/week) or intramuscular (20 mg/week) administration have failed to inhibit neointimal thickening in a porcine coronary stenting model,[34] intramural balloon catheter delivery and stent-based delivery have been explored.

Using a perfusion catheter, Muller et al. found that the tissue activity of methotrexate was high at 2 hours after instillation. The tissue activity decreased from 10.4 µCi/g to 3.9 µCi/g over the first 24 hours, but remained >2.5 µCi/g from 24 hours to 7 days. Compared to the saline treated control group, the mean intimal thickness of the MTX-treated group was not significantly different.[35] With cellulose ester polymer-coated stents, Cox et al. showed that methotrexate had a washout release at the first hour from the stents. Local delivery of methotrexate or heparin was unsuccessful in inhibiting neointimal proliferation in stented porcine coronary arteries.[15] The increased arterial injury by the perforated balloon, lack of biocompatibility of the polymer coating, too rapid drug release, and inadequate tissue concentrations may all have contributed to the failure of these studies. In this study, we found that the release of MTX from the BOBSC-coated stents was slower than from the cellulose ester polymer-coated stents. In the first 24 hours, 50% of the loaded MTX was released and a complete release was observed within 4 weeks. In the over-stretched porcine coronary stenting model, local released MTX could significantly inhibit peristrut inflammation. In-stent neointimal hyperplasia and area stenosis of MTX-loaded stents were also significantly reduced. Improved biocompatibility of the polymer matrix with a relatively slow drug release may account for the efficacy of the BOBSC-coated MTX-loaded stents.

It has been reported that methotrexate could significantly inhibit vascular endothelial cell proliferation in in vitro cell culture.[36] The degree of endothelial cell injury after stenting was related to vascular healing.[37] Furthermore endothelial regeneration could influence vascular thrombosis and neointimal formation after angioplasty.[38] In our study, no influence of MTX on endothelial cell regeneration was observed. The lumen surface of the MTX-loaded stent was completely covered by endothelium at 4 weeks follow-up and no significant difference was noted between the BOBSC-coated stents and the MTX-loaded stents.

Vascular toxicity with incomplete healing has been observed with paclitaxel eluting stents.[39–41] The reduction of SMC numbers and extracellular protein mass in the medial wall may be related to this process. Methotrexate, as a chemotherapy agent, can influence the metabolism of cells and has a cytotoxic effect. Inhibition of SMC proliferation has been presumed as a potential mechanism for its treatment.[42] In this study, we performed an in vitro cell culture analysis and compared the effects of methotrexate on SMC to paclitaxel. The results showed that with concentrations of 10^{-8}–10^{-5} M, MTX had no effect on SMC proliferation and viability. However, a dose-dependent effect with paclitaxel was observed. Paclitaxel significantly inhibited SMC proliferation, but cell viability was also decreased with increased doses of paclitaxel. Therefore, it is not unreasonable to assume that MTX is more safe and has a larger 'therapeutic window' than paclitaxel for local delivery. Antiinflammation and not antiproliferation seems to be the main mechanism to decrease the neointimal hyperplasia.

In summary, the BOBSC coating showed biocompatible behavior in porcine coronary arteries. Loading methotrexate on BOBSC-coated stents could dramatically reduce neointimal formation and area stenosis. No retarded endothelial regeneration and other local vascular toxicity were observed. BOBSC-coated stents with methotrexate could eliminate peristrut inflammation and contribute to prevent in-stent restenosis.

REFERENCES

1. Edelman ER, Rogers C. Pathobiologic responses to stenting. Am J Cardiol 1998; 81:4E–6E.
2. Karas SP, Gravanis MB, Santoian EC, et al. Coronary intimal proliferation after balloon injury and stenting in swine: an animal model of restenosis. J Am Coll Cardiol 1992; 20(2):467–74.
3. De Scheerder I, Wang K, Wilczek K, et al. Local methylprednisolone inhibition of foreign body response to coated intracoronary stents. Coron Artery Dis 1996; 7(2):161–6.

4. Suzuki T, Kopia G, Hayashi S, et al. Stent-based delivery of sirolimus reduces neointimal formation in a porcine coronary model. Circulation 2001; 104(10):1188–93.

5. Sousa JE, Costa MA, Abizaid A, et al. Lack of neointimal proliferation after implantation of sirolimus-coated stents in human coronary arteries: A quantitative coronary angiography and three-dimensional intravascular ultrasound study. Circulation 2001; 103:192–5.

6. Weinblatt ME, Coblyn JS, Fox DA, et al. Efficacy of low-dose methotrexate in rheumatoid arthritis. N Engl J Med 1985; 312(13):818–22.

7. Chao NJ, Schmidt GM, Niland JC, et al. Cyclosporine, methotrexate, and prednisone compared with cyclosporine and prednisone for prophylaxis of acute graft-versus-host disease. N Engl J Med 1993; 329(17):1225–30.

8. Nash RA, Pineiro LA, Storb R, et al. FK506 in combination with methotrexate for the prevention of graft-versus-host disease after marrow transplantation from matched unrelated donors. Blood 1996; 88(9):3634–41.

9. Mease PJ. Tumour necrosis factor (TNF) in psoriatic arthritis: pathophysiology and treatment with TNF inhibitors. Ann Rheum Dis 2002; 61(4):298–304.

10. Gorlick R, Goker E, Trippett T, et al. Intrinsic and acquired resistance to methotrexate in acute leukemia. N Engl J Med 1996; 335(14):1041–8.

11. Huennekens FM. The methotrexate story: a paradigm for development of cancer chemotherapeutic agents. Adv Enzyme Regul 1994; 34:397–419.

12. Hu SK, Mitcho YL, Oronsky AL, Kerwar SS. Studies on the effect of methotrexate on macrophage function. J Rheumatol 1988; 15(2):206–9.

13. Cutolo M, Bisso A, Sulli A, et al. Antiproliferative and antiinflammatory effects of methotrexate on cultured differentiating myeloid monocytic cells (THP-1) but not on synovial macrophages from patients with rheumatoid arthritis. J Rheumatol 2000; 27(11):2551–7.

14. Cutolo M, Sulli A, Pizzorni C, et al. Antiinflammatory mechanisms of methotrexate in rheumatoid arthritis. Ann Rheum Dis 2001; 60(8):729–35.

15. Cox DA, Anderson PG, Roubin GS, et al. Effect of local delivery of heparin and methotrexate on neointimal proliferation in stented porcine coronary arteries. Coron Artery Dis 1992; 3:237–48.

16. Seye CI, Gadeau AP, Daret D, et al. Overexpression of P2Y2 purinoceptor in intimal lesions of the rat aorta. Arterioscler Thromb Vasc Biol 1997; 17:3602–10.

17. De Scheerder IK, Wang K, Kerdsinchai P, et al. The concept of the home-made coronary stent: experimental results and initial clinical experience. Cathet Cardiovasc Diagn 1996; 39:191–6.

18. De Scheerder I, Wang K, Wilczek K, et al. Experimental study of thrombogenicity and foreign body reaction induced by heparin-coated coronary stents. Circulation 1997; 95:1549–53.

19. Schwartz RS, Huber KC, Murphy JG, et al. Restenosis and the proportional neointimal response to coronary artery injury: results in a porcine model. J Am Coll Cardiol 1992; 19:267–74.

20. Fontaine AB, Koelling K, Clay J, et al. Decreased platelet adherence of polymer-coated tantalum stents. J Vasc Interv Radiol 1994; 5:567–72.

21. Palmaz JC. Review of polymeric graft materials for endovascular applications. J Vasc Interv Radiol 1998; 9(1 pt 1):7–13.

22. van der Giessen WJ, van Beusekom HM, Eijgelshoven MH, et al. Heparin-coating of coronary stents. Semin Interv Cardiol 1998; 3(3–4):173–6.

23. van der Giessen WJ, Lincoff AM, Schwartz RS, et al. Marked inflammatory sequelae to implantation of biodegradable and nonbiodegradable polymers in porcine coronary arteries. Circulation 1996; 94:1690–7.

24. De Scheerder IK, Wilczek KL, Verbeken EV, et al. Biocompatibility of polymer-coated oversized metallic stents implanted in normal porcine coronary arteries. Atherosclerosis 1995; 114:105–14.

25. Rogers C, Edelman ER. Endovascular stent design dictates experimental restenosis and thrombosis. Circulation 1995; 91(12):2995–3001.

26. Rectenwald JE, Moldawer LL, Huber TS, et al. Direct evidence for cytokine involvement in neointimal hyperplasia. Circulation 2000; 102(14):1697–702.

27. Feldman LJ, Aguirre L, Ziol M, et al. Interleukin-10 inhibits intimal hyperplasia after

angioplasty or stent implantation in hyper-cholesterolemic rabbits. Circulation 2000; 101(8):908–16.

28. Longo-Sorbello GS, Bertino JR. Current understanding of methotrexate pharmacology and efficacy in acute leukemias. Use of newer antifolates in clinical trials. Haematologica 2001; 86(2):121–7.

29. Cronstein BN, Naime D, Ostad E. The antiinflammatory mechanism of methotrexate. Increased adenosine release at inflamed sites diminishes leukocyte accumulation in an in vivo model of inflammation. J Clin Invest 1993; 92(6):2675–82.

30. Bouma MG, Stad RK, van den Wildenberg FA, Buurman WA. Differential regulatory effects of adenosine on cytokine release by activated human monocytes. J Immunol 1994; 153(9):4159–68.

31. Connolly KM, Stecher VJ, Danis E, et al. Alteration of interleukin-1 production and the acute phase response following medication of adjuvant arthritic rats with cyclosporin-A or methotrexate. Int J Immunopharmacol 1988; 10(6):717–28.

32. Constantin A, Loubet-Lescoulie P, Lambert N, et al. Antiinflammatory and immunoregulatory action of methotrexate in the treatment of rheumatoid arthritis: evidence of increased interleukin-4 and interleukin-10 gene expression demonstrated in vitro by competitive reverse transcriptase-polymerase chain reaction. Arthritis Rheum 1998; 41(1):48–57.

33. Genestier L, Paillot R, Fournel S, et al. Immunosuppressive properties of methotrexate: apoptosis and clonal deletion of activated peripheral T cells. J Clin Invest 1998; 102(2):322–8.

34. Murphy JG, Schwart RS, Edwards WD, et al. Methotrexate and azathioprine fail to inhibit porcine coronary restenosis (abstract). Circulation 1990; 82(suppl): III-429.

35. Muller DW, Topol EJ, Abrams GD, et al. Intramural methotrexate therapy for the prevention of neointimal thickening after balloon angioplasty. J Am Coll Cardiol 1992; 20(2):460–6.

36. Hirata S, Matsubara T, Saura R, et al. Inhibition of in vitro vascular endothelial cell proliferation and in vivo neovascularization by low-dose methotrexate. Arthritis Rheum 1989; 32(9):1065–73.

37. Rogers C, Parikh S, Seifert P, Edelman ER. Endogenous cell seeding. Remnant endothelium after stenting enhances vascular repair. Circulation 1996; 94(11):2909–14.

38. Van Belle E, Tio FO, Chen D, et al. Passivation of metallic stents after arterial gene transfer of phVEGF165 inhibits thrombus formation and intimal thickening. J Am Coll Cardiol 1997; 29(6):1371–9.

39. Farb A, Heller PF, Shroff S, et al. Pathological analysis of local delivery of paclitaxel via a polymer-coated stent. Circulation 2001; 104(4):473–9.

40. Drachman DE, Edelman ER, Seifert P, et al. Neointimal thickening after stent delivery of paclitaxel: change in composition and arrest of growth over six months. J Am Coll Cardiol 2000; 36(7):2325–32.

41. Heldman AW, Cheng L, Jenkins GM, et al. Paclitaxel stent coating inhibits neointimal hyperplasia at 4 weeks in a porcine model of coronary restenosis. Circulation 2001; 103(18):2289–95.

42. Liang GC, Nemickas R, Madayag M. Multiple percutaneous transluminal angioplasties and low dose pulse methotrexate for Takayasu's arteritis. J Rheumatol 1989; 16(10):1370–3.

39

Rapamycin eluting stents

Robert L Wilensky and Bruce D Klugherz

Rapamycin, or sirolimus, is a macrocyclic lactone that inhibits vascular smooth muscle cell proliferation and migration (Figure 39.1). It also possesses immunosuppressive properties and is used clinically to prevent acute renal allograft rejection. Ongoing clinical trials are evaluating its use in preventing cardiac transplant rejection and allograft vasculopathy. Since smooth muscle cell proliferation and chronic inflammation are prominent features of in-stent restenosis, rapamycin has been evaluated as a prophylactic treatment of restenosis. In that in-stent restenosis is a local, self-limited phenomenon and that rapamycin possesses systemic toxic effects, rapamycin may be an ideal anti-restenotic agent to be delivered locally from a stent-based platform.

Rapamycin reduces neointima formation by reducing vascular smooth muscle cell migration,[1] and by inhibiting smooth muscle cell (SMC) progression through the cell cycle, the final common pathway regulating cellular proliferation (Figure 39.2). Upon entry into the SMC rapamycin binds to its cytosolic receptor FKBP12. This complex ultimately inhibits retinoblastoma protein (Rb protein) phosphorylation, the gatekeeper of the cell cycle restriction point. In addition to possibly inhibiting Rb protein phosphorylation directly, the intermediate steps by which rapamycin inhibits phosphorylation include elevation of the cyclin-dependent kinase inhibitor $p27^{Kip1}$ levels and reduction of the levels of some cyclin-dependent kinases (cdks).[2] Rb protein in the constitutive state is hypophosphorylated and bound to the transcription factor E2F. Following a proliferative stimulus Rb is phosphorylated, dissociates from E2F and cellular progression through the G_1–S phase restriction point ensues resulting in DNA synthesis and mitosis. Cdks are cell cycle regulatory proteins, the accumulation and enzymatic activation of which result in Rb phosphorylation.[3] $p27^{Kip1}$ is an important inhibitor of G_1 phase cyclin/cdk complexes and high intracellular levels of $p27^{Kip1}$ inhibit enzymatic activation of cdk2. Finally, the effect of the rapamycin-FKBP12 on Rb phosphorylation may be mediated by a reduction in $p33^{cdk2}$ and $p34^{cdk2}$ activity. The net effect is decreased cellular proliferation via cytostasis rather than cytotoxicity.

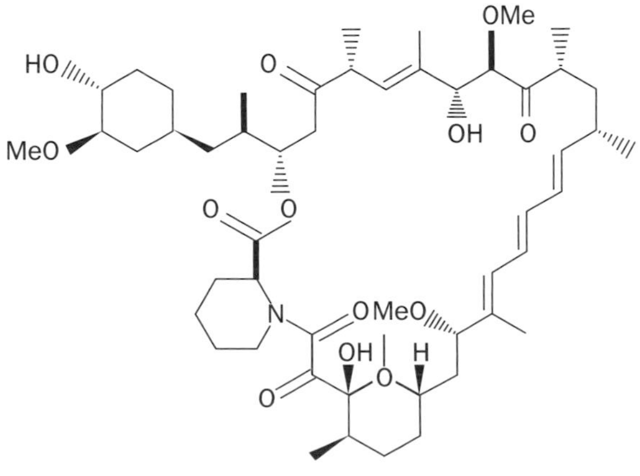

Following oral administration, rapamycin is largely sequestered in erythrocytes resulting in a high blood-to-plasma ratio of 36–49:1.[4–6] The half-life in humans is about 60 hours and rapamycin is metabolized in the liver via

Fig. 39.1 The chemical structure of rapamycin.

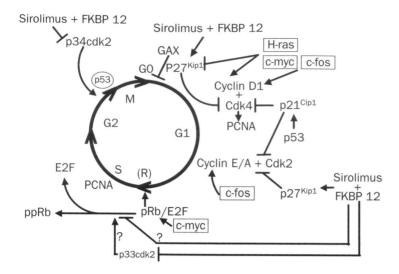

Fig. 39.2 Action of sirolimus on the cell cycle resulting in reduced smooth muscle cell proliferation. Arrows indicate a stimulatory effect and lines indicate an inhibitory effect. (Modified from Braun-Dullaeus RC, Mann MJ, Dzau VJ. Circulation 1998; **98**:82–9[3] with permission from Lippincott Williams & Wilkins.)

cytochrome P450 3A isoforms.[6] Cytopenias represent the major dose-limiting toxicity as thrombocytopenia has been observed in 37% and leukopenia in 39% of renal allograft recipients treated with therapeutic doses of rapamycin.[7] Following renal transplantation a blood level of 5–15 ng/mL is required for adequate prophylaxis against renal transplant tissue rejection.[4]

Blood levels and systemic toxicity may both be reduced using a rapamycin eluting stent. The stent coating consists of a polymer blend with attractive mechanical properties necessary for a biologically safe stent coating (Figure 39.3). It is elastic, easily sterilized, biostable, and non-thrombogenic. The polymer thickness is less than 20 µm and thus the tissue reaction is minimal, since endovascular inflammation is in part determined by polymer mass. Both fast and slow release formulations have been tested in animals and humans and no increased tissue inflammation has been demonstrated. Since sirolimus possesses potent antiinflammatory properties arterial inflammation should be reduced in comparison with other polymer-coated stents.[8]

Following stent deployment in pigs whole blood levels of sirolimus peaked at 1 hour at a level of 0.9 ng/mL. Thereafter, blood levels decreased below the level of quantification by 72 hours (<0.4 ng/mL). Tissue levels of siro-limus were maximal at 14 days and sirolimus remained in the arterial wall for at least 28 days. This persistent elevation of sirolimus tissue levels confers its prolonged effect on vascular SMCs.[9] By 28 days, 32% of the sirolimus loaded on the stent was still bound to the stent and was therefore potentially available for local vascular therapy.

The sirolimus eluting stent has shown efficacy in two animal models of neointimal formation and has demonstrated promising results in early clinical trials. Efficacy studies in the nonatherosclerotic rabbit iliac model have demonstrated a dose-dependent reduction in neointimal area 28 days following stent implantation.[10] Neointimal formation was reduced 23% with the low dose formulation (64 ± 4 µg/stent) and 45% with the high dose formulation (196 ± 9 µg/stent). Efficacy studies in porcine coronary arteries demonstrated a similar, although not dose-dependent, effect with a 30% reduction in the neointimal area at 28 days compared to the uncoated stent group, and a 45% decrease compared to the polymer-coated stent.[11] In addition, preclinical studies have demonstrated that this eluting stent satisfies three important criteria demanded of all potentially efficacious, clinically useful, polymer-coated stent-based drug delivery systems: (1) The biocompatible, non-biodegradable polymer does not cause or exacerbate a local

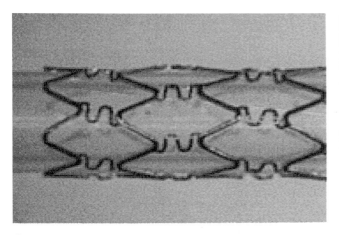

a

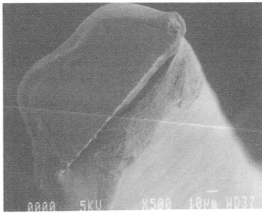

b

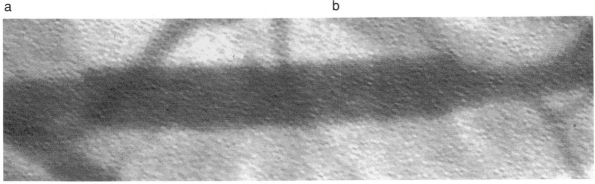

c

Fig. 39.3 (a) Photograph of the stent used for animal studies. (b) Scanning electron micrograph showing a cross-section of a stent strut. Note the thin polymer layer coating the strut. (c) Radiograph of rabbit iliac artery following delivery of a sirolimus eluting stent.

Table 39.1 Studies using sirolimus (rapamycin)

Year	Research model	Delivery modality	Physical properties	Half-life	Metabolism	Study
2000	Human: renal transplant	Oral	Lipophilic	Serum:62 h	Hepatic via cytochrome P450 3A	4,5
2000	Rabbit iliac	Stent	Lipophilic			10
2000	Porcine coronary	Stent	Lipophilic	Stent:68% eluted by 28 d		9,11

inflammatory response; (2) Smooth muscle cell proliferation is inhibited; (3) The combination of drug and coating appears to be non-toxic to the endothelium.

Early clinical observations from patients in São Paolo and Rotterdam have shown that implantation of the rapamycin eluting stent is not associated with increased rates of early or late clinical adverse events.[12,13] In São Paolo 30 patients have undergone stent implantation, 15 patients with a fast release polymer coating and 15 patients with a slow release formulation. In Rotterdam, six patients have undergone stent implantation and angiographic follow-up. None of the 45 patients have suffered clinical restenosis or a long-term major adverse clinical event at 30 day follow-up. Between 30 days and 2 years one subacute occlusion resulting from an edge dissection was noted, one patient had a new stenosis proximal from the drug eluting stent and one patient had a new stenosis distal from the stent.[13–14] Angiographic and intravascular ultrasound studies likewise demonstrated excellent long-term results. By quantitative coronary angiography, a late loss of 0.07 ± 0.29 mm within the lesion and 0.00 ± 0.29 mm within the stent was observed, far less than historical controls. By intravascular ultrasonography the mean percentage volume obstruction at follow-up was 10.7% (range 5–15%) with the mean volume of intimal hyperplasia 15 mm.[3] At 2 year follow-up the lesion late loss was 0.13–0.33 mm with the change in diameter not significantly different than the results observed at 6 months.[13–14]

There have been at least 4 randomized, double-blind, multicenter clinical trials evaluating the efficacy of sirolimus-eluting stents in patients with coronary artery disease. The RAVEL study[15] randomized 238 patients to either a sirolimus-eluting stent or bare metal stent. All patients had a single lesion in a native coronary artery with lesion length <18 mm. The results demonstrated an in-stent restenosis rate of 0% vs 27% in the uncoated stent group. The major adverse clinical event (MACE) rate including target lesion revascularization was

5.5% vs 28.8%. The American pivotal trial SIRIUS enrolled 1058 patients and was designed to evaluate higher-risk lesions than the RAVEL trial.[16] Patients randomized to the sirolimus-eluting stent had an in-stent restenosis rate of 3.2% vs 35.4% for the bare metal stent and the MACE rates were 7.1% and 18.9% respectively. Late luminal loss was 0.17 mm for the sirolimus stent and 1.0 mm for the uncoated stent. E-SIRIUS and C-SIRIUS[17,18] were similar in design to the SIRIUS study, however, mean vessel diameter was smaller in E- and C-SIRIUS and the clinical risk profile was greater in the E-SIRIUS. Both studies confirmed the findings of RAVEL and SIRIUS, demonstrating the superior efficacy of the sirolimus-eluting stent compared to bare metal stents.

REFERENCES

1. Poon M, Marx SO, Gallo R, et al. Rapamycin inhibits vascular smooth muscle cell migration. J Clin Invest 1996; 98:2277–83.

2. Gallo R, Padurean A, Jayaraman T, et al. Inhibition of intimal thickening after balloon angioplasty in porcine coronary arteries by targeting regulators of the cell cycle. Circulation 1999; 99:2164–70.

3. Braun-Dullaeus RC, Mann MJ, Dzau VJ. Cell cycle progression. New therapeutic target for vascular proliferative disease. Circulation 1998; 98:82–9.

4. MacDonald A, Scarola J, Burke JT, Zimmerman JJ. Clinical pharmacokinetics and therapeutic drug monitoring of sirolimus. Clin Therapeut 2000; 22:B101–21.

5. Trepanier DJ, Gallant H, Legatt DF, Yatscoff RW. Rapamycin: distribution, pharmacokinetics and therapeutic range investigations: an update. Clin Biochem 1998; 31:345–51.

6. Brattstrom C, Sawe J, Tyden G et al. Kinetics and dynamics of single oral doses of sirolimus in sixteen renal transplant recipients. Ther Drug Monit 1997; 19:397–406.

7. Groth CG, Backman L, Morales JM, et al. Sirolimus (rapamycin)-based therapy in human renal transplantation: similar efficacy and dif-

ferent toxicity compared with cyclosporine. Sirolimus European Renal Transplant Study Group. Transplantation 1999; 67:1036–42.

8. Attur MG, Patel R, Thakker G, et al. Differential anti-inflammatory effects of immunosuppressive drugs: cyclosporin, rapamycin and FK-506 on inducible nitric oxide synthase, nitric oxide, cyclooxygenase-2 and PGE2 production. Inflamm Res 2000; 49:20–6.

9. Klugherz BD, Llanos G, Lieuallen W, et al. Twenty-eight day efficacy and pharmacokinetics of the sirolimus-eluting stent. Coron Artery Dis, 2002; 13:183–188.

10. Suzuki T, Kopia G, Bailey LR, et al. Stent-based delivery of sirolimus reduces neointimal formation and instent restenosis in a porcine coronary model. Circulation 2001; 104:1188–1193.

11. Abizaid A. Intravascular ultrasound findings after implantation of rapamycin eluting stents in humans. 12th Annual Transcatheter Cardiovascular Therapeutics, Washington DC, October 2000.

12. Serruys, PW. Early clinical observations with the rapamycin (sirolimus) coated velocity stent. 12th Annual Transcatheter Cardiovascular Therapeutics, Washington DC, October, 2000.

13. Sousa JE, Costa MA, Sousa AG, et al. Two-year angiographic and intravascular ultrasound follow-up after implantation of sirolimus-eluting stents in human coronary arteries. Circulation 2003; 104:381–3.

14. Degertekin M, Serruys PW, Foley DP, et al. Persistent inhibition of neointimal hyperplasia after sirolimus-eluting stent implantation: long-term (up to 2 years) clinical, angiographic, and intravascular follow-up. Circulation 2002; 106:1610–13.

15. Morice M-C, Serruys PW, Sousa JE, et al. A randomized comparison of a sirolimus-eluting stent with a standard stent for coronary revascularization. N Engl J Med 2002; 346:1773–80.

16. Moses JW, Leon MB, Popma JJ, et al. A multicenter randomized clinical study of the sirolimus-eluting stent in native coronary lesions: clinical outcomes. Circulation 2002; 106[supplement]: II-392–3.

17. Schofer J, Schluter M. E-SIRIUS: 8-month efficacy results. Presented at the 52nd Annual Scientific Sessions of the American College of Cardiology, Chicago, IL, March, 2003.

18. Schampaert E, Cohen EA, Reeves F, et al. Results from the Canadian multicenter, randomized, double-blind study of the sirolimus-eluting stent in the treatment of patients with de novo coronary artery lesions. Presented at the 52nd Annual Scientific Sessions of the American College of Cardiology, Chicago, IL, March, 2003.

40

Preclinical evaluation of tacrolimus-coated coronary stents

Yanming Huang, Shengqiao Li, Lan Wang, Eric Verbeken, and Ivan De Scheerder

Introduction • **Materials and methods** • **In vivo studies** • **Results** • **Discussion**

INTRODUCTION

In-stent restenosis remains an unresolved problem, which occurs in 10–50% of patients undergoing coronary stenting within the first 3–6 months.[1,2] Neointimal formation is the main contributor to in-stent restenosis.[3,4] Stent-induced arterial injury and peristrut inflammation are involved in the process of neointimal formation by activating cytokines and growth factors, which induce smooth muscle cell dedifferentiation, migration, and proliferation.[5,6] Histopathological studies found that neointimal hyperplasia is principally composed of smooth muscle cells, inflammatory cells, and extracellular matrix.[7,8] Stent-based delivery of antiproliferative and/or antiinflammatory agents have shown beneficial effects on neointimal hyperplasia in experimental studies and clinical trials.[9,10]

Tacrolimus (FK506) is a water-insoluble macrolide immunosuppressant which was discovered in 1984.[11] It has been widely used in reducing the incidence and severity of allograft rejection after organ transplantation.[12] It has also been used to treat other inflammatory conditions, such as atopic dermatitis.[13,14] In this study, we evaluated the efficacy of stent-based delivery of tacrolimus on inflammation and neointimal formation in an over-stretched coronary stent model.

MATERIALS AND METHODS

Stents and stent coating

Stainless steel balloon expandable stents (Jostent™, Germany) were used for these studies. The bare stents, 16 mm long, were dip-coated in a biological polymer (BOBSC coating) or in a polymer/tacrolimus solution (200 µg/stent) for in vivo studies. In addition, bare stents, 18 mm long were dip-coated in a polymer/tacrolimus solution to load 750 µg/stent of tacrolimus for in vitro release analysis.

The surface characteristics of the coated stents were examined by microscopy. The stents were sterilized using ethylene oxide before implantation in porcine coronary arteries.

In vitro drug release studies

Three 750 µg tacrolimus loaded BOBSC-coated stents were placed in vials, containing 1 ml 0.9% NaCl at 37°C. Ultraviolet (UV) absorbance (Cary 4 E spectrophotometer, Varian Inc, CA,

USA) was measured at 205 nm for tacrolimus each day for the first 14 days and after 3 and 4 weeks to determine the tacrolimus release. After every time point, the stents were replaced in a new vial containing NaCl. One control BOBSC-coated stent underwent the same procedure and the UV absorbance values were subtracted from the values of the drug eluting stents.

Impact of tacrolimus on vascular smooth muscle cells (SMCs) in vitro

Smooth muscle cells were isolated from New Zealand White rabbit aorta, passaged and cultured (50 000 cells/well) in six-well plates (Corning).[15] Every third day, 0, 10^{-8}, 10^{-7}, 10^{-6}, and 10^{-5}M tacrolimus or paclitaxel (Bristol-Meyers-Squibb), both dissolved in 20 µl ethanol, was added in combination with medium changes. After 7 days, SMC proliferation was determined by either: (1) cell counting (Coulter Counter) or, (2) protein quantification (BCA Protein Assay Kit, Pierce). Before protein quantification in the latter assay, cell viability was determined using neutral red uptake.[16] A viability index for each concentration was calculated as percentage neutral red from control/percentage total protein from control.

IN VIVO STUDIES

Domestic cross-bred pigs of both sexes, weighing 20–25 kg were used. They were fed with a standard natural grain diet without lipid or cholesterol supplementation throughout the study. All animals were treated and cared for in accordance with the Belgium National Institute of Health Guidelines for the care and use of laboratory animals.

Surgical procedures and stent implantation in coronary arteries were performed according to the method described by De Scheerder et al.[17,18]

Biocompatibility of the polymer coating

Acute study
Five BOBSC-coated stents and five bare stents were randomly implanted in the right and left anterior descending coronary arteries of 5 pigs. The arterial segments were selected to obtain a 1.1:1 stent to artery ratio. The pigs were sacrificed after 5 days to evaluate injury, acute inflammatory response and thrombus formation.

Chronic study
Ten BOBSC-coated stents and 10 bare stents were implanted randomly in a coronary artery of 10 pigs with the same oversizing as in the acute study. Pigs were sacrificed after 4 weeks to evaluate peristrut inflammation and neointimal hyperplasia.

Stent-based tacrolimus delivery

Seventeen BOBSC-coated stents and 17 BOBSC-coated stents loaded with 200 µg tacrolimus were randomly deployed in porcine coronary arteries. The arterial segments were selected to obtain a 1.2:1 stent-to-artery ratio. The pigs were sacrificed after 4 weeks to evaluate the efficacy of local tacrolimus delivery on neointimal hyperplasia.

Tissue processing and histomorphometric analysis

At 5 day or 4 week follow-up, the pigs were sacrificed and the stented coronary artery was perfused with a 10% formalin solution at 80 mmHg. Artery segments were carefully dissected together with a minimum 1 cm vessel segment both proximal and distal to the stent. The segment was fixed in a 10% formalin solution. Each segment was cut into a proximal, middle, and distal stent segment for histomorphometric analysis. The region between the proximal and middle of tacrolimus delivery study was used for immunohistochemical analysis. Tissue specimens were embedded in a cold-polymerizing resin (Technovit 7100, Heraus Kulzer GmbH, and Wehrheim, Germany). Sections, 5 µm thick, were cut with a rotary heavy duty microtome HM 360 (Microm, Walldorf, Germany) equipped with a hard metal knife, and stained with hematoxylin-eosin, elastic, lectin, Movat, and phosphotungstic acid hematoxylin stain. Light microscopic examination was performed with the technician blinded to the type of stent used. Injury of the arterial wall due to stent deployment was evaluated for each stent filament site and graded as described.[19] Inflammatory reaction at every stent filament site was carefully examined searching for inflammatory cells, and scored as follows:

1. sparsely located histiolymphocytic infiltrate around the stent filament;
2. more densely located histiolymphocytic infiltrate covering the stent filament, but no foreign body guanuloma or giant cells;
3. diffusely located inflammatory cells and/or giant cells, also invading the media.

The mean score was calculated as the sum of scores for each filament/number of filaments present.

Morphometric analysis of the coronary segments harvested was performed on 3 slices (proximal, middle and distal stent part) by using a computerized morphometry program (Leitz CBA 8000). The areas of respectively the arterial lumen, the area inside the internal elastic lamina (IEL), and the area inside the external elastic lamina (EEL) were measured. Furthermore, the area stenosis (1 – lumen area/IEL area) and the area of neointimal hyperplasia (IEL area – lumen area) were calculated.

Immunohistochemistry staining

In situ immunohistochemistry was performed on separated sections with monoclonal antibodies against proliferation cell nuclear antigen (PCNA, Dako), macrophages (CD-68, mac-387, 1/300, Serotec), and endothelium (von Willebrand factor – vWf – The Birmingham Site). The PCNA and mac-387 density (number positive cells/mm^2) at 4 stent struts (at 3, 6, 9, and 12 o'clock) were measured as described and the average for each segment was calculated.[20] The vWf staining for each segment was graded as follows:

I. <10% positivity of the lumen circumference

II. between 10% and 50% positivity of the lumen circumference
III. between 50% and 90% positivity of the lumen circumference
IV. >90% positivity of the lumen circumference.

Statistics

Data are presented as mean values ± SD. The in vitro data (protein synthesis and viability assay) were evaluated by means of a one-way analysis of variance (ANOVA) and Dunnett's multiple comparison post-hoc test. For comparison of histomorphometric data between different groups, a non-paired t-test was used. A p-value <0.05 was considered to be statistically significant.

RESULTS

Images of the coated stents

The surface analysis of BOBSC-coated stents is presented in Figure 40.1. Dip-coating resulted in a smooth ultrathin coating (10 μm). Impregnation of the coating with 750 μg tacrolimus did not alter the surface of the coating.

In vitro drug release

Drug release curves showed that after 24 hours, only 28% of the loaded tacrolimus was released

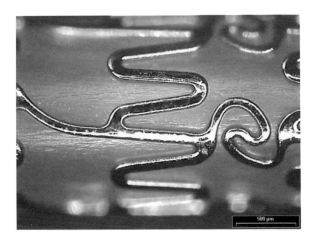

Fig. 40.1 Photograph of a BOBSC-dip-coated stent wire.

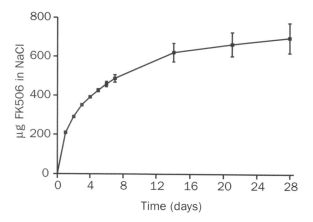

Fig. 40.2 The in vitro tacrolimus (FK506) release curve from three BOBSC-coated stents in 1 mL NaCl at 37°C.

from the stents. After the first 24 hours, the release continuously raised, showing that after 1 week, 65% of the loaded tacrolimus was released. Finally, after 4 weeks of incubation in NaCl at 37°C, almost complete (92%) release was obtained (Figure 40.2).

Effect of tacrolimus on SMC proliferation and cell viability

During SMC culture, tacrolimus did not show any effect on cell proliferation, whereas paclitaxel concentration-dependently reduced both

cell count and protein content. However, neutral red staining showed good SMC survival for tacrolimus with a viability index of 100% at all concentrations, whereas paclitaxel induced >50% cell death at the highest concentration (Figure 40.3).

In vivo biocompatibility of the BOBSC coating

At 5 day follow-up, the bare metallic and BOBSC-coated stents showed a similar histopathological response. The arterial media were intact and mildly compressed. A few inflammatory cells were seen adjacent to the stent filaments (Figure 40.4a). Stent struts with moderate inflammatory reaction were rare. A thin thrombotic mesh covering the stent filaments was observed. The inflammatory and thrombus scores of the coated stents and the bare stents were not significantly different. Arterial injury caused by stent deployment was low and identical for both groups.

At 4 week follow-up, a well organized neointima with a few inflammatory cells was observed. The histopathological reaction of the vessel wall was comparable between the BOBSC-coated and the bare stent group. The mean lumen area, neointimal hyperplasia (bare stents 1.45 ± 0.81 vs coated stents 1.30 ± 0.68, $p>0.05$) and area stenosis (22 ± 14 vs 19 ± 12,

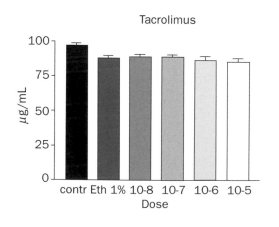

a

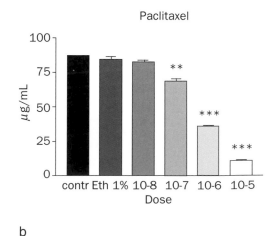

b

Fig. 40.3 Smooth muscle cell (SMC) total protein synthesis assay. SMCs were incubated for 7 days with (a) tacrolimus and (b) paclitaxel. ** $p<0.005$, *** $p<0.0001$ by one-way ANOVA.

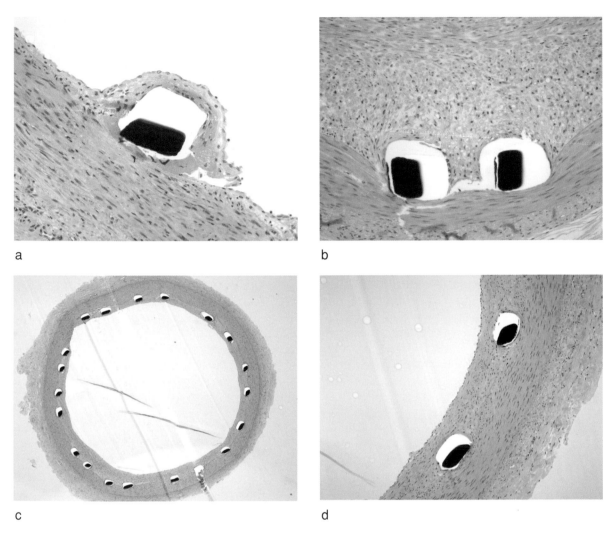

Fig. 40.4 (a) Photomicrograph of a coronary segment stented with a BOBSC-coated stent at 5 days. A few inflammatory cells attached and infiltrated into the thrombus mesh. (b) Photomicrograph of a coronary segment stented with a BOBSC-coated stent at 4 weeks. The media are deeply compressed. Increased neointimal hyperplasia with peristrut inflammation is present. (c,d) Photomicrograph of coronary segment stented with BOBSC-coated tacrolimus loaded stent at 4 weeks showing a decreased peristrut inflammation and neointimal hyperplasia (hematoxylin-eosin stain). (a) and (b) ×200; (c) ×25; (d) ×100.

$p>0.05$) were similar for the two groups. The peristrut inflammation (1.12 ± 0.33 vs 1.03 ± 0.09, $p>0.05$) and arterial injury (0.30 ± 0.43 vs 0.21 ± 0.21, $p>0.05$) of the BOBSC-coated and bare stents were identical. Furthermore, compared to the 5 day follow-up, peristrut inflammation of BOBSC-coated stents did not show an increased response.

Stent-based tacrolimus delivery (Table 40.1)

With an increased stent/artery ratio, the BOBSC-coated stents showed increased arterial injury and inflammatory response. The stent struts showed a moderate compression of the arterial media. Internal elastic lamina disruption and medial laceration were observed. A

Table 40.1   Histomorphometric analysis of tacrolimus-loaded stents at 4 week follow-up

Stent	n	Lumen area (mm²)	Neointimal hyperplasia (mm²)	Area stenosis (%)	Balloon area/IEL area	Inflammation score	Injury score
BOBSC-coated	17	4.57 ± 2.10	2.16 ± 1.34	34 ± 22	1.26 ± 0.16	1.27 ± 0.51	0.48 ± 0.44
Tacrolimus-loaded	17	5.98 ± 1.51*	1.14 ± 0.50**	17 ± 9**	1.22 ± 0.15	1.05 ± 0.08	0.17 ± 0.10**

IEL, internal elastic lamina. Compared to BOBSC-coated stents: *$p<0.05$, **$p<0.01$.

few stent filaments showed a moderate inflammatory reaction, although inflammatory cells in the media and adventitia were rare (Figure 40.4b). In contrast, tacrolimus-loaded stents showed a limited inflammatory response. A few inflammatory cells around the stent filaments were observed. No foreign body granuloma or giant cells were present. The inflammatory score (1.05 ± 0.08 vs 1.27 ± 0.51, $p = 0.088$) and arterial injury (0.17 ± 0.10 vs 0.48 ± 0.44, $p<0.01$) of tacrolimus-loaded stents were lower than the control stents. Furthermore, the neointima of tacrolimus-loaded stents was much thinner. Consistent with the decreased inflammation and arterial injury, both the neointimal thickness (1.14 ± 0.50 vs 2.16 ± 1.34, $p<0.01$) and area stenosis (17 ± 9 vs 34 ± 22, $p<0.01$) of tacrolimus-loaded stents were significantly reduced (Figure 40.4c,d). No intraintimal hemorrhage and focal medial necrosis were observed.

Immunochemistry examination showed a 49.64% reduction of macrophage contents in mac-387 staining in tacrolimus-loaded stents as compared to control stents (5.65 ± 13.28 vs 11.22 ± 19.34 cells/mm², $p>0.05$, Figure 40.5a,b). PCNA staining was more variable in the BOBSC-coated stent group, with one valued as 884.04 cells/mm². Excluding this extreme value, however, the positive cells of PCNA staining were comparable between the two groups (tacrolimus-loaded 92.43 ± 79.67 vs BOBSC-coated 85.46 ± 74.14 cells/mm², $p>0.05$, Figure 40.5c,d). Furthermore, equal vWf staining surrounding the lumen was observed in both groups (tacrolimus-loaded: 3.40 ± 0.51 vs BOBSC-coated: 3.53 ± 0.62, $p>0.05$, Figure 40.5 e,f).

DISCUSSION

In the present study, a porcine coronary stenting model was used to evaluate the biocompatibility of a polymer-coated stent and the efficacy of stent-based tacrolimus delivery to reduce neointimal hyperplasia. Stainless steel bare stents coated with a biological polymer showed a biocompatible response when implanted in porcine coronary arteries. No increased peristrut inflammation and neointimal hyperplasia with coated stents were seen when compared to bare stents. Stent-based tacrolimus delivery significantly reduced neointimal formation, which was associated with a decreased peristrut inflammation and

Fig. 40.5 Quantification of immunochemistry (PCNA) staining of peristrut proliferation, inflammation (macrophages, Mac-387) and endothelium (vWf) in tacrolimus-loaded (left panels) and BOBSC-coated (right panels) stent group. The macrophage contents of BOBSC-coated stents (b) were more pronounced than the tacrolimus-loaded stents (a). The positive cells of PCNA staining (c,d), and vWf staining (e,f) of the two groups were comparable. (a)–(d) ×200; (e) and (f) ×100.

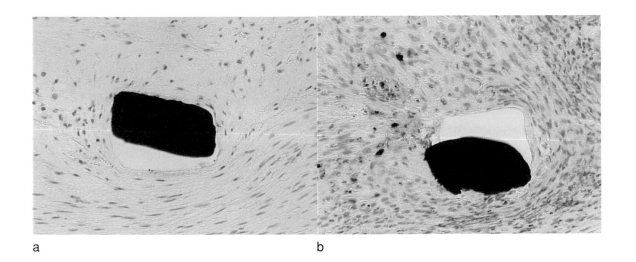

a   b

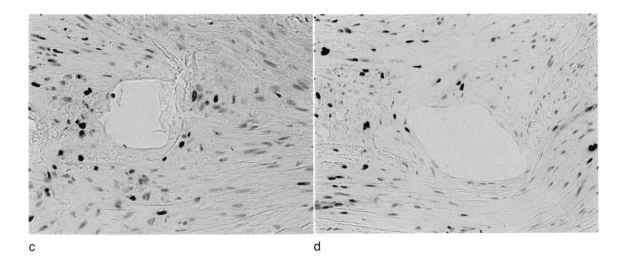

c   d

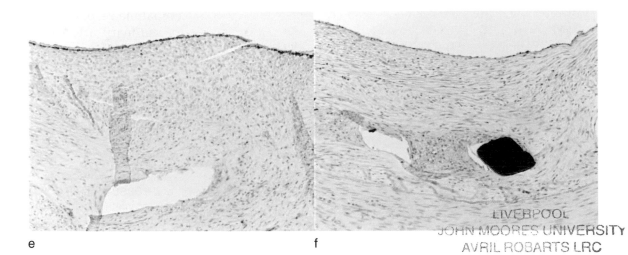

e   f

arterial injury. Our findings demonstrate the feasibility, safety, and efficacy of using tacrolimus eluting stents to prevent in-stent restenosis in a porcine coronary model.

Polymer coatings for local drug delivery

Polymers have been applied to the stent surface as a reservoir for sustained drug release at the stenting site. Drugs can elute from a polymer matrix or be released with the degradation of the polymer coating. Studies have shown that some synthetic polymers, biodegradable or non-biodegradable, result in an important inflammatory and proliferative tissue response.[21,22] These reactions may counteract the biological effect of the local released drug and can contribute to neointimal hyperplasia. Therefore, the polymer matrix is a crucial determinant for the optimal function of a drug eluting stent. Biological polymers, such as fibrin and phosphorylcholine (PC), have the advantage of minimizing the inflammatory response. They may also be beneficial in limiting thrombus formation and neointimal hyperplasia.[23,24] It has been found that fibrin film-coated stents, compared to polyurethane-coated stents, showed a significantly decreased neointimal hyperplasia and foreign body tissue reaction.[24] PC-coated metallic stents did not increase the neointimal formation in a porcine stenting model.[25] In this study, we used a biological polymer to coat the metallic stent surface. At 5 days a few inflammatory cells adjacent to stent struts were observed, which was comparable to the bare metallic stent. No increased fibrin deposition on the stent struts was observed. At 4 week follow-up, the peristrut inflammatory response was still low and no significant difference was observed between 5 day and 4 week follow-up. These results suggest that this biological coating is biocompatible when implanted in coronary arteries. In addition, this coating material slowly dissolves *until 4 weeks* without inducing an inflammatory reaction. The BOBSC-coated stent group did not induce an increased neointimal formation when compared to the bare stent group at 4 weeks. All these data indicate that the BOBSC coating can serve as a suitable coating for local drug delivery.

Tacrolimus eluting stent: possible mechanism for anti-restenosis effects

Tacrolimus is a potent immunosuppressive agent with potent antiinflammatory properties. It is a hydrophobic drug and can easily penetrate the plasma membrane to enter the cytoplasm. Binding to the intracellular FK-binding protein (FK-BP), tacrolimus forms a complex and then binds to calcineurin. This binding inhibits the activation of calcineurin and disrupts the dephosphorylation nuclear translocation of nuclear factor of activated T-cells (NF-AT). Transcription proteins, required for generation of interleukin (IL)-2 and other proinflammatory cytokines, such as IL-3, IL-4, IL-5, IL-6, IL-8 and its receptor, tumor necrosis factor, are inhibited.[14,26,27] With its lipophilic characteristic, suppression of proinflammatory cytokine expression and inhibition of T-cell proliferation, tacrolimus is a potentially interesting drug for stent-based delivery to decrease peristrut inflammation and neointimal hyperplasia.

The lipophilic nature of tacrolimus may enable it to pass easily through the cell membrane and minimize the loss to the blood flow. The BOBSC coating material is able to contain a high dose of tacrolimus keeping a gradient from the stent struts to arterial tissue and facilitating the tissue uptake. To analyze the release characteristics, we loaded a high dose of tacrolimus (750 µg) into the BOBSC matrix. In the first 24 hours, only 28% of the loaded tacrolimus was released and the release period lasted for at least 4 weeks. As the drug release in vivo from stent surface to arterial wall is much slower than the release in vitro, a prolonged tacrolimus release and high arterial tissue concentration in vivo can be assumed.

The role of inflammation in the cascade of neointimal formation has been well documented. The arterial injury and vessel stretch during stenting, focal thrombus formation at the stent struts, and local atherosclerotic lesions can activate and recruit leukocytes, monocytes, and macrophages from the circulating blood and adventitia at the stenting site. Clinical studies have shown that an inflammatory reaction is common in neointimal hyperplasia.[7,8] The number of macrophages and inflammatory markers could predict the rate of restenosis in patients undergoing coronary angioplasty.[28] In addition, a positive relationship has been found between the extent of the inflammatory reaction and the amount of neointimal formation in animal studies.[29] By releasing chemotatic and growth factors, inflammatory cells can regulate the vascular repair and neointimal formation. Antiinflammatory agents delivered using coated stents have shown a beneficial effect on in-stent restenosis in experimental and clinical studies.[30,31]

It has been reported that coronary stent graft (CSG) loaded with a high dose tacrolimus has moderate reduction of neointima in a rabbit iliac artery.[32] In this study, we used an overstretched coronary stent model to increase arterial injury and inflammatory response, and evaluated the effects of tacrolimus on neointimal formation. Our studies demonstrated that local delivery of tacrolimus using BOBSC-coated stents could significantly inhibit the peristrut inflammation. The peristrut macrophage contents of tacrolimus-coated stents were decreased by almost 50% compared to the control stents. In rabbit carotid arteries, ceramic-coated stents loaded with tacrolimus, compared to the uncoated stents, also showed a decreased lymphocyte and macrophage score.[32] Furthermore, compared to BOBSC-coated stents, the neointimal hyperplasia and area stenosis of tacrolimus-loaded stents were significantly reduced, although the PCNA staining positive cells of the two stent groups were comparable. Local released tacrolimus to prevent macrophages and T-cell migration and proliferation, inhibit the release of proinflammatory factors after stenting, and may contribute to these reductions.

Both cytostatic and cytotoxic agents have been used for stent-based delivery. With cytotoxic agents, a delayed healing process has been observed in some drug eluting stents.[33,34] Using chondroitin sulfate- and gelatin-coated stents with paclitaxel, Farb et al. demonstrated

an incomplete healing in the higher dose (42.0 and 20.2 µg) groups.[33] Intimal fibrin deposition and hemorrhage, medial necrosis, and advential inflammation were observed. Although the mechanism of the vascular toxicity of paclitaxel is uncertain, a reduction in cell number and extracellular protein mass was observed. As smooth muscle cells (SMCs) are the dominant cells in the arterial medial layer, we compared the effects of tacrolimus with paclitaxel on SMCs in vitro. No reduction of SMC proliferation by means of a total protein quantification assay was found when SMCs were incubated with tacrolimus in different concentrations from 10^{-8} to 10^{-5}M. Moreover, these SMCs also showed an excellent viability at all concentrations. In contrast, however, a dose-dependent reduction of SMC proliferation and a decreased viability were noted with paclitaxel. These findings suggest that tacrolimus has a higher safety range than paclitaxel. In another study, Lüscher et al (personal communication) found that tacrolimus showed a toxic effect on SMC in vitro cell cultures, however, the tacrolimus concentration to kill 50% of cells was over a hundred times lower than paclitaxel. In our in vivo study, the score of vWf staining of tacrolimus-loaded stents was comparable to the coated control stents, which reflects that local released tacrolimus from the coated stents did not retard the regrowth of endothelium. Furthermore, no medial necrosis, increased adventitial inflammation, and other local arterial toxic effects with tacrolimus-loaded stents were observed.

In conclusion, compared to bare stents, BOBSC-coated stents did not elicit an increased inflammatory response and proliferative tissue reaction. Stent-based tacrolimus delivery using the BOBSC coating could effectively reduce neointimal hyperplasia. This effect relates most probably to its antiinflammatory properties.

REFERENCES

1. Al Suwaidi J, Berger P, Homers DR. Coronary artery stents. JAMA 2000; 284:1826–36.
2. Goldberg SL, Loussararian A, De Gregorio J, et al. Predictors of diffuse and aggressive

intrastent restenosis. J Am Coll Cardiol 2001; 37:1019–25.

3. Hoffmann R, Mintz GS, Dussaillant GR, et al. Patterns and mechanisms of in-stent restenosis. A serial intravascular ultrasound study. Circulation 1996; 94(6):1247–54.

4. Mudra H, Regar E, Klauss V, et al. Serial follow-up after optimized ultrasound-guided deployment of Palmaz-Schatz stents. In-stent neointimal proliferation without significant reference segment response. Circulation 1997; 95(2):363–70.

5. Reidy MA. A reassessment of endothelial injury and arterial lesion formation. Lab Invest 1985; 53:513–20.

6. Ferrell M, Fuster V, Gold HK, et al. A dilemma for the 1990s. Choosing appropriate experimental animal model for the prevention of restenosis. Circulation 1992; 85:1630–1.

7. Grewe PH, Deneke T, Machraoui A, et al. Acute and chronic tissue response to coronary stent implantation: pathologic findings in human specimen. J Am Coll Cardiol 2000; 35:157–63.

8. Farb A, Sangiorgi G, Carter AJ, et al. Pathology of acute and chronic coronary stenting in humans. Circulation 1999; 99:44–52.

9. Sousa JE, Costa MA, Abizaid A, et al. Lack of neointimal proliferation after implantation of sirolimus-coated stents in human coronary arteries: A quantitative coronary angiography and three-dimensional intravascular ultrasound study. Circulation 2001; 103:192–5.

10. De Scheerder I, Huang Y. Anti-inflammatory approach to restenosis. In Rothman MT (ed), Restenosis: Multiple Strategies for Stent Drug Delivery. ReMEDICA: London 2001:13–31.

11. Kino T, Hatanaka H, Hashimoto M, et al. K-506, a novel immunosuppressant isolated from a Streptomyces: I. Fermentation, isolation, and physico-chemical and biological characteristics. J Antibiot 1987; 40:1249–55.

12. Spencer CM, Goa KL, Gillis JC. Tacrolimus. An update of its pharmacology and clinical efficacy in the management of organ transplantation. Drugs 1997; 54:925–75.

13. Alaiti S, Kang S, Fiedler VC, et al. Tacrolimus (FK506) ointment for atopic dermatitis: a phase I study in adults and children. J Am Acad Dermatol 1998; 38:69–76.

14. Zabawski EJ, Costner M, Cohen JB, et al. Tacrolimus: pharmacology and therapeutic uses in dermatology. Int J Dermatol 2000; 39:721–7.

15. Bruijns RH, Bult H. Effects of local cytochalasin D delivery on smooth muscle cell migration and on collar-induced intimal hyperplasia in the rabbit carotid artery. Br J Pharmacol 2001; 134:473–83.

16. Bonin PD, Singh JP, Gammill RB, Erickson LA. Inhibition of fibroblast and smooth muscle cell proliferation and migration in vitro by a novel aminochromone U-67154. J Vasc Res 1993; 30:108–15.

17. De Scheerder IK, Wang K, Kerdsinchai P, et al. The concept of the home-made coronary stent: experimental results and initial clinical experience. Cathet Cardiovasc Diagn 1996; 39:191–6.

18. De Scheerder I, Wang K, Wilczek K, et al. Experimental study of thrombogenicity and foreign body reaction induced by heparin-coated coronary stents. Circulation 1997; 95:1549–53.

19. Schwartz RS, Huber KC, Murphy JG, et al. Restenosis and the proportional neointimal response to coronary artery injury: results in a porcine model. J Am Coll Cardiol 1992; 19:267–74.

20. Farb A, Weber DK, Kolodgie FD, Burke AP, Virmani R. Morphological predictors of restenosis after coronary stenting in humans. Circulation 2002; 105:2974–80.

21. van der Giessen WJ, Lincoff AM, Schwartz RS, et al. Marked inflammatory sequelae to implantation of biodegradable and nonbiodegradable polymers in porcine coronary arteries. Circulation 1996; 94:1690–7.

22. De Scheerder IK, Wilczek KL, Verbeken EV, et al. Biocompatibility of polymer-coated over-sized metallic stents implanted in normal porcine coronary arteries. Atherosclerosis 1995; 114:105–14.

23. Fontaine AB, Koelling K, Clay J, et al. Decreased platelet adherence of polymer-coated tantalum stents. J Vasc Interv Radiol 1994; 5:567–72.

24. Holmes DR, Camrud AR, Jorgenson MA, et al. Polymeric stenting in the porcine coronary artery model: differential outcome of exogenous fibrin sleeves versus polyurethane-coated stents. J Am Coll Cardiol 1994; 24:525–31.

25. Whelan DM, van der Giessen WJ, Krabbendam SC, et al. Biocompatibility of phosphorylcholine coated stents in normal porcine coronary arteries. Heart 2000; 83:338–45.

26. Thomson AW, Bonham CA, Zeevi A. Mode of action of tacrolimus (FK506): molecular and cellular mechanisms. Ther Drug Monit 1995; 17:584–91.

27. Almawi WY, Melemedjian OK. Clinical and mechanistic differences between FK506 (tacrolimus) and cyclosporin A. Nephrol Dial Transplant 2000; 15:1916–18.

28. Moreno PR, Bernardi VH, Lopez-Cuellar J, et al. Macrophage infiltration predicts restenosis after coronary intervention in patients with unstable angina. Circulation 1996; 94:3098–102.

29. Kornowski R, Hong MK, Tio FO, et al. In-stent restenosis: contributions of inflammatory responses and arterial injury to neointimal hyperplasia. J Am Coll Cardiol 1998; 31:224–30.

30. De Scheerder I, Wang K, Wilczek K, et al. Local methylprednisolone inhibition of foreign body response to coated intracoronary stents. Coron Artery Dis 1996; 7(2):161–6.

31. Liu X, Huang Y, De Scheerder I, et al. Study of antirestenosis with the BiodivYsio dexamethasone eluting stent (STRIDE): A multicenter trial. J Am Coll Cardiol 2002; 39:15A (abstract).

32. Wieneke H, Dirsch O, Sawitowski T, et al. Synergistic effects of a novel nanoporous stent coating and tacrolimus on intima proliferation in rabbits. Catheter Cardiovasc Interv 2003; 60:399–407.

33. Farb A, Heller PF, Shroff S, et al. Pathological analysis of local delivery of paclitaxel via a polymer-coated stent. Circulation 2001; 104(4):473–9.

34. Drachman DE, Edelman ER, Seifert P, et al. Neointimal thickening after stent delivery of paclitaxel: change in composition and arrest of growth over six months. J Am Coll Cardiol 2000; 36(7):2325–32.

41

Local delivery of paclitaxel as a stent coating

Alan W Heldman

Introduction • **Paclitaxel** • **Clinical studies of paclitaxel eluting stents**
• **Transition to clinical studies**

INTRODUCTION

Stent restenosis has been a frustrating problem, and is almost entirely due to neointimal proliferation, a scarring response to injury. Certain factors predict the risk of restenosis, including vessel diameter and length of stent, but we are far from being able to detect in advance the one out of four or five patients who will require a repeat intervention after implant of a bare metal stent.

Coronary stents were the first substantial breakthrough in attempts to prevent restenosis following angioplasty. Early clinical trials established that coronary stents reduced the incidence of restenosis by increasing the lumen gain compared to that achieved with angioplasty alone. However, even in those early trials it was evident that the late loss of lumen diameter (the degree of renarrowing that was detected at follow-up angiography) was greater in stented than in non-stented arteries. While stent recoil or compression is not completely insignificant, by far the greatest cause of this lumen loss in stents is neointimal hyperplasia. Restenosis following arterial dilation has three components (Figure 41.1): elastic

recoil, arterial remodeling, and neointimal proliferation. Stents limit the first two, but may exacerbate the third process, so that in-stent restenosis is caused by the proliferation of neointimal cells. In response to injury and to a variety of growth factors, vascular wall cells migrate from outside the stent to within, where proliferation of fibroblastic smooth muscle cells narrows the lumen available for blood flow. This is the principal mechanism of in-stent restenosis, and as a disease of inappropriate cell proliferation, its treatment may draw upon what our colleagues in oncology already know about arresting cell growth.

There is a wide range in degrees of response to vascular injury, and in some sense it is surprising that clinically important in-stent restenosis does not occur more frequently. In most cases, healing occurs in such a way that only mild neointimal ingrowth develops, and durable clinical results are seen in most patients. Smaller diameter and longer stents are indicators of increased risk. With decreasing diameter, stents can accommodate less neointima; it is for this reason that stents that lose diameter after initial expansion (stent recoil)

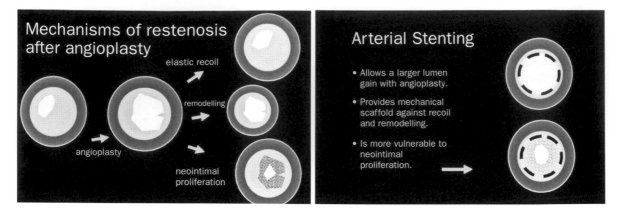

Fig. 41.1 Mechanisms of restenosis after angioplasty and arterial stenting.

have been associated with a higher frequency of restenosis. Other mechanical factors, such as vessel straightening by the stent,[1] may also influence the tendency to restenosis. Some biological markers of a predisposition to neointimal formation have been proposed, including diabetes,[2] female gender,[3] restenosis at another lesion,[4] and allergy to the nickel and molybdenum components of stainless steel stents.[5]

Because of the potential for achieving high concentrations of an agent at the site of injury without systemic side effects, local therapeutics to prevent restenosis have been extensively studied. A wide variety of catheters have been developed to deliver agents to the interventional site. While these devices have conceptually been proven to deliver drug to the vessel wall, none has yet provided convincing evidence of benefit from this form of therapy. In some cases, endothelial barrier function may have limited delivery to the arterial wall, as has been demonstrated for heparin.[6] Extravascular forms of delivery such as periarterial wraps, devices, or drug compounds have been useful in animal models of vascular diseases, providing insights into the mechanisms of drug distribution.[7] Extravascular delivery to the coronaries may even be clinically feasible by an intrapericardial approach using pericardial access tools. However to date, the only clinically useful local delivery strategy has been electromagnetic energy in the form of beta or gamma radiation. Systemic drug therapies to

limit intimal hyperplasia have been generally ineffective, although there is the suggestion that some drugs, such as probucol,[8] and tranilast,[9] may be effective when given orally.

PACLITAXEL

Paclitaxel was discovered in a survey of natural compounds as an antiproliferative agent, originally derived from the bark of the Yew tree. It shifts the dynamic equilibrium between the soluble and insoluble forms of tubulin, producing an abnormally stable population of microtubules. Cell processes depending on the continuous turnover of microtubules are inhibited. As such, paclitaxel has become one of the most important and frequently used chemotherapeutic agents for the treatment of malignant neoplasms, as the active ingredient in the drug Taxol®, which consists of paclitaxel dissolved in an oil vehicle. This formulation is required because paclitaxel is insoluble in water. Indeed, this highly lipophilic character appears to be an important factor in the development of this agent for local prevention of restenosis.

Sollott and colleagues at the Gerontology Research Center of the National Institute of Aging,[10] showed that paclitaxel exerted potent inhibitory effects on proliferation and invasion of rat aortic smooth muscle cells in a Boyden chamber, with an IC50 in the nanomolar range (Figure 41.2). Further, perivascular application

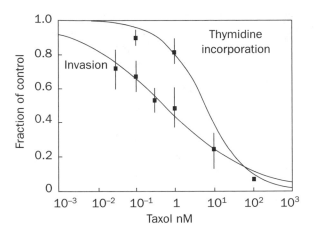

Fig. 41.2 Paclitaxel exhibits potent inhibitory effects on proliferation and invasion of rat aortic smooth muscle cells.

of paclitaxel in a rat carotid injury model limited neointimal proliferation.

Paclitaxel's potent effect at nanomolar range concentrations, and the possibility of delivering adequate amounts to the site of injury with a stent coating suggested that this local delivery strategy was worth testing. The findings of the NIA group were confirmed and extended by the work of Axel and colleagues,[11] in the lab of Dr Karl Karsch. Potent dose-related inhibition of cell proliferation was demonstrated in cultured human aortic smooth muscle cells, with a dose range very similar to that seen with rat cells (Figure 41.3). It was further noted that this effect could be achieved by using either continuous or short-term exposure to the drug. The effect was to inhibit proliferation without cell killing; cell numbers did not fall below those measured before the addition of paclitaxel.

This cytostatic effect of paclitaxel could overcome the stimulatory effects of various growth factors that have been implicated in the initiation of human coronary restenosis, including platelet-derived growth factor (PDGF) and thrombin. Interestingly, endothelial cells were somewhat less sensitive to paclitaxel, and were not significantly inhibited by the short term application of a dose which *did* inhibit smooth muscle cell proliferation.

CLINICAL STUDIES OF PACLITAXEL ELUTING STENTS

A variety of strategies for getting paclitaxel to the vessel wall have been tested in the porcine coronary artery model. For many drugs, polymeric application and delivery coatings have been required for local delivery systems. The challenge of formulating a coating which is free of inflammatory, thrombotic, or restenosis-aggravating effects has driven the development of a large number of candidate polymers as well as nonpolymeric stent-based delivery systems. Simplest among these was to apply drug directly on to the bare metal stent. Early testing of this approach with a simple, crude coating of paclitaxel on a bare stainless steel stent in the porcine coronary model showed powerful dose-dependent inhibition of in-stent neointimal proliferation one month after implantation.[12] At the dose which most effectively limited neointimal growth, other effects were commonly seen, including intramural hemorrhage, inflammation, medial thinning, and tissue retraction away from the stent struts. Nonetheless, there were no thrombotic events in these minipigs, despite antiplatelet treatment with aspirin alone (i.e. without a thienopyridine drug, ticlopidine or clopidogrel). Subsequent refinement of the non-polymeric stent coating technique resulted in a smoother and more uniform drug distribution. Unpublished experiments suggest that the result of such refinement was to reduce or eliminate signs of vessel wall toxicity, indicating a more uniform distribution of drug into the arterial tissue.

Drug distribution: considerations for safety and efficacy

Paclitaxel reduces neointimal hyperplasia both in pig coronary arteries and in rabbit iliac arteries when delivered as a stent coating.[13] Oberhoff and colleagues reported an exploration of paclitaxel locally delivered in another way by a double balloon infusion catheter, and found that this approach did not reduce the neointimal hyperplasia associated with angioplasty and stenting.[14] Taken together these

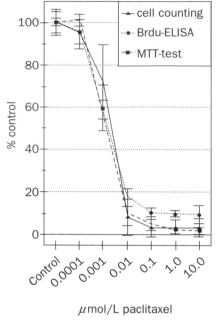

a

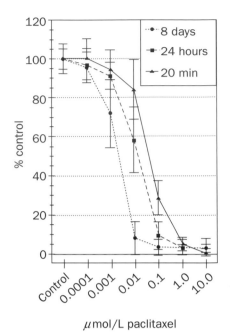

b

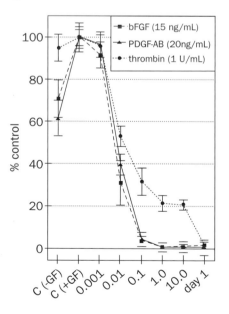

c

Fig. 41.3   Paclitaxel causes dose-related inhibition of cell proliferation in cultured human aortic smooth muscle cells.

different results suggest that the mechanism of drug delivery is a crucial variable, affecting the efficiency of transfer, local pharmacokinetics, the depth of drug delivery, and the relationship between the drug and the site of injury. It is, of course, possible that further refinements to techniques and devices for non-stent based delivery could improve outcomes and reduce the gap between local drug instillation and drug eluting stents. However, in contrast to delivery of hydrophilic drugs, such as heparin, the delivery of highly hydrophobic paclitaxel into arterial tissue is dependent on the duration of contact with the vessel wall,[15] a situation that favors stent-based drug delivery over catheter delivery.

The physical properties of paclitaxel have other important implications for its local delivery. Its intensely hydrophobic nature means that its transfer to the arterial wall will be more efficient than a hydrophilic drug like heparin, as demonstrated experimentally by Baumbach and colleagues.[16] Hwang and colleagues at MIT showed, with an elegant simulation of drug distribution, that the hydrophobic paclitaxel would have very short diffusion distances – so short that even in the space between adjacent stent struts, local tissue concentrations would vary widely, being highest just around the strut.[17] An irregular coating would intensify this effect, the drug concentration in tissue volume immediately adjacent to large clumps of crystalline drug being very high. In contrast, a smooth and uniform non-polymeric coating of paclitaxel directly on the stent's abluminal surface alone resulted in preserved efficacy without the dramatic tissue retraction and other negative effects seen with the early system. This coating technique is now being used in clinical trials of the Cook devices.

An important concern with all antiproliferative therapies has been their effect on the endothelial lining. Endothelial stucture and function would be expected to have important implications for safety and the use of adjunctive drug therapies, particularly of antiplatelet drugs. Re-endothelialization of the injured and stented segment is generally believed to be protective against the risk of stent thrombosis.

Detection of a complete endothelial monolayer (such as with scanning electron microscopy) and of intact barrier function (by the exclusion of dyes) is evidence of re-endothelialization, and is one of the healing processes that might occur along the way to quiescence of the restenosis response.

TRANSITION TO CLINICAL STUDIES

Normal pig coronaries are delicate, nearly transparent thin-walled vessels. In contrast, human coronary disease produces thickened walls, mineralized plaques, fibrous barriers, and dense pools of lipid debris. While the animal studies have informed our thinking about doses for clinical testing, it would not be unreasonable to expect different dose–response relationships in humans. Other differences may also be significant: sources of endothelium for regrowth may be less available or less vigorous in diseased arteries than in normal animals and a cautious approach to prevention of thrombosis is warranted.

Based on our understanding of the very short diffusion and non-uniform distribution of drug within the compartment of the artery wall, the proper expression of dose would be expected to be the *density* of paclitaxel on the abluminal metal surface area of the stent. Early trials of the non-polymeric Cook coating using three rather different stent designs may confirm this expectation. These range from the high metal area Supra-G stent used in the ASPECT study, through the intermediate metal area Logic stent used in the PATENCY study, to the low metal area V-flex used in the ELUTES trial. Taking a different approach, the Boston Scientific program for paclitaxel-eluting stents has focused on polymer-based regulation of drug-release kinetics.

From industrial quarters, tremendous excitement has been generated about drug-coated stents through the lay and financial press. Several compounds hold promise, as do several strategies for getting the drug on to the stent then off again into the vessel wall. A number of research programs for drug-eluting stents have undergone transition from animal studies to clinical testing. Along the way we have seen that different breeds of pig respond differently, and that results are highly sensitive to variables in the experimental protocol. Atherosclerotic human arteries may be more, or less responsive to locally delivered drugs; differences even among our own species relate to different tendencies and mechanisms of restenosis. Gene polymorphisms and metal allergies affect the risk of restenosis,[18] and differences in plaque composition influence the inflammatory response to stenting.[19] We may some day deliver to the arterial wall a drug tailored for an individual patient, or for an individual plaque. Local drug delivery to the arterial wall by stenting is feasible, and holds promise for the reduction of neointimal hyperplasia after injury by another approach than vascular brachytherapy.

Lessons learned from the experience with coronary brachytherapy may prove to be important as we develop and study drug eluting stents. While the effects of radiation are different from those of the antiproliferative drugs, it would not be surprising to find interactions between the angioplasty/stent and the local drug therapy, just as has been seen with brachytherapy. Edge effects ('candy wrapper restenosis') after brachytherapy relate at least in part to the technical demands of precise radiation delivery; it appears to be important to apply the antiproliferative treatment to the entire injured arterial segment, avoiding 'geographic miss'. The increased frequency of late stent thrombosis after brachytherapy suggests that not only restenosis itself, but also vessel wall healing and endothelial function is suppressed by radiation. For brachytherapy, long-term combination antiplatelet therapy with aspirin plus a thienopyridine (clopidigrel or ticlopidine) has become standard. As these drugs are generally well-tolerated, it seems prudent to apply the same standard to trials with antiproliferative drug-coated stents; recent and ongoing clinical trials have protocolized 2–6 months of aspirin plus clopidigrel.

In most other regards, the technique of deploying a drug eluting stent is not much different from the use of any other stent. Some care not to damage the stent coating may be required, and manufacturers should be expected to provide evidence of coating durability. In certain cases, before implantation, drug-coated stents will be challenged by prolonged abrasion against a calcified non-compliant vessel wall. Durability of coatings under these conditions remains to be established, both for polymeric and for non-polymeric approaches. Clinicians will encounter cases of difficult device delivery, vessel tortuosity, and calcification, and extreme conditions beyond those tested in clinical trials. Even with a completely successful coating, stent design and implantation technique will certainly remain important. A stent that is undersized, has been compressed, or which recoils to a smaller diameter will be much more vulnerable to even a small amount of neointimal ingrowth. A uniform coating will go a long way towards minimizing tissue concentration gradients, and the Hwang/Edelman model suggests that the uniformity of stent strut spacing will also be an important variable. In the era of drug eluting stents, stent delivery systems may also be challenged to achieve perfect results every time. Complete apposition of the stent to the vessel wall would be at least as important as ever. Late stent malapposition has been described with rapamycin eluting stents but very rarely with paclitaxel eluting stents. The clinical significance of this phenomenon remains to be seen. While the logistic demands of stenting are less complicated than for brachytherapy, the safety and efficacy of drug eluting stents will be the more important consideration in their clinical development and their comparison to brachytherapy. It is possible that these different strategies will be used for different situations: prevention of vs treatment of in-stent restenosis; native vessels vs vein grafts; large vessels vs small ones.

Stent margin restenosis was not unheard-of even before there was brachytherapy, and particularly given the very short diffusion distance of the hydrophobic drugs, it will undoubtedly prove important that the drug eluting stent covers the entire segment injured by the angioplasty. Edge effects would probably not be the same as we saw with radioactive stents, where the falling-off radiation dose actually stimulated the restenosis process. Rather, we must be vigilant that plain old-fashioned restenosis is not initiated by injury outside the segment protected by the drug delivery device. Side branches too, would not be protected at a distance away from the drug source in the main vessel, and could perhaps even serve as a reservoir of uninhibited vascular cells from which restenosis could appear. Complex coronary anatomy will still challenge interventional technique. Finally, it is clear that we will want to follow the results of the initial trials for the long term, in case catch-up phenomena should occur.

Will we eventually treat all coronary lesions with antiproliferative drug eluting stents, or only selected ones at higher risk for restenosis? Cost of the new devices will undoubtedly influence our ability to provide completely percutaneous multivessel revascularization. Will one drug serve all clinical conditions, or might one drug be best in diabetic patients, for example, and another be best in unstable syndromes? While heparin-coated stents are now available, there is a paucity of evidence to compare these with uncoated devices. In order to understand the utility of drug eluting stents, systematic study in a variety of conditions will be required. Lesion subsets at high risk for recurrence, including small vessels, vein grafts, diffuse stent restenosis, and ostial/bifurcation sites might each require a tailored approach. When we can confidently treat left main coronaries, chronic total occlusions, and diffuse small vessel narrowings safely and with assurance that restenosis will not occur, then coronary angioplasty will finally have achieved its promise.

REFERENCES

1. Gyongyosi M, Yang P, Khorsand A, Glogar D. Longitudinal straightening effect of stents is an additional predictor for major adverse cardiac events. J Am Coll Cardiol 2000; 35(6):1580–9.
2. Lee SG, Lee CW, Hong MK, et al. Predictors of diffuse-type in-stent restenosis after coronary stent implantation. Catheter Cardiovasc Interv 1999; 47(4):406–9.
3. Goldberg SL, Loussararian A, De Gregorio J, et al. Predictors of diffuse and aggressive intra-stent restenosis. J Am Coll Cardiol 2001; 37(4):1019–25.
4. Hoffmann R, Mintz GS, Reineke T, et al. Lesion-to-lesion relationship of the restenosis process after placement of coronary stents. Catheter Cardiovasc Interv 2000; 51(3):266–72.
5. Koster R, Vieluf D, Kiehn M, et al. Nickel and molybdenum contact allergies in patients with coronary in-stent restenosis. Lancet 2000; 356(9245):1895–7.
6. Lovich MA, Philbrook M, Sawyer S, et al. Arterial heparin deposition: role of diffusion, convection, and extravascular space. Am J Physiol 1998; 275(6 pt 2):H2236–42.
7. Lovich MA, Brown L, Edelman ER. Drug clearance and arterial uptake after local perivascular delivery to the rat carotid artery. J Am Coll Cardiol 1997; 29(7):1645–50.
8. Daida H, Kuwabara Y, Yokoi H, et al. Effect of probucol on repeat revascularization rate after percutaneous transluminal coronary angioplasty (from the probucol angioplasty restenosis trial). Am J Cardiol 2000; 86(5):550–2.
9. Tamai H, Katoh O, Suzuki S, et al. Impact of tranilast on restenosis after coronary angioplasty: tranilast restenosis following angioplasty trial (TREAT). Am Heart J 1999; 138:968–75.
10. Sollott SJ, Cheng L, Pauly RR, et al. Taxol inhibits neointimal smooth muscle cell accumulation after angioplasty in the rat. J Clin Invest 1995; 95(4):1869–76.
11. Axel DI, Kunert W, Goggelmann C, et al. Paclitaxel inhibits arterial smooth muscle cell proliferation and migration in vitro and in vivo using local drug delivery. Circulation 1997; 96(2):636–45.
12. Heldman AW, Jenkins GM, Cheng L, et al. Local paclitaxel delivery inhibits neointimal hyperplasia at four weeks in a porcine model of coronary restenosis. Circulation 2001; 103:2289–95.
13. Drachman DE, Edelman ER, Seifert P, et al. Neointimal thickening after stent delivery of paclitaxel: change in composition and arrest of growth over six months. J Am Coll Cardiol 2000; 36(7):2325–32.

14. Oberhoff M, Herdeg C, Al Ghobainy R, et al. Local delivery of paclitaxel using the double-balloon perfusion catheter before stenting in the porcine coronary artery. Catheter Cardiovasc Interv 2001; 53(4):562–8.

15. Creel CJ, Lovich MA, Edelman ER. Arterial paclitaxel distribution and deposition. Circ Res 2000; 86(8):879–84.

16. Baumbach A, Herdeg C, Kluge M, et al. Local drug delivery: impact of pressure, substance characteristics, and stenting on drug transfer into the arterial wall. Catheter Cardiovasc Interv 1999; 47(1):102–6.

17. Hwang CW, Wu D, Edelman ER. Physiological transport forces govern drug distribution for stent-based delivery. Circulation 2001; 104(5):600–5.

18. Koster R, Vieluf D, Kiehn M, et al. Nickel and molybdenum contact allergies in patients with coronary in-stent restenosis. Lancet 2000; 356(9245):1895–7.

19. Farb A, Sangiorgi G, Carter AJ, et al. Pathology of acute and chronic coronary stenting in humans. Circulation 1999; 99(1):44–52.

42

Addition of cytochalasin D to a biodegradable oil stent coating inhibits intimal hyperplasia in a porcine coronary model

Koen J Salu, Yanming Huang, Johan M Bosmans, Xiaoshun Liu, Shengqiao Li, Lan Wang, Eric Verbeken, Hidde Bult, Chris J Vrints, and Ivan K De Scheerder

Introduction • Materials and methods • Results • Discussion • Acknowledgments

INTRODUCTION

Although coronary stents reduce the incidence of restenosis by opposing elastic recoil and late remodeling of the vessel, an excessive neointimal hyperplasia still induces 'in-stent' restenosis in 10–30% of the patients.[1] Local delivery, by the use of polymer-based drug eluting stents, is actually extensively evaluated for the prevention of in-stent restenosis.[2–5] Concern remains, however, about the potential long-term lack of biocompatibility of the polymer stent coatings used in these studies, because many of them have shown in the past to induce an exaggerated tissue response compared to stainless steel stents when implanted in pig coronary arteries.[6,7]

These considerations have generated considerable interest in the development of biocompatible stent coatings as carriers for antiproliferative agents for local drug delivery. Here, we present a new biodegradable oil stent coating, composed of naturally occurring eicosapentaenoic acids (omega-3 fatty acids). The latter have already shown their benefit in reducing restenosis both in experimental,[8] and in clinical studies,[9] partially due to their antiproliferative properties on vascular smooth muscle cells (VSMCs).[10,11] Therefore, it makes them interesting candidates for stent coatings.

A second crucial factor in the development of an 'ideal' drug eluting stent is, as well as biocompatible coatings, the addition of potent antiproliferative and/or antiinflammatory drugs to these coatings. Cytochalasin D is a lipophilic fungal metabolite with high affinity and specificity for actin molecules.[12] It blocks actin monomer addition at the rapidly growing end of actin filaments, thereby interfering with microfilament function.[12] In vitro, this leads to inhibition of cell migration,[13] and proliferation,[14,15] alterations in intracellular signaling,[16] and inhibition of protein synthesis,[17] all important aspects in the pathogenesis of neointimal hyperplasia.[1] Therefore, the present study assesses: (1) the in vivo biocompatibility of this new, stent-based, biodegradable oil coating, and (2) the efficacy of this coating in preventing in-stent restenosis by adding cytochalasin D, both in a porcine coronary model.

MATERIALS AND METHODS

Preparation and loading of the polymer coating

For all experiments, 16 mm balloon-mounted, stainless steel coronary stents (Jostents, Jomed, Germany) with a nominal inflated diameter of 3.0 mm or 3.5 mm were used in all groups. For oil-coating, the bare metal stents were dipped for 1 minute into a basic eicosapentaenoic acid oil solution (Biolog, Global Medical Systems, Zulte, Belgium). After removal, they were allowed to dry in a clean-air cupboard at room temperature for 5 minutes. To prepare cytochalasin D-coated stents, balloon-mounted bare metal stents were dipped into a 20 mg cytochalasin D (Sigma, Belgium)/ml oil solution for 1 minute and afterwards dried in a similar manner. This resulted in a total load of 100 μg cytochalasin D/stent. All stents were sterilized with gamma irradiation (25 kGy) before implantation in porcine coronary arteries. Finally, the surface characteristics of the oil-coated stents were examined by both scanning electron (SEM) and light microscopy, as described by Huang et al.[18]

In vitro cytochalasin D release kinetics

To study the release of cytochalasin D in vitro, three oil-coated stents (3.0–18 mm), containing 100 μg cytochalasin D, were placed in 1 mL 0.9% NaCl at 37°C. Cytochalasin D was measured at an ultraviolet (UV) absorbance of 207 nm (Cary 4E spectrophotometer, Varian, CA, USA) after 1, 2, 3, 4, 7, 14, 21, and 28 days. At each time point, the stents were placed in fresh 1 ml 0.9% NaCl. One control stent (coating-only) underwent the same procedure,

and its UV absorbance values at 207 nm were subtracted from those of the cytochalasin D-loaded stents.

Experimental preparation

The study was approved by the Ethical Committees of both the University of Antwerp and the Catholic University of Leuven. Domestic cross-bred pigs (Sus scrofa) were treated and cared for in accordance with the National Institute of Health Guide for the care and use of laboratory animals. A total of 26 domestic pigs (weight 20–25 kg), fed on a standard natural grain diet without lipid or cholesterol supplements, were used for this study. The pigs were sedated with intravenous azaperone 0.1 mL/h (Janssen Pharmaceutics, Beerse, Belgium) before general anesthesia was induced with intramuscular ketamine (5 mg/kg) and further intravenous ketamine (Parke-Davies, Warner Lambert, Belgium) at a rate of 0.1 mg/kg/h and pancuronium (Organon NV, Oss, Holland) at a rate of 0.4 mg/kg/h. The pigs were intubated and ventilated, adjusted by frequent blood gas monitoring to maintain a minimum PaO_2 of 100 mmHg and physiological $PaCO_2$ and pH values. Continuous electrocardiography, pressure, and temperature monitoring were performed throughout the procedure. An external carotid artery was surgically exposed and an 8 Fr intraarterial sheath was introduced over a 0.035 inch guidewire.

Heparin 5000 IU and 250 mg acetyl salicylic acid (aspirin) were administered intravenously as a bolus. Furthermore, 400 IU/h heparin was given as a continuous infusion during the procedure. The right (RCA) and left coronary artery (LAD) were visualized using an 8 Fr left Judkins 2.5 catheter and iohexol (Nycomed, Oslo, Norway) was used as the contrast agent. Coronary stents were then implanted (8 atm for 30 sec) with a 3.5–18 mm balloon for the RCA and a 3.0–18 mm balloon for the LAD artery, so that a balloon-to-vessel ratio between 1.0:1 and 1.2:1 was obtained. Randomly, one artery was used for treatment and the other as the control vessel. The stents were deployed using a deployment pressure of 8 atm with an inflation time of 30 sec. All selected arteries underwent a control angiogram after administration of a bolus of 200 mg nitroglycerin to evaluate successful deployment of the stent. Finally, the carotid arteriotomy was repaired and the dermal layers were closed using standard techniques. No antiplatelet agents or additional anticoagulants were administered during follow-up.

Measurements

A first study consisted of the random placement of 30 stents (15 oil-coated and 15 bare) to evaluate the biocompatibility of the biodegradable oil-coating in 15 pigs. The pigs were sacrificed at 5 days (10 stents) and 4 weeks (20 stents) respectively. A second study consisted of the random implantation of 11 control (oil-coating only) and 100 μg cytochalasin D-loaded (n = 11) stents in the coronary arteries of 11 additional pigs. Follow-up period was 4 weeks to evaluate the efficacy of local cytochalasin D delivery with this coating on in-stent neointimal hyperplasia.

Histopathology and morphometry

Five days or 4 weeks after implantation, the pigs were sacrificed using an intravenous bolus of 20 mL saturated potassium chloride. The stented arteries were pressure fixed using a 10% formalin solution at 80 mmHg. Coronary segments were carefully dissected together with a 1 cm vessel segment both proximal and distal to the stent. The segment was fixed in a 10% formalin solution for 7 days and then divided into three or four blocks containing the proximal, one or two middle, and distal regions of the stent. The proximal, one middle, and the distal region were embedded in the cold-polymerizing resin Technovit 7100 (Heraeus Kulzer GmbH, Wehrheim, Germany). From each stent implanted in seven, at random chosen, animals of both studies, a separate middle part was embedded in Technovit 9100, allowing immunohistochemistry. Histological sections (5 μm) were cut with a Tungsten Wolfram Carbide metal knife (Rotary heavy-duty microtome HM 360, Microm, Walldorf, Germany) and stained with hematoxylin-eosin, elastin (Verhoeff's-von Giesson), and Movat's pentachrome. An experienced pathologist who was blinded to the treatments performed light microscopic examination. Injury of the arterial wall was evaluated for every stent filament, and graded according to Schwartz et al.[19] Inflammation at each stent filament was examined on hematoxylin-eosin stained according to Kornowsky et al.[20] The mean score was calculated as the sum of scores for each filament/number of filaments. Luminal thrombus appearance was examined on hematoxylin-eosin stained sections as previously described.[21] The presence of focal fibrin deposition, intra-intimal hemorrhage, and focal media necrosis was examined at every strut using Movat's pentachrome according to Farb et al.,[22] and quantified as percentage positive struts.

The cross-sectional areas of lumen, intima, and media, were determined on all three segments (proximal, middle, and distal) by means of stereological point counting,[23] using a square grid (0.09 mm^2 per point, final magnification ×4). Subsequently, the internal elastic lamina (IEL) area, external elastic lamina (EEL) area, and percentage area stenosis were calculated, using the following equations: IEL area = lumen area + intima area (= area within the internal elastic lamina), EEL area = IEL + media area (= area within the external elastic lamina), and percentage area stenosis = (IEL area − lumen area)/IEL area. Finally, the balloon-to-vessel ratio for each vessel was calculated as the balloon diameter at nominal pressure/IEL diameter of the mid segment. The latter parameter was obtained by a computer-assisted analysis system (PC-image software for Windows, Foster Findlay Associates).

Finally, in situ immunohistochemistry was performed on separate middle sections with monoclonal antibodies against proliferation cell nuclear antigen (PCNA, Dako), macrophages (CD-68, mac-387, 1/300, Serotec) and endothelium (von Willebrand factor − vWf −

The Birmingham Site). The mac-387 density (number positive cells/mm^2) at four stent struts (at 3, 6, 9, and 12 o'clock) was measured as described by Farb et al.,[24] and the average for each segment was calculated. To evaluate possible antiproliferative effects, a proliferation index (number of PCNA-positive cells/total number of cells) was calculated at four stent struts (at 3, 6, 9, and 12 o'clock) and the average for each segment was calculated. Only fully stained PCNA positive cells were taken into account as described by Carter et al.[25] The vWf staining for each segment was graded as follows:

I.   <10% positivity of the lumen circumference
II. between 10% and 50% positivity of the lumen circumference
III. between 50% and 90% positivity of the lumen circumference
IV. >90% positivity of the lumen circumference.

Statistics

Data are presented as mean ± standard of the mean, n represents the number of arteries or stents. Morphometrical data, injury scores, and inflammatory scores between the two groups were analyzed using a factorial ANOVA, using segment (proximal, middle, distal) as within stent factor and treatment (bare or coating; coating or cytochalasin) as between stent factor. Immunohistopathological data were compared using an unpaired Student's t-test. A two-tailed p-value < 0.05 was considered to be statistically significant. Statistical analysis was carried out, using the SPSS 10.0 statistical package.

RESULTS

Scanning electron (SEM) and light microscopy images of the coated stents

Using SEM, the thickness of the coating covering the stent filaments measured 10 μm. The oil-coated stent surface was smooth without cracking or peeling, and the oil film was homogeneously distributed over the stent wires. Expanding the stent and loading cytochalasin D into the biodegradable oil did not affect the surface characteristics (Figure 42.1).

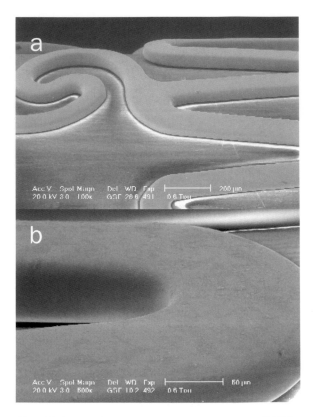

Fig. 42.1 (a) Scanning electron microscope (SEM) images of an unexpanded oil-coated stent loaded with 100 μg cytochalasin D after sterilization. (b) The coated stent surface resembled a smooth thin layer, without cracking or peeling of the oil film.

Evaluation of the in vivo biocompatibility of the oil coating

At 5 day follow-up, histopathology showed that the polymer-coated stents and the bare stents elicited an identical histopathological response. The stent filaments showed a good alignment to the vascular wall without rupture of the internal elastic membrane. The media were mildly compressed. Arterial injury induced by stent implantation was not significantly different between the two groups. A thin fibrin layer covering the stent filaments was observed. The vascular segment without stent filaments appeared normal without the presence of edge effects. No significant differences in inflammatory score and thrombus score between coated stents and bare stents were observed (Figure 42.2).

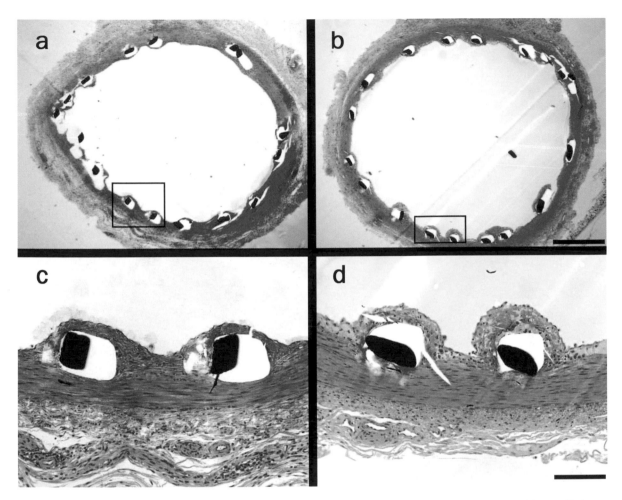

Fig. 42.2 Photomicrographs of cross-sections of stented porcine coronary vessel segments (RCA) at 5 day follow-up (hematoxylin-eosin stain). *Left*: Bare metal stents. *Right*: Oil-coated stents at the right. (c) and (d) High power fields of (a) and (b), as indicated by the rectangles. Scale bar (b), 500 μm; (d) 50 μm.

At 4 week follow-up, the neointima of both oil-coated and bare stents was well organized and consisted of extracellular matrix with SMCs (Figure 42.3a–d, Table 42.1). A few inflammatory cells were adjacent to the stent filaments and a peristrut inflammation score of more than 2 was only found in one bare stent. This was probably due to a higher arterial injury in this particular stent, despite equivalent balloon-to-vessel ratios in both groups (bare: 1.08 ± 0.02 vs oil coating: 1.13 ± 0.03, $p>0.05$, $n = 10$) were observed. Therefore, both the mean inflammation score and arterial injury score were slightly, but statistically significant, lower in the oil-coated stents com-

pared to the bare metal stents. Mean intimal hyperplasia was also slightly lower in the oil-coated group. As the IEL area was not significantly different between both groups, this resulted in larger lumen area and lower area stenosis values in the oil-coated stents as compared to bare stents. Immunohistopathological analysis revealed an equal distribution of fibrin-positive stent struts (bare: 24.6 ± 7.6 vs oil coating: $23.5 \pm 6.3\%$, $p>0.05$, $n = 10$) and of vWf staining covering the lumen circumference (bare: 3.1 ± 0.2 vs oil-coating: $3.2 \pm 0.3\%$, $p>0.05$, $n = 7$) in both groups. The mac-387 staining around stent struts was, however, reduced in the oil-coating group as

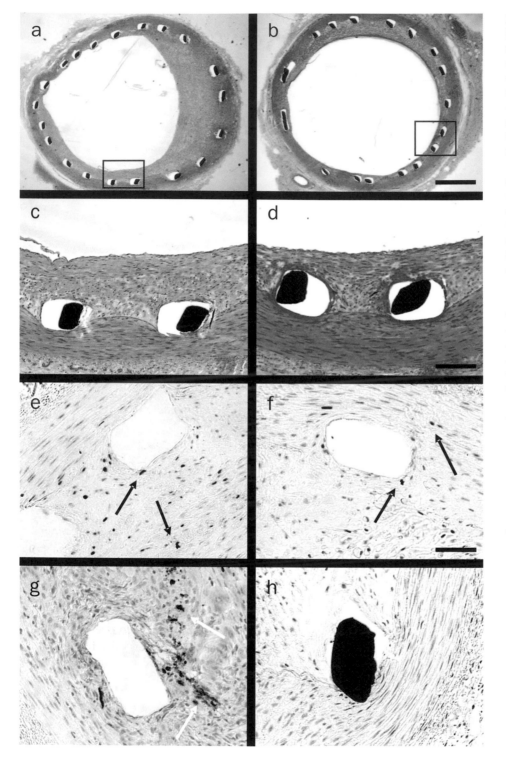

Fig. 42.3 (a)–(d) Photomicrographs of cross-sections of stented porcine coronary vessel segments (RCA) at 4 week follow-up (hematoxylin-eosin stain). *Left*: Bare metal stents. *Right*: Oil-coated stents. (c) and (d) High power fields of (a) and (b), as indicated by the rectangles. Scale bar (b) 500 μm; (d) 50 μm. (e)–(h) representative photomicrographs of PCNA (e and f) and mac-387 stained (g and h) sections of bare (*left*) and oil-coated (*right*) stents after 4 weeks implantation in porcine coronary arteries. Scale bar (f) 25 μm. Black arrows in (e) and (f) indicate PCNA-positive cells. White arrows in (g) indicate mac-387 positive leukocytes.

Table 42.1   Histomorphometric analysis of the biocompatibility of the oil coating

	Bare (n = 10)	Oil coating (n = 10)
Lumen area (mm^2)	5.65 ± 0.15	5.93 ± 0.28*
Intimal area (mm^2)	1.48 ± 0.10	1.25 ± 0.12
IEL area (mm^2)	7.13 ± 0.19	7.17 ± 0.20
Area stenosis (%)	21 ± 1	19 ± 2
Injury score	0.36 ± 0.09	0.21 ± 0.04**
Inflammatory score	1.15 ± 0.07	1.02 ± 0.01**

IEL, internal elastic lamina. Data are represented as mean ± standard error of the mean. *$p<0.05$, **$p<0.01$ vs bare by factorial ANOVA. No differences were seen within segments for all parameters in both groups.

compared to the bare group (7.8 ± 4.4 vs 27.6 ± 12.6 cells/mm^2, $p>0.05$, $n = 7$), which was also true for the proliferation index (2.0 ± 0.6 vs 5.4 ± 2.3%, $p>0.05$, $n = 7$) (Figure 42.3e–h). Finally, edge effects, luminal thrombus formation, intraintimal hemorrhages and focal medial necrosis around stent struts were not observed in both groups.

In vitro release kinetics of cytochalasin D eluting stents

The release of cytochalasin D from three polymer-coated stents is shown in Figure 42.4. For the 100 μg cytochalasin D loaded stents, 31 ± 2% of the total amount was released within the first 24 hours. Hereafter, the release slowed down, with only 56 ± 8% release after 1 week and 87 ± 15% after 4 week follow-up.

In vivo evaluation of the safety and efficacy of local cytochalasin D delivery

Control angiograms obtained 15 minutes after stent implantation showed that all deployment procedures were successful and that all stented vessels were patent. All 11 pigs survived for 4 weeks.

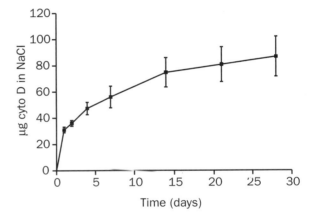

Fig. 42.4 The in vitro accumulation of 100 μg cytochalasin D released from 3.0–18 mm coated stents in 1 ml NaCl at 37°C. Data are represented as mean ± standard error of the mean ($n = 3$).

Morphometry and histopathology
After 4 week follow-up, very low injury scores (<0.5) were found in both groups as internal elastic lamina disruption and medial laceration by stent filaments were rare. However, despite equivalent balloon-to-vessel ratio values in both groups (oil-coating: 1.12 ± 0.03 vs cytochalasin D: 1.18 ± 0.02, $p>0.05$, $n = 11$), higher injury scores (>1) were found in two oil-coated stents as compared to all other stents in this experiment. Therefore, the mean injury score

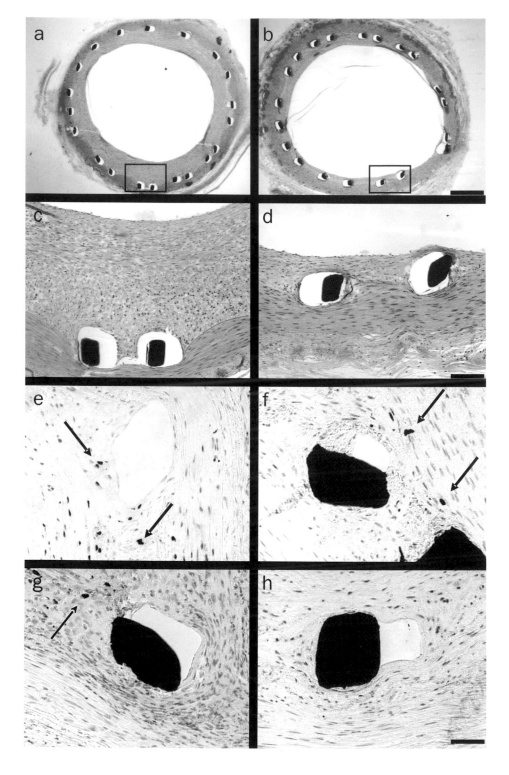

Fig. 42.5 (a)–(d) Photomicrographs of cross-sections of stented porcine coronary vessel segments (RCA) at 4 week follow-up (hematoxylin-eosin stain). *Left*: Oil-coated stents. *Right*: Cytochalasin D eluting stents. (c) and (d) High power fields of (a) and (b), as indicated by the rectangles. Scale bar (b) 500 μm, (d) 50 μm. (e)–(h) Representative photomicrographs of PCNA (e) and (f) and mac-387 stained (g) and (h) sections of oil-coated (*left*) and cytochalasin D-eluting (*right*) stents after 4 weeks implantation in porcine coronary arteries. Scale bar (f) 25 μm. Black arrows in (e) and (f) indicate PCNA-positive cells. Arrow in (g) indicates mac-387 positive leukcocytes.

Table 42.2 **Histomorphometric analysis of the efficacy of cytochalasin D-coated stents**

	Oil coating (n = 11)	Cyto D (n = 11)
Lumen area (mm²)	4.96 ± 0.34	5.26 ± 0.15
Intima area (mm²)	1.92 ± 0.25	1.17 ± 0.09**
IEL area (mm²)	6.88 ± 0.15	6.42 ± 0.15
Area stenosis (%)	29 ± 4	18 ± 1**
Injury score	0.44 ± 0.09	0.18 ± 0.03**
Inflammatory score	1.30 ± 0.11	1.03 ± 0.01**

IEL, internal elastic lamina. Data are represented as mean ± standard error of the mean; $**p<0.01$ vs oil coating by factorial ANOVA. No differences were seen within segments for all parameters in both groups.

was slightly, but statistically significant, less in cytochalasin D-coated stents (Figure 42.5a–d, Table 42.2). These two particular oil-coated stents also showed a modest inflammatory response around stent filaments (>2) as compared to all the other stents, which exerted only low inflammatory responses in their vessel wall. Compared to the control group, cytochalasin D-loaded stents therefore showed a significant decreased inflammatory response. More importantly, neointimal hyperplasia in cytochalasin D-loaded stents was limited and predominantly localized around the stent filaments, resulting in significantly smaller in-stent neointimal hyperplasia and percentage area stenosis in the cytochalasin D-treated vessels compared to control vessels. The lumen area was also, although not statistically significant, larger in cytochalasin D-coated stents. Edge effects, (sub)acute occlusive thrombus formation, intraintimal hemorrhage, and focal necrosis around stent struts were not observed. Fibrin-positive stent struts were equally distributed in both groups (oil-coating: 23.5 ± 4.8 vs cytochalasin D: 16.9 ± 5.7%, $p>0.05$, $n = 10$). Finally, immunohistopathological examination showed reductions in both mac-387 staining (5.3 ± 2.7 vs 18.0 ± 7.5 cells/mm², $p>0.05$, $n = 7$) and PCNA index (2.7 ± 0.5 vs 4.0 ± 1.4%, $p>0.05$, $n = 7$) in cytochalasin D-

coated stents as compared to control stents. Finally, equal vWf staining surrounding the lumen was observed in both groups (oil-coating: 3.3 ± 0.2 vs cytochalasin D: 3.4 ± 0.1, $p>0.05$, $n = 7$) (Figure 42.5e–h).

DISCUSSION

Our results show that biodegradable oil-coated stents induce a histopathological response of the vessel wall comparable to bare stainless steel stents. Peristrut inflammation was not raised after 5 day and at 4 week follow-up in the oil-coated stent group. Also, the neointima formation was not greater when compared to bare stents. Moreover, adding 100 µg cytochalasin D to this biocompatible stent coating, significantly reduced neointimal hyperplasia. This study demonstrated the feasibility, efficacy, and safety of local cytochalasin D delivery by means of a biocompatible stent coating to prevent in-stent restenosis.

Biocompatible coatings: a crucial interface of drug eluting stents

Here, we present a new, highly biocompatible stent coating, which can be applied to a metallic stent surface to serve as a matrix for efficient slow release, local drug delivery. This oil coating consists of naturally occurring eicosapentaenoic acids. Depending on the amount of loading and the actual constitution, this oil coating degrades in a biological manner over approximately 1 month. Eicosapentaenoic acids are omega-3-fatty acids, which are well known for their antiatherosclerotic effects, due to their antiinflammatory and antiproliferative properties.[26–28] Histopathologic evaluation of this oil coating in a porcine coronary stent model showed identical tissue response 5 days post implantation as compared to bare stainless steel stents. Injury scores, peristrut inflammation scores, and thrombus formation were comparable to control. This low inflammatory response was sustained at 4 week follow-up, resulting in even, statistically significant, lower inflammatory scores in the oil-coated stent group. However, this was only due to the fact that in one bare stent a somewhat higher arterial injury (>1) was observed as compared to the other bare stents, which also resulted in higher inflammatory responses (>2). Nevertheless, a slight reduction in mac-387 staining was still observed in the oil-coated stents as compared to bare stents, as the outlier in the bare stent group was no part of the limited number of sections in the immunohistochemistry analysis. Eicosapentaenoic acids have, however, indeed been shown to exert antiinflammatory effects in vitro. They alter the metabolism of adhesion molecules such as vascular cell adhesion molecule-1 (VCAM-1) and intracellular adhesion molecule-1 (ICAM-1), and inflammatory mediators like interleukins and tumor necrosis factor-α (TNF-α).[28–30] They also compete with arachidonic acid and thereby inhibit the production of leukotrienes-4.[26–28] All these cell factors might play a role in the chemoattraction of polymorphonuclear leukocytes and monocytes. By inhibiting this cascade, eicosapentaenoic acids might thus have contributed to the fact that no greater neointima was observed as compared to the bare stents. This is important, as it shows that this oil coating is inert and thus does not elicit a hyperproliferative and inflammatory response as seen in the past with many other polymer drug carriers.[6]

As the injury score is directly correlated with the vascular neointimal response,[19,20] the reduced injury score could also have contributed to the slightly lower intimal hyperplasia observed in the oil-coated stents at 4 week follow-up. However, this difference was thus solely due to one outlier in the bare stent group. This outlier exerted an averaged intimal area of 1.75 mm^2, which did not markedly influence the mean intimal area of all the other bare stents (1.45 ± 0.10 mm^2). Therefore, the oil-coated stents still showed a slightly lower intimal area as compared to the bare stents. Besides possible antiinflammatory properties, this was perhaps also due to possible antiproliferative effects by the oil coating itself, as a lower proliferation index was observed in the oil-coated stents as compared to the bare stents. Indeed, eicosapentaenoic acids are known to inhibit VSMC proliferation in vitro, suggesting a possible beneficial role in reducing neointimal formation.[10] Finally, edge effects, (sub)acute thrombus formation, intraintimal hemorrhages, and focal medial necrosis around stent struts were not observed in either group and also the fibrin deposition around stent struts was equally distributed in both groups. In summary, these results suggest that this new biodegradable oil coating alone can perhaps reduce the antiinflammatory and antiproliferative cascade following stent implantation and that it induces no delayed healing or local toxic vascular reactions as compared to stainless steel stents.

In vitro release kinetic studies showed that, by adding a drug (here, 100 µg cytochalasin D) to this coating, about 90% of the initial dose was gradually released during a 4 week follow-up period. This thus compares favorably with the approximately 1 month in vivo biodegradation of the oil coating. Moreover, this sustained release pattern is of clinical interest, because in humans, intimal hyperplasia develops over a time interval of 4 to 8 weeks.[1] Figure 42.4 also shows the small (<20%) but intrinsic variability of the dip-coating technique concerning the drug stent loading. Indeed, the limited approach of dipping stents into a particular drug solution does not allow the same low variability as more technically advanced methods of drug loading, such as polymer spray-coating on coronary stents.[31] Nevertheless, these data confirm that this biocompatible coating has also the capacity to include high amounts of drugs that are potentially interesting to block the neointimal hyperplasia cascade after stent implantation and therefore can be used as an efficient vehicle for local drug delivery.

Cytochalasin D: potential drug to prevent in-stent restenosis

Since in-stent restenosis is the result of a complex vascular healing process, in which several cell types (i.e. platelets, inflammatory cells, SMCs, and fibroblasts) play a pivotal role, drugs with pleiotropic effects on various cell types are preferable, as already proved by the success of paclitaxel eluting stents.[4,32] Cytochalasins are lipophilic, cell-permeable fungal metabolites that inhibit the polymerization of actin into microfilaments, which are, as well as microtubuli, important compounds in the cytoskeleton. The literature has shown that cytochalasins can inhibit important cell processes in neointimal formation, as cell migration and proliferation, protein synthesis and intracellular signaling.[12–17] Recently, we showed a benefit from direct stent coating with only 2 µg cytochalasin D, the most potent cytochalasin, in suppressing to some extent in-stent restenosis in pig coronary arteries.[33] Therefore, cytochalasin D seemed an interesting candidate for inhibiting neointimal formation using a more sustained release stent platform.

Inclusion of 100 µg cytochalasin D in the oil film, showed a significant benefit by morphometrical analysis: 39% less intimal hyperplasia and 38% less area stenosis in the treated group was seen compared to the control group. As well as inhibitory effects on migration and proliferation of SMC,[3,34] and fibroblasts,[13,14,16,34,35] which are essential mechanisms in reducing neointimal formation, cytochalasin D displays also important antiinflammatory effects. In vitro, it impairs the migration of neutrophils

and monocytes[36–38] and also phagocytosis by macrophages and their fusion to giant cells.[39,40] In vivo, local delivery of cytochalasin D using osmotic minipumps, opposes the diapedesis of leukocytes from the lumen to the deeper layers of the media and the adventitia of the rabbit carotid artery.[13] Moreover, also with direct stent coating, a reduced inflammation score was seen in cytochalasin D-treated vessels.[33] The present study confirms this antiinflammatory effect of cytochalasin D, as shown by the reduced inflammation scores and mac-387 staining around cytochalasin D-coated stent filaments. The reduced inflammatory response could thus have been an additional mechanism of cytochalasin D in effectively suppressing neointimal hyperplasia as well as its antiproliferative characteristics. The latter were also confirmed in this study, as the PCNA index was reduced around cytochalasin D stent struts as compared with oil-coated-only stents.

This should, however, be interpreted with caution, as in analogy to the first experiment, there were also higher histological injury scores (>1) found in two stents of the oil-coating group as compared to the other stents in this group, which was also reflected in greater inflammatory responses (inflammation score >2). These two outliers influenced the mean injury scores and inflammatory scores in the oil-coated stents, as these two parameters were significantly larger as compared to the cytochalasin D eluting stents. Also, this finding probably explains that despite the fact that these stents were implanted in separate animals and smaller vessels, the difference in vessel wall response in this group of oil-coated stents as compared to the oil-coated stents in the first experiment. The increased intimal hyperplasia observed in the oil-coated stents could thus simply result from the observed higher injury score. However, the two outliers did not exert, also in this second experiment, significantly higher neointima formation (0.92 mm^2 and 0.94 mm^2) as compared to the other stents in this group (2.14 ± 0.29 mm^2). Therefore, the reduced mac-387 staining and PCNA index around cytochalasin D eluting stent struts, where the outliers were also no part of the randomly chosen sections, might thus suggest possible anti-restenotic properties by this actin-skeleton inhibitor.

Edge effects, (sub)acute luminal thromboses, intraintimal hemorrhages and focal medial necrosis were not seen during the 4 week follow-up in both groups and also focal fibrin deposition around stent struts was equally distributed in both groups, suggesting that local cytochalasin D delivery causes no toxic vascular reactions or delayed healing. Finally, vWf staining showed almost complete coverage of the lumen in both groups, suggesting that local cytochalasin D administration in itself, causes no deleterious effects on the regeneration of the endothelium.

Limitations of the study and conclusions

In this study, normal porcine coronary arteries were used to evaluate the biocompatibility of a new biodegradable oil coating and the effect of stent-based cytochalasin D delivery on neointima formation and inflammation. We used an artificial model, using native porcine coronary arteries, which are not representative of human coronary, lipid-rich atherosclerotic, lesions. Therefore, it remains uncertain whether this beneficial effect on inflammation and neointimal hyperplasia of both the coating and the cytochalasin D delivery, remains in these latter lesions. Also larger and long-term (3–6 month) safety and efficacy studies should be performed to evaluate whether the effect of both the coating and cytochalasin D remains or only reflects a delay in vessel wall healing. Finally, this study also exerts some methodological limitations. First, quantitative coronary angiographic analysis (QCA) was not performed, and therefore clinically relevant parameters, such as late lumen loss and minimal lumen diameter at follow-up, were not measured. Second, only one cytochalasin D dose was evaluated and further optimal dose-finding studies are therefore warranted. Finally, immunohistochemistry was only partially used and should be applied in larger future studies.

Despite these limitations, this new biodegradable oil stent coating showed good biocompatible behavior in porcine coronary arteries, comparable to regular bare metal stents. Loading 100 µg cytochalasin D to these stents could significantly reduce neointimal formation and percentage area stenosis at 4 week follow-up. Edge effects, (sub)acute thrombus formation, retarded endothelial regeneration, and local vascular toxicity were not observed. Eicosapentaenoic oil-coated stents loaded with cytochalasin D can reduce peri-strut inflammation and could therefore contribute to the prevention of in-stent restenosis.

ACKNOWLEDGMENTS

The authors wish to thank Mr. David De Coux, Mrs. Tony Stassen and Mrs. Rita van den Bossche for technical assistance and Mrs. Liliane Van den Eynde for secretarial help. Prof. Dr IK De Scheerder is holder of the Andreas Grüntzig Chair for Interventional Cardiology, sponsored by Medtronic AVE Inc.

REFERENCES

1. Virmani R, Farb A. Pathology of in-stent restenosis. Curr Opin Lipidol 1999; 10:499–506.
2. Honda Y, Grube E, de La Fuente LM, et al. Novel drug-delivery stent: intravascular ultrasound observations from the first human experience with the QP2-eluting polymer stent system. Circulation 2001; 104:380–3.
3. Morice MC, Serruys PW, Sousa JE, et al. A randomized comparison of a sirolimus-eluting stent with a standard stent for coronary revascularization. N Engl J Med 2002; 346:1773–80.
4. Grube E, Silber S, Hauptmann KE, et al. TAXUS I: six- and twelve-month results from a randomized, double-blind trial on a slow-release paclitaxel-eluting stent for de novo coronary lesions. Circulation 2003; 107:38–42.
5. Sousa JE, Costa MA, Abizaid A, et al. Lack of neointimal proliferation after implantation of sirolumus-coated stents in human coronary arteries. A quantitative coronary angiography and three-dimensional intravascular ultrasound study. Circulation 2000; 103:192–5.
6. De Scheerder IK, Wilczek KL, Verbeken EV, et al. Biocompatibility of polymer-coated

oversized metallic stents implanted in normal porcine coronary arteries. Atherosclerosis 1995; 114:105–14.

7. van der Giessen WJ, Lincoff AM, Schwartz RS, et al. Marked inflammatory sequelae to implantation of biodegradable and nonbiodegradable polymers in porcine coronary arteries. Circulation 1996; 94:1690–7.

8. Faggin E, Puato M, Chiavegato A, et al. Fish oil supplementation prevents neointima formation in nonhypercholesterolemic balloon-injured rabbit carotid artery by reducing medial and adventitial cell activation. Arterioscler Thromb Vasc Biol 2000; 20:152–63.

9. Maresta A, Balduccelli M, Varani E, et al. Prevention of postcoronary angioplasty restenosis by omega-3 fatty acids: main results of the Esapent for Prevention of Restenosis ITalian Study (ESPRIT). Am Heart J 2002; 143:E5.

10. Shiina T, Terano T, Saito J, Tamura Y, Yoshida S. Eicosapentaenoic acid and docosahexaenoic acid suppress the proliferation of vascular smooth muscle cells. Atherosclerosis 1993; 104:95–103.

11. Pakala R, Pakala R, Sheng WL, Benedict CR. Eicosapentaenoic acid and docosahexaenoic acid block serotonin-induced smooth muscle cell proliferation. Arterioscler Thromb Vasc Biol 1999; 19:2316–2322.

12. Cooper JA. Effects of cytochalasin and phalloidin on actin. J Cell Biol 1987; 105:1473–8.

13. Bruijns RH, Bult H. Effects of local cytochalasin D delivery on smooth muscle cell migration and on collar-induced intimal hyperplasia in the rabbit carotid artery. Br J Pharmacol 2001; 134:473–83.

14. Carter SB. Effects of cytochalasins on mammalian cells. Nature 1967; 213:261–4.

15. Aubin JE, Osborn M, Weber K. Inhibition of cytokinesis and altered contractile ring morphology induced by cytochalasins in synchronized PtK2 cells. Exp Cell Res 1981; 136:63–79.

16. Rubtsova SN, Kondratov RV, Kopnin PB, et al. Disruption of actin microfilaments by cytochalasin D leads to activation of p53. FEBS Lett 1998; 430:353–7.

17. Ornelles DA, Fey EG, Penman S. Cytochalasin releases mRNA from the cytoskeletal framework and inhibits protein synthesis. Mol Cell Biol 1986; 6:1650–62.

18. Huang Y, Wang L, Verweire I, et al. Optimization of local methylprednisolone delivery to inhibit inflammatory reaction and neointimal hyperplasia of coated coronary stents. J Invasive Cardiol 2002; 14:505–13.

19. Schwartz RS, Huber KC, Murphy JG, et al. Restenosis and the proportional neointimal response to coronary artery injury: results in a porcine model. J Am Coll Cardiol 1992; 19:267–74.

20. Kornowski R, Hong MK, Tio FO, et al. In-stent restenosis: contributions of inflammatory responses and arterial injury to neointimal hyperplasia. J Am Coll Cardiol 1998; 31:224–30.

21. De Scheerder I, Wang K, Zhou XR, et al. Neointimal hyperplasia and late pathologic remodeling in a porcine coronary stent model. J Invas Cardiol 1999; 11:9–12.

22. Farb A, Heller PF, Shroff S, et al. Pathological analysis of local delivery of paclitaxel via a polymer-coated stent. Circulation 2001; 104:473–9.

23. Salu KJ, Knaapen MWM, Bosmans JM, et al. A three-dimensional quantitative analysis of restenosis parameters after balloon angioplasty: comparison between semi-automatic computer-assisted planimetry and stereology. J Vasc Res 2002; 39:437–46.

24. Farb A, Weber DK, Kolodgie FD, et al. Morphological predictors of restenosis after coronary stenting in humans. Circulation 2002; 105:2974–80.

25. Carter AJ, Laird JR, Farb A, et al. Morphologic characteristics of lesion formation and time course of smooth muscle cell proliferation in a porcine proliferative restenosis model. J Am Coll Cardiol 1994; 24:1398–405.

26. Mehta J, Lopez LM, Wargovich T. Eicosapentaenoic acid: its relevance in atherosclerosis and coronary artery disease. Am J Cardiol 1987; 59:155–9.

27. Leaf A, Weber PC. Cardiovascular effects of n-3 fatty acids. N Engl J Med 1988; 318:549–57.

28. Kris-Etherton PM, Harris WS, Appel LJ. Fish consumption, fish oil, omega-3 fatty acids, and cardiovascular disease. Circulation 2002; 106:2747–57.

29. Abe Y, El Masri B, Kimball KT, et al. Soluble cell adhesion molecules in hypertriglyceridemia and

potential significance on monocyte adhesion. Arterioscler Thromb Vasc Biol 1998; 18:723–31.

30. Endres S, von Schacky C. n-3 polyunsaturated fatty acids and human cytokine synthesis. Curr Opin Lipidol 1996; 7:48–52.

31. Heldman AW, Cheng L, Jenkins GM, et al. Paclitaxel stent coating inhibits neointimal hyperplasia at 4 weeks in a porcine model of coronary restenosis. Circulation 2001; 103:2289–2295.

32. Gershlick AH, De Scheerder I, Chevalier B, et al. Local drug delivery to inhibit coronary artery restenosis. Data from the ELUTES (EvaLUation of pacliTaxel Eluting Stent) clinical trial. Circulation 2001; 104:II-416 (abstract).

33. Salu KJ, Yanming H, Bosmans JM, et al. Direct cytochalasin D stent coating inhibits neointimal formation in a porcine coronary model. Circulation 2001; 104:II-506 (abstract).

34. Numaguchi K, Eguchi S, Yamakawa T, et al. Mechanotransduction of rat aortic vascular smooth muscle cells requires RhoA and intact actin filaments. Circ Res 1999; 85:5–11.

35. Böhmer RM, Scharf E, Assoian RK. Cytoskeletal integrity is required throughout the mitogen stimulation phase of the cell cycle and mediates the anchorage-dependent expression of cyclin D1. Mol Biol Cell 1996; 7:101–11.

36. Anderson SI, Hotchin NA, Nash GB. Role of the cytoskeleton in rapid activation of CD11b/CD18 function and its subsequent downregulation in neutrophils. J Cell Sci 2000; 113:2737–45.

37. Kielbassa K, Schmitz C, Gerke V. Disruption of endothelial microfilaments selectively reduces the transendothelial migration of monocytes. Exp Cell Res 1998; 243:129–41.

38. Suria H, Chau LA, Negrou E, et al. Cytoskeletal disruption induces T cell apoptosis by a caspase-3 mediated mechanism. Life Sci 1999; 65:2697–707.

39. Newman SL, Mikus LK, Tucci MA. Differential requirements for cellular cytoskeleton in human macrophage complement receptor- and Fc receptor-mediated phagocytosis. J Immunol 1991; 146:967–74.

40. DeFife KM, Jenney CR, Colton E, Anderson JM. Disruption of filamentous actin inhibits human macrophage fusion. FASEB J 1999; 13:823–32.

43

Vascular endothelial growth factor (VEGF) eluting stents

Neil Swanson and Anthony Gershlick

Introduction • **VEGF: Functions and delivery** • **Conclusions**

INTRODUCTION

At angioplasty or stent implantation, significant damage is unavoidably done to the endothelial lining of the vessel. It is thought that the loss of the protective endothelial lining of the artery is one of the key stimuli to the smooth muscle cell proliferation that is the hallmark of the restenotic lesion. This is probably due to the loss of the endothelial cell products, such as nitric oxide (NO) and prostacycline, which normally inhibit smooth muscle cell growth. An intact endothelium also acts as a physical barrier to platelets that will otherwise adhere to the subendothelial layers of the vessel wall. As well as potentially causing vessel thrombosis, these platelets produce factors that stimulate smooth muscle cells, leading to restenosis. For a delayed period, endothelial function around a stent is impaired compared to the recovery seen after angioplasty alone.[1] The lack of endothelial recovery is exacerbated in patients receiving vascular brachytherapy,[2] and this may be the cause of the 'late thrombosis' seen in up to 11% of these patients.[3]

VEGF: FUNCTIONS AND DELIVERY

Vascular endothelial growth factor is an endogenous peptide with potent angiogenic properties and acts as a cell-specific stimulant to endothelial cell proliferation (see Figure 43.1).

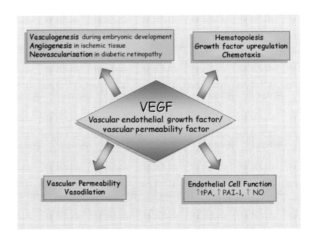

Fig. 43.1 Diagram showing the multiple actions of VEGF. VEGF was initially described as 'vascular permeability factor'. tPA, tissue plasminogen activator; PAI-I, plasminogen activator inhibits.

Table 43.1   Studies using VEGF or VEGF plasmid bound to polymer-coated stents

Year	Study	Results
1999	VEGF plasmid bound to a stent[6]	29 ± 18% reduction in intimal thickness ($p<0.016$) in rabbit iliac model
2000	In vitro VEGF protein elution from Supra G stent in perfusion circuit[7]	Biexponential elution over 9 d, 17% of initial VEGF residual at 5 d
2000	VEGF protein-coated stent effects in cell culture[8]	Human endothelial cell (HUVEC) growth stimulated by 10% after 3 d culture ($p<0.05$). Benefit maintained despite preliminary washout of superficial VEGF from polymer

Delivery of exogenous VEGF has been reported to accelerate re-endothelialization and to attenuate the development of intimal hyperplasia of damaged arteries.[4] Similar work using a local drug delivery balloon has shown that a plasmid engineered to code for VEGF also leads to increased endothelialization and decreased intimal hyperplasia when administered to a stented rabbit iliac vessel.[5]

Work in our laboratory has shown that VEGF protein can be absorbed into the polymer coating of a stent and that gradual elution of VEGF from the stent will stimulate endothelial cells. This and other work with VEGF plasmids is summarized in Table 43.1.

CONCLUSIONS

In vitro work with VEGF eluting stents has shown that the drug can be delivered in a sustained fashion. This prolonged release of VEGF is in contrast to the bolus approach that is seen with balloon catheter delivery systems. VEGF plasmid will also release VEGF slowly although VEGF release will only occur *after* transfected cells have begun to synthesize the protein. The transfection efficiency of plasmid based techniques may be as low as 0.12% of targeted cells.[5] In cell culture, VEGF-eluting stents have a positive effect but this has not been demonstrated as yet in vivo. VEGF plasmid-coated stents have shown benefit in vivo. Ongoing work is examining the effects on

stent endothelialization and intimal hyperplasia of a VEGF protein eluting stent in an animal model.

No clinical trials of VEGF eluting stents have been performed although VEGF has been delivered via intracoronary catheter to patients in a clinical trial.[9] This examined the angiogenic properties of the agent rather than any effect on restenosis. No ill-effects were seen in a series of 10 patients who received VEGF plasmid infusion into the coronaries after angioplasty.[10]

A VEGF eluting stent is likely to be of most use in patients who have had brachytherapy as this procedure, and, to a lesser degree, stents in general, have a sustained adverse effect on endothelial recovery after angioplasty.

REFERENCES

1. van Beusekom HM, Whelan DM, Hofma SH, et al. Long-term endothelial dysfunction is more pronounced after stenting than after balloon angioplasty in porcine coronary arteries. J Am Coll Cardiol 1998; 32(4):1109–17.
2. Hehrlein C, Gollan C, Donges K, et al. Low-dose radioactive endovascular stents prevent smooth muscle cell proliferation and neointimal hyperplasia in rabbits. Circulation 1995; 92(6):1570–5.
3. Waksman R. Late thrombosis after radiation. Circulation 1999; 100:780–2.
4. Asahara T, Bauters C, Pastore C, et al. Local delivery of vascular endothelial growth factor

accelerates reendothelialization and attenuates intimal hyperplasia in balloon-injured rat carotid artery. Circulation 1995; 91(11):2793–801.

5. Van Belle E, Tio FO, Chen D, et al. Passivation of metallic stents after arterial gene transfer of phVEGF165 inhibits thrombus formation and intimal thickening. J Am Coll Cardiol 1997; 29(6):1371–9.

6. Mir-Akbari H, Sylven C, Lindvall B, et al. PhVEGF coated stent reduces restenosis intimal hyperplasia. XXIst Congress of the European Society of Cardiology 1999; 1536 (abstract).

7. Swanson N, Baron J, Hogrefe K, et al. Novel delivery of vascular endothelial growth factor delivery using polymer-coated stents: loading and elution characteristics. Heart 2000; 83(suppl 1): P28 (abstract).

8. Swanson N, Hogrefe K, Javed Q, et al. VEGF-eluting coronary stents stimulate endothelial growth *in vitro*. J Submicrosc Cytol Pathol 2000; 32(3):419-B087 (abstract).

9. Henry TD. VIVA (vascular endothelial growth Factor in ischemia for vascular angiogenesis). Clin Cardiol 1999; 22:369 (abstract).

10. Laitinen M, Hartikainen J, Hiltunen MO, et al. Catheter-mediated vascular endothelial growth factor gene transfer to human coronary arteries after angioplasty. Hum Gene Ther 2000; 11(2):263–70.

44

An advanced antisense for local vascular delivery for prevention of restenosis

Nicholas Kipshidze, Patrick Iversen, Jeffrey W Moses, Patrick W Serruys, and Martin B Leon

Introduction • Preclinical safety and efficacy studies • Clinical studies • Medtronic program • Acknowledgment

INTRODUCTION

Antisense oligomers are polymers designed to interfere with the information transfer from gene to protein.[1–3] Such compounds may have a therapeutic advantage by specifically targeting genetic sequences that are critical to disease processes. The clinical applicability of antisense technology however, has been limited due to a relative lack of target specificity, slow uptake across the cell membranes, and rapid intracellular degradation of the oligonucleotide.[4] The only randomized study in humans with c-myc antisense demonstrated no reduction in restenosis after stent implantation when arteries were pretreated with the drug.[5]

The recently introduced AVI-4126 (Resten-NG) belongs to a family of molecules known as the phosphorodiamidate morpholino oligomers (PMO). These oligomers are comprised of (dimethylamino) phosphinylideneoxy-linked morpholino subunits. The morpholino subunits contain a heterocyclic base recognition moiety of DNA (A,C,G,T) attached to a substituted morpholine ring system (Figure 44.1). In general, PMO are capable of binding to RNA in a sequence specific fashion with sufficient avidity to be useful for the inhibition of the translation of mRNA into protein in vivo, a

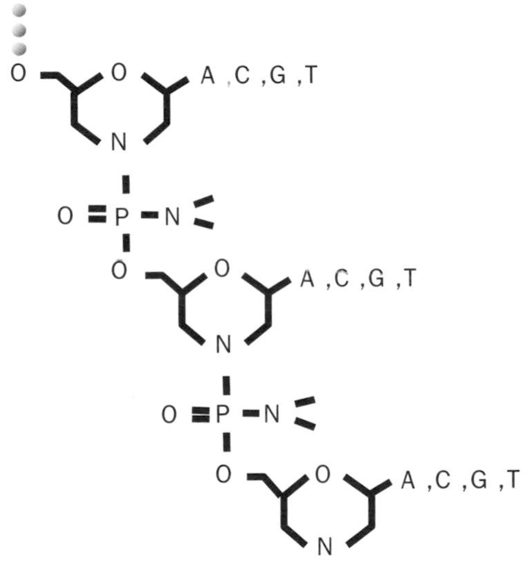

Fig. 44.1 Properties of gene-targeted technologies.

result commonly referred to as an 'antisense' effect. Although the PMO share many similarities with other substances capable of producing antisense effects, such as DNA, RNA, and their analogous oligonucleotide analogs like the phosphorothioates (PSO), there are important differences. Most importantly, the PMO are uncharged and resistant to degradation under biological conditions. The neutral character of the PMO chemistry for antisense oligomers avoids a variety of potentially significant limitations observed with PSO chemistry. The PMO are resistant to the nucleases found in serum and liver extracts,[1] and exhibit a high degree of specificity and efficacy both in vitro and in cell culture.[2-5] The antisense mechanism of action appears to be through the PMO hybrid duplex with mRNA to inhibit translation.[2,6] Finally, PMO have demonstrated antisense activity against the c-myc pre-mRNA in living human cells.[7] The combination of efficacy, potency, and lack of non-specific activities of the PMO chemistry compelled us to re-examine the approach to antisense to c-myc for the prevention of restenosis following percutaneous coronary intervention.

The drug substance is very inert chemically. It dissolves in water to give a solution with a neutral pH. It is decomposed with acid below pH 4 and with alkali above pH 11. AVI-4126 is very stable to extremes of temperature and is resistant to degradation in plasma.

AVI-4126 is an antisense phosphorodiamidate morpholino oligomer (PMO) with sequence complementary to the translation initiation start site of the c-myc mRNA. The mechanism of action of AVI-4126 involves the interference with ribosomal assembly thus preventing translation of c-myc and the interference with intron 1-exon 2 splicing of the c-myc pre-mRNA preventing appropriate translation of the c-myc mRNA. The IC_{50} for inhibition of c-myc is 0.3 μM in cell culture. The cellular response to AVI-4126 is diminished cell growth associated with arrest of cells in the G_0/G_1 phase of the cell cycle. Inhibition of c-myc would also interfere with expression of downstream genes such as those associated with cellular adhesion, the cell cycle, and connective tissue matrix remodeling.

PRECLINICAL SAFETY AND EFFICACY STUDIES

Local delivery in a rabbit atherosclerotic restenosis model

Twenty-five male, New Zealand, white, atherosclerotic rabbits maintained on a diet of 0.25% cholesterol were anesthetized, a Transport Catheter™ inserted into the iliac artery and percutaneous transluminal coronary angioplasty (PTCA) performed (8 atm for 30 sec, ×3). The endoluminal delivery of saline or 0.5 mg of AVI-4126 to the PTCA site was at 2 atm via the outer balloon for 2 minutes. The area of the intima and media was determined by planimetry. Quantitative angiography from these animals shows the maximal luminal diameter (MLD) at the time of harvest (60 days after PTCA) was significantly greater in the antisense-treated group than in the control animals. The morphometric analysis confirms the angiography in demonstrating significantly greater lumen area than in the control. The intimal area was also significantly smaller in the AVI-4126-treated animals. We also observed positive remodeling of the vessel. Vessel area was significantly greater ($p<0.05$) in the treated animals. An additional late follow-up (6 months) study was also conducted which also demontrated sustained reduction of neointimal thickness with complete wound healing at long-term follow-up. There was no aneurysm formation in any treated animals.

Local delivery in a pig coronary stent restenosis model

We evaluated the long-term influence of intramural delivery of advanced c-myc antisense on neointimal hyperplasia following stenting in a pig model. In acute experiments different doses (from 500 μg to 5 mg) of AVI-4126 (Resten-NG) ($n = 11$) or saline ($n = 14$) were delivered to the stent implantation site with Infiltrator™ delivery system. Animals were sacrificed at 2 h, 6 h, and 18 h after interventions, and excised vessels were analyzed for c-myc expression by Western blot. In chronic experiments ($n = 20$) saline or 1 mg, 5 mg, and 10 mg of Resten-NG was delivered at same fashion and animals were sacrificed at 28 days following intervention.

Western blot analysis demonstrated inhibition of c-myc expression and was dose-dependent. Morphometry showed that the intimal area was $3.88.5 \pm 1.04$ mm^2 in the control. There was statistically significant reduction of intimal areas in 5 mg and 10 mg groups (2.01 ± 0.66 and 1.95 ± 0.91, respectively, $p<0.001$), but no significant reduction in the 1 mg group (2.81 ± 0.56, $p>0.5$) compared to control. This study demonstrated that intramural delivery of advanced c-myc neutrally charged antisense morpholino compound completely inhibits c-myc expression and dramatically reduces neointimal formation in a dose-dependent fashion in a porcine coronary stent restenosis model, while allowing for complete vascular healing.

PC-coated stent-based delivery in a porcine coronary model

The efficacy of stent coating technologies led us to re-examine the potential efficacy of a neutrally charged c-myc antisense approach for the prevention of restenosis following coronary stenting.

PC stents were loaded with AVI-4126 using soak-trap (ST) and dry-trap (DT) methods. Twelve pigs underwent AVI-4126 PC coronary stent implantation (three stents/animal). At 2–6 hours post procedure, three pigs were sacrificed and stented segments were analyzed by Western blot for c-myc expression. In chronic experiments, six pigs (27 stent sites)

were sacrificed at 28 days following intervention and vessels were perfusion-fixed. High performance liquid chromatography (HPLC) analysis of plasma showed minimal presence of the antisense oligomer, suggesting no systemic release of AVI-4126. Western blot analysis of the stented vessels demonstrated inhibition of c-myc expression at 2 and 6 hours after procedure. Quantitative histologic morphometry showed that the neointimal area was significantly reduced in the ST group compared with control (2.3 ± 0.7 vs 3.9 ± 0.7, mm^2, respectively, $p = 0.0077$) (Table 44.1). Immunostaining and electron microscopy demonstrated complete endothelialization, without fibrin deposition, thrombosis, or necrosis in all groups.

Control arteries exhibited a substantial neointima consisting mostly of stellate and spindle-shaped cells, in a loose extracellular matrix. The neointima from treated arteries with antisense-loaded stent implantation was significantly smaller in size (Figure 44.2). In general, the neointima of the ST and DT-coated stents consisted of SMCs, matrix proteoglycans, and minimal focal regions of residual fibrin adjacent to the stent struts (Figure 44.3). Focal medial necrosis or intimal hemorrhage was an infrequent observation within any of the control or drug-coated stents. A semiquantitative

Table 44.1 Histomorphometric results in porcine coronary arteries 28 days following stent implantation

	Control	Soak-trap	Dry-trap	p-value
Number	6	6	6	
Vessel area	9.4 ± 1.1	10.2 ± 1.8	9.6 ± 1.1	ns
Luminal area	3.4 ± 0.9	5.2 ± 0.9*	4.1 ± 1.3	0.0496
Intima area (IA)	3.9 ± 0.8	2.30 ± 1.1*	3.1 ± 0.1	0.0077
Stent strut area (SSA)	7.4 ± 0.8	7.59 ± 1.59	7.3 ± 0.8	ns
Medial area	2.1 ± 0.4	2.34 ± 0.58	2.4 ± 0.4	ns
IA/Injury score	2.1 ± 0.7	1.2 ± 0.27	2.1 ± 0.5	0.0099
Injury score	1.8 ± 0.4	1.79 ± 0.25	2.0 ± 0.7	ns

* $p = 0.001$ (ANOVA post test with Bonferroni correction); ns, not significant.

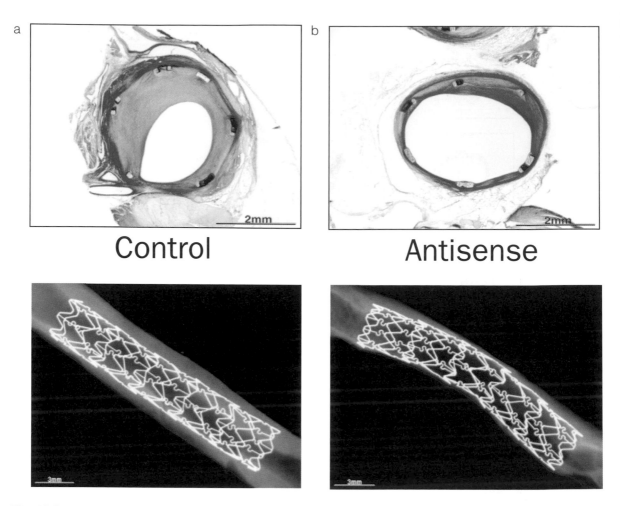

a

b

Control

Antisense

Fig. 44.2 (a) Control arteries have a substantial neointima in a loose extracellular matrix. (b) Antisense-treated arteries have significantly smaller neointima.

histological grading system demonstrated similar SMC colonization in all groups and minimal residual fibrin deposition for the ST-eluting stents. However DT and control PC stents had higher intimal fibrin scores (Table 44.2).

Most importantly, there was no difference in the appearance of re-endothelialization (Figure 44.4). The transmission electron microscopy (TEM) revealed a virtually normal appearance of endothelium (Figure 44.5). A semiquantitative histological grading system demonstrated similar SMC colonization in all groups and minimal residual fibrin deposition for the ST eluting stents. However, DT and control PC stents had higher intimal fibrin scores (Table 44.2).

We also observed less inflammation after implantation of the antisense-loaded stent (Figure 44.6). In general, the neointima of the ST- and DT-coated stents consisted of smooth muscle cells (SMC), matrix proteoglycans, and minimal focal regions of residual fibrin adjacent to the stent struts. Focal medial necrosis or intimal hemorrhage was infrequent observation within any of the control or drug-coated stents.

Its favorable influence on hyperplasia (reduction of intima by 40%) in the absence of endothelial toxicity may represent an advantage over more destructive methods, such as brachytherapy,[16] or cytotoxic inhibitors.[17] Indeed recently local antiproliferative strategies including pharmacologic stent coatings (paclitaxel, rapamycin, etc.) have demonstrated inhibition

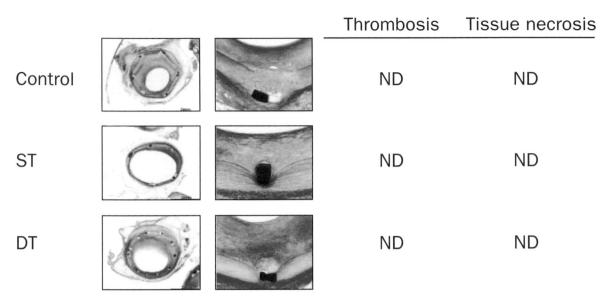

	Thrombosis	Tissue necrosis
Control	ND	ND
ST	ND	ND
DT	ND	ND

Fig. 44.3 Neointimal histopathology of control, soak-trap (ST), and dry-trap (DC) arteries. ND, no difference.

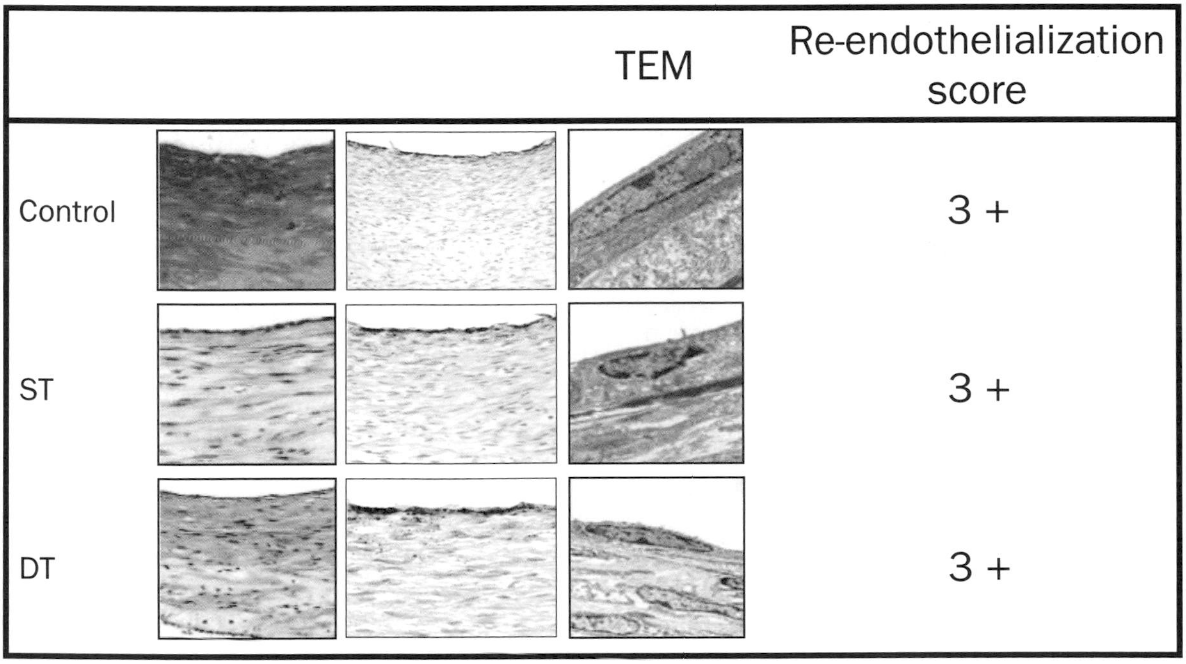

	TEM	Re-endothelialization score
Control		3 +
ST		3 +
DT		3 +

Fig. 44.4 Re-endothelialization histopathology of control, ST, and DT arteries.

of SMC proliferation in vitro, reduced neointimal thickening in animal models of restenosis, and produced promising results in the pilot clinical studies.[18–21] However, questions remain concerning the re-endothelialization process after

stent implantation with certain cytotoxic compounds which could put patients at risk for late stent thrombosis and cause late complications.[22,23] In contrast to other chemotherapeutics (paclitaxel, actinomycin D) Resten-NG inhibits

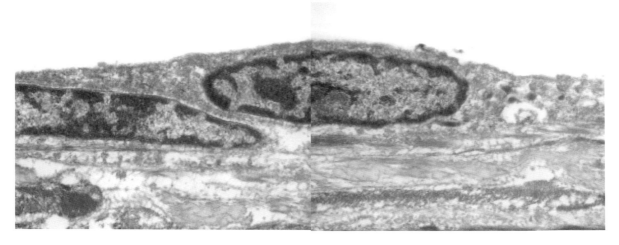

Fig. 44.5 The antisense stent does not seem to affect the endothelium. It appears normal.

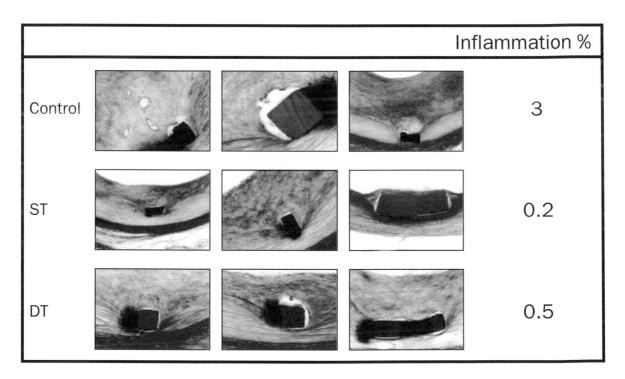

Fig. 44.6 Histopathology of control, ST, and DT stents. The antisense stent seems to cause less inflammation.

cell cycle in the G_1 phase. Compounds that inhibit cell cycle in the early phase are often less toxic. Therefore, Resten-NG as well as rapamycin fit this description. In addition, advanced antisense can also inhibit the cell cycle at multiple points so it may be effective regardless of what stage of cell growth the drug is applied (Figure 44.7).

This study showed that vascular healing was completed at 4 weeks in both treatment groups and was no different than in control stents. Interestingly, we observed less adventitial fibrosis in ST-loaded stents then in control stents (Table 44.2).

In addition, c-myc is an early activated oncogene and stent-loading technology will

Table 44.2   Antisense histopathology

| | Treatment groups | | | |
	Control	Dry-trap	Soak-trap	p-value
Intimal SMC	3.00	3.00	3.00	ns
Intimal vascularity	0.67 ± 0.49	0.42 ± 0.44	0.21 ± 0.33	ns
Intimal fibrin	0.25 ± 0.39	0.33 ± 0.20	0.19 ± 0.29	ns
Adventitial fibrosis	0.83 ± 0.30	0.96 ± 0.51	0.46 ± 0.46	ns

SMC, smooth muscle cell; ns, not significant.

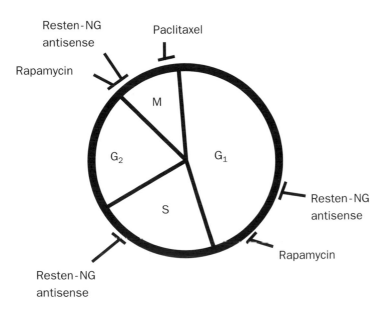

Fig. 44.7 The Resten-NG (AVI-4126) antisense inhibits the cell cycle.

therefore be relatively simple because the antisense needs to be released primarily in the first 24–48 hours after intervention. In contrast sirolimus (rapamycin) is a cell cycle inhibitor that affects late genes and may need to be released from the stent for a much longer period of time.[18,24] This limitation is similarly true for paclitaxel and its derivatives.[17,23,25] Therefore, a stent-coating technique may be appropriate for the antisense compound.

A significant fraction may also be retained by membrane lipids and remain there as a depot for more prolonged release. On the other hand, the presence of calcified material and variations in the lipid content of plaque in diseased human vessels may alter the drug distribution pattern and reduce its efficacy.

Another concern from the standpoint of therapeutics is whether adequate tissue levels of antisense can be maintained over the period of a few days. A more extended period of antisense availability (weeks, months) may, however, induce rebound effect.

CLINICAL STUDIES

Phase I: Dose-escalating safety study

A Phase I study was conducted to evaluate the safety and pharmacokinetic properties of AVI-4126 (Resten-NG) at five dose levels (1 mg,

3 mg, 10 mg, 30 mg, 90 mg) administered intravenously. Six subjects were tested at each dose level. Safety laboratory assessments (chemistry, hematology, urinalysis) were performed at baseline, and 24 h, 48 h, 72 h, 1 week and 2 weeks post dose. Adverse experiences were collected on an ongoing basis from the time of dosing to discharge from the study at 2 week follow-up.

The most frequent adverse events reported included lower extremity aches and headache. The majority of adverse events were graded as mild in intensity and were generally self-limiting. Serum complement C3a was measured. Four subjects had elevated C3a greater than twice the upper limit of normal (ULN) (normal = 0–400 ng/mL), including two subjects at the 3 mg dose level, one subject in the 10 mg cohort, and one subject in the 90 mg dose group. Three of the four elevations occurred at 24 h post dose and one occurred at 0.5 h post dose. In the light of pharmacokinetic studies of the investigated compound, elevations of C3a at 24 h post dose are unlikely to be related to administration of AVI-4126, but rather to spurious assay results. Further, there was no concurrent clinical symptomatology accompanying the elevated C3a, which is expected with elevated split complement levels.

Phase II: The AVAIL trial

Objectives

The purpose of the study is to evaluate the safety of AVI-4126, and to determine if intraluminal delivery of AVI-4126 in patients with de novo stenosis or in-stent restenosis reduces the restenosis rate when compared to patients in the control arm. The objectives of this study are:

1. *To evaluate the safety of AVI-4126 administered intramurally with the Infiltrator® delivery system to a restenosed stent site.* Safety will be evaluated by comparing the incidence of adverse events in patients receiving AVI-4126 (Arm A and Arm B) to those patients in the control arm (Arm C).
2. *To evaluate the effectiveness of AVI-4126 when administered intramurally with the Infiltrator® delivery device to the site of a restenosed stent lesion.* The effectiveness of AVI-4126 will be

evaluated by comparing the angiographic and intravascular ultrasound (IVUS) analysis at baseline to 6 months (or time of restenosis whichever occurs first) of AVI-4126 3 mg, AVI-4126 10 mg, and control arm in respect to: (1) the late loss index; (2) percentage diameter stenosed; (3) minimal luminal diameter; and (4) binary restenosis rate.
3. *To evaluate the clinical benefit of AVI-4126.* Clinical benefit will be assessed by comparing three treatment groups for the incidence of major adverse cardiovascular events (MACE).

Rationale for dose selection

The dose has been selected based on preclinical and clinical studies of AVI-4126. Efficacy studies of AVI-4126 in rabbit and pig models of arterial restenosis involved local delivery of AVI-4126 at 0.5 mg and 1 mg per vessel. Intravenous administration of AVI-4126 in a Phase I clinical study ranged from 1 mg to 90 mg. As there were no dose-limiting events in this dose-escalation study, a mid dose level was selected for intramural arterial delivery to provide the most efficacious dose with minimal safety risk.

Study design

This is a Phase II randomized, evaluator-blinded three-arm study. It will be conducted at up to five investigation sites. The patients will be scheduled for angiography and angioplasty following confirmed stenosis or in-stent restenosis. Patients will receive study treatment (AVI-4126 3 mg, AVI-4126 10 mg, or the Infiltrator® catheter alone) following angiographic procedures. The patient will return for physical examinations and safety evaluations at 1 month, 3 months, and 6 months post study treatment. The final angiographic and IVUS measurement outcomes will occur at the 6 month visit unless ischemic changes warrant earlier angiographic evaluation.

Study population

Patients with known prior implantation of an intracoronary stent undergoing angiography are candidates for this study. An accrual of approximately 120 patients is expected in order to result in 100 total evaluable patients into the study. There will be a minimum of 30 patients assigned to each arm of the study. Patients are considered to be evaluable for efficacy who receive the assigned study treatment and undergo a follow-up angiography and IVUS to determine the primary outcome measurements. Non-evaluable patients will be replaced, including those: (1) where the PTCA or Infiltrator® catheter advancement was a failed procedure; (2) who were randomized and did not receive study treatment or the Infiltrator® catheter.

Patients who provide an informed consent, are willing to participate in the required study procedures, and meet the inclusion and exclusion criteria may be considered for this study. The following criteria must be met in order to enroll a patient into the study.

Inclusion criteria

1. Patient in the range: ≥18 and <80 years of age.
2. Patient undergoing planned treatment for first-time implantation of a stent as a result of stenosis, or planned treatment of an in-stent restenotic lesion.

3. Patient is an acceptable candidate for coronary artery bypass surgery.
4. The target in-stent lesion will have a minimum occlusion of 50%.
5. Target vessel diameter at the target lesion site will be >2.5 mm and <4.0 mm, as indicated by angiography.
6. Target lesion will be ≤15 mm in length as measured by angiography.
7. A woman of childbearing potential has agreed to take part in the study and is currently practicing acceptable birth control methods.
8. Patient must have given written informed consent.
9. Patient agrees and is able to return for the scheduled study visits.

Study status

Although the enrollment was complicated because of the learning curve required for the use of the Infiltrator® catheter, and its limited flexibility to navigate coronary arteries, five US centers were able to enroll patients. There have been no AVI-4126-related serious adverse events. There was also a reduction in the restenosis rate in the high dose versus control (Figure 44.8, preliminary dat).

	Group A (3 mg)	Group A (10 mg)	Group C (Control)
Restenosis	66.7% (4/6)	11.1% (1/9)	40.0% (2/5)

➤No MACE observed linked to the antisense compound

➤No adverse events linked to the antisense compound

Fig. 44.8 The AVAIL trial: 6 month angiographic follow-up.

ACKNOWLEDGMENT

The authors wish to thank Cathy Kennedy for manuscript preparation and copyediting.

REFERENCES

1. Speir E, Epstein SE. Inhibition of smooth muscle cell proliferation by an antisense oligodeoxynucleotide targeting the messenger RNA encoding proliferating cell nuclear antigen. Circulation 1992; 86:538–47.

2. Simons M, Edelman ER, DeKeyser JL, et al. Antisense c-myb oligonucleotides inhibit arterial smooth muscle cell accumulation in vivo. Nature 1992; 359:67–70.

3. Gunn J, Holt CM, Francis SE, et al. The effect of oligonucleotides to c-myb on vascular smooth muscle cell proliferation and neointima formation after porcine coronary angioplasty. Circ Res 1997; 80:520–31.

4. Zalewski A, Shi Y, Mannion JD, et al. Synthetic DNA-based compounds for the prevention of coronary restenosis: current status and future challenges. In: Clinical trials of genetic therapy with antisense DNA and DNA vectors. Eric Wickstrom (ed.), Marce Dekker 1998:363–93.

5. Serruys P, Kutryk MJB, Bruining N, et al. Antisense oligonucleotide against c-myc administered with the Transport delivery catheter for the prevention of in-stent restenosis. Results of the randomized ITALICS trial [Scientific Sessions Abstracts]. Circulation 1998; 98(17) (suppl): I-1–I-1016.

6. Stein C, Cheng Y. Antisense oligonucleotides as therapeutic agents – Is the bullet really magical? Science 1993; 261:1004–12.

7. Shocman RL, Hartig R, Huang Y, et al. Fluorescence microscopic comparison of the binding of phosphodiester and phosphothioate oligodeoxyribonucleotides to subcellular structures, including intermediate filaments, the endoplasmic reticulum and the nuclear interior. Antisense Nucleic Acid Dev 1997; 7:291.

8. Hudziak RM, Barofsky E, Barofsky DF, et al. Resistance of morpholino phosphorodiamidate oligomers to enzymatic degradation. Antisense. Nucleic Acid Drug Dev 1996; 6:267–72.

9. Summerton J, Stein D, Huang B, et al. Morpholino and phosphorothioate antisense oligomers compared in cell-free and in-cell systems. Antisense Nucleic Acid Drug Dev 1997; 7:63–75.

10. Taylor MF, Paulaskis JD, Weller DD, et al. In vivo efficacy of morpholino modified oligomers directed against tumor necrosis factor-a mRNA. J Biol Chem 1996; 29:17452–5.

11. Summerton J, Weller D. Morpholino antisense oligomers: design, preparation and properties. Antisense Nucleic Acid Drug Dev 1997; 7:63–70.

12. Larrouy B, Boiziau C, Toulme J. RNAse H is responsible for non-sequence specific inhibition of in vitro translation by 2'-O-alkyl chimeric oligonucleotides: High affinity or selectivity, a dilemma to design antisense oligomers. Nucleic Acids Res 1995; 23:3434–40.

13. Walder J. Role of RNAse H in the action of antisense oligonucleotides. In Biotechnology International. Century Press: London; 1992:67–71.

14. Kipshidze N, Keane E, Stein D, et al. Local delivery of c-myc neutrally charged antisense oligonucleotides with transport catheter inhibits myointimal hyperplasia and positively affects vascular remodeling in the rabbit balloon injury model. Catheter Cardvasc Interv 2001; 54(2):247–56.

15. Kipshidze NK, Kim H-S, Iversen P, et al. Intramural coronary delivery of advanced antisense oligonucleotides reduces neointimal formation in the porcine stent restenosis model. J Am Coll Cardiol 2002; 39:1686–91.

16. Sheppard R, Eisenberg MJ. Intracoronary radiotherapy for restenosis. N Engl J Med 2001; 344(4):295–7.

17. Herdeg C, Oberhoff M, Baumbach A, et al. Local paclitaxel delivery for the prevention of restenosis: biological effects and efficacy in vivo. JACC 2000; 35(7):1969–76.

18. Sousa JE, Costa MA, Abizaid A, et al. Lack of neointimal proliferation after implantation of sirolimus-coated stents in human coronary arteries: A quantitative coronary angiography and three-dimensional intravascular ultrasound study. Circulation 2001; 103(2):192–5.

19. Sousa JE, Morice MC, Serruys PW, et al. The RAVEL Study: A randomized study with the Sirolimus coated BX velocity balloon-expandable stent in the treatment of patients with de novo native coronary artery lesions. Circulation 2001; 104(suppl): 104II-463 (abstract).

20. Moses JW, Leon MB, Popma JJ, et al. Sirolimus-eluting stents versus standard stents in patients with stenosis in a native coronary artery. N Engl J Med 2003; 349:1315–23.

21. Stone GW, Ellis SG, Cox DA, et al. A polymer-based, paclitaxel-eluting stent in patients with coronary artery disease. N Engl J Med 2004; 350:221–31.

22. Liistro F, Colombo A. Late acute thrombosis after paclitaxel eluting stent implantation. Heart 2001; 86:262–4.

23. Virmani R, Liistro F, Stankovic G, et al. Mechanism of late in-stent restenosis after implantation of a paclitaxel derivate-eluting polymer stent system in humans. Circulation 2002; 106:2649–51.

24. Suzuki T, Kopia G, Hayashi S et al. Stent-based delivery of sirolimus reduces neointimal formation in a porcine coronary model. Circulation 2001; 104:1188–93.

25. Farb A, Heller Phillip F, Shroff S, et al. Pathological analysis of local delivery of paclitaxel via a polymer-coated stent. Circulation 2001; 104:473–9.

45

Stent-based gene delivery

Bruce D Klugherz, Robert J Levy, and Robert L Wilensky

Introduction • Studies • Conclusions

INTRODUCTION

Catheter-based vascular gene therapy is a promising approach to mitigate restenosis following percutaneous intervention, but it suffers from several limitations. These include: variable delivery efficiency using catheter-based techniques,[1] systemic biodistribution of DNA,[2] and short-lived intramural gene expression due to non-chromosomal transfection with either plasmid DNA or adenoviral vectors.[3] Direct gene delivery from a stent may overcome some of these limitations as stents provide an implanted metallic surface upon which a porous, non-erodable or a hydrolyzable polymeric stent coating may be applied. A gene vector can be incorporated in the coating and the surface coating modified to provide controlled vector release. As stents scaffold the injured arterial segment, the chosen gene may be delivered directly to the site of anticipated restenosis in a sustained release fashion. And since intervention cardiologists already incorporate stents into daily practice, clinical integration of a well-engineered gene delivery stent will not be difficult.

STUDIES

Successful endovascular polymeric gene delivery using bioresorbable porous matrices adsorbed with a solution of lacZ-carrying adenoviral vectors was first reported in 1996.[4] Transduction of the arterial wall was observed following matrix deployment in rabbit carotid arteries. However, a lack of sustained virus delivery and systemic virus distribution were also observed and may limit the clinical application.

Recently, successful arterial wall transfection using a controlled-release polymeric coating on a conventional metallic stent was reported by our group.[5] DNA emulsions were prepared by mixing plasmid DNA with the biodegradable copolymer polylactic-polyglycolic acid (PLGA). Within the emulsion, DNA was homogeneously dispersed. The emulsions were then applied to Crown stents (Cordis, Johnson & Johnson, Figure 45.1). Ex vivo balloon expansion of the

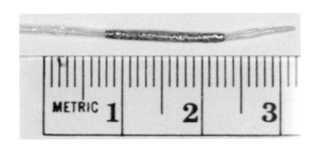

Fig. 45.1 A Crown stent showing emulsion coating.

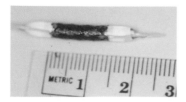

Fig. 45.2 Ex vivo balloon expansion shows a web-like stretching of the emulsion coating across the stent fenestrations.

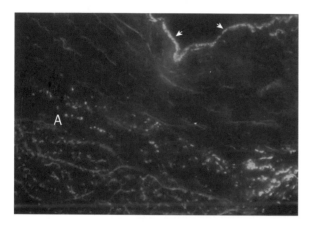

Fig. 45.3 Transfection of endothelial cells (arrows) and focal adventitial transfection (A) 7 days after delivery of GFP plasmid DNA into a non-atherosclerotic porcine coronary artery.

coated stents resulted in a web-like stretching of the coating across the stent fenestrations (Figure 45.2). There was no apparent fragmentation of the coating. In vitro, the coated stent released DNA for more than seven days, during which time the eluted DNA remained capable of transfecting cultured smooth muscle cells. Seven days following deployment of coated stents in porcine coronary arteries, gene expression was observed in approximately 1% of cells in the vessel wall. Figure 45.3 shows transfection of endothelial cells and focal adventitial transfection 7 days after delivery of green fluorescent protein (GFP) plasmid DNA into a non-atherosclerotic porcine coronary artery. Although systemic DNA distribution was not observed, DNA was occasionally detected in the pulmonary parenchyma using PCR, suggesting transit of microemulsions con-taining DNA through the coronary capillary and venous beds, and into the pulmonary vasculature. This study proved the concept that stent-based gene delivery was feasible as the PLGA-coated stent provided consistent trans-fection efficiency, sustained DNA delivery, and minimal systemic biodistribution.

More recently, the use of an *adenoviral* vector for stent-based gene delivery has been reported by our group.[6] Using a monoclonal antibody-tethered adenovirus covalently linked to a col-lagen coating, tight association of virus to the coating was demonstrated. Site-specific gene expression was observed in both cell culture and in pig coronary arteries, with no detectable vector DNA in distal organ systems. The major-ity of transduced cells were in the neointimal and medial layers. Transduction in vivo was more efficient than it had been with plasmid DNA.

These results hold promise for the future of stent-based endovascular gene therapy. The plasmid DNA and adenovirus-tethered coated stent experiments described above were com-pleted using conventional pharmacothera-pies (aspirin, ticlopidine, and unfractionated heparin) and conventional angioplasty equip-ment. The coated stents were hand-crimped on balloons, and once mounted were easily delivered by experienced interventionists. Nonetheless, a number of challenges remain.

First, many polymer coatings exacerbate inflammation of the arterial wall, thereby con-tributing to greater neointimal formation. Both biodegradable and biostable polymer matrices in contact with the injured arterial wall promote inflammatory cellular infiltration.[7] By minimizing the quantity of the stent coating, the inflammatory response can be curtailed.[8] However, the quantity of loaded DNA would also be limited. Formulation of a coating from endogenous proteins, such as collagen,[9] or fibrin,[10] as the matrix for gene delivery may also enhance biocompatibility.

Identification of the appropriate vector for gene delivery from a stent presents an additional challenge. The principal advantage of plasmid DNA eluted from a stent lies in its retention of functional integrity despite necessary preparatory steps including exposure to organic solvents and air-drying, either of which would be deleterious to adenoviruses. The principal disadvantage of plasmid DNA is its relative inefficiency in cellular transfection.[11] Whether transfection of 1% of cells, as was observed in our experiments with plasmid DNA, is sufficient to attenuate neointimal formation following stenting remains to be determined.

In contrast, adenoviral vectors are associated with more efficient transduction,[12] an obvious advantage over plasmid DNA. The principal concerns with these vectors are the potential to exacerbate the local inflammatory response,[13] resulting from host immunity to adenovirus, and systemic viral toxicity. The latter concern may prove less relevant with a stent-based delivery strategy which localizes gene delivery.

Finally, the gene(s) of choice to prevent in-stent restenosis remain(s) uncertain. Several candidate genes have shown promise in animal models using techniques including catheter-based, adventitial,[14] or pericardial delivery.[15] Among these, genes encoding cytostatic cell cycle regulatory proteins, such as the retinoblastoma protein,[16] or cytotoxic proteins, such as herpesvirus thymidine kinase,[17] are particularly attractive.

CONCLUSIONS

Stent-based gene delivery is a therapeutic strategy in its infancy. This technique holds promise for overcoming the weaknesses inherent in catheter-based gene delivery. Identification of the optimal formulation for stent coating, the most efficient and biosafe vector, and the most efficacious gene product to overexpress represent the hurdles for the future.

REFERENCES

1. Willard JE, Landau C, Glamann DB, et al. Genetic modification of the vessel wall: comparison of surgical and catheter-based techniques for delivery of recombinant adenovirus. Circulation 1994; 89:2190–7.
2. March KL, Madison JE, Trapnell BC. Pharmaco-kinetics of adenoviral vector-mediated gene delivery to vascular smooth muscle cells: modulation by poloxamer 407 and implications for cardiovascular gene therapy. Hum Gene Ther 1995; 6:41–53.
3. Verma IM, Somia N. Gene therapy – promises, problems, and prospects. Nature 1997; 389:239–42.
4. Ye YW, Landau C, Meidell RS, et al. Improved bioresorbable microporous intravascular stents for gene therapy. ASAIO J 1996; 42:M823–M827.
5. Klugherz BD, Jones PL, Cui X, et al. Gene delivery from a DNA controlled-release stent in porcine coronary arteries. Nature Biotechnol 2000; 18:1181–4.
6. Song C, Klugherz B, DeFelice S, et al. Antibody tethered stent-based adenoviral vector delivery in pig coronaries. Circulation 2000; 102 (suppl II):566.
7. van der Giessen WJ, Lincoff AM, Schwartz RS, et al. Marked inflammatory sequellae to implantation of biodegradable and nonbiodegradable polymers in porcine coronary arteries. Circulation 1996; 94:1690–7.
8. Alt E, Haehnel I, Beilharz C, et al. Inhibition of neointima formation after experimental coronary artery stenting. A new biodegradable stent coating releasing hirudin and the prostacyclin analogue iloprost. Circulation 2000; 101:1453–8.
9. Chandler LA, Doukas J, Gonzalez AM, et al. FGF2-targeted adenovirus encoding platelet-derived growth factor-B enhances *de novo* tissue formation. Mol Ther 2000; 2:153–60.
10. McKenna CJ, Camrud AR, Sangiorgi G, et al. Fibrin-film stenting in a porcine coronary injury model: efficacy and safety compared with uncoated stents. J Am Coll Cardiol 1998; 31:1434–8.
11. Kullo IJ, Simari RD, Schwartz RS. Vascular gene transfer: from bench to bedside. Arterioscler Thromb Vasc Biol 1999; 19:196–207.
12. Flugelman MY, Jaklitsch MT, Newman KD, et al. Low level in vivo gene transfer into the arterial wall through a perforated balloon catheter. Circulation 1992; 85:1110–17.
13. Newman KD, Dunn PF, Owens JW, et al. Adenovirus-mediated gene transfer into normal rabbit arteries results in prolonged vascular cell activation, inflamation, and neointimal hyperplasia. J Clin Invest 1995; 96:2955–65.

14. Rios CD, Ooboshi H, Piegors D, et al. Adenovirus-mediated gene transfer to normal and atherosclerotic arteries: a novel approach. Arterioscler Thromb Vasc Biol 1995; 15:2241–5.

15. Lamping KG, Rios CD, Chun JA, et al. Interpericardial administration of adenovirus for gene transfer. Am J Physiol 1997; 272:H310–H317.

16. Chang MW, Barr E, Seltzer J, et al. Cytostatic gene therapy for vascular proliferative disorders with a constitutively active form of the retinoblastoma gene product. Science 1995; 267:518–22.

17. Guzman RJ, Hirschowitz EA, Brody SL, et al. *In vivo* suppression of injury-induced vascular smooth muscle cell accumulation using adenovirus-mediated transfer of the herpes simplex virus thymidine kinase gene. Proc Natl Acad Sci USA 1994; 91:10732–6.

46

Catheter-based local heparin delivery

Aaron V Kaplan and Antonio L Bartorelli

Introduction • Heparin as an agent rationale • The LocalMed infusion sleeve • Acute infarct angioplasty • 'Bail-out' stenting • Restenosis • Conclusions

INTRODUCTION

Direct vascular delivery of heparin (local heparin) in the setting of percutaneous coronary interventions (PCI) is among the most extensively studied local delivery strategies. A local heparin approach has been employed to evaluate the safety and feasibility of specific local delivery catheters and protocols as well as its efficacy in reducing acute complications and restenosis following PCI. The central role of heparin in the systemic anticoagulation of patients undergoing PCI along with its well characterized antithrombotic and antiproliferative properties,[1] make local heparin strategy well suited for this role. This chapter will review the rationale, preclinical data and clinical results from studies utilizing this strategy with particular emphasis on its use in patients undergoing coronary stenting.

HEPARIN AS AN AGENT RATIONALE

Heparin is a complex mixture of acidic sulfated mucopolysaccharides with diverse biologic properties. Heparin inhibits thrombin primarily by potentiating the effects of antithrombin III and secondly by the inactivation of coagulation factors, IX, X, XI, and XII.[2] In addition, heparin has properties that make it a good candidate as an antirestenotic agent. Heparin has been shown to inhibit smooth muscle cell proliferation and migration, and has a suppression effect on matrix-degrading-protease expression.[3,4]

The antithrombotic impact of heparin delivered locally has been evaluated in a porcine model.[5] In the presence of ^{111}In-platelets, carotid arteries underwent balloon over-stretch injury followed by local heparin or vehicle. Animals were maintained for 30 minutes or 12 hours prior to sacrifice at which time the arteries were harvested. A 57% and 39% reduction in platelet deposition was observed at 30 minutes and 12 hours, respectively.

As reviewed elsewhere in this text, a limitation of local drug delivery catheters is a low transfer efficiency, which has been measured to be between 0.1% and 10% in animal studies and in patients following balloon angioplasty, with the remainder of agent delivered into the arterial lumen.[6,7] This is a serious liability when delivering agents with high systemic toxicity. With agents, such as heparin, which is required systemically, delivery via one of the local delivery catheters provides a means of providing systemic anticoagulation as well as achieving markedly higher concentrations at the site of drug delivery.

THE LocalMed INFUSION SLEEVE

The majority of clinical work evaluating the local delivery of heparin has been performed with the Infusion Sleeve (LocalMed, Palo Alto, California USA). The Infusion Sleeve was designed to provide the operator with a versatile platform to define the optimal conditions for local heparin delivery.[8]

The Infusion Sleeve is a multilumen catheter consisting of a proximal infusion port, a proximal hub, a main catheter shaft, and a distal infusion region with multiple side holes (Figure 46.1). The catheter has a central lumen for dilatation catheter and guidewire access, as well as four separate outer lumens for drug delivery. Side holes in each of the drug delivery lumens are located within the infusion region

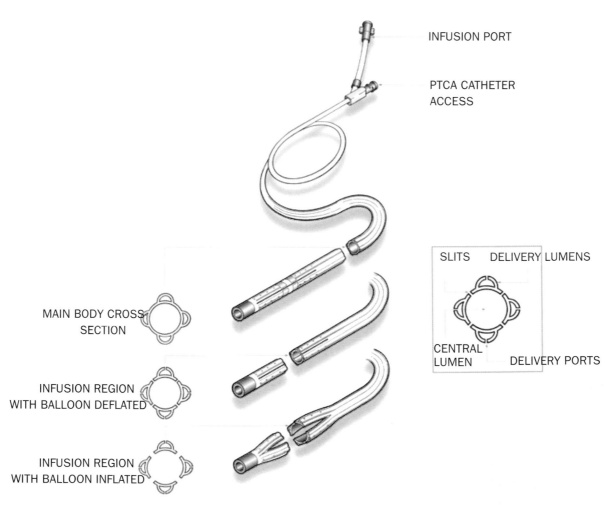

Fig. 46.1 Schematic drawing of the Infusion Sleeve. The catheter consists of a multilumen extrusion with a large central lumen surrounded by four drug delivery tubes in a clover-leaf pattern. The drug delivery tubes run the entire length of the catheter and have microperforations near the distal tip. In addition, there are slits at the distal end within the webs between the drug delivery tubes, which allow for radial expansion. PTCA, percutaneous transluminal coronary angioplasty.

near the distal tip of the Infusion Sleeve. Radiopaque markers are also located in each drug delivery lumen within the infusion region. Agent travels through the proximal infusion port and the outer infusion lumens and exits via side holes (nine 40 μm diameter holes per drug delivery lumens). The Infusion Sleeve is designed to track over standard dilatation balloon catheters. During drug delivery, the Infusion Sleeve is aligned with the underlying balloon. The Infusion Sleeve has been designed to provide independent control of the apposition of the drug delivery elements

against the arterial wall: this is determined by the inflation pressure of the underlying percutaneous transluminal coronary angioplasty (PTCA) balloon, and agent delivery into the arterial wall (determined by the infusion pressure of the drug delivery elements).

The Infusion Sleeve is used clinically in the following manner (Figure 46.2). Before the procedure, the Infusion Sleeve is loaded on to a standard balloon dilatation catheter of the operator's choice. PTCA is performed in the usual fashion with the Infusion Sleeve retracted within the guide. After angioplasty

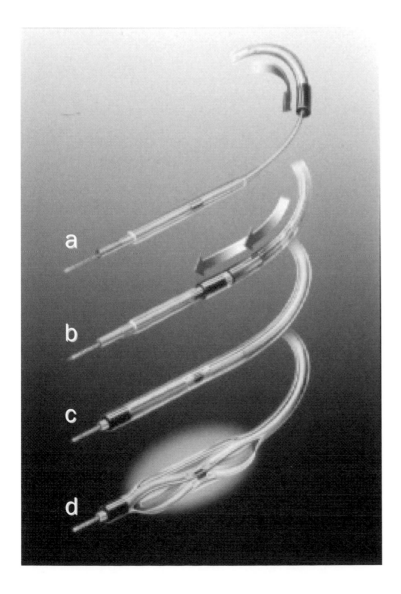

Fig. 46.2 Infusion Sleeve configurations. (a) Retracted configuration: the Infusion Sleeve is retracted proximal to the PTCA balloon. PTCA and stenting are performed in this configuration. (b) and (c) The Infusion Sleeve is advanced with its infusion region aligned with the deflated PTCA balloon. (d) Balloon inflation in the aligned configuration allows the infusion region of the drug delivery tubes to be brought into apposition with the arterial wall; local delivery is then performed under specific apposition and infusion conditions.

the Infusion Sleeve is advanced over the dilatation catheter, aligning the infusion region of the Infusion Sleeve with the balloon of the PTCA catheter. The balloon is then inflated bringing the infusion elements in contact with the arterial wall after which drug delivery is performed under specific infusion conditions. After drug delivery, the balloon is deflated and the Infusion Sleeve retracted back into the guide. The unsheathed PTCA balloon is then available to perform additional angioplasty, or the Infusion Sleeve/PTCA balloon catheter assembly can simply be removed.

Heparin delivery via the Infusion Sleeve has been evaluated in the setting of primary acute infarct angioplasty, 'bail-out' stenting, and in elective patients to prevent restenosis following stent implantation.

Feasibility and safety

The initial safety and feasibility of the Infusion Sleeve catheter was demonstrated in a series (n = 95) performed at Red Cross Hospital in Frankfurt and the Centro Cardiologico 'Monzino' in Milan. The Milan group subsequently evaluated a local heparin strategy in the setting of stent placement in elective patients (n = 33).[9] In this study, the Infusion Sleeve was successfully tracked and heparin delivered in 94% of patients. Stent placement was successful in all cases (Figure 46.3). Ten dissections were observed after PTCA and prior to heparin delivery. Sequential evaluation of angiograms following heparin infusion in these 10 patients demonstrated that 7 dissections remained unchanged, 2 worsened, and 1 improved with local heparin infusion. Six month follow-up was obtained in all 33 patients; 30 (91%) of them were asymptomatic and had a negative exercise treadmill test. Angiographic restenosis (≥50% stenosis) was observed in 4 (12.5%) of the 32 patients who underwent follow-up angiography. These data demonstrated the safety and feasibility of this strategy and provided an understanding of the technology that allowed for evaluation in specific clinical and anatomic settings.

ACUTE INFARCT ANGIOPLASTY

The role of a local heparin strategy in the setting of acute infarct angioplasty was investigated in the Local PAMI Pilot Study. Local PAMI, a prospective, multicenter series, studied the impact of local heparin in acute infarct patients undergoing primary angioplasty.[10] A total of 120 patients with standard definition of acute myocardial infarction (AMI) underwent angioplasty using standard techniques, after which heparin (4000 U) was delivered locally. Stent placement was reserved for patients with suboptimal angiographic results.

After initial lesion dilatation, heparin was successfully delivered in 120 (99.2%) of the 121 patients enrolled in the study. Core lab evaluation of serial angiograms demonstrated a change in TIMI flow in 15 (12.5%) patients, 11 improving and 4 deteriorating. A change in dissection score was noted in 13 (10.8%) patients, 4 improving and 9 worsening. Stents were deployed in 30 (25%) patients. Procedural success (NHLBI definition, with successful heparin infusion and TIMI 2 flow) was achieved in 118 (98.3%) patients. TIMI 3 flow was documented in 115 (96.6%) patients. The combined endpoint of death, reinfarction, recurrent ischemia or stroke was observed in 8 (6.7%) patients during the index hospitalization. Infarct artery revascularization for restenosis, defined as patients undergoing repeat percutaneous coronary intervention (PCI) or coronary artery bypass graft (CABG) after 30 days and during the 6 month follow-up period occurred in 8.3% and 4.2% of the patients, respectively.

These data demonstrate that local heparin therapy with provisional stenting in AMI patients is safe, feasible, and associated with a low rate of revascularization of the infarct-related artery. It is intriguing to speculate regarding the very low clinical restenosis rate observed following local heparin delivery. This reduction in restenosis may be specific to patients with high thrombus burden, as is the case in AMI patients. Such speculation

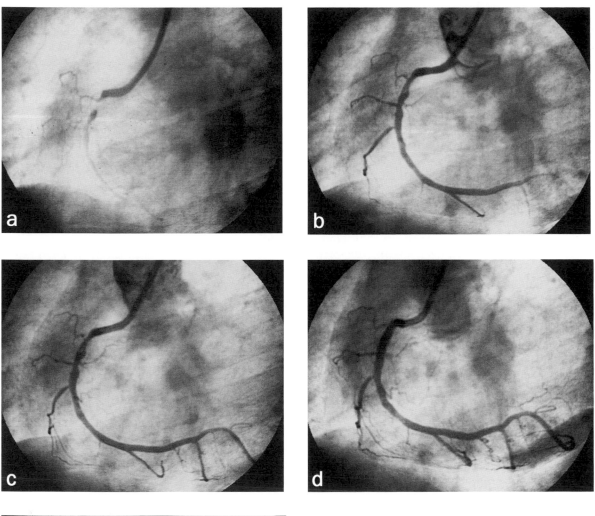

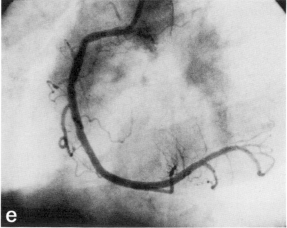

Fig. 46.3 Case example of local heparin delivery prior to coronary stent implantation. (a) Chronic total occlusion of the proximal segment of the right coronary artery. (b) Post-PTCA angiogram demonstrating recanalization of the vessel with residual stenosis. (c) No change in the angiographic appearance of the vessel is visible following local delivery of 4 mL of concentrated heparin (1000 U/mL) via the infusion sleeve pressurized at 100 psi. (d) Final angiographic result after implantation of a 3.5 mm Palmaz-Schatz stent. (e) Six month angiographic follow-up showing excellent long-term outcome.

is hazardous without adequate randomized studies to rigorously test this hypothesis.

'BAIL-OUT' STENTING

Bail-out stenting for major dissection and threatened closure is associated with a high rate of ischemic complications.[11,12] The role of local heparin infusion in patients with suboptimal angioplasty in which bail-out stenting was planned was evaluated in a pilot prospective randomized study.[13] The study had two phases. Phase I, in which 20 patients were randomized to either low (40 psi) or high (100 psi) pressure delivery. Phase II in which 37 patients were randomized in a 2:1 design to receive local heparin at high (100 psi) pressure delivery or standard therapy. The Infusion Sleeve catheter was successfully tracked to the index lesion and heparin delivered in all but one patient.

Coronary angiography did not show any significant change in the number, severity, and length of coronary dissections following local heparin infusion. A total of 79 stents were deployed in 56 lesions. One patient treated, who was assigned to the high (100 psi) pressure infusion group, experienced perforation, which was noted >30 minutes after heparin delivery following initiation of glycoprotein IIb/IIIa inhibitor infusion and stent placement. This complication was treated successfully with prolonged inflation, heparin reversal, and platelet infusion.

No significant differences were observed in the composite endpoint of death, myocardial infarction, CABG, urgent repeat angioplasty, and stent thrombosis (at 30 days). However, a trend towards a higher rate of myocardial infarction was noted in each arm of Phase I and in the local infusion group of Phase II.

The size and design of this small randomized pilot study makes it difficult to draw definite conclusions on local delivery of antithrombotic therapy during bail-out stenting. However, it suggests a cautious approach with the clinical use of local heparin delivery in the presence of major coronary dissections.

RESTENOSIS

Percutaneous coronary intervention (PCI) has recently undergone fundamental changes with the incorporation of stents into the clinical armamentarium. It is estimated that stents were used in more than 80% of cases performed in the United States in 1999. Stents have been shown to reduce both acute complications, as well as late restenosis.[14,15] Stents have provided the interventionist with a means to treat large dissections, leading to a dramatic reduction in acute abrupt closure and the rate of emergency surgery.[16] The mechanical scaffold provided by stents is also responsible for the prevention of arterial recoil and negative geometric remodeling, which make up a significant component of restenosis. The benefit of stent placement within the coronary vasculature has been demonstrated primarily in discrete lesions in large vessels. As new more trackable and longer stents become available, allowing for the treatment of lesions in smaller vessels and diffuse disease, the benefit of stent placement may be reduced. Multiple studies have demonstrated that stent placement increases late lumen loss, mainly due to neointimal proliferation.[17] Furthermore, the treatment of restenosis within a stented artery (i.e. in-stent restenosis), presents the interventionist with a far more difficult problem than 'old fashioned' restenosis. Therefore, the benefit of a local delivery strategy may be the greatest in the prevention of in-stent restenosis. Platelet deposition and thrombus are considered among the initial steps in neointimal proliferation. Local heparin delivery at the site of balloon injury significantly reduced platelet deposition in the initial 12 hours in a porcine carotid model.[5] Therefore, local heparin delivery may provide a simple, easy and attractive antirestenotic strategy. Its impact on prevention of in-stent restenosis was formally studied in the HIPS Trial (Heparin Infusion Prior to Stenting), an open labeled, multicenter, prospective, randomized, and core laboratory-evaluated trial comparing heparin delivery utilizing an intracoronary or intramural strategy

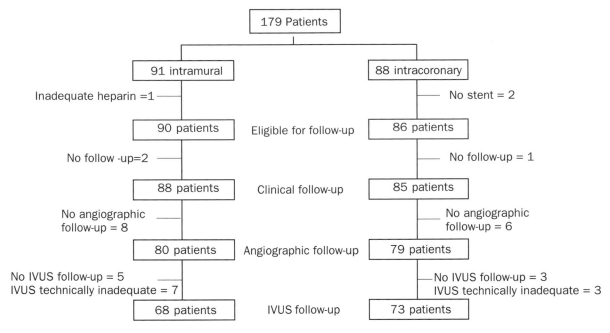

Fig. 46.4 Patient enrollment and follow-up in the HIPS study.

(Figure 46.4).[18] A total of 179 patients were randomly assigned to receive 5000 U of heparin delivered as an intracoronary infusion (control group) or intramural via the Infusion Sleeve (local group) after initial balloon dilatation and prior to stent (J&J, PS-153) placement. Patients were monitored for procedural events and underwent clinical, angiographic, and intravascular ultrasound (IVUS) follow-up at 6 months. Control and local group patients were evenly matched with respect to baseline clinical and angiographic criteria. A trend toward increased prevalence of diabetes mellitus in the local group was noted. There was no difference in the incidence of acute arterial injury, as monitored by angiographic dissections, acute closure or decrease in TIMI grade flow. At follow-up there was no difference in the major adverse event rate between local and control groups. Six month follow-up showed no difference in the angiographic in-stent restenosis and in the in-stent volumetric analysis as measured by intravascular ultrasound. However, the HIPS study sample size, patient selection, and excellent long-term results of elective stent implantation in large coronary arteries guided, in part, by IVUS may have masked a positive biological effect of local heparin delivery.

CONCLUSIONS

Local vascular delivery of heparin using a dedicated local drug delivery catheter has been shown to be feasible and safe in patients undergoing angioplasty/stent percutaneous coronary interventions, electively or in the acute infarct setting. However, this alternative route of heparin administration does not appear to be effective in reducing in-stent restenosis. Nevertheless, the concept of site-specific intracoronary delivery of agents such as heparin is an attractive strategy to prevent in-stent restenosis following percutaneous interventions. Further refinement in delivery technology as well as identification of new agents coupled with further clinical evaluation will be required before this approach is appropriately incorporated into routine clinical practice.

REFERENCES

1. Clowes AW, Karnovsky MJ. Suppression by heparin of smooth muscle cell proliferation in injured arteries. Nature 1977; 265:625–6.
2. Roden L. Highlights in the history of heparin. In Lane DA, Lindhal V (eds), Heparin: Chemical and Biological Properties: Clinical Applications. CRC Press: Boca Raton, FL 1989:1–8.
3. Reilly CF, Koindy MS, Brown KP, et al. Heparin prevents vascular smooth muscle cell progression through G1 phase of the cell cycle. J Biol Chem 1989; 264:6990–5.
4. Snow AD, Bolender RP, Wight TN, et al. Heparin modulates the composition of the extracellular matrix domain surrounding arterial smooth muscle cells. Am J Pathol 1990; 137:313–30.
5. Moura A, Lam JYT, Hébert D, et al. Intramural delivery of agent via a novel drug delivery sleeve: histologic and functional evaluation. Circulation 1995; 92:2299–305.
6. Camenzind E, Bakker WH, Reijs A, et al. Site-specific intracoronary heparin delivery in humans after balloon angioplasty: A radioisotopic assessment of regional pharmacokinetics. Circulation 1997; 96:154–65.
7. Azrin MA, Mitchel JF, Fram DB, et al. Decreased platelet deposition and smooth cell proliferation after intramural heparin delivery with hydrogel-coated balloons. Circulation 1994; 90:433–41.
8. Kaplan AV. Infusion sleeve catheter. Semin Interv Cardiol 1996; 1:36–8.
9. Bartorelli AL, De Cesare N, Kaplan AV, et al. Local heparin delivery prior to coronary stent implantation: Acute and six-month clinical and angiographic follow-up. Catheter Cardiovasc Diag 1997; 42:313–20.
10. Esente P, Kaplan AV, Ford JK, et al. Local intramural heparin delivery during primary angioplasty for acute myocardial infarction: Results of the local PAMI study. Catheter Cardiovasc Diagn 1999; 47:237–42.
11. Hermann HC, Buchbinder M, Clemen MW, et al. Emergent use of balloon-expandable coronary artery stenting for failed percutaneous transluminal coronary angioplasty. Circulation 1992; 86:812–19.
12. Schömig A, Kastrati A, Mudra H, et al. Four-year experience with Palmaz-Schatz stenting in coronary angioplasty complicated by dissection with threatened or present vessel closure. Circulation 1994; 90:2716–24.
13. Tanguay JF, Cantor WJ, Krukoff MW, et al. Local heparin delivery post-PTCA: A multicenter randomized pilot study. Catheter Cardiovasc Interv 2001; 49:461–7.
14. Fischman DL, Leon MB, Baim DS, et al. A randomized comparison of coronary stent placement and balloon angioplasty in the treatment of coronary artery disease. N Engl J Med 1994; 331:496–501.
15. Serruys PW, de Jaegere P, Kiemeneij F, et al. A comparison of balloon-expandable stent implantation with balloon angioplasty in patients with coronary artery disease. N Engl J Med 1994; 331:489–95.
16. Lincoff AM, Topol EJ, Chapekis AT, et al. Intracoronary stenting compared with conventional therapy for abrupt vessel closure complicating coronary angioplasty: a matched case-control study. J Am Coll Cardiol 1993; 21:866–75.
17. Mudra H, Regar E, Klauss V, et al. Serial follow-up after optimized ultrasound-guide deployment of Palmaz-Schatz stents: In-stent neointimal proliferation without significant reference segment response. Circulation 1997; 95:363–70.
18. Wilensky RL, Tanguay JF, Shigenori I, et al. Heparin infusion prior to stenting (HIPS) trial: Final results of a prospective, randomized, controlled trial evaluating the effects of local vascular delivery on intimal hyperplasia. Am Heart J 2000; 139:1061–70.

Local delivery of low molecular weight heparins

R Stefan Kiesz, M Marius Rozek, and Jack L Martin

Introduction • Studies • Conclusions

INTRODUCTION

Restenosis following coronary stent implantation remains an important and costly therapeutic problem. Since intimal smooth muscle cell (SMC) proliferation is largely the culprit,[1–4] various attempts to inhibit this process have been studied.[5–10] Modulation of the stimuli for neointimal hyperplasia by appropriate pharmacologic agents would, in theory, permit vessel wall healing after coronary stent implantation without an exaggerated, obstructive proliferative response. Until recently, local drug delivery, using various agents and different methods of administration, has failed to affect restenosis rate after stenting (see further the discussion in Chapter 29).[11,12] This may be related to the agent studied, and the design of the delivery device, as well as the timing of drug delivery with respect to stenting. Arterial injury triggers thrombus formation with release of growth factors known to stimulate neointimal proliferation: platelet-derived growth factor (PDGF), transforming growth factor (TGF)-β, fibroblast growth factor (FGF) and others.[13–15]

STUDIES

Enoxaparin has been shown to inhibit smooth muscle cell proliferation at high tissue concentrations.[16–18] However, it has not reduced the incidence of angiographic restenosis or clinical events after successful coronary angioplasty when administered systemically.[19] In a baboon angioplasty model low molecular weight heparin (LMWH) blocked serum-induced but not PDGF-induced SMC proliferation and migration, suggesting heparin sensitive and insensitive pathways. If the assumption that human SMC are less sensitive to growth inhibition by heparin is true, one may consider the possibility that in-stent restenosis may be reduced by local prevention of early prothrombotic events. Enoxaparin is a potent inhibitor of factor Xa and thrombin.[20,21] The strategy of local delivery of enoxaparin during predilation was specifically designed to modulate the magnitude of thrombin-mediated and thrombus-mediated stimuli for neointimal proliferation. The purpose of enoxaparin delivery during predilation is to have an antithrombotic agent in place at the time of the initial balloon deflation, when the injured vessel wall was first exposed to circulating prothrombotic elements. This hypothesis was tested in an atherosclerotic rabbit model where 10 mg of enoxaparin delivered during iliac angioplasty reduced neointimal proliferation as evidenced by reduced BRDU uptake compared with conventional angioplasty.[18]

In humans, this strategy has been applied in a small, preliminary PILOT registry,[22] and the recently completed prospective, randomized multicenter POLONIA study. Patients were selected with de novo lesions, which contain tissue factor (factor VIIa) and other procoagulant molecules.[23,24] The investigators postulated that the local drug delivery of a small volume of highly concentrated enoxaparin at the time of initial injury (predilation) with subsequent compression of the treated wall segment by the expanded stent would result in a sufficient local concentration and retention of enoxaparin to prevent subacute stent closure and to decrease intimal hyperplastic response. This is an important consideration, since animal studies using a rabbit model for intramural delivery of enoxaparin with the Transport catheter without subsequent stenting revealed poor retention of the agent.[18] This strategy, if effective, would reduce late luminal loss, and ultimately, the restenosis rate.

In the PILOT registry, 10 mg of enoxaparin was delivered with the Transport catheter during predilation in 25 patients before the insertion of Palmaz-Schatz stents. In this non-randomized study the late loss of 0.46 ± 0.1 mm compared favorably with a contemporary population treated with the same stent deployment techniques in the Stress III trial.[25]

In the POLONIA study, local drug delivery of 10 mg of enoxaparin was also performed with the Transport catheter and all patients received the balloon expandable, stainless steel NIR stent. The local drug delivery group received reduced systemic anticoagulation with 2500 U of intravenous unfractionated heparin, the control group received $\geq$10 000 U of systemic heparin to achieve activating clotting time (ACT) >300 seconds. The study population, other procedural details, and results are described in Tables 47.1 and 47.2. This study demonstrated that local delivery of enoxaparin during predilation and prior to coronary stent implantation reduces late luminal loss and restenosis as compared with a conventional stent implantation strategy and systemic heparinization. The late luminal loss and restenosis rates in the control arm correspond well with the findings from other studies, where less than 3.0 mm vessels stenting was performed with the early generation

---

Table 47.1 Procedural data in local drug delivery (LDD) and systemic heparinization (SH) groups

	LDD group (n = 50)	SH group (n = 50)	p-value
Stent deployment pressures (atm)	14.0 ± 2.8	15.0 ± 2.9	ns
Number of stents deployed	54	53	
Baseline ACT (sec)	106.2 ± 37.6	129.4 ± 49.8	ns
Final ACT (sec)	146.9 ± 39.8	381.9 ± 182.2	0.000001
Procedure total time (min)	70.5 ± 31.8	66.1 ± 30.5	ns
Total sheath time (min)	122.9 ± 66.6	384.5 ± 94.4	0.00001

atm, atmospheres; act, activated clotting time; ns, not significant.

Table 47.2 Technical data of local drug delivery with the Transport catheter in 50 patients	
Balloon support pressure (atm)	3.3 ± 0.4
Enoxaparin infusion time (sec)	85.9 ± 41.2
Enoxaparin infusion pressure (psi)	49.1 ± 6.9

atm, atmospheres; psi, pounds per square inch.

stents.[26,27] On the other hand, observed luminal loss and the restenosis rate in the local drug delivery group compares favorably with the results of small vessel stenting.[26,27] The incidence of subacute closure in this vessel category ranges from 2.5%–3.6% with full systemic heparinization.[26,27] In the local drug delivery group there was no subacute closure events, despite the lack of full systemic heparinization. This may suggest local, persistent antithrombotic effect of enoxaparin.

CONCLUSIONS

Our findings are in contrast to those of the IMPRESS study where local delivery of nadroparin did not affect restenosis when delivered after stent implantation.[28] There are several major methodological differences between the POLONIA and IMPRESS trials. In addition to delivering drug during initial predilation, the POLONIA strategy used a device, which uncouples the drug delivery pressure from the dilating pressure. Moreover the studies employed different low molecular weight heparins, which differ chemically and pharmacologically.

We must stress that the findings of the POLONIA study require confirmation by a larger trial. The precise anti-restenosis mechanism of enoxaparin, although not fully elucidated, is likely the combination of a reduction of thrombotic events, downregulation of thrombotic growth factor generation, and perhaps a direct inhibitory effect on smooth muscle cell proliferation. These data suggest that local drug delivery may constitute a viable therapeutic option to prevent restenosis after coronary stent implantation. Thus, there is a need for a large, randomized trial

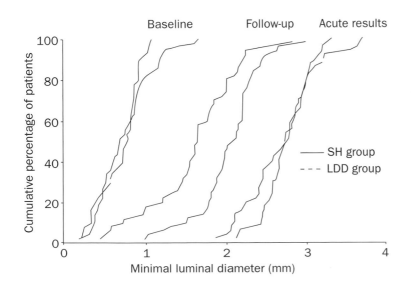

Figure 47.1 Cumulative distribution of minimal diameter before, immediately after stenting and at 6 months of angiographic follow-up. ——, patients randomized to systemic heparinization (SH); ......, patients randomized to local drug delivery (LDD), and reduced systemic heparinization.

Table 47.3   Clinical outcomes in local drug delivery (LDD) vs systemic heparinization (SH) groups

	LDD group	SH group	p-value
Acute results			
MI	0	2%	ns
Death	0	0	ns
Subacute closure	0	2%	ns
Emergent CAGB	0	0	ns
Emergent PTCA	0	2%	ns
Angina	4%	10%	ns
6 month FU			
MI	0	0	ns
Death	0	0	ns
CABG	0	2%	ns
TLR	8%	22%	0.0499
Angina	12%	24%	ns

MI, myocardial infarction; CABG, coronary artery bypass surgery; TLR, target lesion revascularization; PTCA, percutaneous transluminal coronary angioplasty; ns, not significant.

and further development of active antiproliferative agents as well, as improved drug delivery devices.

REFERENCES

1. Pickering J, Weir L, Jekanowski J, et al. Proliferative activity in peripheral and coronary atherosclerotic plaque among patients undergoing percutaneous revascularization. J Clin Invest 1993; 91:1469–80.

2. Dussaillant GR, Mintz GS, Pichard AD, et al. Small stent size and intimal hyperplasia contribute to restenosis: a volumetric intravascular ultrasound analysis. J Am Coll Cardiol 1995; 26:720–4.

3. Painter JA, Mintz GS, Wong SC, et al. Serial intravascular ultrasound studies fail to show evidence of chronic Palmaz-Schatz stent recoil. Am J Cardiol 1995; 75:398–400.

4. Carter AJ, Laird JR, Kufs WM, et al. Coronary stenting with a novel stainless steel balloon-expandable stent: determinants of neointimal formation and changes in arterial geometry after placement in an atherosclerotic model. J Am Coll Cardiol 1996; 27:1270–7.

5. Forrester J, Fishbein M, Helfanat R, Fagin J. A paradigm for restenosis based on cell biology: clues for the development of new preventive therapies. J Am Coll Cardiol 1991; 17:758–69.

6. Ferns G, Raines E, Sprugel K, et al. Inhibition of neointimal smooth muscle cell acummulation after angioplasty by an antibody to PDGF. Science 1991; 235:1129–32.

7. Wilensky RL, March KL, Gradus-Pizlo I, et al. Vascular injury, repair, and restenosis after percutaneous transluminal angioplasty in the atherosclerotic rabbit. Circulation 1995; 92:2995–3005.

8. Waksman R, Robinson KA, Crocker IR, et al. Intracoronary radiation before stent implantation inhibits neointima formation in stented porcine coronary arteries. Circulation 1995; 92:1383–6.

Table 47.4   Quantitative coronary angiography results in local drug delivery (LDD) and systemic heparinization (SH) groups

	LDD group (n = 50)	SH group (n = 50)	p-value
Baseline			
Ref vessel	2.94 ± 0.29	2.92 ± 0.29	ns
MLD	0.77 ± 0.33	0.67 ± 0.25	ns
Stenosis	73.84 ± 11.03	77.11 ± 8.83	ns
Lesion length	10.93 ± 4.32	10.22 ± 3.96	ns
Acute results			
Ref vessel	3.00 ± 0.29	2.92 ± 0.29	ns
MLD	2.80 ± 0.37	2.67 ± 0.38	ns
Residual stenosis	6.5 ± 10.0	8.0 ± 12.9	ns
Acute gain	2.03 ± 0.42	2.00 ± 0.47	ns
6 month FU	(*n* = 50)	(*n* = 49)	
Ref vessel	2.91 ± 0.24	2.83 ± 0.28	ns
MLD	2.02 ± 0.39	1.59 ± 0.54	0.00002
Stenosis	30.5 ± 13.0	43.8 ± 18.2	0.00006
Late loss	0.76 ± 0.42	1.07 ± 0.49	0.0009
Loss index	0.38 ± 0.21	0.55 ± 0.25	0.0004
Net gain	1.27 ± 0.50	0.92 ± 0.55	0.003
Restenosis	10%	24%	0.049

MLD, minimal luminal diameter; ns, not significant.
Acute luminal gain is the minimal luminal diameter immediately after the procedure minus the diameter before the procedure.
Late luminal loss is the minimal luminal diameter immediately after the procedure minus the diameter at follow-up.
Net luminal gain is the minimal luminal diameter at follow-up minus the minimal luminal diameter before the procedure.
Late loss index is the late luminal loss divided by the immediate luminal gain.

9. Waksman R. Local catheter-based intracoronary radiation therapy for restenosis. Am J Cardiol 1996; 78:23–8.
10. Farb A, Sangiorgi G, Carter AJ, et al. Pathology of acute and chronic coronary stenting in humans. Circulation 1999; 99:44–52.
11. Wilensky R, Tanguay J-F, Ito S, et al. The Heparin Infusion Prior to Stenting (HIPS) Trial: Procedural, in-hospital, 30 day, and six month clinical, angiographic and IVUS results. J Am Coll Cardiol 1998; 31:457A.
12. Serruys P, Kurtyk M, Bruining N, et al. Antisense oligonucleotide against c-myc administered with the transport delivery catheter for the prevention of in-stent restenosis. Results of the Randomized ITALICS Trial. Circulation 1998; 98:I-363.
13. Dinbergs ID, Brown L, Edelman ER. Cellular response to transforming growth factor-beta1 and basic fibroblast growth factor depends on release kinetics and extracellular matrix interactions. J Biol Chem 1996; 271:29822–9.

14. Unterberg C, Meyer T, Wiegand V, et al. Proliferative response of human and minipig smooth muscle cells after coronary angioplasty to growth factors and platelets. Basic Res Cardiol 1996; 91:407–17.

15. Skaletz-Rorowski A, Schmidt A, Breithardt G, Buddecke E. Heparin-induced overexpression of basic fibroblast growth factor, basic fibroblast growth factor receptor, and cell-associated proteoheparan sulfate in cultured coronary smooth muscle cells. Arterioscler Thromb Vasc Biol 1996; 16:1063–9.

16. Hammerle H, Betz E, Herr D. Human endothelial cells are stimulated and vascular smooth muscle cells are inhibited in their proliferation and migration by heparins. Vasa J Vasc Dis 1991; 20:207–15.

17. Taylor A, Ao P, Fletcher J. Inhibition of intimal hyperplasia and occlusion in Dacron graft with heparin and low molecular weight heparin. International Angiology 1995; 14:375–80.

18. Hong MK, Wong SC, Barry JJ, et al. Feasibility and efficacy of locally delivered enoxaparin via the Channeled Balloon catheter on smooth muscle cell proliferation following balloon injury in rabbits. Catheter Cardiovasc Diagn 1997; 41:241–5.

19. Faxon DP, Spiro TE, Minor S, et al. Low molecular weight heparin in prevention of restenosis after angioplasty. Results of Enoxaparin Restenosis (ERA) Trial. Circulation 1994; 90:908–14.

20. Gikakis N, Khan MM, Hiramatsu Y, et al. Effect of factor Xa inhibitors on thrombin formation and complement and neutrophil activation during in vitro extracorporeal circulation. Circulation 1996; 94:II341–6.

21. Gikakis N, Rao AK, Miyamoto S, et al. Enoxaparin suppresses thrombin formation and activity during cardiopulmonary bypass in baboons. J Thorac Cardiovasc Surg 1998; 116:1043–51.

22. Deutsch E, Kiesz R, Martin J, et al. Preliminary experience with a novel stent design (NIRside) for unprotected distal left main disease. Circulation 1997; 96:I-710.

23. Toschi V, Gallo R, Lettino M, et al. Tissue factor modulates the thrombogenicity of human atherosclerotic plaques. Circulation 1997; 95:594–9.

24. Gertz SD, Fallon JT, Gallo R, et al. Hirudin reduces tissue factor expression in neointima after balloon injury in rabbit femoral and porcine coronary arteries. Circulation 1998; 98:580–7.

25. Fischman DL, Savage MP, Penn I, et al. Clinical outcome after stent implantation with high pressure deployment and reduced anticoagulation: Late follow-up from the STRESS III Trial. Circulation 1998; 17:I-159.

26. Elezi S, Kastrati A, Neumann FJ, et al. Vessel size and long-term outcome after coronary stent placement. Circulation 1998; 98:1875–80.

27. Savage MP, Fischman DL, Rake R, et al. Efficacy of coronary stenting versus balloon angioplasty in small coronary arteries. Stent Restenosis Study (STRESS) Investigators. J Am Coll Cardiol 1998; 31:307–11.

28. Schielle F, Seronde M, Gupta S, et al. Local delivery of low molecular heparin after stent implantation to prevent neointimal proliferation. Results of the intravascular ultrasound sub-study. JACC 1999; 33:85A.

48

Local delivery of steroids before coronary stent implantation

Bernhard Reimers and Antonio Colombo

Introduction • **Methods** • **Results** • **Discussion** • **Limitations of the study** • **Conclusions**

INTRODUCTION

In this chapter we present a clinical pilot study on local drug delivery of steroids before stent treatment of coronary arteries. This study was performed to evaluate the feasibility and safety of intrawall delivery of long acting methylprednisolone before stent implantation and to test the efficacy of this treatment in reducing intimal hyperplasia in lesions at high risk for restenosis.

Despite recent advances in interventional cardiology, restenosis remains a major problem affecting 15–50% of patients undergoing percutaneous coronary interventions.[1,2] The main causes of restenosis have been identified as acute elastic recoil of the vessel, late arterial remodeling, and neointimal hyperplasia.[3,4] Coronary stents have been a mainstay in attenuating acute and chronic vessel recoil but facilitate the development of neointimal hyperplasia,[5] due to smooth muscle cell proliferation.[6–8] This process involves the recruitment of cells of the monocyte/macrophage line as a prominent feature. This line produces several factors that have been shown to increase smooth muscle proliferation and collagen synthesis.[9,10] Steroids have been shown in vitro to reduce those processes.[11–13] Two randomized trials with systemic treatment of methylprednisolone prior to balloon angioplasty did not reduce restenosis,[14,15] but coronary stents were not used in these studies and the active drug concentration in the vessel wall might have been rather low. More recent studies evaluating steroid effects on neointimal hyperplasia gave contradictory results.[16–18]

The present pilot study was based on these preclinical results and it was performed to test the efficacy of local intrawall delivery of long-acting steroids before elective stent implantation in reducing neointimal hyperplasia with subsequent reduction of the angiographic restenosis rate. In addition, the safety and feasability of a new local drug delivery device were tested. This new delivery balloon holds a design that has the potential to effectively deliver a drug into the vessel wall by direct injection.[19–21]

METHODS

Between January 1996 and July 1996 a total of 309 patients (449 lesions) were treated with coronary stent implantation. Of these, 24 patients (40 lesions) were prospectively selected to be treated with local drug delivery before stent implantation. Inclusion criteria were >18 years of age, no child bearing female, no clinical history of diabetes or other metabolic disorders, and ability to understand and sign an informed consent form. In all cases elective stent implantation was planned. Lesions considered at high risk for restenosis (long lesions: ≥20 mm length and/or small vessels: reference diameter <3.0 mm) were selected by the operator to be included in this registry. In this pilot evaluation, a significant decrease of restenosis compared with a matched historical control group would have justified further investigation of the presented approach. Written consent for the study was obtained after the possible benefits and risks were well explained. The study protocol was approved by the local ethics committee.

Study drug

Methylprednisolone acetate (Depo-Medrol, Upjohn, Puurs, Belgium), a long-acting corticosteroid available in vials containing 40 mg in 1 cc of drug suspension, was delivered intramurally. Every 40 mg of methylprednisolone acetate correspond to 36 mg of methylprednisolone. According to the manufacturer, the pharmaceutical effect starts within the first 6 hours and lasts for 7–14 days. For intramuscular or local administration dosages of 40–120 mg of methylprednisolone acetate once a week are recommended (Pharmaceutical information, Upjohn, Puurs, Belgium).

Local drug delivery device

A new delivery device (Barath Infiltrator® catheter; InterVentional Technologies, Letterkenny, Ireland) was used (Figure 48.1). This is a

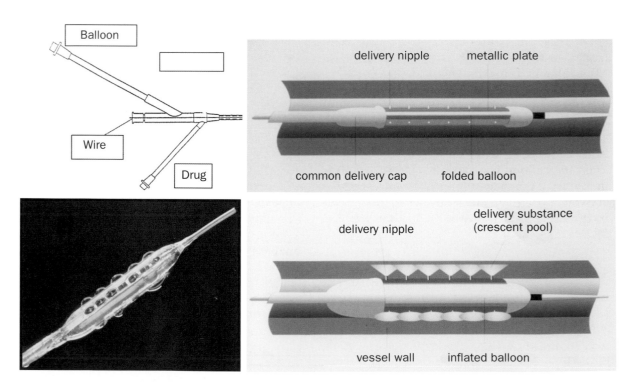

Fig. 48.1 Representation of the Infiltrator™ local drug delivery device.

three-lumen balloon catheter with one lumen for balloon inflation, one lumen for drug infusion, and one lumen for an over-the-wire system guidewire insertion. The balloon length is 15 mm with two radiopaque markers. The balloon is available in different diameters ranging from 2.0 mm to 4.0 mm (0.5 mm increments). The balloon carries 21 metallic microports distributed in three lines that run parallel to the balloon axis, each line having seven microports of 0.010 inch height and 0.004 inch exit width. The balloon is inflated to 3–4 atmospheres to permit microport penetration into the vessel wall. The 0.5 cc drug can be injected intramurally during a short inflation of 10–15 seconds.

Drug delivery

Intrawall drug delivery was performed after predilatation with adequately sized angioplasty balloons. The delivery balloon has been chosen with a balloon/artery ratio of approximately 1. The drug infusion lumen of the catheter was carefully filled with drug suspension avoiding the presence of air. The flow of suspension out of all the microports was controlled with a 2.5 cc syringe containing the drug attached to the infusion lumen. The catheter was then advanced over a 0.014 inch guidewire and positioned at the lesion site. The balloon was inflated at 3–4 atm under fluoroscopic observation for 10–15 sec during which 0.5 cc of the drug was slowly injected by hand. Then the balloon was deflated and withdrawn in the usual manner. In long lesions drug delivery was repeated in different sites up to 4 times in the same vessel in order to treat the entire diseased segment.

Stent implantation

Before stent implantation all patients were treated with acetylsalicylic acid (aspirin) 325–500 mg. A bolus of 100 U/kg of heparin was given after sheath insertion and repeat boluses of 2500 U heparin were given as needed to maintain the activated clotting time >250 sec. Different types of stents were used: 15

beStents (Medtronic, Inc., San Diego, CA), 13 NIR stents (Boston Scientific, Maple Grove, MN), 4 coronary Palmatz-Schatz stents (Johnson & Johnson Interventional System, Warren, NJ), 4 Gianturco-Roubin II stents (Cook, Bloomington, IN), 6 Micro II stents (Advanced Vascular Engineering, Richmond, Canada), and 4 Wallstents (Schneider, Bülach, Switzerland). The stent type was chosen by the operator. Stents were either hand crimped on a percutaneous transluminal coronary angioplasty (PTCA) balloon or positioned with a dedicated delivery system. Following stent deployment, further high pressure dilatations ($\geq$14 atm) were performed within the stent to obtain a close to zero angiographic residual stenosis. In 23 lesions (64%) stents were placed with intracoronary ultrasound guidance (Microview, 3.2F Monorail, CardioVascular Imaging System, CA). Multiple stents were implanted to cover the entire diseased segment ensuring minimal overlap and no gaps.

Patients did not receive any heparin or oral anticoagulants after the procedure and the sheaths were removed 2–6 hours later with an activated clotting time $\leq$150 sec. Ticlopidine 250 mg twice a day was given for 2 months and aspirin 325 mg once daily indefinitely. No further treatment with systemic steroids was given.

Angiographic analysis

Coronary angiograms were obtained in a routine manner. Patients received intracoronary isosorbide-dinitrate prior to initial and post-procedure angiograms to achieve maximal vasodilation. The vessels and lesions were analyzed using a computerized quantitative analysis system (QCA-CMS Version 3.0, MEDIS, Leiden, The Netherlands) according to previously described and validated edge detection algorithms taking the catheter for calibration.[22] Measurements included: the interpolated reference diameter, the minimal lumen diameter, the percentage diameter stenosis and the lesion length. Measurements were obtained at baseline, after stent implantation, and at follow-up. Lesions were characterized according to the modified American Heart Association (AHA)/Canadian Cardiovascular Society (CCS) classification.

Definitions

Drug delivery success was defined as the delivery of a minimum of 20 mg (0.5 cc) methylprednisolone acetate at the lesion site. Primary stent success was defined as stent implantation at the target lesion with ≤ 30% residual stenosis without the occurrence of Q-wave myocardial infarction, urgent coronary bypass surgery, or death. Q-wave infarction was defined by the presence of a new pathological Q-wave in association with creatine kinase elevation twice or more the normal value. Non-Q wave infarction was present in case of cardiac enzyme elevation equal to or greater than 2-fold the normal value without occurrence of a new Q-wave. Target lesion revascularization included lesion-related bypass surgery or repeat angioplasty. Recurrence of angina included the presence of CCS class II–IV angina and/or positive exercise test during the follow-up period. Stent restenosis was defined as ≥ 50% diameter stenosis at the stented site or at the edges proximally or distally. Diffuse restenosis was defined as a ≥50% lumen narrowing of ≥10 mm length while restenoses <10 mm were defined as focal.

Follow-up

Cardiac enzymes were determined at 6 and 12 hours after the procedure in all patients. A platelet count was performed at weeks 2 and 4. Clinical follow-up at 2 weeks, 3 months, and 6 months was performed in an outpatient clinic or by phone call. Angiographic follow-up was scheduled at 5–6 months after the procedure.

Matching process

Matching was based on principles derived from the Rotterdam Thoraxcenter group.[23] (1) The angiographic dimensions of matched lesions are assumed to be 'identical'. (2) The observed differences between the two matched lesions after stenting must be within the range of the quantitative angiographic analysis system's reproducibility.

Of the 413 lesions in which treatment with local drug delivery was not performed, 249 lesions with angiographic follow-up were eligible for matching. It was possible to match 24 out of 36 treated lesions (treament group) with 24 out of 249 not treated lesions (control group). Matching was performed by a computerized program written in dBase language that iteratively scanned the two databases chronologically, and selected for each lesion in the treatment group the first lesion encountered in the control group, which satisfied the selection criteria. The following angiographic and procedural selection variables for individual lesion matching were:

(1) vessel treated
(2) vessel reference diameter ± 0.5 mm
(3) baseline minimum lumen diameter ± 0.4 mm
(4) post-stenting minimum lumen diameter ± 0.4 mm
(5) diabetes
(6) type of stent (slotted tube, coil stent, combination of both)
(7) number of stents deployed ± 1.

Statistical analysis

Data were analyzed using the SAS statistical software package. Categorical variables are presented as absolute numbers (%). Continuous variables are presented as mean ± SD. Differences between groups were evaluated by Chi-square analysis or Fisher's exact test for categorical variables, and Student's *t*-test for continuous variables. Probability values <0.05 were considered to be significant.

RESULTS

Patient and lesion characteristics are shown in Table 48.1. The incidence of AHA/ACC type C lesions was 47% and in 25% of cases total occlusions were treated. The mean reference diameter of treated vessels was 2.85 mm and lesion length was 13.6 mm.

Table 48.1 Patient and lesion characteristics, and procedural data of the 21 patients (36 lesions) with successful drug delivery	
Age (yrs)	58 ± 2
Men	16 (76%)
Ejection fraction (%)	56 ± 10
Unstable angina	8 (38%)
Treated vessel	
LAD	11 (31%)
LCX	9 (25%)
RCA	13 (36%)
Venous graft	3 (8%)
Multivessel disease	15 (71%)
Lesions/patient	1.5 ± 0.4
Lesion type[a]	
B 1	3 (8%)
B 2	16 (45%)
C	17 (47%)
Total occlusions	9 (25%)
Restenosic lesions	4 (11%)
Stents implanted	46
Stents per lesion	1.3 ± 0.6
Stented segment length (mm)	30.1 ± 18.8
≥20 mm long stents	23 (64%)
Balloon/artery ratio	1.2 ± 0.2
Mean final inflation pressure (atm)	16.4 ± 3.1
IVUS guidance	23 (64%)

LAD, left anterior descending artery; LCX, left circumflex artery; RCA, right coronary artery; atm, atmospheres; IVUS, intravascular ultrasound. [a]According to modified AHA/ACC criteria. Values are given as mean ± SD or in percentages.

Drug delivery

Drug delivery was successfully performed in 36 lesions (21 patients) (90%). In the remaining four lesions, attempts to advance the delivery catheter to the lesion site failed. In two of these lesions it was also impossible to cross the lesion with a stent. A mean of 60 ± 21 mg (range 20–80 mg) of methylprednisolone acetate were delivered per lesion. The total amount of drug never exceeded 120 mg in the single patient (mean per patient 98 ± 23 mg). Complications during and immediately after drug delivery such as prolonged chest pain, persistent ST changes, vessel occlusion, vessel dissection, or slow flow were not observed. Steroid induced pharmacological side effects were not observed.

Stenting procedure

Primary stent success was obtained in all 36 lesions where the drug was successfully delivered. Long stents (≥20 mm) were used in 64% of cases and the resulting mean stented segment length was 30.1 ± 18.8 mm. Mean final inflation pressure was 16.1 ± 3.1 atm and the balloon artery ratio was 1.2 ± 0.2. Procedural details are shown in Table 48.2. The residual diameter stenosis after stenting was 5.1 ± 9.1%. Quantitative angiographic and intracoronary ultrasound results are shown in Table 48.3.

Procedural and in-hospital complications

Two non-Q wave myocardial infarctions occurred. One due to side branch occlusion, and the other to thrombus embolization during pre-interventional intracoronary ultrasound (IVUS) examination. The maximum creatine kinase rises were 460 U/L and 540 U/L, respectively.

Clinical follow-up at 6 months

One (3%) subacute stent thrombosis occurred 5 weeks after stent implantation but did not result in a myocardial infarction. In this patient, a bifurcational lesion of the left circumflex artery and the obtuse marginal branch, treated with two 40 mm long stents, occluded. Stents

Table 48.2 Angiographic and intravascular ultrasound results

	Baseline	After stent	Follow-up
Angiographic analysis (n = 36)			
Mean reference diameter (mm)	2.85 ± 0.44	3.04 ± 0.37	3.00 ± 0.38
Minimal lumen diameter (mm)	0.78 ± 0.54	2.87 ± 0.38*	1.64 ± 0.74**
Diameter stenosis (%)	73 ± 18	5 ± 9*	45 ± 25**
Acute lumen gain (mm)		2.10 ± 0.53	
Late loss (mm)			1.24 ± 0.70
Loss index			0.61 ± 0.36
Lesion length (mm)	13.6 ± 9.1		9.7 ± 6.5
Intravascular ultrasound analysis (n = 23)			
Minimal lumen diameter (mm)	1.92 ± 0.45	2.98 ± 0.43*	
Luminal cross-sectional area (mm²)	2.93 ± 1.36	7.05 ± 1.77*	
Vessel cross-sectional area (mm²)	12.42 ± 2.15		
Plaque (%)	76.85 ± 7.97		

Values are given as means ± SD. *$p<0.001$ vs original lesion; **$p<0.001$ vs after stent.

were successfully reopened with repeat balloon angioplasty. Recurrence of angina and/or positive exercise test was observed in 12 out of 21 patients with successful drug delivery (57%). Myocardial infarction and death did not occur during the time of follow-up.

Angiographic follow-up

Angiographic follow-up was performed in all 36 lesions with successful delivery of methylprednisolone acetate at a mean of 4.5 ± 1.7 months. Twelve patients (57%) were restudied before the scheduled time for clinical indications. A ≥50% diameter stenosis at follow-up was present in 14 of 36 lesions (39%). In one case (3%), a small aneurismatic dilatation at the side of drug delivery and stent implantation was observed. Repeat target lesion revascularization was performed in 15 lesions (42%). In 14 patients reintervention consisted in repeat percutaneous angioplasty and one patient underwent coronary bypass surgery. One lesion

with angiographical 43% diameter stenosis observed within the stent was treated with repeat balloon angioplasty at early follow-up in a patient with recurrent angina. Quantitative angiographic results are shown in Table 48.3. IVUS evaluation was not performed at follow-up. Representative examples of treated lesions with different angiographic outcome are shown in Figures 48.2–48.5.

Comparison with matched lesions

It was possible to match 24 out of 36 treated lesions (67%) (= treatment group) with 24 lesions out of 249 eligible not treated lesions (= control group). Patient and lesion characteristics, procedural, and follow-up results of both groups are shown in Table 48.4. The only significant difference between the groups was the lesion length which was longer in the treatment group compared to the control group (8.5 ± 5.0 mm vs 15.1 ± 9.9 mm, $p = 0.002$). The angiographic restenosis rates were 38% in the

Table 48.3   Results of clinical and angiographical follow-up of 21 patients (36 lesions) with successful drug delivery

In hospital	
Non-Q wave myocardial infarction	2 (8%)
6 months clinical follow-up	
Subacute stent thrombosis	1 (3%)
Recurrence of angina and/or	
positive stress test	12 (57%)
Target lesion revascularization	15 (42%)
Repeat angioplasty	14 (39%)
Coronary bypass surgery	1 (3%)
Death, Myocardial infarction	0 (0%)
Angiographic follow-up	
Obtained	36 (100%)
Months	4.5 ± 1.7
≥ 50% diameter stenosis	14 (39%)
Diffuse restenosis (≥10 mm length)	21 (58%)

Values expressed in mean ± SD or percentages.

treatment group (9 out of 24 lesions) and 33% in the control group (8 out of 24 lesions) ($p = 0.5$).

DISCUSSION

Mechanisms of stent restenosis

The restenotic process after coronary stenting is mainly caused by neointimal proliferation within and adjacent to the stent while acute recoil and late remodeling, which are observed following balloon angioplasty, have been virtually eliminated by the scaffolding properties of the stent itself.[4,5,24] The proliferative process which is generally completed within 12 weeks is probably caused by deep mechanical injury during balloon inflation,[25] but might be more pronounced after stent implantation as a response to metal, early thrombus formation, and permanent vessel wall strain.[24,26] Animal studies have reported on the pathogenesis of stent-induced neointimal hyperplasia which is more intense and of longer duration compared to balloon injury-induced neointimal hyperplasia.[6]

Why steroids again?

In previous studies systemic steroid administration failed to reduce restenosis after balloon

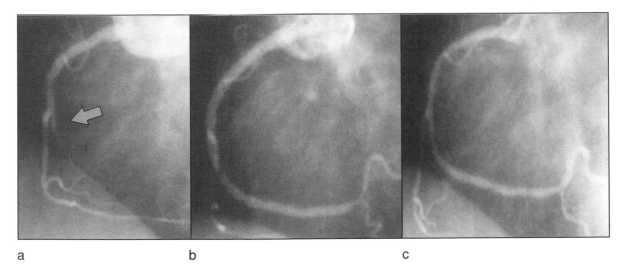

a   b   c

Fig. 48.2   (a) A total occlusion of the right coronary artery reopened and treated at three sites with 20 mg of methylprednisolone acetate (total 60 mg) before implantation of three stents (b). (c) Angiographic result after 4 months with mild restenosis.

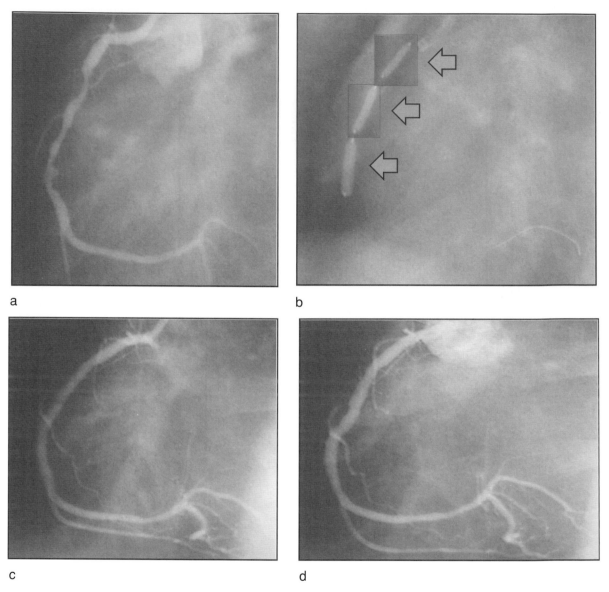

Fig. 48.3 (a) A diffusely diseased right coronary artery before treatment. (b) During inflation of the drug delivery device in three different sites. (c) Final procedural result after implantation of two 32 mm long slotted tube stents (d) at 4 month follow-up angiography.

angioplasty.[14,15] However, assuming cell proliferation as the main cause of stent restenosis, antiproliferative drugs might have the potential to modify this process. The efficient reduction of stent restenosis using low dose γ-irradiation by inhibiting neointima proliferation confirms the importance to stop or reduce the proliferative process.[27] Localized endothe-

lial injury during angioplasty induces the migration of mononuclear cells to the sites of injury where they are probably transformed to macrophages and foam cells, which release vasoactive substances that influence platelet aggregation and proliferation of exposed vascular smooth muscle.[6–10,28] Glucocorticoids reduce the migration of mononuclear cells,[13,29]

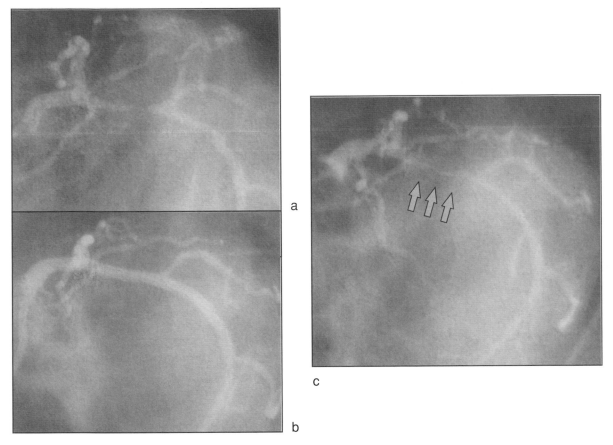

Fig. 48.4   (a) A left circumflex artery at baseline. (b) After delivery of 30 mg prednisolone acetate and after elective implantation of a 32 mm slotted tube stent. (c) At 3 month follow-up angiography with diffuse, critical in-stent restenosis.

and inhibit immune processes by diminishing the role of lymphocytes in perpetuating injury.[30] A direct action of steroids on platelets has not been shown.[31]

In the present study, steroids were delivered locally with the intent to obtain higher local concentration of the drug in the vessel wall compared to systemic drug administration. The Infiltrator injects microliter quantities of compound directly into the vessel wall. Its delivery efficiency defined as *volume deposited intrawall/volume delivered* is around 90% as shown in an animal study.[20] In a recent evaluation of the Infiltrator device using loaded low molecular weight heparin at the time of delivery, 80–85% of the radiolabeled volume was present at the delivery site but only 4% of the delivered drug was shown to persist more than 5 hours in the treated area.[32] Thus, one can conclude that the heparin was delivered into the wall but migrated rapidly out of the wall. This relatively low percentage, however, compares well with reported data of other devices. Further evaluations of different drug compounds and their retention time in the vessel wall should be performed to clearly determine the delivered quantity of the drug and how long it acts locally before migrating.

A long-acting steroid compound was chosen to assure a minimum drug action of a minimum of 7 days after a single administration. This approach of local administration of long-acting steroids is commonly and successfully used for many articular and periarticular inflammatory

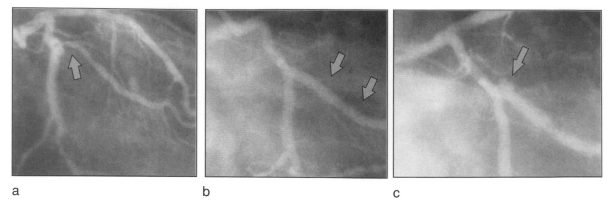

a   b   c

Fig. 48.5 (a) An obtuse marginal branch before treatment. (b) After elective implantation of a 39 mm proximal and a 20 mm distal stent implanted for dissection. (c) At 3 month follow-up angiography where a moderate aneurysmatic dilatation (arrow) can be observed. This patient presented at the follow-up angiography with a subocclusive restenosis of a stented diagonal branch without aneurysmatic dilatations.

Table 48.4 Patient and lesion characteristics, angiography results, and follow-up of 24 lesions (16 patients) treated with intrawall delivery of long-acting steroids (= treatment) compared with 24 matched, not treated lesions (= control; 21 patients)

	Treatment	Control	p-value
Age (yrs)	58 ± 11	55 ± 7	0.05
Ejection fraction (%)	58 ± 12	57 ± 10	0.54
Unstable angina	8 (38%)	8 (38%)	
Diabetes	0	0	
Treated vessel			
LAD	9 (37%)	9 (37%)	
LCX	5 (21%)	5 (21%)	
RCA	9 (37%)	9 (37%)	
Venous graft	1 (4%)	1 (4%)	
Multivessel disease	15 (71%)	13 (62%)	0.47
Lesion type[a]			0.08
A	0	1 (4%)	
B 1	1 (4%)	6 (29%)	
B 2	11 (46%)	10 (42%)	
C	12 (50%)	6 (25%)	
Total occlusions	5 (21%)	3 (13%)	0.44
Restenotic lesions	4 (17%)	2 (8%)	0.37

Table 48.4 *Continued*

	Treatment	Control	p-value
Stents/lesion	1.3 ± 0.2	1.4 ± 0.3	0.09
Stented segment length	29.1 ± 16.9	24.3 ± 13.7	0.07
≥20 mm long stents	16 (67%)	12 (50%)	0.35
Mean final inflation pressure (atm)	16.7 ± 2.9	16 ± 3.3	0.53
IVUS guidance	16 (67%)	16 (67%)	
Follow-up angiography at months	4.2 ± 1.4	5.6 ± 1.8	0.13
Mean reference diameter (mm)			
Pre	2.91 ± 0.44	2.81 ± 0.39	0.22
Post	3.05 ± 0.42	3.05 ± 0.46	0.34
Follow-up	2.93 ± 0.41	2.88 ± 0.49	0.21
Minimal lumen diameter (mm)			
Pre	0.86 ± 0.46	1.00 ± 0.52	0.29
Post	2.92 ± 0.41	2.95 ± 0.44	0.38
Follow-up	1.56 ± 0.69	1.59 ± 0.86	0.16
Diameter stenosis (%)			
Pre	70 ± 14	66 ± 16	0.30
Post	3 ± 10	2 ± 11	0.31
Follow-up	48 ± 21	44 ± 25	0.28
Lesion length (mm)	15.1 ± 9.9	8.5 ± 5.0	0.02*
≥50% diameter stenosis at follow-up	9 (38%)	8 (33%)	0.53
Target lesion revascularization	9 (38%)	8 (33%)	0.53

LAD, left anterior descending artery; LCX, left circumflex artery; RCA, right coronary artery; atm, atmospheres; IVUS, intravascular ultrasound. [a]According to modified AHA/ACC criteria. Values are given as mean ± SD or in percentages. *$p<0.05$.

processes.[33] Coronary aneurysm formation after chronic steroid therapy combined with other antiinflammatory agents have been reported.[34] In the present study, one case of a moderate aneurysmatic dilatation of the treated segment at 4 months after local steroid delivery was observed. The aneurysm was of small size and located proximally to the stent and was possibly due to enlargement of a proximal localized wall rupture (pseudoaneurysm).

In the large randomized studies evaluating systemic short-term steroid administration before coronary balloon angioplasty, aneurysms were not observed.[14,15]

Lesions at high risk of restenosis

In this study, the length of the lesion (13.6 ± 9.1 mm) and the stented segment length were particularly long (30.1 ± 18.8 mm) and the vessel reference diameter relatively small (2.85 ± 0.44 mm). Since lesion and stent length and vessel diameter are powerful angiographic predictors of stent restenosis,[35] the present lesion cohort can be considered at high risk for restenosis with a predicted restenosis rate of 43% (CI = 20–69). This high risk subgroup was chosen because a significant decrease in angiographic restenosis, below the lower limit of the predicted restenosis rate could have justified further evaluations on a larger patient cohort in a randomized fashion.

Persistent high restenosis rate

The resulting angiographic restenosis rate of 39% can be considered a failure to reduce restenosis with local long acting steroid administration before coronary stenting. One may also hypothesize that steroids may be of some advantage if we assume that angiographic restenosis for vessels treated with long or multiple stents is reported to be between 30% and 63%.[35–37] However, in the comparison with matched lesions treated in the same period of time at the same institution using the same procedural approach there was no significant difference in restenosis rate.

Several explanations for the inefficacy of steroids are possible:

1. The mechanisms of in-stent proliferation may be different than those influenced by steroids. Despite the fact that animal and in vitro studies clearly showed an antiproliferative effect of steroids,[11,12] this was not observed in the present study. Steroids do inhibit the monocyte/macrophage line which secretes platelet-derived growth factors (PDGF) but platelets are relatively unaffected by steroids.[31] Therefore, early in-stent platelet aggregation leading to early platelet-rich thrombi formation,[38] may remain unaffected by steroids.

2. Different types of steroid administration using different dosages have been studied to reduce restenosis. Both the following: a pulse infusion of 1 g of methylprednisolone before balloon angioplasty,[14] and systemic administration of 125 mg methylprednisolone followed by 60 mg prednisone daily for one week,[15] did not reduce restenosis after balloon angioplasty. The per patient dose (mean 98 mg methylprednisolone acetate) in the present study was far lower, but the local concentration is supposed to be high using a local drug delivery device that is reported to have 90% delivery efficiency and no luminal washout.[19,20] An additional systemic pulse dose, which is known to inhibit mononuclear cell function for 1 month,[13] was not given and might have altered the results of the present study.

3. Pepine et al. observed a beneficial effect of steroids after balloon angioplasty in angiographically less severe lesions with probably less plaque volume.[14] In the present study, severe lesions (mean pre-stent diameter stenosis 73 ± 18%) in diffusely diseased vessels were treated and therefore data on the effect on less severe lesions are not available. However, diffuse coronary disease with high plaque volume is afflicted by the highest restenosis rates and would profit most from an efficient restenosis reducing agent.

A recently published study evaluated sustained local delivery of dexamethasone with an eluting stent in a porcine model.[18] In that study neointimal hyperplasia was not reduced by documented high doses of steroids at the lesion site, a result that appears to be confirmed by our results.

Drug delivery device

The local drug delivery catheter Infiltrator® appeared to be safe, confirming a previous clinical experience.[19] The two non-Q-wave infarctions are explained by side branch occlusion and plaque embolization and cannot be connected to the use of the drug delivery device. The feasibility of the procedure seemed acceptable with a delivery success of 90% in diffusely diseased vessels and with not always favorable anatomy for lesion crossing. Time of inflation and drug delivery are short, adding only a few minutes to the duration of the procedure. The drug was delivered in all cases following predilatation with currently used angioplasty balloons, which obviously facilitated the crossing of the device.

LIMITATIONS OF THE STUDY

This is a prospective but not randomized pilot study on a small patient population without a direct control group. The choice of the drug compound (long-acting steroids) and the dose were empiric as no previous clinical studies are available. Local and systemic drug concentration after delivery were not measured. Many different types of stents were implanted. This was due to the heterogenic lesion morphology and might have influenced the outcome. The very high risk for restenosis of the lesions selected may be beyond the therapeutic potentials of this approach. Therefore, definite conclusions of the efficacy of steroids to reduce stent restenosis cannot be drawn. Results, however, are not very encouraging.

CONCLUSIONS

Local drug delivery of long-acting steroids before coronary stenting did not reduce the angiographic restenosis rate and the incidence of target lesion revascularization compared to a matched control group. However, due to the small number of studied patients, the not randomized study design, and the not controlled effective local drug concentration we cannot definitely exclude an antiproliferative effect of steoids to reduce in-stent restenosis. The local drug delivery catheter used in this study appeared to be safe with an acceptable feasibility.[39]

REFERENCES

1. Landau C, Lange RA, Hillis LD. Percutaneous transluminal coronary angioplasty. N Engl J Med 1994; 330:981–3.
2. Bittl JA. Advances in coronary angioplasty. N Engl J Med 1996; 332: 1290–302.
3. Post M, Borst C, Kuntz RE. The relative importance of arterial remodeling compared with intimal hyperplasia in lumen narrowing after balloon angioplasty: a study in the normal rabbit and the hypercholesteremic Yucatán micropig. Circulation 1994; 89:2816–21.
4. Kuntz RE, Gibson CM, Nobuyoshi M, Baim DS. Generalized model of restenosis after conventional balloon angioplasty, stenting and directional atherectomy. J Am Coll Cardiol 1993; 21:15–25.
5. Hoffmann R, Mintz GS, Dussaillant GR, et al. Patterns and mechanisms of in-stent restenosis. A serial intravascular ultrasound study. Circulation 1996; 94:1247–54.
6. Karas SP, Gravanis MB, Santonian EC, et al. Coronary intimal proliferation after balloon injury and stenting in swine: An animal model of restenosis. J Am Coll Cardiol 1992; 20:467–74.
7. Austin GE, Ratcliff NB, Hollman J, et al. Intimal proliferation of smooth muscle cells as an explanation for recurrent coronary artery stenosis after percutaneous transluminal coronary angioplasty. J Am Coll Cardiol 1985; 6:369–75.
8. O'Brien ER, Alpers CE, Stewart DK, et al. Proliferation in primary and restenotic coronary atherectomy tissue: Implications for antiproliferative therapy. Circ Res 1993; 73:223–31.
9. Jonasson L, Holm J, Skalli O, et al. Regional accumulations of T cells, macrophages, and smooth muscle cells in the human atherosclerotic plaque. Arteriosclerosis 1986; 6:131–8.
10. Weiss HJ, Hawiger J, Ruggeri Z, et al. Fibrinogen-independent platelet adhesion and thrombus formation on subendothelium mediated by glycoprotein IIa-IIIb complex at high shear rate. J Clin Invest 1989; 83:288–97.
11. Villa AE, Guzman LA, Chen W, et al. Local delivery of dexamethasone for prevention of neointimal proliferation in a rat model of balloon angioplasty. J Clin Invest 1994; 93:1243–9.
12. Voisard R, Seitzer U, Baur R, et al. Corticosteroid agents inhibit proliferation of smooth muscle cells from human atherosclerotic arteries in vitro. Int J Cardiol 1994; 43:257–67.
13. Macdonald RG, Panush RS, Pepine CJ. Rationale for use of glucocorticoids in modification of restenosis after percutaneous transluminal angioplasty. Am J Cardiol 1987; 60:56B–60B.

14. Pepine CJ, Hirshfeld JW, Macdonald RG, et al. (M-HEART Group). A controlled trial of corticosteroids to prevent restenosis after coronary angioplasty. Circulation 1990; 81:1753–61.

15. Stone GW, Rutherford BD, McConahay DR, et al. A randomized trial of corticosteroids for the prevention of restenosis in 102 patients undergoing repeat coronary angioplasty. Catheter Cardiovasc Diagn 1989; 18:227–31.

16. Berk BC, Gordon JB, Alexander RW. Pharmacologic roles of heparin and glucocorticoids to prevent restenosis after coronary angioplasty. J Am Coll Cardiol 1991; 17:111B–117B.

17. Guzman LA, Labhastwar V, Song C, et al. Single intraluminal infusion of biodegradable polymeric nanoparticles matrixed with dexamethasone decreases neointimal formation after vascular injury. Circulation 1995; 92(suppl):I-293 (abstract).

18. Lincoff AM, Furst JG, Ellis SG, Tuch RJ, Topol EJ. Sustained local delivery of dexamethasone by a novel intravascular eluting stent model to prevent restenosis in the porcine coronary injury model. J Am Coll Cardiol 1997; 29:808–16.

19. Pavlides G, Barath P, Maginas A, et al. Intramural drug delivery by direct injection within the arterial wall: First clinical experience with a novel intracoronary delivery-infiltrator-system. Catheter Cardiovasc Diagn 1997; 41:287–92.

20. Barath G, Popov A, Dillehay G, et al. Infiltrator angioplasty balloon catheter: A device for combined angioplasty and intramural site specific treatment. Catheter Cardiovasc Diagn 1997; 41:333–341.

21. Mitchel J, Pedersen C, Fram D, et al. Local delivery of heparin at coronary angioplasty sites with the infiltrator catheter: Enhanced intramural drug deposition. J Am Coll Cardiol 1997; 28(suppl A):187A (abstract).

22. Zwet PMJ, van der Reiber JHC. A new approach to the quantification of complex lesion morphology: the gradient field transform; basic principles and validation results. J Am Coll Cardiol 1994; 24:216–24.

23. Umans VA, Keane D, Quaedvlieg P, Serruys PW. Matching to guide the design and predict the outcome of randomized atherectomy trials. Am Heart J 1995; 130:1135–43.

24. Painter JA, Mintz GS, Wong SC, et al. Serial intravascular ultrasound studies fail to show evidence of chronic Palmaz-Schatz stent recoil. Am J Cardiol 1995; 75:398–400.

25. Robinson KA. Pig coronary artery model of post-angioplasty restenosis. In Waksman R, King SB, Crocker IR, Mould RF (eds), Vascular Brachitherapy. Nucletron: Veenendaal, The Netherlands 1996:30–40.

26. Edelman ER, Rogers C. Hoop dreams: Stent without restenosis. Circulation 1996; 94:1199–202.

27. Waksman R, Robinson KA, Crocker IR, et al. Endovascular low dose irradiation inibits neointima formation after coronary artery balloon injury in swine: a possible role for radiation therapy in restenosis prevention. Circulation 1995; 91:1533–9.

28. Liu MW, Roubin GS, King SB. Restenosis after coronary angioplasty: Potential biologic determinants and role of intimal hyperplasia. Circulation 1989; 79:1374–87.

29. Parillo JE, Fuci AS. Mechanism of glucocorticoid action on immune processes. Annu Rev Pharmacol Toxicol 1979; 19:179–201.

30. Krane SM, Amento EP. Glucocorticoids and collagen disease. Adv Exp Med Biol 1984; 171:61–71.

31. Makila UM. The effects of betamimetics and glucocorticoids on fetal vascular prostacyclin and platelet thromboxane synthesis in humans. Prostaglandins Leukot Med 1984; 16:11–17.

32. Camenzind E, Bakker W, van Haskamp E, et al. First quantification of intramural heparin delivery in man using the nipple-Catheter (Infiltrator) following coronary balloon angioplasty. Circulation 1997; 96(suppl)I:529 (abstract).

33. Brandt KD. Management of osteoarthritis. In Kelley WN, et al. (eds), Textbook of Rheumatology, 3rd edn. Saunders: Philadelphia 1989: 1501–12.

34. Rab ST, King SB III, Roubin GS, et al. Coronary aneurysms after stent placement: a suggestion of altered vessel wall healing in the presence of anti-inflammatory agents. J Am Coll Cardiol 1991; 18:1524–8.

35. Ellis SG, Savage M, Fishman D, et al. Restenosis after placement of Palmaz-Schatz stents in native coronary arteries. Circulation 1992; 86:1836–44.

36. Strauss BH, Serruys PW, de Scheerder IK, et al. Relative risk analysis of angiographic predictors of restenosis within the coronary Wallstent. Circulation 1991; 84:1636–43.

37. Kobayashi Y, De Gregorio J, Kobayashi N, et al. Stented segment length as an independent predictor of restenosis. J Am Coll Cardiol 1999; 34:651–9.

38. Rogers C, Edelman ER. Endovascular stent design dictates experimental restenosis and thrombosis. Circulation 1995; 91:2995–3001.

39. Reimers B, Moussa M, Akiyama T, et al. Persistent high restenosis after local intrawall delivery of long-acting steroids before coronary stent implantation. J Invasive Cardiol 1998; 10:323–31.

49

Clinical studies with the Carbostent

Antonio L Bartorelli and Daniela Trabattoni

Introduction • The ANTARES study • The SAFE study • Conclusions

INTRODUCTION

The Sorin Carbostent is a new generation stent with a unique cellular design developed to avoid stress concentration and elastic distortion, which may stimulate exuberant intimal proliferation and long-term in-stent restenosis. Another peculiar feature of this stent is a turbostratic carbon permanent coating (Carbofilm™), which has demonstrated high hemocompatibility and non-thrombogenic properties.

The first clinical study with the Carbostent, an open prospective trial, was conducted in two Italian centers to evaluate safety and efficacy of this innovative stent.[1] Between April 1988 and January 1999, 112 patients underwent coronary revascularization with the Carbostent at the Centro Cardiologico 'Monzino' in Milan and at the Division of Cardiology of the Careggi hospital in Florence. The mean age was 61 ± 9.8 years and 82% were men. The proportion of patients with unstable angina was 55.4% (IIIb, 27.5%; IIIc, 9.6%). Lesions were moderately complex according to ACC/AHA classification (A, 18.2%; B1, 43.9%; B2, 31.8%; C, 6.1%) with a mean length of 12.5 ± 7.2 mm (<15 mm, 72%; 15–20 mm, 15.2%; >20 mm, 12.8%), and were located mainly in vessels ≥ 2.9 mm (82.1%). A total of 153 Carbostents were implanted for different indications (elec-

tive in 80.3% of the cases, for suboptimal results in 14.4% and for 'bail out' in 5.3%) at a variety of coronary sites (LAD, 47.7%; RCA, 38.6%; LCx, 13.6%; Left main, 0.6%) using high pressure dilations (15 ± 2.4 atm). The final balloon size was 3.53 ± 0.6 mm and no routine intravascular ultrasound (IVUS) guidance was used. Single-and multiple-vessel stenting was performed in 84% and 16% of patients, respectively, with a stent/patient ratio of 1.4 ± 0.7 and a stent/lesion ratio of 1.1 ± 0.3. Procedural and angiographic success was achieved in 100% of the cases, obtaining a final mean lumen diameter of 3.2 ± 0.4 mm, corresponding to a percentage diameter stenosis of 3.8 ± 7.4. All patients received acetylsalicylic (aspirin) and ticlopidine as antithrombotic therapy and no episode of acute or subacute stent thrombosis occurred. The only in-hospital adverse cardiac event was one non-Q wave myocardial infarction (major adverse cardiac event – MACE rate = 0.9%). No other clinical events were observed in the first 30 days of clinical follow-up. The 6 month angiographic follow-up of this initial study with the Carbostent, obtained in 108 patients, favorably compared with that of previous stent trials. Quantitative coronary analysis (QCA) showed an overall restenosis rate of 11% with a mean loss index of 0.29 ± 0.28; in lesion subsets at higher restenosis

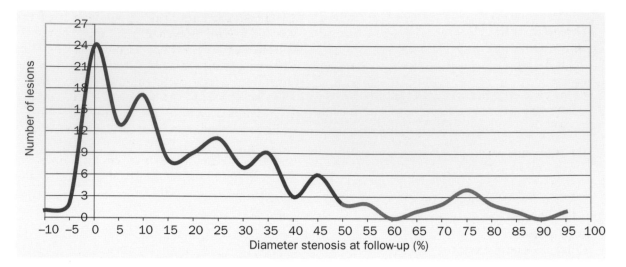

Fig. 49.1 Frequency distribution of percentage diameter stenosis at 6-month angiographic follow-up following Carbostent implantation. The graph shows the existence of two different groups of coronary stenoses, one consisting of the majority of lesions with a peak at a diameter stenosis of 0%, and the other formed by few lesions with a peak at a diameter stenosis of 75%.

risk, such as lesions longer than 15 mm ($n = 37$) and small vessels ($n = 29$), restenosis was 16% and 6.9%, respectively. In addition, statistical analysis from angiographic measurements suggested the existence of a bimodal response after Carbostent implantation: one presented by most patients and characterized by no or minimal late loss, and a subsequent very low loss index (0.21 ± 0.16), and the other, observed in a few patients, with marked neointimal proliferation (loss index $= 0.92 \pm 0.26$) (Figure 49.1).

Therefore, in this initial clinical experience with the Carbostent, an exuberant pattern of neointimal in-stent proliferation was observed in only few cases, while the majority of the patients showed minimal proliferative response. In conclusion, the Carbostent advanced design and innovative features resulted in a remarkably high procedural and angiographic success, with very low incidence of major adverse cardiac events and no stent subacute thrombosis. Moreover, the very modest restenosis rate observed at 6 month angiographic follow-up may reflect a lower tendency to stimulate neo-

intimal proliferation compared to other currently available stents.

THE ANTARES STUDY

Although significantly reduced, stent thrombosis is still associated with major clinical events, such as death, myocardial infarction, or emergency revascularization, in virtually all cases.[3] The effect of stent coatings in preventing early thrombotic occlusion remains to be proved. The Carbofilm™ (turbostratic carbon thin film) coating of the Carbostent provides high biocompatibility and was developed to further reduce the risk of stent thrombosis.[4]

The *Aspirin Alone Treatment After Carbostent Stenting* (ANTARES) study was a prospective, observational single-center pilot study in which aspirin monotherapy was used after the intracoronary placement of the Carbostent.[5] The aim of the study was to assess whether the Carbofilm coating of the Carbostent could prevent platelet-mediated stent thrombosis. This study enrolled 110 consecutive patients (73.6% men,

Table 49.1   ANTARES study exclusion criteria

Clinical
- Oral anticoagulation unrelated to stent procedure
- Ticlopidine therapy before stenting
- Contraindications/allergy to aspirin
- Documented peptic ulcer or gastric bleeding in the previous 6 months
- Depressed LV function (EF<40%)
- Q or non-Q wave myocardial infarction within the prior 48 hours

Angiographic
- Target lesion in a venous bypass graft
- Bifurcation lesion
- Lesion located in the only remaining vessel
- Unprotected left main lesion
- Massive thrombus
- Heavily calcified lesion

mean age 61 ± 9 years) who met prespecified clinical and angiographic inclusion criteria and were treated with aspirin monotherapy after Carbostent implantation. Exclusion criteria of the ANTARES study are listed in Table 49.1. Post-stenting inclusion criteria were a post-procedural diameter stenosis <10% by visual estimate associated with TIMI flow grade 3 and no angiographic evidence of thrombus, dissection, and proximal or distal stenosis limiting in- or outflow. Stable angina (75.5%), unstable angina (18.2%), and silent ischemia (6.3%) were clinical indications for coronary revascularization. Patients received 10 000 U of heparin and no glycoprotein IIb/IIIa inhibitors or post-procedural heparin. Complex lesion characteristics were present in 39 out of 128 (30.5%) lesions (Figure 49.2). Mean lesion length was 15.6 ± 7.53 mm and 32% of the lesions were >15 mm (range 16–52 mm). Small coronary vessels were treated in 28% of the cases. A total of 165 Carbostents were used in 129 coronary lesions. Single vessel stenting was performed in 97 (88%) patients and multivessel stent placement in

13 (12%) patients. The mean length of the stented segment was 21 ± 13 mm (range 9–95 mm). Procedural and clinical success was achieved in all patients. There were no stent thromboses or other major adverse cardiac events. Two (1.8%) non-Q-wave myocardial infarctions and two (1.8%) vascular complications were the only events. These results suggest that, in addition to limit longer-term restenosis, the Carbofilm coating and the other unique features of the Carbostent may minimize the risk of thrombosis.

THE SAFE STUDY

The ANTARES study was conducted in a single center and with a relatively small number of selected patients. The lack of a control group represented another limitation. The SAFE (*Sorin* and *Aspirin Following Elective Stenting*) study is an appropriately designed and randomized trial conducted in 15 Italian centers, which is currently comparing two antithrombotic regimens, aspirin alone versus combined ticlopidine and aspirin (Figure 49.3). This study is evaluating whether coronary implantation of the Carbostent will lead to the equivalent incidence of endpoints in the two groups, clinically confirming the thrombo-resistance of the Carbofilm coating. A total of 1400 patients, with single vessel or multivessel disease (1–3 native coronary arteries with a reference diameter >2.5 mm and ≤2.5 mm length), will be randomized to the two antithrombotic regimens following successful Carbostent implantation. The study sample size has been based on the reported incidence of thrombotic events using aspirin and ticlopidine which ranges between 0.5% and 1.5% in previous stent studies. Therefore, a one-side equivalence testing approach will be used, assuming a stent thrombosis rate in the aspirin and ticlopidine group of 0.5% and a clinical equivalence tolerability of 1%. Inclusion and exclusion criteria that have to be met by the patients are similar to those of the ANTARES study. The primary endpoint of the SAFE study is the occurrence of stent thrombosis within 30 days

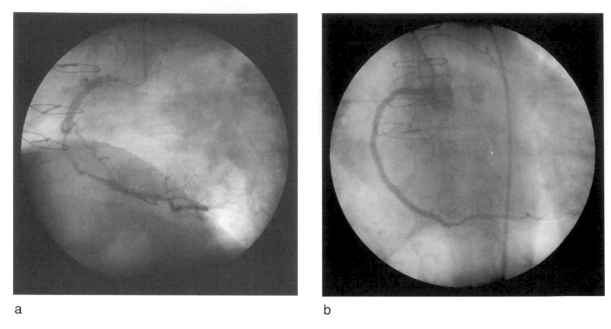

a   b

Fig. 49.2 Diffusely diseased segment of the right coronary artery (45 degree right anterior oblique projection) of a patient enrolled in the ANTARES study. (a) Before stenting. (b) After implantation of five Carbostents (three 15 mm and two 25 mm long stents).

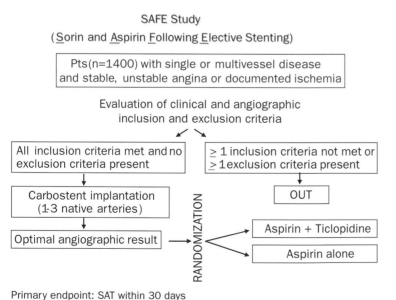

Fig. 49.3 The SAFE study design.

Primary endpoint: SAT within 30 days
Secondary endpoints: Vascular/bleeding complications, MACE at 6 months

from Carbostent implantation. Secondary endpoints are bleeding complications and the occurrence of MACE at 6 months.

CONCLUSIONS

The confirmation that the Carbofilm coating may significantly reduce the thrombotic potential of the stent surface will have important clinical implications. The Carbostent may improve the safety profile of coronary stenting, in particular when treating patients at high risk for thrombosis. Moreover, the introduction of brachytherapy for in-stent restenosis prevention has brought back the problem of thrombosis, especially when a new stent is implanted.[6] Therefore, a thrombo-resistant stent may improve the safety of vascular radiation therapy and other anti-restenotic strategies, which have an impact on the re-endothelization process, such as antiproliferative stent coatings.[7] Finally, aspirin monotherapy combined with a non-thrombogenic stent may simplify post-implant management, avoiding the risk of serious side effects associated with the use of adenosine 5'-diphosphate (ADP) receptor inhibitors.[8,9]

REFERENCES

1. Antoniucci D, Bartorelli A, Valenti R, et al. Clinical and angiographic outcome after coronary arterial stenting with the Carbostent. Am J Cardiol 2000; 85:821–5.

2. Mak KH, Belli G, Ellis SG, Moliterno DJ. Subacute stent thrombosis: Evolving issues and current concepts. J Am Coll Cardiol 1996; 27:494–503.

3. Paccagnella C, Majni G, Ottavaiani G, et al. Properties of a new carbon film for biomedical applications. Int J Artif Organs 1986; 9:127–30.

4. Bartorelli AL, Fabbiocchi F, Montorsi P, et al. Aspirin-alone treatment after Carbostent stenting: the ANTARES study. Am J Cardiol 16 (suppl 8A):18i (abstract).

5. Cenni E, Arciola CR, Ciapetti G, et al. Platelet and coagulation factor variations induced in vitro by polyethylene terephtalate (Dacron) coated with pyrolytic carbon. Biomaterials 1995; 16:973–6.

6. Costa MA, Sabate M, van der Giessen WJ, et al. Late coronary occlusion after intracoronary brachytherapy. Circulation 1999; 100:789–92.

7. Sousa JE, Costa MA, Abizaid A, et al. Lack of neointimal proliferation after implantation of Sirolimus-coated stents in human coronary arteries. A quantitative coronary angiography and three-dimensional intravascular ultrasound study. Circulation 2001; 103:192–5.

8. Bennet C, Weinberg P, Rozenberg-Ben-Dror, et al. Thrombotic thrombocytopenic purpura associated with ticlopidine: A review of 60 cases. Ann Intern Med 1998; 128:541–4.

9. Dillon WC, Eckert GJ, Dillon CJ, Ritchie ME. Incidence of thrombocytopenia following coronary placement using abciximab plus clopidogrel or ticlopidine. Catheter Cardiovasc Interv 2000; 50:426–30.

50

Gold-coated stents

Jörg Rodermann, Nicolaus Reifart

Introduction   •   **The Niroyal™**   •   **Conclusions**

INTRODUCTION

The complications of coronary stenting, including thrombosis and restenosis allow room for significant improvement in product performance.[1] Several animal and clinical observations revealed a possible proliferative effect of stainless steel, e.g. by release of nickel ions.[2] Thus surface modification of stents may provide a solution to these adverse effects.

One approach that has been discribed was using pure gold as a biocompatible and hemocompatible coating material. The expected benefits were the reduction of intimal hyperplasia or excessive tissue growth at the stent-site, a decreased thrombosis rate and an improved fluoroscopic visibility. The background for these expectations were the results of several in vitro studies that showed decreased neointimal proliferation[3–5] and platelet activation[6] and it was of particular interest to know whether these properties of gold coating could be translated into a meaningful clinical benefit for patients treated with gold coated stainless steel stents.

However, several clinical trials[7–10] did not correspond with the expected results and two gold-coated stainless steel stents were taken off the market because of their inferior performance compared with uncoated stents. There are some indications, however, that the reason for these failures is the complex process that is required to complete gold plating. Inferior coating technology may result in variable adherence of the gold layer to the stainless steel surface and in cracking or peeling of the gold layer during the stent expansion. The incompletely coated stent then presents as a bimetallic 'battery' that might even enhance proliferation. Boston Scientific improved the coating process to avoid the described problems. Another new approach was an additional thermal processing after gold coating.[11]

THE NIROYAL™-STENT

The NIROYAL™ (Boston Scientific) was the last available gold coated stainless steel stent on the market. The stent differed from previous gold-coated stents in that it featured high purity and a two-step plating process to ensure complete coating and to eliminate pores, flakes and cracks with stent expansion, exposing the underlying material. However, even gold processed to 99.99% purity retains other base metals and might alter tissue reactions.

Among the benefits of the NIROYAL stent, optimal radiopacity was most evident.[12] This is important whereever precise placement is warranted: multiple-stenting, bifurcation-stenting and ostial lesion-stenting.

In 1998 a non randomized, prospective multi-center trial as a registry[8] was conducted. These registry results indicated comparable acute and long-term outcomes of the NIROYAL™ and the NIR™ stent (stainless steel).

The randomized NUGGET (NIR Ultimate Gold-Gilded Equivalency Trial) study was performed with a stent produced by an improved gold-coating process to demonstrate equivalency in the minimal lumen diameter (MLD) at six month post procedure of the NIR™ stent and the NIROYAL™ stent. It was a prospective, multi-center, randomized, controlled clinical study including 603 patients at 21 sites in 14 countries. The results were an increase in percent diameter stenosis of the NIROYAL™-stent, a smaller MLD, a higher late loss and similar MACE rates[10] compared to the NIR™ stent.

CONCLUSIONS

While gold coating appeared superior to uncoated stainless steel stents in vitro, the clinical results were disappointing. This might have been due to an insufficiant coating process resulting in an incomplete gold-coverage after stent expansion. Even the later performed NUGGET-trial, a comparison between the NIROYAL™-stent with an improved gold-coating technology and the NIR™-stainless-steel-stent, showed a superiority of the NIR™-stainless-steel stent at 6 months. The concept of improved visibility requested by operators should not be abandoned but might be combined with other technologies (i.e. drug-eluting coatings, other alloys/metals).

REFERENCES

1. Alt E, Pasquantonio J, Fliedner T, et al. Effect of endovascular stent design on experimental restenosis. J Am Coll Cardiol 1997; 24(2):953–75.
2. Köster R, Vieluf D, Kiehn M. et al. Nickel and molybdenum contact allergies in patients with coronary in-stent restenosis. Lancet 2000; 356:1895–7.
3. Tanigawa N, Sawada S, and Kobayah M. Reaction of the aortic wall to six metallic stent materials. Acada Radio 1997; 2:379–84.
4. Nikolaychik V, Sahota H, Keelen Jr MH, et al. Influence of different stent materials on endotheliasation in vitro. J Invas Cardiol 1999; 11:410–15.
5. Rogers C, Edelman ER. Endovascular stent design dictates experimental restenosis and thrombosis. Circulation. 1995; 91:2995–3001.
6. Bethien C, Gutensohn K, Bau J, et al. Gold coating of coronary stents: a flow cytometric analysis of platelet activation in a pulsed flowting model. Thromb Hämost 1997; 105:426.
7. Kastrati A, Schomig A, Dirschinger J, et al. Increased risk of restenosis after placement of gold-coated stents. Circulation. 2000; 101:2478–83.
8. Cremonesi A, Benit E, Carlier et al. Multicenter registry to evaluate the efficacy of the NIROYAL™ stent in denovo or restenotic coronary stenosis. J Invas Cardiol 2000; 12:225–32.
9. vom Dahl J, Haager PK, Grube E, et al. Effects of gold coating of coronary stents on neointimal proliferation following stent implantation Am J Cardiol 2002; 89:801–5.
10. Reifart N, Morice MC, Silber S, et al. The NUGGET-trial (NIR ultimate gold-gilded equivalence trial). Catheter Cardiovasc Interv 2004; 62:18–25.
11. Edelman E, Seifert P, Groothuis A et al. Gold coated NIR-stents in porcine coronary arteries. Circulation. 2001; 103:429–34.
12. Fischell T. Visible stents: All that glitters. is it gold? J Invas Cardiol 2000; 12(5):233–5.

51

Heparin-coated stent trials

Sjoerd H Hofma, Patrick W Serruys, Willem J van der Giessen

Effects of heparin on blood coagulation and cellular proliferation • Methods of heparin-coating • Heparin coated stents in acute myocardial infarction • Conclusions

EFFECTS OF HEPARIN ON BLOOD COAGULATION AND CELLULAR PROLIFERATION

Heparin is a highly sulphated linear polysaccharide that was discovered in 1916 as an anticoagulant. Heparin binds to antithrombin III, thereby inducing a conformational change. This results in inhibition of thrombin and other serine proteases involved in the blood clotting cascade immediately after administration. The actions of heparin on neointimal proliferation are complex. This was demonstrated by Edelman et al.[1] They found an increase of intimal hyperplasia after arterial injury in the rat model when heparin was administered once daily. Twice daily administration had different effects depending on the time-interval of dosing but very significant reduction in intimal hyperplasia was seen with continuous administration. Clowes et al. showed that heparin should be administered for 4–7 days in order to have an antiproliferative effect after injury.[2]

Therefore, the need for continuous heparin administration for 7 days after stent implantation provides the rationale for a heparin-coated stent.

METHODS OF HEPARIN-COATING

There are several ways to attach heparin to the stent surface. These include: adsorption of benzylkonium alcohol solution,[3,4] ionic bonding,[5,6] dispersion in polymer,[7–9] surface grafting,[10–12] covalent coupling of functionalized surface with mid- or end-point attachment[13–17] and heparin—polymer block copolymers.[18]

The first methods result in a weak binding and heparin will be lost within a short time span. Most research and all clinical trials have been performed with covalently bound heparin-coated stents.

The Palmaz-Schatz- and BX-stent with Hepacoat™

In the early development of heparin coatings, a reduction of heparin activity was frequently seen after covalent attachment of the molecules to the surface. Larm et al.[19] immobilized heparin fragments with end-point attachment on materials coated with polyethylamine. By this method heparin activity was preserved after attachment. Based on this principle, the Carmeda BioActive Surface coating (CBAS, Carmeda AB, Stockholm) was developed and applied to extracorporeal systems. This coating was used as a base for the heparin-coated Palmaz-Schatz stent. However, in a demanding environment, such as the porcine coronary model, this coating was not sufficient to eliminate stent occlusion. Elimination of subacute stent thrombosis could be shown with higher-activity heparin coating (12–20 pmol anti-thrombin III binding activity per stent; Hepacoat™, J & J Cordis, Warren, NJ).[20]

In the early 1990s, stents were still implanted with a strict anti-coagulant regime and prolonged heparinization. In four phases of Benestent-II pilot, using this heparin-coated PS stent, anti-coagulant regime was reduced and finally coumadin and postprocedural heparin were replaced by aspirin and ticlopidin. Stent thrombosis did not occur and bleeding complications dropped to 0%.[21]

The BENESTENT-II trial randomized 827 patients to heparin-coated stent implantation or standard balloon angioplasty. The patients were more challenging with 45% unstable angina pectoris. Stent thrombosis occurred in only one patient (0.2%).[22] This is well below the 1–2% of stent thrombosis seen in contemporary trials. Restenosis rates at 6 months were 16% in the heparin-stent group. Similar restenosis rates have been achieved with non-coated stents. Data suggest no reduction of neointimal hyperplasia within the stent in comparison to uncoated stents.[20–22]

The heparin-coated Palmaz-Schatz stent has also been used in chronic total occlusion (TOSCA) and acute myocardial infarction (Stent-PAMI trial). In the TOSCA trial 410 patients with chronic total occlusion of a native coronary artery were randomized to heparin-coated stent vs balloon angioplasty. The incidence of MACE after 6 months was similar with both strategies (PTCA: 23.6 vs stent: 23.3%) but restenosis rate was reduced from 70% in the PTCA group to 55% in the stent group.[23] Evaluating the 721 patients with stable and unstable angina pectoris as well as acute myocardial infarction who have been treated with a heparin-coated Palmaz-Schatz stent in the Benestent-II pilot, the Benestent-II trial and PAMI trials, the incidence of subacute stent thrombosis (SAT) was extremely low (incidence of 0.12%!).

A recent registry from a single, large cardiac center evaluated primary thrombotic outcome (defined as angiographically documented SAT and/or sudden unexplained cardiac death (SCD)) in 337 patients receiving 543 BX velocity Hepacoat stents and 939 patients receiving 1688 bare-metal stents. SAT or SCD was seen in 3.03% of procedures in the bare-metal stent group and 0.58% in the heparin-coated stent group. 96% of SAT within 30 days occurred in patients with an acute coronary syndrome.[24]

Hep@net Registry and HOPE

This internet-based registry compares the Hepacoat BX-Velocity stent with the bare BX-velocity stent. Last data available on www.TCTMD.com show 0.5% stent thrombosis with the Hepacoat (n=1062) vs 1.2% with the bare stent (n=1301) P= 0.14. Enrollment in this registry is continuing. In another registry, the HOPE Registry (Hepacoat and an antithrOmbotic regimen of asPirin alone) 200 patients were stented with the BX Velocity stent with Hepacoat. SAT rate was acceptable with 1% at 30 days despite only aspirin use post procedure and no ticlid or clopidogrel. However, IIb/IIIa-inhibitor use was 55% in this study.[25]

The Hepamed™-coated Wiktor stent and beStent

The conditioning layer of the coating of the Hepamed coating (Medtronic Bakken Research Center, Maastricht, NL) is completely covalently coupled.[26] This makes this coating potentially more stable than Hepacoat™. In addition, the heparin molecules are neither fragmented nor enriched with the active antithrombin binding site, resulting in a predictable heparin layer on the stent, but with a lower antithrombin binding capacity per picomole of attached heparin. Therefore, additional heparin has been added.

In the MENTOR trial the Wiktor stent with Hepamed coating was implanted in 132 patients. A subacute occlusion rate of 0.8% was seen despite the fact that 43% of patients had unstable angina. The 6-month event-free survival was 85% and angiographic restenosis rate was 22%.[27] The Wiktor Stent with Hepamed coating has also been studied in saphenous vein bypass grafts. In 50 patients, 55 stents were placed in lesions in very old vein grafts (11.7 +/- 3.9 years). MACE free survival was 86% at 6 months and angiographic restenosis rate was 22%. This is a favourable result for this challenging patient subset.[28]

A randomized , multicenter trial has been initiated in Scandinavia (Stents in Small Coronary Arteries, SISCA), comparing the efficacy of the Hepamed coated beStent (Medtronic Instent, Minneapolis MN, USA) with balloon angioplasty in 145 patients with stable angina pectoris due to a de novo lesion with a reference diameter between 2.1 and 3.0 mm. There were no differences between the groups regarding early events (mean reference diameter 2.4 mm). Event-free survival at 6-month follow-up was significantly better with the heparin-coated stent than with balloon angioplasty (90.5% vs 76.1%, respectively; $P = 0.016$).[29]

This clinical benefit was maintained at 1 year follow-up with no change in eventfree survival between 6 months and 1 year.[30]

The Corline™ coated Jostent

In the Corline coating a single modified polymeric amine conditioning layer is used. Unfractionated heparin is linked with specific covalent bounds to form a macromolecular heparin conjugate. The anti-thrombin activity per cm^2 may be lower than in the Hepacoat and Hepamed coatings. However, in the Corline coating unfractionated heparin is used as opposed to fragmented heparin in the Hepacoat. Theoretically, important properties of the heparin molecule, like antiproliferative actions, which are not necessarily associated with the antithrombin binding site, may be retained.

A small pilot study using this stent was performed in Russia. The stent was implanted in 46 patients with 93.4% acute angiographic succes. However, follow-up was limited to the in-hospital phase.[31]

The Corline coating has been used in the only trial that has been initiated thus far to compare heparin-coated with bare stents (COAting of STents : COAST trial). In this study the Jomed stent was compared side-to-side with the Corline Jo stent in a three-armed study of 588 patients. Patients with stable or unstable angina pectoris due to single or multiple stenoses were included when the reference diameter of the

coronary artery was between 2.0 and 2.6 mm, thus providing additional information on performance of coated and non-coated stents in small arteries. COAST, however, lacks the power to discriminate between the (sub)acute thrombosis rates, even when the incidence of stent thrombosis in these small vessels would have been as high as 5%. In COAST, patients were randomized to balloon angioplasty (n=195), bare stent (n=196) or heparin-coated stent (n=197). In the balloon angioplasty arm 27% (n=53) of patients crossed over to recieve a stent, which is a considerably higher percentage than usually seen in trials in larger (mean diameter 3.0 mm) vessels. Only 3 patients in the bare stent arm and 4 patients in the heparin-coated stent arm crossed over to recieve balloon angioplasty. In a per-protocol analysis 6-month restenosis rates were 32%, 27% and 30%, for balloon, stent and heparin-coated stent groups respectively. The 'intention to treat'results are summarized in the Table 51.1. There were no statistical differences between the groups. The only suspected stent thrombosis occurred in the heparin-coated arm.[32]

Wõhrle et al.[33] reported a non-randomized study in which 368 stents were implanted in 303 lesions from 278 patients, comparing uncoated and Corline heparin-coated Jomed stents. More patients included in this study were high risk than in any of the studies cited above, since > 60% had multivessel disease, 8% total occlussion, 17% of patients had acute infarction and 19% of lesions were restenotic lesions, equally divided over both groups. No benefit of heparin coating could be detected on the incidence of stent thrombosis, myocardial infarction, restenosis rate or re-intervention rate.[33]

HEPARIN COATED STENTS IN ACUTE MYOCARDIAL INFARCTION

The heparin-coated Palmaz-Schatz stent was used in the Stent-PAMI trial.[34] In this trial patients with acute myocardial infarction (AMI) were randomized to angioplasty alone (448 patients) or angioplasty with stenting (452 patients). Abciximab was only used in 5.8% of stented patients and 4.5% in the angio-

Table 51.1   Clinical trials with heparin-coated stents

Year/ref	Trial	Coating	Study	Patients	6 or 7 months MACE	6 months Restenosis
1996[21]	**Benestent II pilot**	**Hepacoat**	4-phased registry; AP/UAP	n = 207; angio success 98%	14%	13%
1998[22]	**Benestent II randomized**	**Hepacoat**	Balloon vs HC-stent; AP/UAP	Balloon n = 410 Stent n = 413	19% 13% p = 0.013	31% 16% p < 0001
1999	**Stent-PAMI pilot**	**Hepacoat**	Registry; acute MI	n = 101; angio success 96%	19%	18%
1999[34]	**Stent-PAMI randomized**	**Hepacoat**	Balloon vs. HC-stent; acute MI	Balloon n = 448 Stent n = 452	20% 13% p < 0,01	34% 20% p < 0.001
1999[23]	**TOSCA**	**Hepacoat**	Randomized; Total occlusion	Balloon n = 208 Stent n = 202	24% 23% ns	70% 55% p = 0.001
2000[27]	**Mentor**	**Hepamed coating**	Registry AP/UAP	n = 132	15 %	22 %
2001[33]		**Corline coating**	Alternating cohorts of 50 coated or uncoated	Bare 133 HC 144	25.7 25.2 ns	30.3 33.1 ns
2001[29]	**SISCA**	**Hepamed coating**	Randomized; AP, small vessels	Balloon n = 71 Stent n = 74	23.9 9.5 p = 0.016	18.8 9.7 p = 0.15
2003[32]	**COAST**	**Corline coating**	Randomized; AP/UAP, small vessels	Balloon n = 195 Coated stent n = 197 Bare stent n = 196	15.4 11.7 ns 11.7	32.2 29.6 ns 24.8
1998[31]	**Russian Pilot**	**Corline coating**	Feasibility	Stent n = 46 93.4% angio succes	No follow-up	No follow-up
1999[35]	**South Korean study**	**Corline coating**	Registry Acute MI	Stent n = 102	13.7%	17.2 %
2004[36]		**Hepacoat**	Registry, AMI primary and rescue	Bare n = 114 HC n = 124	21.1% 16.1%	14.9% 10.5%

AMI, acute myocardial infraction; AP, angina pectoris; UAP, unstable angina pectoris; NA, not available.

plasty group. The combined primary endpoint at 6 months of death, reinfarction, disabling stroke, or target-vessel revascularization was significantly lower in the stent group (12.6% vs 20.1% for PTCA, $p<0.01$). At 1 month and at 6 months no significant difference was seen in reinfarction. This suggests no lower thrombotic occlusion rate with a heparin-coated stent. Restenosis rate at 6.5 months was 20.3 % for the stent group vs 33.5% for the PTCA alone group ($P<0.001$).

Recently, a study comparing 124 patients receiving a heparin-coated stent (HepaCoat BX Velocity, Cordis, NJ) for acute myocardial infarction with 114 patients receiving a bare stent showed reductions in stent thrombosis (0.8% vs 6.1%, $p=0.03$) and recurrent MI (4% vs 10.5%, $p=0.05$) at 30 days, but no significant effect on 180-day outcome (composite outcome death/MI/TVR 16.1% vs 21.1%).[36]

A South-Korean group reported a registry of 102 patients with acute MI treated with 111 Corline heparin-coated stents.[35] Postprocedural heparin or abciximab was not used. Mortality at 6 months was 6.0%, 1 patient with recurrent infarction was seen and revascularisation rate was only 8%. Restenosis rate at 6 months was 12.7%. This registry lacked a control group, which is especially regretted since the outcome was quite good, even in the absence of abciximab.

CONCLUSIONS

The high thrombotic occlusion rate of stents in the early nineties prompted research to develop a heparin-coated stent.

The very low incidence of less than 0.2% sub-acute thrombosis after implantation of a heparin-coated stent in the setting of stable angina, unstable angina and even acute myocardial infarction holds promise. However, whether this is truly the result of the heparin coating or of improved interventional techniques is difficult to distinguish. Though apparent in 'real-world registries', a trial directly comparing Corline-coated versus non-coated stents showed no benefit in small (mean diameter 2.4 mm) arteries (COAST). In the

meantime it seems justified to use a heparin-coated stent in situations of high thrombus burden or high platelet reactivity. Adverse effects of this choice have at least never been seen. Another niche may be treatment of patiens with known aspirin or clopidogrel intolerance.

No significant reduction of in-stent restenosis has been demonstrated compared to bare metal stents.

REFERENCES

1. Edelman ER, Karnovsky MJ. Contrasting effects of the intermittent and continuous administration of heparin in experimental restenosis. Circulation 1994; 89:770–6.
2. Clowes AW, Reidy MA, Clowes MM. Kinetics of cellular proliferation after arterial injury,I: smooth muscle growth in the absence of endothelium. Lab Invest 1983; 49:327–33.
3. Breckwoldt WL, Belkin M, Gould K, et al. Modification of the thrombogenicity of a self-expanding vascular stent. J Invest Surg 1991; 4:269–78.
4. Cavender J, Anderson P, Roubin G. The effect of heparin bounded tantalum stents on thrombosis and neointimal proliferation. Circulation 1992; 82(suppl III):III-541 (abst).
5. Tanzawa H, Mori Y, Harumiya N, et al. Preparation and evaluation of a new athrombogenic heparinized hydrophilic polymer for use in cardiovascular system. Trans Am Soc Artif Intern Organs 1973; 19:188–94.
6. Grode GA, Anderson SJ, Grotta HM, Falb RD. Nonthrombogenic materials via a simple coating process. Trans Am Soc Artif Intern Organs 1969; 15:1–6.
7. Miyama H, Harumiya N, Mori Y, Tanzawa H. A new antithrombogenic heparinized polymer. J Biomed Mater Res 1977; 11:251–65.
8. Heyman PW, Cho CS, McRea JC, et al. Heparinized polyurethanes:in vitro and in vivo studies. J Biomed Mater Res 1985; 19:419–36.
9. Cox D, Anderson P, Roubin G, et al. Effect of local delivery of heparin and methotrexate on neointimal proliferation in stented porcine coronary arteries. Coron Artery Dis 1992; 3:237–48.

10. Jozefowicz M, Jozefowicz J. Heparin-containing and heparin-like polymers. Polymers in Medicine. New York: Plenum Press, 1986.

11. Labarre D, Jozefowicz M, Boffa MC. Properties of heparin-poly(methyl methacrylate) copolymers. II. J Biomed Mater Res 1977; 11:283–95.

12. Lagergren HR, Eriksson JC. Plastics with a stable surface monolayer of cross-linked heparin: preparation and evaluation. Trans Am Soc Artif Intern Organs 1971; 17:10–12.

13. Schmer G. The biological activity of covalently immobilized heparin. Trans Am Soc Artif Intern Organs 1972; 18:321–24.

14. Hennink WE, Feijen J, Ebert CD, Kim SW. Covalently bound conjugates of albumin and heparin: synthesis, fractionation and characterization. Thromb Res 1983; 29:1–13.

15. Hennink WE, Kim SW, Feijen J. Inhibition of surface induced coagulation by preadsorption of albumin-heparin conjugates. J Biomed Mater Res 1984; 18:911–26.

16. Miura Y, Aoyagi S, Kusada Y, Miyamoto K. The characteristics of anticoagulation by covalently immobilized heparin. J Biomed Mater Res 1980; 14:619–30.

17. Larm O, Larsson R, Olsson P. A new non-thrombogenic surface prepared by selective covalent binding of heparin via a modified reducing terminal residue. Biomater Med Devices Artif Organs1983; 11:161–73.

18. Vulic I, Pijpers A, Okano T, et al. Heparin containing block copolymers. Part I: surface characterization. J Mater Sci 1993; 4:353–65.

19. Larm O, Larsson R, Olsson P. A new non-thrombogenic surface prepared by selective covalent binding of heparin via a modified reducing terminal residue. Biomater Med Devices Artif Organs 1983; 11:161–73.

20. Hardhammar PA, van Beusekom HMM, Emanuelsson HU, et al. Reduction in thrombotic events with heparin coated Palmaz-Schatz stents in normal porcine coronary arteries. Circulation 1996; 93:423–30.

21. Serruys PW, Emanuelsson H, van der Giessen W, et al. Heparin coated Palmaz-Schatz stents in human coronary arteries. Early outcome of the BENESTENT-II pilot study. Circulation 1996; 93:412–2.

22. Serruys PW, van Hout B, Bonnier H, et al. Randomized comparison of implantation of heparin coated stents with balloon angioplasty in selected patients with coronary artery disease (Benestent II). Lancet 1998; 352:673–81.

23. Buller CE, Dzavik V, Carere RG et al. Primary stenting versus balloon angioplasty in occluded coronary arteries: the Total Occlusion Study of Canada (TOSCA). Circulation 1999; 111(3):236–42.

24. Gupta V, Aravamuthan BR, Baskerville S, et al. Reduction of subacute stent thrombosis (SAT) using heparin-coated stents in a large-scale, real world registry. J Invasive Cardiol. 2004; 1 6(6):304–10.

25. Mehran R, Aymong ED, Ashby DT, et al. Safety of an aspirin-alone regimen after intracoronary stenting with a heparin-coated stent: final results of the HOPE (HEPACOAT and an Antithrombotic Regimen of Aspirin Alone) study. Circulation 2003; 108:1078–83.

26. Blezer R, Cahalen L, Cahalan PT, et al. Heparin coating of tantalum coronary stents reduces surface thrombin generation but not factor IXa generation. Blood Coagul Fibrinol 1998; 9:435–40.

27. Vrolix MCM, Legrand VM, Reiber JHC, et al. Heparin coated Wiktor stents in human coronary arteries (MENTOR trial). Am J Cardiol 2000; 86:385–89.

28. Van Langenhoven G, Vermeersch P, Serrano P, et al. Saphenous vein graft disease treated with the Wiktor Hepamed stent: procedural outcome, in-hospital complications and six-month angiographic follow-up. Can J Cardiol. 2002; 16(4):473–80.

29. Moer R, Myreng Y, Mølstad P, et al. Stenting In Small Coronary Arteries (SISCA) Trail. A randomized comparison between balloon angioplasty and the heparin-coated bestent. J Am Coll Cardiol 2001; 38:1598–603

30. Moer R, Myreng Y, Molstad P, et al. Clinical benefit of small vessel stenting: one-year follow-up of the SISCA trial. Scand Cardiovasc J 2002; 36(2):70–2.

31. Savchenko AP, Matchin Iu G, Smirnov MA, Liakishev AA. Use of heparin coated "Jo Stent M" in patients with ischemic heart disease:first results. Vestn Rentgenol Radiol 1998; 5:4–8.

32. Haude M, Thomas F.M, Konorza, et al. Heparin-Coated Stent Placement for the Treatment of Stenoses in Small Coronary Arteries of Symptmatic Patients. Circulation 2003; 107:1265–70.

33. Wöhrle J, Al-Kayer I, Grötzinger U, et al. Comparison of the heparin coated and the uncoated version of the JOMED stent with regard to stent thrombosis and restenosis rates.Eur Heart J 2001; 22:1808–16.

34. Grines CL, Cox DA, Stone GW, et al. Coronary angioplasty with or without stent implantation for acute myocardial infarction. N Engl J Med 1999; 341:1949–56.

35. Shin EK, Sohn MS, Son JW, et al. Efficacy of heparin coated stent in the early setting of acute myocardial infarction. Cathet cardiovasc Intervent 2001; 52:306–12.

36. Lev EI, Assali AR, Teplisky I, et al. Comparison of outcomes up to six months of Heparin-Coated with noncoated stents after percutaneous coronary intervention for acute myocardial infarction. Am J Cardiol. 2004; 93(6):741–3.

52

The Blue Medical 50% TEMPO coronary stent: preclinical studies and the first clinical pilot trial

Xiaoshun Liu, Yanming Huang, and Ivan De Scheerder

Introduction • Material and methods • Results • Material and methods • Results • Discussion • Summary

INTRODUCTION

The success of coronary stenting is plagued by high restenosis rates of up to 67%, depending on issues, such as patient and lesion related factors, the indication and technique of stent deployment, and others.[1–3] In-stent restenosis is considered as being a local increase of the biological response to vessel wall injury, which involves a cascade of cellular and molecular responses. Among others, oxygen free radicals, induced by the inflammatory response, induced by the implantation of a foreign body may play an important role in the formation of the neointimal hyperplasia and in-stent restenois. Free radical driven reactions, such as oxidative phosphorylation, lipid peroxidation, and DNA scission can be toxic for the cell function, resulting in cell necrosis.

Antioxidants were found to be vital in the preservation of endothelium-dependent functions and to have beneficial effects on cell proliferation and arterial remodeling.[4,5] Systemic administration of antioxidants, such as vitamin E and omega-3 fatty acids, has shown beneficial effects on restenosis in animal studies,[6] and small clinical trials after percutaneous coronary interventions (PCI).[7,8] However, these effects were not demonstrated in large scale randomized trials.[9,10]

Drug eluting stents may provide a sufficient amount of antioxidants, by means of using a stent platform coated with a biodegradable polymer conjugated with a drug, therefore acting as a free radical scavenger at the treated vessel site. The Blue Medical 50% TEMPO-coated coronary stent is a new generation coronary device characterized by its unique coating and the use of an antioxidant. The coating is a novel class of polymers, comprising naturally occurring amino acids and other non-toxic 'building blocks'.[11] The drug, tempamine (4 amino-2,2,2,6,6-tetramethyl-piperidine-N-oxyl), is conjugated to the biodegradable polymer, thus being the active part of the coating agent or coating material. Tempamine can penetrate through the cell membrane and can act both intra- and extracellularly.[12] The in vivo half-life of the tempamine is about 3.5 minutes in mice,[13] therefore, gradual exposure is essential in order to prevent overdosage and ensure a longer treatment window.

The objective of this study was to test the hypothesis that a potent antioxidant, tempamine, conjugated to a biodegradable polymer may react as a free radical scavenger, thereby modulating the coronary arterial response to injury and prevent neointimal hyperplasia and restenosis.

Preclinical study

The aim of this study was to evaluate the safety and efficiency of the Blue Medical 50% TEMPO-loaded coronary stent in a porcine coronary artery over-stretched injury model. Post-implantation injury, inflammatory response, and in-stent neointimal hyperplasia are compared with the non-coated stent.

MATERIAL AND METHODS

The Blue Medical TEMPO coated coronary stent is a 316 L stainless steel stent characterized by its particular polyester amide (PEA) coating and an antioxidant substance, tempamine, conjugated to the PEA coating.

The copolymer, a biodegradable functional co-PEA, was prepared using naturally occurring α-amino acids (L-leucine and L-lysine) and other non-toxic building blocks, such as 16-hexanediol and sebacic acid. This copolymer (PEA coating) has unique properties for stent coating, including its ability to conjugate drugs and elastic film-forming characteristics desirable for stent coating.[11]

Tempamine is conjugated to the biodegradable polymer. The active part of the coating agent or coating material is thus tempamine. The biological and chemically active part of the tempamine molecule is a nitroxyl group (N*O, the asterisk means an electron) that is an integrated part of pyperidine ring. The nitroxyl group is considered to be a stable radical. This group acts as a spin trap or spin label. During the biodegrading process of the polymer, tempamine is gradually and (constantly) exposed to the surface and able to react and neutralize

oxygen free radicals, see (1) and (2). This enables lengthening biochemical treatment to a more regular dose. The nitroxyl radical can interact (neutralize) with endogenous free radicals, such as superoxide and ascorbyl radicals (it undergoes redox reaction while it neutralizes other potentially toxic-free radicals). The mode of action can be described as:

$$N^*\text{–}O + {^*O}^{2-} + H+ \rightarrow N\text{–}OH + O_2 \qquad (1)$$
$$N\text{–}OH + {^*O}^{2-} + H+ \rightarrow N^*\text{–}O + H_2O_2^* \qquad (2)$$

The Blue Medical Tempo stent is available in different sizes and versions (small vessel: 2.0–2.5–2.75 mm; standard vessel: 2.5–3.0–3.5 mm; large vessel: 3.5–4.5–5.0 mm and lengths (10–14–18–22–28 mm). In this study, 3.0 mm and 3.5 mm diameter and 14/18 mm in length were used.

Stent implantation

All the animals were treated and cared for in accordance with the Belgian National Institute of Health Guide for the care and use of laboratory animals. Domestic cross-bred pigs of both sexes weighing 20–25 kg were used. They were fed with a standard natural grain diet without lipid or cholesterol supplementation throughout the study. Surgical procedure and stent implantation in the coronary arteries were performed according to the method described by De Scheerder et al.[14] The guiding catheter was used as a reference to obtain a stent-to-artery ratio of 1.1–1.2:1.

In this study, bare stents ($n = 9$) and 50% TEMPO loaded ($n = 9$) stents were randomly implanted in coronary arteries of nine pigs. All stent implantation procedures were successful and the pigs survived until the end of the 6 week study. One pig was sacrificed after 5 days to evaluate acute inflammatory response and thrombus formation. The remaining pigs were sacrificed after 6 weeks to evaluate peri-strut inflammation and neointimal hyperplasia.

Quantitative coronary angiography (QCA)

Angiographic analysis of stented vessel segments was performed before stenting, immediately after, and at follow-up, using the polytron

1000® system as described previously by De Scheerder et al.[15] The diameters of the vessel segments were measured before, immediately after stent implantation, and at follow-up.

Histopathology and morphometry

Coronary segments were carefully dissected together with a 1 cm minimal vessel segment both proximal and distal to the stent. The segments were fixed in a 10% formalin solution. Each segment was cut into a proximal, middle, and distal stent segment for histomorphometric analysis. Tissue specimens were embedded in a cold-polymerizing resin (Technovit 7100, Heraus Kulzer GmbH, and Wehrheim, Germany). Sections, 5 μm thick, were cut with a rotary heavy duty microtome HM 360 (Microm, Walldorf, Germany) equipped with a hard metal knife and stained with hematoxylin-eosin, elastic stain and phosphotungstic acid hematoxylin stain. Light microscopic examination was performed by an experienced pathologist who was blinded to the type of stent used. Injury of the arterial wall due to stent deployment (and eventually inflammation induced by the polymer) was evaluated for each stent filament and graded as described by Schwartz et al.[16]

Grade 0: internal elastic membrane intact, media compressed but not lacerated
Grade 1: internal elastic membrane lacerated
Grade 2: media visibly lacerated; external elastic membrane compressed but intact
Grade 3: Large laceration of the media extending through the external elastic membrane or stent filament residing in the adventitia.

Inflammatory reaction at each stent filament was carefully examined, investigated for inflammatory cells, and scored as followed:

1. sparsely located histolymphocytes surrounding the stent filament
2. more densely located histolymphocytes covering the stent filament, but no lymphogranuloma and/or giant cells formation found

3. diffusely located histolymphocytes, lymphogranuloma and/or giant cells, also invading the media.

Mean score = sum of score for each filament/number of filaments present.

Morphometric analysis of the coronary segments harvested was performed using a computerized morphometry program (Leitz CBA 8000). Measurements of the lumen area, lumen area inside the internal elastic lamina (IEL), and lumen inside the external elastic lamina (EEL) were performed. Furthermore, area stenosis and neointimal hyperplasia area were calculated.

Statistics

Data are presented as mean value ± SD. For comparison among different groups, a nonpaired t-test was used. A p-value ≤ 0.05 was considered to be statistically significant.

RESULTS

Quantitative coronary angiography (QCA)

The results of the QCA analysis are shown in Table 52.1. The selected arterial segments and recoil ratio of 50% TEMPO-coated groups were similar to the bare control group. The balloon size of 50% TEMPO group was lower than the bare group, however, no significant difference of stent-to-artery ratio was observed.

Histomorphometry

A representative photomicrograph of a vessel segment at 5 day follow-up is shown in Figure 52.1. Residual polymer material was detected around the stent filaments. The inflammatory response of 50% TEMPO-coated and bare stents was low (1.00 ± 0.00 vs 1.03 ± 0.07). A few inflammatory cells were seen adjacent to the stent filaments. A thin thrombotic mesh covering the stent filaments was observed. The internal elastic membrane was beneath the stent filaments and the media were moderately compressed. Arterial injury

Table 52.1 The NOBLESSE I Study: QCA and morphometry variables

	Control (n = 9)[a]	50% TEMPO (n = 9)[a]	p
QCA variables			
Pre stenting (mm)	2.63 ± 0.30	2.66 ± 0.23	0.815
Balloon size (mm)	3.17 ± 0.26	3.02 ± 0.11	0.131
Post stenting (mm)	3.09 ± 0.28	2.92 ± 0.14	0.123
Recoil (%)	2.51 ± 2.34	3.37 ± 1.83	0.398
Stent:Artery ratio	1.21 ± 0.9	1.14 ± 0.69	0.855
Morphometry variables	(n = 8)	(n = 8)	
Lumen area (mm^2)	4.21 ± 2.31	4.18 ± 0.64	0.972
Area stenosis (%)	35 ± 23	23 ± 7	0.18
Neointimal hyperplasia (mm^2)	1.80 ± 0.77	1.26 ± 0.38	0.097
Balloon area/IEL area	1.26 ± 0.34	1.31 ± 0.15	0.765

[a]One pig had follow-up at 5 days and was included. Values are mean ± SD. QCA, quantitative coronary angiography.

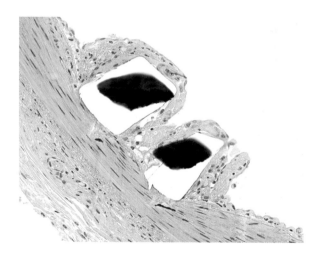

Fig. 52.1 Representative photomicrograph of a vessel segment stented with a 50% TEMPO-coated stent at 5 days. The media are compressed. Sparse inflammatory cell infiltrate invading mural thrombi are seen (hematoxylin-eosin stain, ×200).

caused by stent deployment was low and identical for the 50% TEMPO-coated and bare stents.

Representative photomicrographs of vessel segments at 6 weeks follow-up are shown in Figure 52.2 a,b and data are quantified in the bar chart (Figure 52.2c) and Table 52.1. In the 50% TEMPO-coated stent group, stent struts compressed the arterial medial layer. Some TEL was lacerated. Only a few sections showed a disruption of arterial media and/or EEL. Compared to the bare stent group, the mean injury scores of 50% TEMPO-coated stent group were decreased (0.39 ± 0.20 vs 0.62 ± 0.41, p = 0.14). Furthermore, 50% TEMPO-coated stent groups showed a mild inflammatory response. A few inflammatory cells were observed around the stent struts. Only a few stent struts showed a moderate inflammatory response. The mean inflammatory scores of 50% TEMPO-coated stent groups were lower than the bare stent group (1.02 ± 0.03 vs 1.08 ± 0.14, p, not significant). The neointimal hyperplasia of the 50% TEMPO-coated group was lower than the bare stent group (1.26 ± 0.77 vs 1.80 ± 0.38, p = 0.0097).

The first clinical pilot trial – NOBLESSE I (Nitric Oxide through Biodegradable Layer Elective Study for Safety and Efficacy Reduction of in-stent resteonosis) is described below.

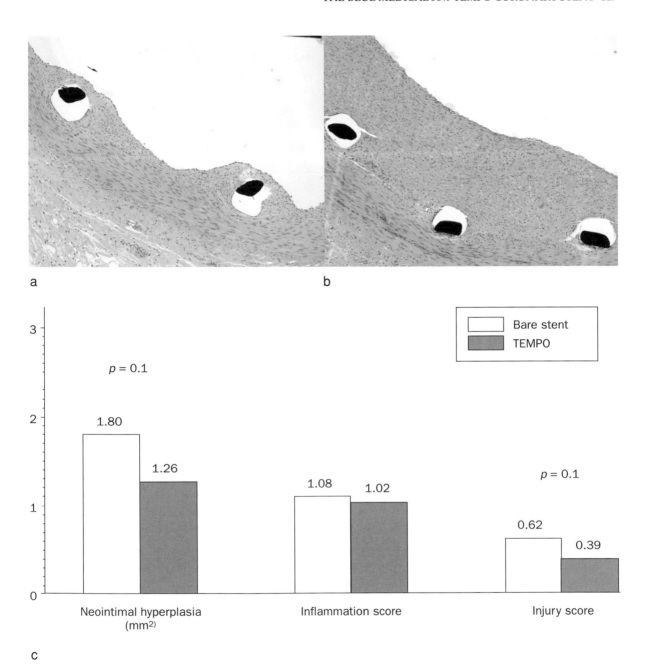

Fig. 52.2 Representative photomicrographs of vessel segments stented with 50% TEMPO (a) and bare stents (b) at 6 weeks. The peristrut inflammation of 50% TEMPO is comparable to the bare stent. The neointimal hyperplasia of the coated stents is limited. (Hematoxylin-eosin stain; a, b, ×100). (c) Bar graphs showing the histomorphometric parameters of the study groups at 6 weeks.

The aim of this study was to assess the safety and efficacy of the Blue Medical 50% Tempo-loaded stent deployment in the treatment of patients with de novo lesions in native coronary arteries of ≥2.75 mm for the preservation of vessel patency.

MATERIAL AND METHODS

In this study, Blue Medical 50% TEMPO-coated coronary stents of 3.0 mm and 3.5 mm in diameter and 14 mm and 18 mm in length were used.

Study design

This study was a prospective, multicenter, multinational phase III feasibility and safety trial performed at three medical centers. Patients with stable angina pectoris (Canadian Cardiovascular Society (CCS) class I–III) or documented ischemia due to a single de novo lesion in a native coronary artery were included. Eligible patients were required to agree to undergo the 4 month angiographic follow-up and 1 year clinical follow-up and had to be over 18 years old and not pregnant or lactating. Additional eligibility criteria were the de novo lesion in the coronary artery with a reference vessel between 2.75 mm to 3.50 mm in diameter and lesion stenosis between 70% and 99% (visually estimated) and <15 mm long and could be treated with a single 18 mm stent.

Patients were excluded if they had an unstable angina pectoris (Braunwald class 1–3), an acute or recent myocardial infarction, diabetes mellitus, severe congestive heart failure, severe valvular heart disease, a cerebral stroke <4 months prior to the procedure, clinical signs of cardiogenic shock at the time of procedure, bleeding diathesis in whom anticoagulation or antiplatelet medication was contraindicated. Patients were also not eligible if they had evidence of extensive thrombosis within the target lesion, a bifurcate lesion, a side branch >2 mm in diameter originating from the target lesion, a previous percutaneous transluminal coronary angioplasty (PTCA), a coronary stent implanted previously or an intolerance for aspirin, clopidine, ticlopidine, heparin, stainless steel or contrast media.

The ethical committee at each study site approved the study protocol and all patients gave written informed consent.

Medication

All patients were premeditated with aspirin 100 mg/d orally more than 2 days before the intervention or 250 mg IV when the indication for enrollment was given during the procedure. Heparin 50–150 U/kg body weight, after insertion of sheath and weight adjusted, was administrered as needed to maintain an active clotting time (ACT) of more than 300 seconds. Intracoronary nitrates 0.2 mg was administered before the baseline and before the final reference angiogram. After stent implantation, aspirin, at least 100 mg per day orally, was continued indefinitely. A loading dose of 300 mg clopidogrel was administered before procedure, followed by 75 mg per day for 4 weeks. Alternatively, ticlopidine 250 mg twice daily was prescribed for 4 weeks. During the follow-up angiography, heparin 50–100 U/kg body weight, after insertion of sheath, was given at the discretion of the operator. Nitrates (0.2 mg) was given prior to the first reference view.

Procedure

Standard angioplasty was performed via femoral approach. Guiding catheters were used (6Fr, 7Fr or 8Fr). Initial angiograms were performed in two orthogonal projections or, if not possible, in two different non-orthogonal views perpendicular to the investigated arterial segment. Under the same angiographic conditions, the same projections were performed during the follow-up studies.

Predilation of the target lesion could be performed according to established practice with a conventional balloon catheter type at the operator's decretion. Direct stenting was also allowed. An appropriately sized stent (3.0 or 3.5 mm in diameter by 14 mm or 18 mm in length) was selected and was deployed at the target lesion to achieve a stent diameter-to-reference diameter ratio of 1.1:1 and the appropriate stent length to fully cover the lesion. The placement was confirmed by a fluoroscopic test injection. In the instance of a suboptimal stent apposition, additional high pressure or larger balloon inflation was performed. Procedural success was defined as successful implantation of the study device and a remaining diameter stenosis less than 30%.

Quantitative coronary angiographic (QCA) analysis

Preprocedural, post-stent and 4 month follow-up QCA measurements were carried out offline by a specially trained investigator who was not involved in the angioplasty procedure. It was performed using a computer-assisted auto-mated arterial contour detection system (AWOS V 4.01, Siemens AG, Erlangen, Germany), which has been validated in vitro and in vivo.[17] Each lesion was analyzed in two approximate orthogonal projections selected to maximally avoid superimposition and vessel foreshortening. The distal end of the catheter was used for calibration in each analyzed projection. Reference and minimal luminal diameter (MLD), as well as the degree of percentage diameter stenosis (DS) before angioplasty, after stent implantation, and at 4 month follow-up were studied. All measurements were assessed in both obtained views and averaged. Acute gain, late loss, and loss index were subsequently calculated. Acute gain was defined as the difference between the post- and preprocedural MLD, while late loss was calculated by subtracting the MLD at follow-up from the post-procedural. Loss index was defined as late loss divided by acute gain.

Clinical follow-up

All patients were required to return to the investigative site or their primary cardiologist for a clinical visit 30 days and 60 days post procedural to monitor any acute clinical event. All subjects were asked to return to the investigative site for a repeated coronary angiography at 4 months ± one week. If a patient with recurrent chest pain associated with scintigraphic or electrocardiogram (ECG) evidence of myocardial ischemia or had a positive exercise stress test at any time up to the follow-up, a repeated angiography was performed. All patients were contacted by telephone by the investigative site at 12 months ± one week for evaluation.

Study endpoints

The primary endpoints were percentage of in-stent stenosis of the luminal diameter and late loss at 4 months follow-up as determined by QCA. The second endpoints were a composite of major cardiac events (MACE), defined as death, myocardial infarction, coronary artery bypass graft (CABG), and target lesion revascularization of the target lesion at 30 day, 60 day, 4 month, and 12 month follow-up, binary restenosis rate of the target lesion at 4 month follow-up and acute and (sub)acute study stent thrombosis.

Statistics

Categorical data are summarized using count and percentage. The Kolmogorov-Smirnov test was used to prove Gaussian distribution allowing for calculation of the means and standard deviations. Samples with non Gaussian distribution were described by median and range. Discriminate variables were evaluated with the two-side exact Fisher test. For comparison of subgroups, the unpaired two-tailed student's t-test was used. Results were considered statistically significant at a p-value less than 0.05.

RESULTS

Between August 2002 and June 2003, 45 patients were enrolled. Baseline demographic characteristics are summarized in Table 52.2. Overall, 64% of the patients were men, and the mean age was 61 with a range of 37–86. Lesion characteristics are summarized in Table 52.2. The target vessel was the left anterior descending coronary in 42%, the right coronary artery vessel in 36%, and the left circumflex artery in 22% of the patients. The treated lesions were class A (13.3%), B1 (48.5%) or B2 (37.8%) according to the American College of Cardiology and American Heart Association classification. Nearly all (98%) patients had a TIMI flow grade 3. Of the patients 57% underwent a direct stenting and 18 mm long stents were implanted in 49% of the cases.

One stent implantation resulted in a distal dissection, treated by an additional coated stent implantation. The procedure success rate was 98%. All patients were discharged from the hospital within 1.69 days (range: 1–5 days) without any MACE. Two patients were

Table 52.2 The NOBLESSE I study: lesion characteristics	
	NOBLESSE I (n = 45) (%)
Male	64.44%
Mean age (years)	61.31 ± 11.29 (37–86)
Target vessels	
LAD	42.22
RCA	35.56
LCX	22.22
ACC/AHA classification[a]	
A	13.33
B1	48.49
B2	37.78
C	0
Lesion length (mm)	9.02 (4–15)
Direct stenting	57.14
Stent deployment pressure	12.61 ± 3.24
Maximum inflation pressure	15.95 ± 3.02
Number of inflations	2.27 ± 1.71
14 mm long stent used	51.11
18 mm long stent used	48.89

[a]According to American College of Cardiology/American Heart Association classification. Values are mean ± SD or (%); LAD, left anterior descending artery; RCA, right coronary artery; LCX, left circumflex artery.

excluded because of the violation of the inclusion and/or exclusion criteria; one with a long (>15 mm) diffuse lesion which was not covered by the study stent, another because the stent was deployed proximal to the lesion.

Clinical follow-up

During the 30 day and 60 day follow-up, no MACE was observed. Between 60 day and 4 month follow-up, no death or myocardial infarction (MI) occurred, one patient had a recurrence of angina pectoris, and angiography showed a significant in-stent restenosis, which required a revascularization (TLR) 93 days after the procedure. At 4 month follow-up, angina states of the patients were significantly improved (only two patients had New York Heart Association (NYHA) 1). Two patients underwent a TLR because of in-stent restenosis resulting in a MACE-free rate of 93.3%. A 12 month clinical follow-up was available for 14 patients, no further MACE was observed.

Angiographic outcome

A 4 month angiographic follow-up rate was obtained in 98% (one patient did not come back for the 4 month follow-up). The angiographic results are summarized in Table 52.3. Mean

Table 52.3   The NOBLESSE I study: quantitative coronary angiography (QCA) data

	NOBLESSE I (n = 42)
Before procedure	
RVD (mm)	3.01 ± 0.29
MLD (mm)	1.07 ± 0.35
%DS	64.01 ± 12.20
After procedure	
RVD (mm)	3.03 ± 0.24
MLD (mm)	2.78 ± 0.22
%DS	8.40 ± 4.01
Acute gain (mm)	1.71 ± 0.42
Follow-up	
RVD (mm)	3.00 ± 0.23
MLD (mm)	2.09 ± 0.53
%DS	30.37 ± 17.03
Late loss (mm)	0.69 ± 0.52
Loss index	0.39 ± 0.30
Binary restenosis rate (%)	9.52

RVD, reference vessel diameter; MLD, minimal luminal diameter; DS, diameter stenosis.

reference vessel diameter was 3.01 ± 0.29 mm. MLD increased from 1.07 ± 0.35 at baseline to 2.78 ± 0.22 after the procedure, and diameter stenosis decreased from $64.01 \pm 12.20\%$ before PCI, to $8.40 \pm 4.01\%$ after stent implantation The acute gain was 1.71 ± 0.42 mm. At 4 month follow-up, the MLD and DS% were 2.09 ± 53 mm and $30.37 \pm 17.03\%$, respectively. The late loss was 0.69 ± 0.52. Four patients developed an in-stent restenosis, resulting in a binary restenosis rate of 9.52%.

QCA data of direct stenting vs indirect stenting

Of the patients, 57% underwent direct stenting in this study. There were no significant differences between reference vessel diameters. The target lesion was shorter in the direct stenting group (9.94 ± 2.31 vs 8.17 ± 2.42, $p = 0.02$). The target lesion was less severe in the direct stenting group (MLD: 0.86 ± 0.24 vs 1.23 ± 0.33, DS%: $71.64 \pm 8.73\%$ vs $58.29 \pm 11.38\%$, $p<0.001$), resulting in a significant low acute gain (1.91 ± 0.32 vs 1.56 ± 0.43, $p = 0.006$). The MLD was similar after stenting. The MLD at follow-up was larger in the direct stenting group resulting in a lower late loss, however, this difference was not significant (1.98 ± 0.54 vs 2.18 ± 0.53, $p = 0.24$). (See Table 52.4.)

DISCUSSION

This was a first clinical trial using a Blue Medical 50% TEMPO coronary stent loaded with an antioxidant compound, tempamine, to

Table 52.4   The NOBLESSE I study: QCA data on direct stenting vs indirect stenting

	NOBLESSE I (n = 42)		
	Indirect stenting (n = 18)	Direct stenting (n = 24)	p-value
Before procedure			
RVD (mm)	3.0 ± 0.32	2.98 ± 0.26	0.47
MLD (mm)	0.86 ± 0.24	1.23 ± 0.33	<0.001
%DS	71.64 ± 8.73	58.29 ± 11.38	<0.001
Lesion length	9.94 ± 2.31	8.17 ± 2.42	0.02
After procedure			
RVD (mm)	3.02 ± 0.20	3.04 ± 0.26	0.74
MLD (mm)	2.78 ± 0.17	2.79 ± 0.26	0.88
%DS	7.96 ± 4.04	8.73 ± 4.05	0.55
Acute gain (mm)	1.91 ± 0.32	1.56 ± 0.43	0.006
Follow-up			
RVD (mm)	3.01 ± 0.23	3.00 ± 0.23	0.91
MLD (mm)	1.98 ± 0.54	2.18 ± 0.53	0.24
%DS	33.94 ± 17.41	27.69 ± 16.60	0.24
Late loss (mm)	0.79 ± 0.53	0.61 ± 0.51	0.25
Loss index	0.42 ± 0.29	0.36 ± 0.32	0.53
Binary restenosis rate	11.11	8.33	NS

QCA, quantitative coronary angiography; RVD, reference vessel diameter; MLD, minimal luminal diameter; DS, diameter stenosis.

treat patients with de novo single vessel coronary disease. The absence of the MACE at 30 days and 60 days and a low late loss, percentage diameter stenosis, and binary restenosis rate at 4 month angiographic follow-up suggest a beneficial effect of this novel treatment modality to prevent in-stent restenosis.

The MACE rate in this study was extremely low, no death or MI was observed during the 4 month follow-up. Three patients underwent a TLR, however, only one was clinically symtomatic.

Direct stenting with a drug eluting stent

The use of direct stenting provides a way to reduce procedural costs, shorten procedural and fluoroscopy time, and lower material consumption. However, it is still under debate due to some of its limitations, such as a lower procedural success, especially in the complicated lesion subsets, such as calcified lesions. Immediate and long-term clinical and angiographic outcomes appear to be similar to stenting with predilation.[18,19] But, in the analysis of early outcomes, direct stenting was associated with a trend towards reduction of in-hospital death, myocardial infarction, and target lesion revascularization.[20] Direct stenting may reduce plaque embolization or enhanced trauma caused by balloon predilatation.[19]

Since one of the main features of the drug eluting stents is to provide a significant amount of agent directly to the target lesion, direct stenting may be particularly interesting in this domain. It provides the therapeutic drug to the target site at the very beginning of the injury therefore blocking the restenosis cascade. In the current study, direct stenting was performed in 57% of cases. The studied lesions in this study were less severe (MLD: 1.23 ± 0.33 vs 0.86 ± 0.24; DS%: $58.29 \pm 11.38\%$ vs $71.64 \pm 8.73\%$, $p<0.001$) in the direct stenting group. The MLD post stenting, which was shown to be the only angiographic predicator of the lumen loss after stenting was almost identical in the two groups. Nevertheless, the direct stenting group showed a trend towards better results at 4 month follow-up (MLD: 1.98 ± 0.54 vs 2.18 ± 0.53, $p = 0.24$; Late loss: 0.79 ± 0.53 vs 0.61 ± 0.51) (Figures 53.3, 53.4). With the increased use of drug eluting stents, a randomized study comparing direct stenting and conventional stenting is needed.

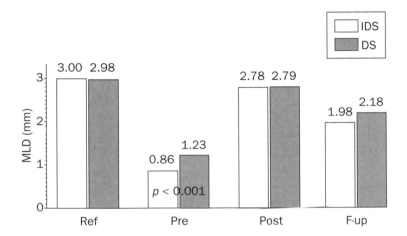

Fig. 52.3 Quantitative coronary analysis (QCA) comparison of the direct stenting and indirect stenting. IDS, indirect stenting; DS, direct stenting; MLD, mean luminal diameter; Ref, reference vessel diameter; Pre, minimum luminal diameter before stenting; Post, minimum luminal diameter after stenting; F-up, minimum luminal diameter at 4 month follow-up.

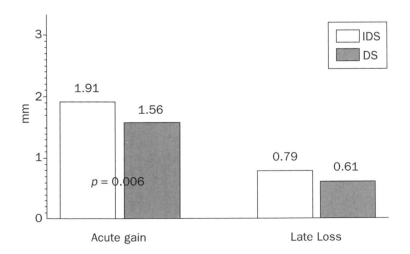

Fig. 52.4 Quantitative coronary analysis (QCA) comparison of the patient underwent direct stenting and indirect stenting. IDS, indirect stenting; DS, direct stenting. Acute gain = minimum luminal diameter post stent – minimum luminal diameter before stenting. Late loss = minimum liminal diameter post stent – minimum luminal diameter post stent – minimum luminal diameter at 4 month follow-up.

Limitations

The NOBLESSE I was neither a randomized nor a blinded trial and had only a small study population. Since the development of the neointimal hyperplasia peaks between the first 3–6 months after the stent implantation and can be retarded by drug eluting stents (DES), the angiographic evaluation at 4 months may underestimate the diameter stenosis as well as the restenosis rate. However, the polymer was estimated to be fully degraded within 2 months, and the 4 month angiographic follow-up was also conducted in some very promising drug eluting stent trials such as the sirolimus-FIM study.[21] A 12 month clinical and IVUS follow-up and a 2 year angiographic follow-up are planned. Patients who underwent direct stenting in this study had less severe target lesions thus the trend towards a better angiographic result at 4 months may be washed out by this bias selection.

SUMMARY

Preclinical studies in a porcine coronary model showed good biocompatibility without additional inflammatory response or increased thrombus formation. Histopathological data showed a lower mean injury score, peristrut inflammatory score, and a lower neointimal hyperplasia of the 50% TEMPO-coated stents compared to the bare stents at 6 weeks.

In this first clinical pilot trial, the absence of acute and (sub)acute thrombosis and MACE at 30 day and 60 day follow-up suggest that implantation of the Blue Medical 50% TEMPO coronary stent is feasible and safe. QCA data at 4 months showed a low late loss and binary restenosis rate, thus suggesting a beneficial effect on neointimal hyperplasia and in stent restenosis in patients with de novo single vessel disease.

REFERENCES

1. Marso SP, Ellis SG, Raymond R. Intracoronary stenting: an overview for the clinician. Cleve Clin J Med 1999; 66(7):434–42.

2. Al Suwaidi J, Berger PB, Holmes DR Jr. Coronary artery stents. JAMA 2000; 284(14):1828–36.

3. Ikeda S, Bosch J, Banz K, Schneller P. Economic outcomes analysis of stenting versus percutaneous transluminal coronary angioplasty for patients with coronary artery disease in Japan. J Invasive Cardiol 2000; 12(4):194–9.

4. Anderson TJ, Meredith IT, Yeung AC, et al. The effect of cholesterol-lowering and antioxidant therapy on endothelium-dependent coronary vasomotion. N Engl J Med 1995; 332(8):488–93.

5. Kuzuya M, Naito M, Funaki C, et al. Probucol prevents oxidative injury to endothelial cells. J Lipid Res 1991; 32(2):197–204.

6. Lafont AM, Chai YC, Cornhill JF, et al. Effect of alpha-tocopherol on restenosis after angioplasty in a model of experimental atherosclerosis. J Clin Invest 1995; 95(3):1018–25.

7. Gapinski JP, VanRuiswyk JV, Heudebert GR, Schectman GS. Preventing restenosis with fish oils following coronary angioplasty. A meta-analysis. Arch Intern Med 1993; 153(13):1595–601.

8. DeMaio SJ, King SB III, Lembo NJ, et al. Vitamin E supplementation, plasma lipids and incidence of restenosis after percutaneous transluminal coronary angioplasty (PTCA). J Am Coll Nutr 1992; 11(1):68–73.

9. Tardif JC, Cote G, Lesperance J, et al. Probucol and multivitamins in the prevention of restenosis after coronary angioplasty. Multivitamins and Probucol Study Group. N Engl J Med 1997; 337(6):365–72.

10. Johansen O, Brekke M, Seljeflot I, et al. N-3 fatty acids do not prevent restenosis after coronary angioplasty: results from the CART study. Coronary Angioplasty Restenosis Trial. J Am Coll Cardiol 1999; 33(6):1619–26.

11. Lee SH, Szinai I, Carpenter K, et al. In-vivo biocompatibility evaluation of stents coated with a new biodegradable elastomeric and functional polymer. Coron Artery Dis 2002; 13(4):237–41.

12. Swartz HM, Sentjurc M, Morse PD II. Cellular metabolism of water-soluble nitroxides: effect on rate of reduction of cell/nitroxide ratio, oxygen concentrations and permeability of nitroxides. Biochim Biophys Acta 1986; 888(1):82–90.

13. Komarov AM, Joseph J, Lai CS. In vivo pharmacokinetics of nitroxides in mice. Biochem

Biophys Res Commun 1994; 201(2):1035–42 (PMID: 8002974).

14. De Scheerder IK, Wilczek KL, Verbeken EV, et al. Biocompatibility of polymer-coated oversized metallic stents implanted in normal porcine coronary arteries. Atherosclerosis 1995; 114(1):105–14.

15. De Scheerder IK, Wang K, Kerdsinchai P, et al. The concept of the home-made coronary stent: experimental results and initial clinical experience. Catheter Cardiovasc Diagn 1996; 39:191–6.

16. Schwartz RS, Huber KC, Murphy JG, et al. Restenosis and the proportional neointimal response to coronary artery injury: results in a porcine model. J Am Coll Cardiol 1992; 19(2):267–74.

17. De Scheerder IK, Wang K, Kerdsinchai P, et al. Clinical and angiographic outcome after implantation of a home-made stent for complicated coronary angioplasty. Catheter Cardiovasc Diagn 1997; 42(3):339–47.

18. Baim DS, Flatley M, Caputo R, et al. PRE-Dilatation vs Direct Stenting In Coronary Treatment (PREDICT) Trial. Comparison of PRE-dilatation vs direct stenting in coronary treatment using the Medtronic AVE S670 Coronary Stent System (the PREDICT trial). Am J Cardiol 2001; 88(12):1364–9.

19. Burzotta F, Trani C, Prati F, et al. Comparison of outcomes (early and six-month) of direct stenting with conventional stenting (a meta-analysis of ten randomized trials). Am J Cardiol 2003; 91(7):790–6.

20. Loubeyre C, Morice MC, Lefevre T, et al. A randomized comparison of direct stenting with conventional stent implantation in selected patients with acute myocardial infarction. J Am Coll Cardiol 2002; 39(1):15–21.

21. Sousa JE, Costa MA, Abizaid A, et al. Lack of neointimal proliferation after implantation of sirolimus-coated stents in human coronary arteries: A quantitative coronary angiography and three-dimensional intravascular ultrasound study. Circulation 2001; 103(2): 192–5.

53

Dexamethasone: mode of action, preclinical, and clinical studies

Ivan De Scheerder, Xiaoshun Liu, Yanming Huang, and Eric Verbeken

INTRODUCTION

In-stent restenosis, mainly caused by an abundant neointimal hyperplasia, remains the major limitation of coronary stent implantation. Mural thrombi, inflammatory response, smooth muscle cell (SMC) dedifferentiation, migration and proliferation, and furthermore extracellular matrix formation, all participate in the pathogenesis of neointimal hyperplasia. Changing any of these factors could have an impact on neointimal hyperplasia. Systemic delivery of drugs has been unsuccessful in reducing restenosis. Indeed, local drug delivery via infusion devices has introduced additional complexity to the procedure and may not deliver sufficient medication to the injury site. Drug eluting stents, however, can deliver an adequate amount of medication to the injury site for a sufficient period of time, and have been proposed as an alternative approach to decrease neointimal hyperplasia. Some preliminary studies have shown very promising results.[1,2]

MODE OF ACTION OF DEXAMETHASONE

The role of inflammation in atherosclerosis and restenosis has been widely discussed in recent literature.[3–6] Inflammation is an inevitable consequence of angioplasty, as injury to the vessel wall and the introduction of a foreign object (stent) both elicit an adverse host response. Whilst the injury is somewhat dictated by the procedure used or the type of stent selected, the subsequent host response can be controlled by use of antiinflammatory compounds. The corticosteroids, including dexamethasone, methylprednisolone, and hydrocortisone, are a well-documented group of steroidal drugs. Indeed, dexamethasone itself has been approved by the Federal Drug Administration (FDA) since 1958 and is extensively used in inflammation management. In animal models, local delivery of such corticosteroids has been shown to reduce inflammation markers caused by percutaneous transluminal coronary angioplasty (PTCA) and stenting procedures (Figure 53.1).[7,8]

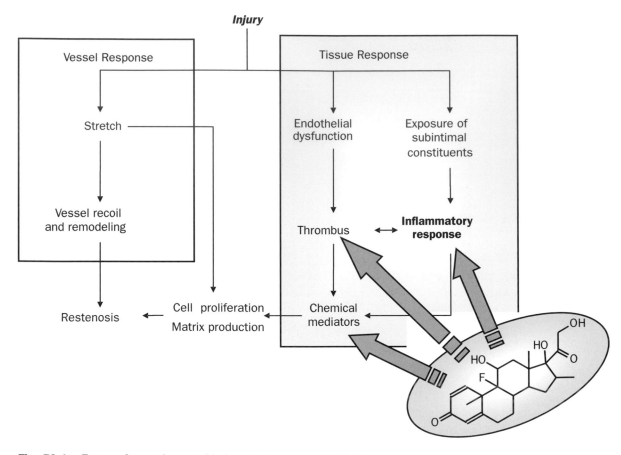

Fig. 53.1 Targets for corticosteroids in response to vessel injury.

The inflammatory response consists of both innate (non-specific) and acute (specific) reactions. The innate reactions are induced by release of plasma and cell-derived mediators. Increased vessel permeability results in the exudation of fluid into the injured tissue, which contains components from the complement, coagulation, fibrinolytic, and kinin cascades, that stimulate the release of a host of chemical inflammatory mediators; cellular events are induced by endothelial, mast, and macrophage cells present in the tissue, and platelets and leukocytes from the blood. The acute reactions are a consequence of more specific activation of B- and T-lymphocytes by antigens that migrate to the lymph nodes.

Dexamethasone is a glucocorticoid that readily crosses target cell membranes (1) and binds to the intracytoplasmic glucocorticoid receptor complex (2), causing the dissociation of two protein subunits (3), and the subsequent activation of the complex.[9] The activated complex can migrate to the nucleus where it binds to glucocorticoid response elements (GRE) (4) (receptors) in the DNA, resulting in the modification of protein synthesis (5), thereby inhibiting inflammatory responses (Figure 53.2). A transcription activator protein (AP-1) can also interact with the activated complex to bring about modification of collagenase and interleukins. Cytokines are affected through a similar process (6) as their genes possess several GREs.[10] Glucocorticoids also have an effect on the prostaglandin synthesis pathway, which is responsible for production of the lipid inflammatory mediators. The primary antiinflammatory action is inhibition of the induction of cyclooxygenase-2 (COX-2),[11]

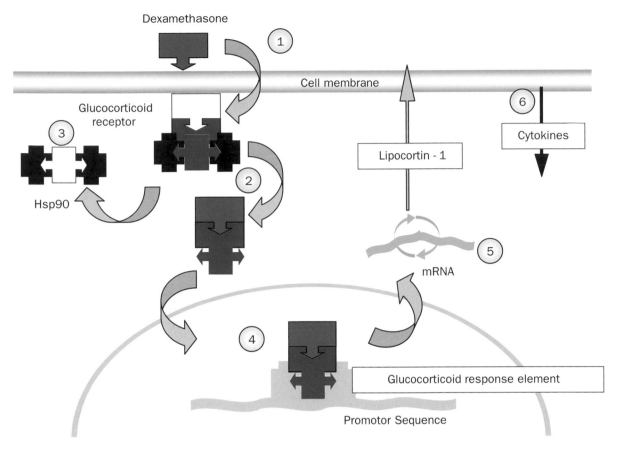

Fig. 53.2 Molecular mode of action for dexamethasone.

by the AP-1-glucocorticoid complex. COX-2 is generally undetectable in most tissues but increases its expression during acute inflammation or in response to cytokine stimulation-producing prostaglandins found at sites of inflammation.

PRECLINICAL EVALUATION OF STENT-MEDIATED DELIVERY OF CORTICOSTEROIDS

Continuous administration of hydrocortisone or dexamethasone, either systemically or from periadventitial polymers, has been shown to reduce reactive intimal hyperplasia in rabbit and rat models of restenosis.[7,12] Evidence to support the inhibitory effects of corticosteroids to the foreign body response when delivered from a stent were described in a study of methyl prednisolone impregnated in Wiktor

stents coated with polyorganophosphazene,[13] and stents coated with a fluorinated poly-methacrylate by a variety of methods.[14] Local drug delivery of dexamethasone from a poly(L-lactic acid) coated tantalum wire stent in a porcine model did not result in a reduction of intimal hyperplasia.[8] The positive effects from the drug may however, have been offset by the adverse effects from the polymer, as it has been shown that biodegradable polymers can cause increased inflammation and neointimal thickening in a porcine model.[15] Indeed, when Strecker stents, coated with pure polylactide or a polylactide copolymer containing a 10-fold higher dose of dexamethasone than the previous study, were evaluated in a canine femoral model, significantly less neointimal hyperplasia compared to uncoated stents was reported.[16] Furthermore, only 20% of the dexamethasone

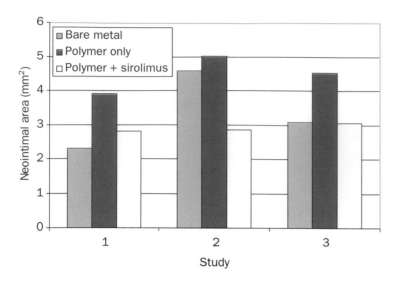

Fig. 53.3 Comparison of neointimal area for bare metal, polymer-coated and polymer-coated + sirolimus stents in preclinical studies reported by Cordis Corp.[17]

was released over the first 24 hours, with sustained delivery over 40 days. Adverse effects induced by polymer coatings are not however, limited to biodegradable materials.[15] Analysis of the preclinical data from three separate porcine studies of sirolimus delivery from polymer-coated stents shows that the powerful effects of the drug are necessary to overcome the increase in neointimal area induced by the polymer alone (Figure 53.3).[17]

In order to separate the antiinflammatory effects of the drug from potential adverse reactions to the polymer coatings employed as delivery vehicles, preclinical studies in a porcine coronary model were performed using the Bio*divYsio* Matrix LO drug delivery stent, which has been shown in many studies to cause no coating-related inflammatory reaction.[18–21] The stent is characterized by a biocompatible coating capable of absorbing a range of therapeutic agents for subsequent delivery to the vessel wall.[22] Drug loadings of $0.9~\mu g/mm^2$ of dexamethasone (low dose delivery) and ~2.5 $\mu g/mm^2$ for both dexamethasone (high dose delivery) and methyl prednisolone (MP) were used in this preclinical study. Results of this study showed only scarce leukocytes, macrophages, and giant cells in the neointima in all samples studied, supporting other investigations,[19] which show

that phosphorylcholine (PC)-coated stents demonstrate a minimal inflammatory response at 5 days follow-up, even in an oversized injury model (Figure 53.4). Even with the lower than normal results obtained in the control stents, it was observed that local release of dexamethasone or methyl prednisolone further decreased the severity of the inflammatory response, the inflammatory score of the methyl prednisolone group being significantly lower than that of the control group (Figure 53.5a).

Steroids have also been shown to inhibit the formation of platelet-activating factor and may exert an antiplatelet effect.[23] The occurrence of thrombus surrounding the stent filaments in the dexamethasone and methyl prednisolone groups was also lower than the control (Figure 53.5b). As the early inflammatory reaction after angioplasty may have potent promoting effects on neointimal formation, reduction of these processes by delivery of a corticosteroid might be expected to have an effect on the early neointimal hyperplasia. Certainly, the number of macrophages in arteries healing after coronary intervention has been shown to correlate with the amount of tissue growth.[24] This was further supported by this study (see Table 53.1), with early neointimal hyperplasia and area stenosis of the

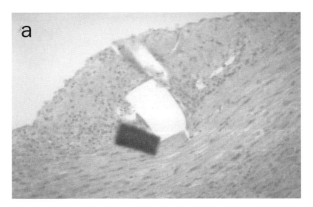

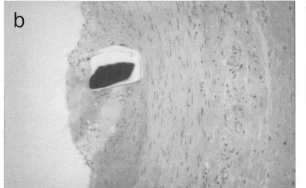
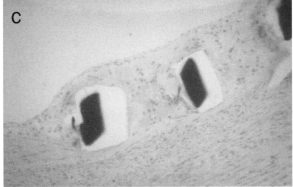

Fig. 53.4 Photomicrograph of a vessel segment stented with (a) a bare stent, (b) a dexamethasone-loaded stent, and (c) a methylprednisolone-loaded stent, all at 5 day follow-up. The histolymphocytic reaction surrounding the stent filaments was reduced by the local steroid delivery in (b) and (c) (hematoxylin-eosin stain). LDD, low dose delivery; HDD, high dose delivery: MP, methyl prednisolone.

dexamethasone and methyl prednisolone groups being significantly lower compared to those of the control group.

The inflammatory response at 4 week follow-up was still low, but higher than the 5 day time point with all stent groups being statistically equivalent. Endothelialization of the drug-loaded stents was identical to the control and hence unaffected by the presence of the drug (Figure 53.6).

The conclusion of the study was that local doses of the corticosteroids dexamethasone and methyl prednisolone delivered from BiodivYsio Matrix LO stents were safe for human clinical evaluation.[25] Furthermore, it was demonstrated that use of these drugs might be effective in decreasing the inflammatory response and potentially neointimal hyperplasia, without affecting the rate of endothelialization of the stent.

CLINICAL EVALUATION OF STENT-MEDIATED DELIVERY OF DEXAMETHASONE: STRIDE

The aim of the STudy of anti-Restenosis with the BIodivYsio Dexamethasone Eluting stent (STRIDE) was to evaluate the safety and efficacy of the BiodivYsio Matrix LO stent loaded with dexamethasone. The primary objective was to evaluate the proportion of patients having a clinical restenosis 6 months after receiving the dexamethasone-loaded stent. The secondary objectives were to evaluate the safety and the 6 month quantitative coronary angiography (QCA) endpoints after receiving the dexamethasone-loaded stent.

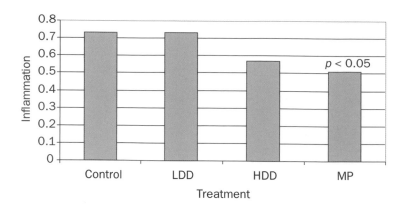

a

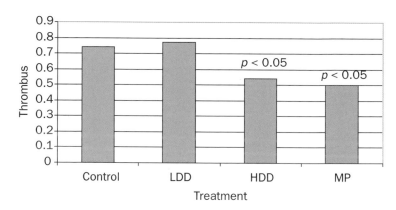

b

Fig. 53.5 Effects of corticosteroid delivery from the Bio*divYsio* Matrix LO stent on (a) inflammation and (b) thrombus.

Table 53.1   Acute 5 day data for corticosteroids delivered from the Bio*divYsio* Matrix LO stent

Stent	Lumen area (mm²)	IEL area (mm²)	EEL area (mm²)	Neointimal hyperplasia (mm²)	Area stenosis (%)
Control	7.94 ± 0.49	8.74 ± 0.44	10.44 ± 0.39	0.80 ± 0.16	9 ± 2
Dexamethasone	9.02 ± 0.49***	9.70 ± 0.49**	11.47 ± 0.69***	0.68 ± 0.12*	7 ± 1*
Methylprednisolone	8.34 ± 0.68	8.89 ± 0.73	10.26 ± 0.16	0.54 ± 0.16**	6 ± 2***

IEL, internal elastic lamina; EEL, external elastic lamina. $n = 12$, *$p<0.05$, **$p<0.01$, ***$p<0.001$ compared to control.

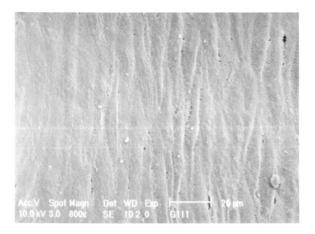

Fig. 53.6 Scanning electron micrograph (SEM) showing complete endothelialization of the drug-loaded stent.

Study design

This multicenter trial was performed at eight interventional cardiovascular centers in Belgium. Symptomatic patients with documented myocardial ischemia with de novo coronary lesions >2.75 mm and <4.0 mm in diameter, with stenosis >50%, and length <15 mm long were recruited.

Procedure

All patients were premedicated with acetylsalicylic acid (aspirin) (160 mg/d) orally. Oral ticlopidine 500 mg was given before PTCA. Standard balloon angioplasty was performed via the femoral approach. Heparin (100 U/kg), after insertion of the arterial sheath, was weight adjusted and administered as needed to maintain an activated clotting time (ACT) of approximately 250–300 seconds. Intracoronary nitroglycerin 100–200 µg was administered immediately prior to baseline angiography, post-stent deployment, and after final postdilatation angiography. Initial angiograms were performed in two orthogonal projections or, if not possible, in two different non-orthogonal views perpendicular to the investigated arterial segment. Under the same angiographic conditions, the same projections were repeated

during the follow-up studies. After predilatation, angiography was performed and evaluated. An appropriately sized Bio*divYsio* Matrix LO stent was selected and immersed in a solution of 15 mg/mL dexamethasone yielding approximately 0.5 µg/mm^2 of stent. The stent mounted on balloon was allowed to rest in the sterile solution for a minimum of 5 min and then was left to air-dry in the sterile field for 5 min. Then the dexamethasone loaded Bio*divYsio* matrix LO stent was deployed at the treatment site. In the case of a suboptimal stent apposition, additional high pressure or upsized balloon inflations were performed. Procedural success was defined as a less than 10% diameter stenosis (DS) after stent implantation. After stent implantation, aspirin was continued indefinitely and ticlopidine (250 mg/d) was prescribed for 28 days in all cases.

Quantitative coronary angiographic (QCA) analysis

Preprocedural, post-PTCA, post-stent and 6 month follow-up QCA measurements were performed off-line using a computer-assisted automated arterial contour detection system (AWOS V 4.01, Siemens AG, Erlangen, Germany), which has been validated in vitro and in vivo. Each lesion was analyzed in two approximately orthogonal projections selected to maximally avoid superimposition and vessel foreshortening. The distal end of the guiding catheter was used for calibration in each analyzed projection. The in-lesion segment was defined as the stent plus 5 mm proximal and 5 mm distal to the edge or the nearest side branch. In-stent and in-lesion restenosis were defined as >50% DS at follow-up, located within the stent and target lesion, respectively. Reference and minimal luminal diameters (MLD), as well as the degree of percentage diameter stenosis before and after angioplasty, after stent implantation and at 6 month follow-up were studied. All measurements were assessed in both obtained views and averaged. Acute gain, late loss and net gain were subsequently calculated. Acute gain was defined as the difference between the post- and preprocedural MLD, while late loss and net gain were calculated by subtracting the MLD at control from the postprocedural and preprocedural MLD, respectively.[26]

Clinical follow-up

All patients were asked to return to the investigative site or their primary cardiologist for a clinical visit 4 weeks post procedure to monitor acute clinical events. All patients were contacted by telephone by the investigative site at 3 months +1 week for a safety evaluation. All subjects were required to return to the inves-

tigative site for a repeat coronary angiography whether they were experiencing symptoms or not. If a patient had a positive exercise stress test at any time up to and including the required follow-up, a repeat angiogram was performed.

RESULTS

From 16 January to 5 June 2001, 71 patients from eight study sites were included. Table 53.2 represents the baseline clinical characteristics of the study population. The mean age was 61.9 with a range of 42–82 years; 21% were females; 63% of the patients had hypercholesterolemia;

Table 53.2 Baseline clinical characteristics		
	n	%
Study population	71	
Female/Male	12/56	21/79
Mean age	61.9 (range 42–82)	
Risk factors		
Family history CHD	24	34
Hypercholesterolemia	45	63
Hypertension	40	56
Peripheral vascular disease	5	7
Previous stroke	5	7
Previous MI	30	42
Previous PTCA	11	15
Smoking state	–	–
Never smoked	16	23
Current smokers	24	34
Ex-smokers	25	35
Stable angina	29	42
Unstable angina	27	38
Silent ischemia	13	19

Values are mean ± SD or n (%). CHD, coronary heart disease; MI, myocardial infarction; PTCA, percutaneous transluminal coronary angioplasty.

56% had hypertension; 42% had a previous myocardial infarction (MI); 46% had two or more than two vessel disease; 31% had lesion type B2 or C; 28% had unstable angina pectoris. Five patients were excluded from further analysis because of obvious protocol violations: one patient received a study stent to treat a no-reflow phenomenon after balloon dilatation, one patient had a documented acute myocardial infarction within 72 hours of the study procedure, one patient had a long tandem lesion (35 mm), treated by one study stent, overlapping with a long non-study stent, in one patient, the study stent was implanted in a significantly diseased bifurcation of the Lad/Diagonal, covering a diagonal >2 mm. Finally, one patient with multiple vessel disease underwent a staged PTCA procedure.

Acute and 30 days clinical follow-up

All the stents were implanted successfully. One patient had recurrent angina pectoris, requiring a non-target vessel revascularization at 15 days.

Follow-up at 3 months

The 3 month follow-up was available for all the remaining patients. Two additional major adverse cardiac events (MACE) occurred: one patient suffered a myocardial infarction not related to the target vessel, and another patient had recurrence of symptoms due to progression of his coronary disease and was referred for coronary bypass graft (CABG).

Angiographic results

The angiographic characteristics of the stented coronary segments are presented in Table 53.3. Of the patients, 46% had at least 2 vessel disease; 30% of stents were placed in right coronary artery, 41% in the left anterior descending artery (LAD), and 20% in the circumflex coronary artery. Quantitative coronary analysis is summarized in Table 53.3. The mean lesion length was 9.99 mm with a range of 4–23.5 mm. The mean reference diameter at baseline was 2.95 ± 0.52 mm. Minimal luminal diameter and diameter stenosis before the procedure were 1.03 ± 0.35 mm and $64.75 \pm 11.81\%$, respectively. Six-month follow-up angiographic data have been collected and are awaiting analysis.

Selected case studies at 6 months

Figure 53.7 shows a coronarogram of the left coronary artery showing a severe eccentric lesion of the mid LAD. The lesion was pretreated with a 12 mm/3.0 mm balloon and stented with a 16 mm/3.5 mm study stent. At 6 month follow-up the treated vessel segment was still fully patent. Figure 53.8 shows a coronarogram of the left coronary artery showing a subtotal, eccentric lesion of the circumflex artery. The lesion was pretreated with a 12 mm/2.5 mm balloon and stented with a 16 mm/3.0 mm study stent. Six-month follow-up coronarogram revealed a moderate restenosis in the treated segment.

DISCUSSION AND CONCLUSIONS

Coronary stenting is still hampered by subacute in-stent early thrombosis and later in-stent restenosis. Although largely prevented by improved stent implantation and adjunctive treatment with thienopyridines (ticlopidine or clopidogrel), subacute thrombotic stent occlusion still occurs in less than 2% of cases and is often associated with significant morbidity and mortality. The median time of thrombosis occurrence is one day with virtual elimination of events on day 2 after the stent implantation.[27] In patients undergoing intravascular brachytherapy an increased incidence of subacute and even late thrombotic stent occlusion have been reported. This was explained by the retarded regrowth of endothelial cells after intravascular brachytherapy. Also, drug eluting stents are considered at risk for increased incidence for subacute and late stent thrombosis since the drug used to inhibit neointimal hyperplasia may also affect endothelial cell regrowth. In this pilot trial, no increased incidence of subacute thrombosis was observed despite the lack of prolonged administration

Table 53.3 Angiographic characteristics		
	n	%
Disease state		
Single vessel disease	38	54
2 vessel disease	20	29
3 vessel disease	10	14
4 vessel disease	2	3
Vessels treated		
RCA	21	30
LAD	29	41
CX	14	20
First obtuse marginal	4	6
Ramus intermedius	2	3
Lesion classification[a]		
A	15	21
B1	34	48
B2	19	27
C	3	4
Lesion length	9.99 (range: 4–23.5 mm)	

[a] According to American College of Cardiology Classification/American Heart Association (ACC/AHA) classification. Values are mean ± SD or n (%). RCA, right coronary artery; LAD, left anterior descending artery; CX, left circumflex artery.

of ticlopidine. We await the 6 month angiographic data in order to assess whether the drug has had any effect on the extent of neointimal hyperplasia that has occurred in these patients.

Implantation of a dexamethasone loaded Bio*divYsio* Matrix LO stent to treat de novo coronary lesions is feasible and safe. In particular, there was no increased incidence of subacute or late stent thrombosis, notwithstanding the absence of prolonged antiaggregation treatment in this study. Clinical event rate and clinically driven revascularization need was low. This study, however, was a pilot study that was neither blinded, nor randomized, and without a control group. It was performed in a small selected group of patients. Two further randomized studies are therefore planned to further investigate the effects of dexamethasone delivery on late loss (EMPEROR, Table 53.4) and in patients with acute coronary syndromes (DESCEND, Table 53.5).

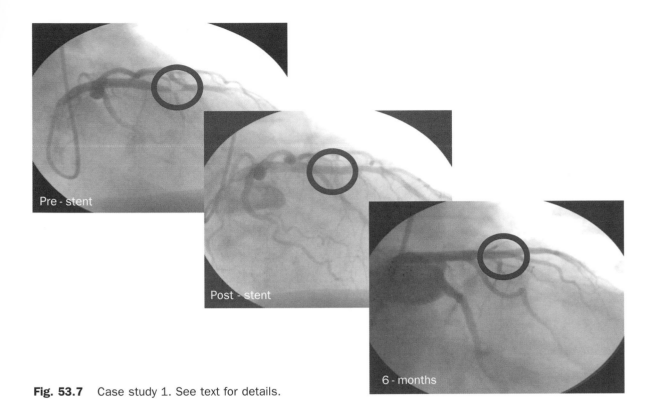

Fig. 53.7 Case study 1. See text for details.

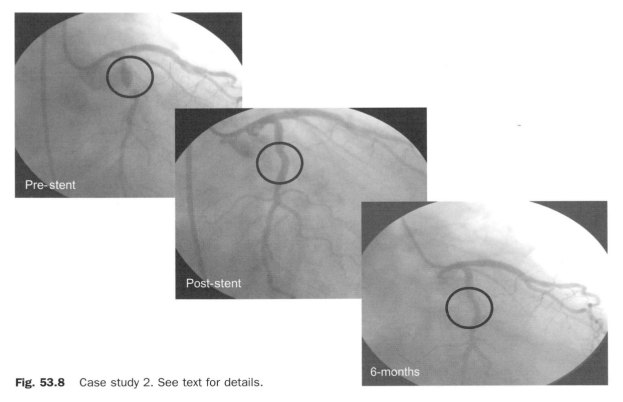

Fig. 53.8 Case study 2. See text for details.

Table 53.4   The structure of the EMPEROR trial[a]

Purpose	Comparative evaluation of lumen loss (MLD after stent placement – MLD at follow-up) 6 months after stent implantation between coronary lesions treated by 9α-f-16-methylprednisolone (dexamethasone) – loaded Bio*divYsio* Matrix stents and Bio*divYsio* standard OC PC-coated stents
Trial phase	Phase II
Structure	Multicenter, prospective, randomized clinical study
Enrollment	420 subjects with proven CAD and angiographic follow-up in at least 330 patients
Clinical sites	Approximately 20 sites in Germany, February 2002
Principal investigators	PD Dr med. R. Hoffmann, Universitätsklinikum, Aachen der RWTH, Germany

[a] Evaluation of 9α-Fluoro-16-MethylPrednisolone Eluting stents on the Reduction Of Restenosis.
MLD, minimal luminal diameter; oc, open cell; PC, phosphorylcholine; CAD, Coronary heart disease.

Table 53.5   The structure of the DESCEND trial[a]

Purpose	To evaluate the safety and efficacy of the Bio*divYsio* Matrix PC coated stent loaded with dexamethasone in patients with acute coronary syndromes
Trial phase	Phase II
Structure	Multicenter, prospective, randomized clinical study
Enrollment	160 patients with angiographic follow-up (80 randomized to receive a standard Bio*divYsio* stent and 80 to a Bio*divYsio* Matrix stent preloaded with dexamethasone)
Clinical sites	Approximately four sites in the UK, April 2002
Principal investigators	Dr Peter M Schofield, Papworth Hospital, Cambridge, UK

[a] The Dexamethasone Eluting Stent in aCuteE coroNary synDromes.

REFERENCES

1. Sousa JE, Costa MA, Abizaid A, et al. Lack of neointimal proliferation after implantation of sirolimus-coated stents in human coronary arteries: A quantitative coronary angiography and three-dimensional intravascular ultrasound study. Circulation 2001; 103:192–5.

2. Honda Y, Grube E, de la Fuente LM, et al. Novel drug-delivery stent; Intravascular ultrasound observations from the first human experience with the QP2-eluting polymer stent system. Circulation 2001; 104:380–3.

3. Simon DI, Chen Z, Seifert P, et al. Decreased neointimal formation in *Mac-1*$^{-/-}$ mice reveals a role for inflammation in vascular repair after angioplasty. J Clin Invest 2000; 105:293–300.

4. Libby P, Simon DI. Inflammation and thrombosis – the clot thickens. Circulation 2001; 103:1718–20.

5. von Hundelshausen P, Weber KSC, Huo Y, et al. RANTES deposition by platelets triggers monocyte arrest on inflamed and atherosclerotic endothelium. Circulation 2001; 103:1772–7.

6. Baker CSR, Gupta S. Chemokines: the link between inflammation, restenosis and atherosclerosis? Int J Cardiol 2001; 80:107–8.

7. Villa AE, Guzman LA, Chen W, et al. Local delivery of dexamethasone for prevention of neointimal proliferation in a rat model of balloon angioplasty. J Clin Invest 1994; 93:1243–9.

8. Lincoff AM, Furst JG, Ellis SG, et al. Sustained local delivery of dexamethasone by a novel intravascular eluting stent to prevent restenosis in the porcine coronary injury model. J Am Coll Cardiol 1997; 29(4):808–16.

9. Barnes PJ, Adcock I. Anti-inflammatory actions of steroids: molecular mechanisms. TiPS 1993; 14:436–41.

10. Boumpas DT, Paliogianni F, Anastassiou ED, Balow JE. Glucocorticosteroid action on the immune system: molecular and cellular aspects. Clin Exp Rheumatol 1991; 9:413–23.

11. Yucel-Lindberg T, Ahola H, Nilsson S, et al. Interleukin-1 beta induces expression of cyclooxygenase-2 mRNA in human gingival fibroblasts. Inflammation 1995; 19(5):549–60.

12. Beck BC, Gordon JB, Alexander RW. Pharmacologic roles of heparin and glucocorticoids to prevent restenosis after coronary angioplasty. J Am Coll Cardiol 1991; 17:111B–117B.

13. De Scheerder I, Wang K, Wilczek K, et al. Local methylprednisolone inhibition of foreign body response to coated intracoronary stents. Coron Artery Dis 1996; 7:161–6.

14. De Scheerder I, Huang Y, Schacht E. New concepts for drug eluting stents. 6th Local Drug Delivery Meeting and Cardiovascular Course on Radiation and Molecular Strategies, Geneva, Switzerland, 27–29 January 2000.

15. Van der Giessen WJ, Lincoff MA, Schwartz RS, et al. Marked inflammatory sequelae to implantation of biodegradable and nonbiodegradable polymers in procine coronary arteries. Circulation 1996; 94:1690–7.

16. Strecker EP, Gabelmann A, Boos I, et al. Effect on neointimal hyperplasia of dexamethasone released from coated metal stents compared to non-coated stents in canine femoral arteries. Cardiovasc Intervent Radiol 1998; 21:487–96.

17. WO 01/87342 A2. Falotico R, Kopia GA, Llanos GH, Sierierka J, assigned to Cordis Corp, 2001.

18. Lewis AL, Tolhurst LA, Stratford PW. Analysis of a phosphorylcholine-based polymer coating on a coronary stent pre- and post-implantation. Biomaterials 2002; 23:1697–706.

19. Whelan DM, van der Giessen WJ, Krabbendam SC, et al. Biocompatibility of phosphorylcholine coated stents in normal porcine coronary arteries. Heart 2000; 83(3):338–45.

20. Galli M, Bartorelli A, Bedogni F, et al. Italian BiodiviYsio open registry (BiodiviYsio PC-coated stent): Study of clinical outcomes of a PC-coated coronary stent. J Invasive Cardiol 2000; 12:452–8.

21. Zheng H, Barragan P, Corcos T, et al. Clinical experience with a new biocompatible phosphorylcholine-coated coronary stent. J Invasive Cardiol 1999; 11:608–14.

22. Lewis AL, Vick TA, Collias ACM, et al. Phosphorylcholine-based polymers for stent drug delivery. J Mater Sci, Mater Med 2001; 12:865–70.

23. Parente L, Fitzgerald MF, Flower RJ, De Nucci G. The effect of glucocorticoids on lyso-PAF formation in vitro and in vivo. Agents Actions 1986; 17(3–4):312–13.

24. Moreno PR, Bernadi VH, Lopez-Cuellar J, et al. Macrophage infiltration predicts restenosis after coronary intervention in patients with unstable angina. Circulation 1996; 94(12):3098–102.

25. De Scheerder, I, Huang Y. Anti-inflammatory approach for restenosis. In Rothman MT (ed), Restenosis: Multiple Strategies for Stent Drug Delivery. ReMedica Books: London 2001:13–32.

26. Popma JJ, Basshore TM. Qualitative and quantitative angiography. In Topol EJ (ed), Textbook of Interventional Cardiology, 2nd edn. WB Saunders: Philadelphia 1994: 1052–68.

27. Cutlip DE, Baim DS, Kuntz RE, et al. Stent thrombosis in the modern era: A pooled analysis of multicenter coronary stent clinical trial. Circulation 2001; 103:1967–71.

54

17β-Estradiol eluting stents: a potential therapy in the prevention of restenosis

Gishel New, Nicholas Kipshidze, Alexander S Abizaid, and Antonio Colombo

Introduction • Background • Mechanisms of action of estrogen • Delivery • Clinical studies • Conclusions • Summary

INTRODUCTION

Restenosis remains the final frontier in interventional cardiology. In the best series, in-stent restenosis still occurs in 20–30% of lesions.[1] Epidemiological studies have suggested that women taking estrogen post menopause develop less restenosis post angioplasty.[2] Previous studies suggest that estrogen may work through several mechanisms to inhibit atherosclerosis and possibly restenosis.[3,4] The systemic use of estrogen is limited due to the possible hyperplastic effects on breast and uterine tissue and feminizing effects in males. However, experimental work with the local intracoronary administration of estrogen to the lesion site looks promising.[5] Our preliminary work using local delivery of estrogen via a drug eluting stent to prevent restenosis looks encouraging. Clinical trials are currently underway in Europe and South America to determine whether estrogen eluting stents inhibit restenosis.

BACKGROUND

Estrogen is a naturally occurring sex hormone. In females, estrogen is produced by the ovary, adrenal cortex, and adipose tissue. In males, estrogen is derived from the testes and from the peripheral conversion of androgens in extraglandular tissue. Estradiol-17β is the most potent form of circulating estrogen (Figure 54.1). The level of plasma estradiol in normal men is less than 180 pmol/L and in females it varies depending on the menstrual cycle (follicular: 0.07–2.6 nmol/L; luteal: 0.7 nmol/L).

The cardioprotective effects of estrogen have been know for many years. The incidence of coronary artery disease (CAD) in premenopausal women is considerably less than that of males,[6] however after the menopause, it increases ultimately equaling or even exceeding that of males.[7] Numerous observational studies have shown that postmenopausal women taking hormone replacement therapy (HRT) have a reduced risk of cardiovascular system (CVS) disease.[2,8,9] Although some controversy exists surrounding the lack of an effect in clinical trials to date, a large volume of in vitro and in vivo data suggest that estrogen can retard atherosclerosis and inhibit restenosis. As mentioned, potential side effects of the systemic use of estrogen are limiting. However, local delivery via a drug eluting stent may be a practical alternative for prevention and treatment of restenosis.

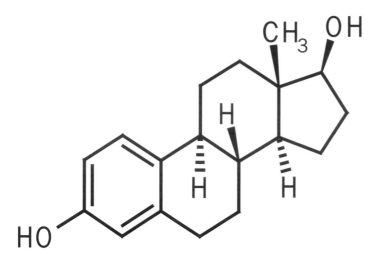

Fig. 54.1 The chemical structure of 17β-estradiol.

MECHANISMS OF ACTION OF ESTROGEN

A number of mechanisms may account for the effects of estrogen on the cardiovascular system. Endogenous and exogenous estrogen is known to improve lipid metabolism in experimental and clinical studies. The use of estrogen in postmenopausal women reduces total and low density lipoprotein (LDL) cholesterol and increases high density lipoprotein (HDL) cholesterol.[10] Estrogens can inhibit LDL oxidation and LDL uptake into the vessel wall, an important step in the atherogenic process.[11] However, the effects of estrogen on lipoproteins do not fully account for the estimated benefit, and other important mechanisms may prevail.[12]

Estrogen retards the atherosclerotic process in animal models.[13–17] Williams' and Clarkson's groups in the 1980s demonstrated the development of less plaque in monkeys fed with high cholesterol diets and treated with estrogen.[15,18] Clinical case-controlled studies also found that estrogen replacement therapy in postmenopausal women was associated with less atherosclerotic lesions at angiography compared with women not taking estrogen.[19–22]

At the cellular level, the typical mode of action of estrogen is via the classical steroid-hormone receptor-binding pathway. Estrogen receptors are present on the cell surfaces of blood vessels of both males and females.[23–25]

Estrogen can directly affect both the structure and function of the blood vessel wall.[3] Endothelial cells that comprise the inner layer of the blood vessel wall provide an important connection between the circulation and the underlying smooth muscle layer. In health, the purpose of the endothelium is to maintain vascular tone and to provide an antithrombotic, antiproliferative, and antiinflammatory surface. Alterations in the structure and function of normal endothelial cells are thought to be an important early step in atherogenesis.[26] Protection of the endothelium may therefore prevent this process. Estrogen has been shown to induce proliferation and migration of endothelial cells in response to injury, thereby maintaining endothelial cell integrity.[27–29] Estrogen has been shown to accelerate regrowth of the endothelium in response to injury,[7,30,31] and attenuate impaired endothelial function in both sexes.[32–34] Estrogen can also have a direct effect on vasomotion in both males and females.[35,36] Most of this effect is mediated via the endothelial cell and L-arginine nitric oxide pathways,[36–39] although some non-nitric oxide and non-endothelial vasodilator responses have also been demonstrated with the use of estrogen.[40,41]

The smooth muscle cell layer is responsible for the normal contraction and dilatation of the arterial wall. Smooth muscle cells also secrete many substances including collagen and elastin that are important for maintaining vascular tone. Abnormal proliferation and migration of smooth muscle cells as well as changes in production of collagen and elastin occur in 'response to injury', such as with atherosclerosis,[26] and following balloon angioplasty.[42] The pathophysiology of restenosis following angioplasty involves neointimal hyperplasia and negative vessel remodeling and neointimal hyperplasia. In stenting, neointimal hyperplasia alone accounts for restenosis.[43]

Many in vitro,[44–46] and in vivo models,[45,47–50] have shown that estrogen can inhibit this growth and migration of smooth muscle cells.[51–55] This effect of estrogen may be mediated by the estrogen-receptor (ER) pathway,[56] and via the improvement of nitric oxide endothelial responses after endothelial cell damage that occurs during angioplasty.

Recent work by Chandrasekar et al. has shown that intracoronary estrogen delivered to the arterial wall can inhibit smooth muscle cell proliferation in the pig following angioplasty.[57] This group randomized 19 juvenile pigs to an intracoronary infusion of 600 μg of 17β-estradiol, infusion of vehicle alone, or no infusion prior to angioplasty. At 1 month, the estradiol-treated group had significantly less intimal proliferation compared to the two control groups (see Figure 54.2). Immunohistochemistry studies also demonstrated significantly less smooth muscle cell proliferative activity compared with control groups.

This same group subsequently demonstrated that this effect of estrogen on the smooth muscle layer is associated with enhanced regrowth of the endothelium and restoration of endothelial function via the expression of endothelial cell Nitric Oxide Synthase (eNOS). This suggests that estrogen works via accelerated repair of the endothelium and subsequently diminishes the smooth muscle cell hyperplastic response.[5] This dual action of protecting the endothelium while preventing smooth muscle cell hyperplasia may prove this naturally occurring hormone as superior to the rapidly increasing library of non-selective 'antiproliferative drugs' that are being coated on stents for the prevention of restenosis.

Furthermore, estrogen may have other additional cardiovascular effects in preventing restenosis and ischemic events. Estrogen has been shown to improve myocardial ischemia,[58] alter adhesion molecule expression,[59] increase intrinsic fibrinolytic activity,[60] and decrease reperfusion injury after myocardial infarction.[61–63] These effects may participate in the reduction in coronary events associated with estrogen, and it is also possible that the first three observations could also benefit restenosis.

DELIVERY

17β-Estradiol from the Bio*divYsio* Matrix LO stent

Recently, drug eluting stents have been tested to prevent restenosis.[64–69] Large clinical trials

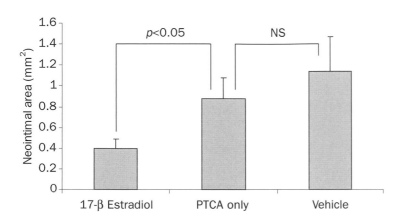

Fig. 54.2 An example of neointimal response after balloon dilatation. Intracoronary injection of 600 mg of 17β-estradiol reduced neointima formation. PTCA, percutaneous transluminal coronary angioplasty; NS, not significant.

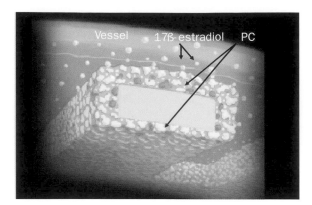

Fig. 54.3 Schematic representation of a double layer phosphorylcholine (PC) polymer coated with 17β-estradiol, showing its release into the vessel wall. 17β-Estradiol has a low molecular weight, is hydrophobic and lipophilic, making it pharmacokinetically suitable for loading on a stent delivery system.

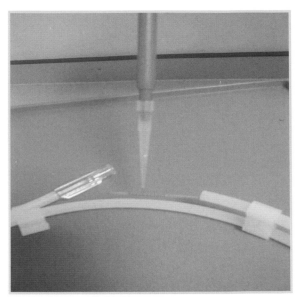

Fig. 54.4 Method of drug impregnation into a Bio*divYsio* stent delivery system. Following immersion of the stent into a solution of 17β-estradiol for 5 minutes, 10 μL of the same solution is then pipetted on to the stent.

using different agents demonstrated high efficacy in the prevention of restenosis.[70–72] However, late stent thrombosis may remain an issue as these agents may also retard regrowth of the endothelium. Indeed, some malapposition has been observed on intravascular ultrasound (IVUS) in some trials, the significance of which remains to be determined.[73] Estrogen with its dual action of accelerating endothelial repair and inhibiting smooth muscle cell proliferation may avoid this problem.

The Bio*divYsio* Matrix LO stent is able to load estradiol by a simple immersion in the drug solution (Figure 54.3). Where higher doses were desired, a dipping and pipetting method was used (Figure 54.4). Table 54.1 summarizes

the dosage obtained for the different stent sizes, and Figure 54.5 shows the release profile of the drug when measured in vitro by simple release into a large volume of phosphate buffered saline (PBS) solution.

A preclinical study in a high injury porcine coronary model using 17β-estradiol eluting PC-coated stents (Abbott/Biocompatibles) demonstrated reduction in neointimal formation by 40% in comparison with control stents (Figure 54.6) and may have a potential benefit in the prevention and treatment of in-stent restenosis.

Table 54.1	Dosage of estradiol per stent size			
Stent size and design	*Surface area (mm²)*	*Avg dosage (μg/stent)*	*Std Dev (μg/stent)*	*Avg dose (mg/mm²)*
11 mm OC	61.56	156	9	2.54
15 mm OC	80.40	204	12	2.54
18 mm OC	99.24	252	15	2.54

OC, open cell.

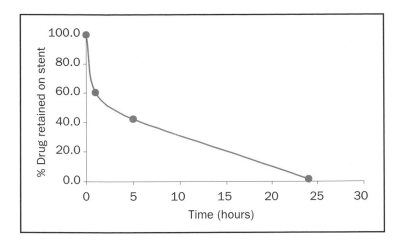

Fig. 54.5 Release kinetics of 17β-estradiol Bio*divYsio* stent delivery system. Complete drug release is achieved at 24 hours. Average dose per stent is 252 ± 15 μg.

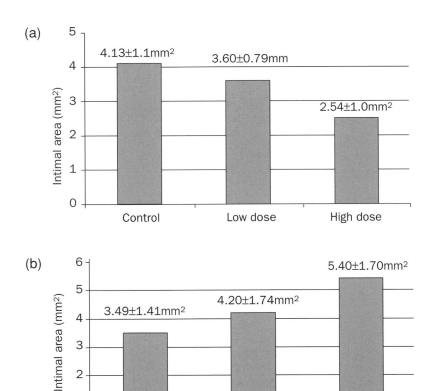

Fig. 54.6 Porcine coronary artery 30 days after severely oversized Bio*divYsio* stent injury. Note the significant difference in neointimal formation (a) between the high dose treated 17β-estradiol and the control group.

EASTER (São Paolo)

  1 center 35 patients each with de novo lesions
  6 month angiographic and IVUS follow-up
  Primary endpoint: Binary restenosis
  Secondary endpoints: MACE, IVUS

EASTER (Italy)

  5 centers, 200 patients randomized trial (100 each arm vs Bio*divYsio*)
  6 month angiographic follow-up
  Primary endpoint: Binary restenosis
  Secondary endpoints: MACE, SAT

Fig. 54.7   The EASTER trial in Brazil and Italy. Quantative coronary angiography by core lab.

CLINICAL STUDIES

There are currently two clinical studies completed with estradiol release from the Bio*divYsio* Matrix LO stent, both called EASTER (Estrogen And Stents To Eliminate Restenosis). The first is a single-center pilot study in Brazil, whilst the second in a randomized trial against the non-drug loaded Bio*divYsio* stent (Figure 54.7).

Study design

The Brazilian study was a prospective trial of patients who were scheduled to undergo elective percutaneous intervention for single, short, de novo lesions in native coronary arteries.

Each patient received one 18 mm stent (3.0–3.5 mm in diameter). All lesions were predilated. Stents were deployed at high pressure (>14 atm) and the need for post dilatation was guided by intravascular ultrasound (IVUS).

All patients received aspirin (325 mg) at least 12 hours before the procedure (and 325 mg/d, indefinitely), and clopidogrel (300 mg at least 6 h prior to stent implantation and 75 mg daily continued for 60 days). All patients underwent angiographic and IVUS follow-up at 6 months. The patients returned for clinical assessment at 30 days, and 6 and 12 months in which physicians were blinded to the angiographic and ultrasonographic data.

Results

The mean age of the patients was 61 ± 12 years. A total of 21 patients (70%) were males. Systemic hypertension was the most frequent coronary risk factor, involving 15 patients (49%), followed by smoking in 10 patients (33%) and dyslipidemia in eight (27%), whereas only three patients (10%) were diabetics. Eleven patients (37%) had a prior history of myocardial infarction (MI). The procedure was successful in all patients. There were no in-hospital events, including no elevation of cardiac enzymes, post procedure. One patient underwent target lesion revascularization at 6 month follow-up due to symptomatic angiographic restenosis. All other patients were asymptomatic at 6 month angiographic follow-up (Table 54.2). There was no stent thrombosis or other MACE (major adverse

Table 54.2 Results of the EASTER trial	
Death	0%
Q-wave MI	0%
TLR	3.3%
Non-TLR (other vessel)	3.3%
Event-free survival	93.4%

MI, myocardial infarction; TLR, target lesion revascularization.

Table 54.3 The EASTER trial: QCA at 6 months (in stent) (*n* = 29)		
	Post intervention	*6 month follow-up*
Reference (mm)	2.76 ± 0.56	
MLD (mm)	2.44 ± 0.52	1.89 ± 0.57
Diameter stenosis (%)	13.6 ± 10.4	28.2 ± 14.8
Late loss (mm)		0.54 ± 0.44
Binary restenosis		(2) 6.6%
Lesion length = 9.1 ± 2.4		

QCA, quantitative coronary angiography; MLD, minimal luminal diameter.

Table 54.4 The EASTER trial: QCA at 6 months (in segment) (*n* = 29)		
	Post intervention	*6 month follow-up*
MLD (mm)	2.04 ± 0.43	1.76 ± 0.56
Diameter stenosis (%)	23.4 ± 10.9	30.5 ± 14.9
Late loss (mm)		0.31 ± 0.38

QCA, quantitative coronary angiography; MLD, minimal luminal diameter.

cardiovascular events including death, MI, stroke or target vessel revascularization) up to 12 month clinical follow-up.

The angiographic results are shown in Tables 54.3 and 54.4. Mean lesion length was 9.1 ± 2.4 mm. Two patients developed in-stent restenosis. One patient with a 60% lesion was asymptomatic with a negative non-invasive stress test and did not undergo repeat revascularization. There was no restenosis at the stent edge segments, and in-segment late loss was only 0.31 mm.

The neointimal hyperplasia volume amounted to 32.3 ± 16.4 mm^3 with a stent volume of 143.7 ± 43.7 mm^3, resulting in a mean neointimal volume obstruction of 23.5 ± 12.5%. No patient had ≥50% volume obstruction by IVUS. There was no evidence of stent malapposition or echo lucent images ('black hole').

CONCLUSIONS

This study represents the first human experience with 17β-estradiol eluting stents for the prevention of restenosis. Clinical outcomes up to 1 year follow-up suggest that the use of 17β-estradiol, PC-coated eluting stents is safe and feasible, with a low incidence of restenosis and without associated local or systemic toxicity. Only one (out of 30) patients required target vessel revascularization. The angiographic and IVUS follow-up results at 6 months demonstrated a low amount of intimal hyperplasia and late loss, which compares favorably with previous studies testing the same PC-coated Bio*divYsio* stents without estradiol (DISTINCT trial) and other bare metal stents.[74] In addition, there was minimal in-segment late loss and no edge restenosis, suggesting an anti-restenotic effect of estradiol despite the suboptimal stent elution.

Whether similar results are reproducible in a larger population with more complex lesion morphology in a randomized trial remains to be tested. At 1 year follow-up, these results appear to be sustained. A second phase of EASTER with preloaded 17b-estradiol eluting stents was recently completed in Italy and results are pending.

SUMMARY

These observations suggest that vasculoprotective agents, such as estradiol, may provide an alternative approach to antiproliferative agents in the prevention of restenosis, and warrant further investigation with a large, randomized, multicenter trial, utilizing more sophisticated stent platforms.

REFERENCES

1. Serruys PW, de Jaegere P, Kiemeneij F, et al. A comparison of balloon-expandable-stent implantation with balloon angioplasty in patients with coronary artery disease. Benestent Study Group. N Engl J Med 1994; 331:489–95.

2. Grady D, Rubin SM, Petitti DB, et al. Hormone therapy to prevent disease and prolong life in postmenopausal women. Ann Intern Med 1992; 117:1016–37.

3. White MM, Zamudio S, Stevens T, et al. Estrogen, progesterone, and vascular reactivity: potential cellular mechanisms. Endocr Rev 1995; 16:739–51.

4. Mendelsohn ME, Karas RH. The protective effects of estrogen on the cardiovascular system. N Engl J Med 1999; 340:1801–11.

5. Chandrasekar B, Nattel S, Tanguay JF. Coronary artery endothelial protection after local delivery of 17beta-estradiol during balloon angioplasty in a procine model: a potential new pharmacologic approach to improve endothelial function. J Am Coll Cardiol 2001; 38:1570–6.

6. Lerner DJ, Kannel WB. Patterns of coronary heart disease morbidity and mortality in the sexes: a 26-year follow-up of the Framingham population. Am Heart J 1986; 111:383–90.

7. White CR, Shelton J, Chen SJ, et al. Estrogen restores endothelial cell function in an experimental model of vascular injury. Circulation 1997; 96:1624–30.

8. Grodstein F, Stampfer MJ, Manson JE, et al. Postmenopausal estrogen and progestin use and the risk of cardiovascular disease. N Engl J Med 1996; 335:453–61.

9. Stampfer MJ, Colditz GA, Willett WC, et al. Postmenopausal estrogen therapy and cardiovascular disease. Ten-year follow-up from the nurses' health study [see comments]. N Engl J Med 1991; 325:756–62.

10. Effects of estrogen or estrogen/progestin regimens on heart disease risk factors in postmenopausal women. The Postmenopausal Estrogen/Progestin Interventions (PEPI) Trial. The Writing Group for the PEPI Trial. JAMA 1995; 273:199–208.

11. Sack MN, Rader DJ, Cannon RO. Oestrogen and inhibition of oxidation of low-density lipoproteins in postmenopausal women. Lancet 1994; 343:269–70.

12. Barrett-Connor E, Bush TL. Estrogen and coronary heart disease in women. JAMA 1991; 265:1861–7.

13. Hough JL, Zilversmit DB. Effect of 17 beta estradiol on aortic cholesterol content and metabolism in cholesterol-fed rabbits. Arteriosclerosis 1986; 6:57–63.

14. Adams MR, Kaplan JR, Manuck SB, et al. Inhibition of coronary artery atherosclerosis by 17-beta estradiol in ovariectomized monkeys. Lack of an effect of added progesterone. Arteriosclerosis 1990; 10:1051–7.

15. Williams JK, Adams MR, Klopfenstein HS. Estrogen modulates responses of atherosclerotic coronary arteries. Circulation 1990; 81:1680–7.

16. Subbiah MT. Effect of estrogens on the activities of cholesteryl ester synthetase and cholesteryl ester hydrolases in pigeon aorta. Steroids 1977; 30:259–65.

17. Haarbo J, Leth-Espensen P, Stender S, et al. Estrogen monotherapy and combined estrogen-progestogen replacement therapy attenuate aortic accumulation of cholesterol in ovariectomized cholesterol-fed rabbits. J Clin Invest 1991; 87:1274–9.

18. Hamm TE, Jr., Kaplan JR, Clarkson TB, et al. Effects of gender and social behavior on the development of coronary artery atherosclerosis in cynomolgus macaques. Atherosclerosis 1983; 48:221–33.

19. Sullivan JM, Vander Zwaag R, Lemp GF, et al. Postmenopausal estrogen use and coronary atherosclerosis. Ann Intern Med 1988; 108:358–63.

20. McFarland KF, Boniface ME, Hornung CA, et al. Risk factors and noncontraceptive estrogen use in women with and without coronary disease. Am Heart J 1989; 117:1209–14.

21. Gruchow HW, Anderson AJ, Barboriak JJ, et al. Postmenopausal use of estrogen and occlusion of coronary arteries. Am Heart J 1988; 115:954–63.

22. Hong MK, Romm PA, Reagan K, et al. Effects of estrogen replacement therapy on serum lipid values and angiographically defined coronary artery disease in postmenopausal women [see comments]. Am J Cardiol 1992; 69:176–8.

23. Lin AL, McGill HC, Jr, Shain SA. Hormone receptors of the baboon cardiovascular system. Biochemical characterization of myocardial cytoplasmic androgen receptors. Circ Res 1981; 49:1010–16.

24. Karas RH, Patterson BL, Mendelsohn ME. Human vascular smooth muscle cells contain functional estrogen receptor. Circulation 1994; 89:1943–50.

25. Losordo DW, Kearney M, Kim EA, et al. Variable expression of the estrogen receptor in normal and atherosclerotic coronary arteries of premenopausal women. Circulation 1994; 89:1501–10.

26. Ross R. The pathogenesis of atherosclerosis: a perspective for the 1990s. Nature 1993; 362:801–5.

27. Kim-Schulze S, McGowan KA, Hubchak SC, et al. Expression of an estrogen receptor by human coronary artery and umbilical vein endothelial cells. Circulation 1996; 94:1402–7.

28. Morales DE, McGowan KA, Grant DS, et al. Estrogen promotes angiogenic activity in human umbilical vein endothelial cells in vitro and in a murine model. Circulation 1995; 91:755–63.

29. Venkov CD, Rankin AB, Vaughan DE. Identification of authentic estrogen receptor in cultured endothelial cells. A potential mechanism for steroid hormone regulation of endothelial function. Circulation 1996; 94:727–33.

30. Krasinski K, Spyridopoulos I, Asahara T, et al. Estradiol accelerates functional endothelial recovery after arterial injury. Circulation 1997; 95:1768–72.

31. Brouchet L, Krust A, Dupont S, et al. Estradiol accelerates reendothelialization in mouse carotid artery through estrogen receptor-alpha but not estrogen receptor-beta. Circulation 2001; 103:423–8.

32. Gilligan DM, Quyyumi AA, Cannon RO. Effects of physiological levels of estrogen on coronary vasomotor function in postmenopausal women. Circulation 1994; 89:2545–51.

33. Gerhard MD, Creager SJ, Roddy M, et al. Long term estradiol therapy improves endothelium-dependent vasodilation of forearm resistance vessels in postmenopausal women. Circulation 1997; 96(suppl):I-420 (abstract).

34. Reis SE, Wu CW, Counihan PJ, et al. Estrogen has an acute beneficial effect on coronary vasoreactivity in men. Circulation 1995; 92:I-249 (abstract).

35. Blumenthal RS, Heldman AW, Brinker JA, et al. Acute effects of conjugated estrogens on coronary blood flow response to acetylcholine in men. Am J Cardiol 1997; 80:1021–4.

36. Guetta V, Quyyumi AA, Prasad A, et al. The role of nitric oxide in coronary vascular effects of estrogen in postmenopausal women. Circulation 1997; 96:2795–801.

37. Kawano H, Motoyama T, Kugiyama K, et al. Menstrual cyclic variation of endothelium-dependent vasodilation of the brachial artery: Possible role of estrogen and nitric oxide. Proc Assoc Am Physicians 1996; 108:473–80.

38. Rosselli M, Imthurn B, Keller PJ, et al. Circulating nitric oxide (nitrite/nitrate) levels in postmenopausal women substituted with 17beta-estradiol and norethisterone acetate. A two-year follow-up study. Hypertension 1995; 25:848–53.

39. Collins P, Shay J, Jiang C, et al. Nitric oxide accounts for dose-dependent estrogen-mediated coronary relaxation after acute estrogen withdrawal. Circulation 1994; 90:1964–8.

40. Thompson LP, Weiner CP. Long-term estradiol replacement decreases contractility of guinea pig coronary arteries to the thromboxane mimetic U46619. Circulation 1997; 95:709–14.

41. Sullivan J, Sudhir K, Ko E, et al. Physiological concentrations of estradiol attenuate endothelin-1-induced coronary vasoconstriction in vivo. Circulation 1997; 96:3626–32.

42. Hanke H, Strohshneider T, Oberhoff M, et al. Time course of smooth muscle cell proliferation in the intima and media of arteries following experimental angioplasty. Circulation 1990; 67:651–9.

43. Mintz GS, Popma JJ, Hong MK, et al. Intravascular ultrasound to discern device-specific effects and mechanisms of restenosis. Am J Cardiol 1996; 78:18–22.

44. Bhalla RC, Toth KF, Bhatty RA, et al. Estrogen reduces proliferation and agonist-induced calcium increase in coronary artery smooth muscle cells. Am J Physiol 1997; 272:H1996–2003.

45. Hanke H, Hanke S, Finking G, et al. Different effects of estrogen and progesterone on experimental atherosclerosis in female versus male rabbits. Quantification of cellular proliferation by bromodeoxyuridine. Circulation 1996; 94:175–81.

46. Morey AK, Pedram A, Razandi M, et al. Estrogen and progesterone inhibit vascular smooth muscle proliferation. Endocrinology 1997; 138:3330–9.

47. Sullivan TR, Jr, Karas RH, Aronovitz M, et al. Estrogen inhibits the response-to-injury in a mouse carotid artery model. J Clin Invest 1995; 96:2482–8.

48. Iafrati MD, Karas RH, Aronovitz M, et al. Estrogen inhibits the vascular injury response in estrogen receptor alpha-deficient mice. Nat Med 1997; 3:545–8.

49. Foegh ML, Zhao Y, Farhat M, et al. Oestradiol inhibition of vascular myointimal proliferation following immune, chemical and mechanical injury. Ciba Found Symp 1995; 191:139–45 (discussion 145–9).

50. Akishita M, Ouchi Y, Miyoshi H, et al. Estrogen inhibits cuff-induced intimal thickening of rat femoral artery: effects on migration and proliferation of vascular smooth muscle cells. Atherosclerosis 1997; 130:1–10.

51. Dai-Do D, Espinosa E, Liu G, et al. 17beta-estradiol inhibits proliferation and migration of human vascular smooth muscle cells:

similar effects in cells from postmenopausal females and in males. Cardiovasc Res 1996; 32:980–5.

52. Chen SJ, Li H, Durand J, et al. Estrogen reduces myointimal proliferation after balloon injury of rat carotid artery. Circulation 1996; 93:577–84.

53. Oparil S, Chen SJ, Chen YF, et al. Estrogen attenuates the adventitial contribution to neointima formation in injured rat carotid arteries. Cardiovasc Res 1999; 44:608–14.

54. Bakir S, Mori T, Durand J, et al. Estrogen-induced vasoprotection is estrogen receptor dependent: evidence from the balloon-injured rat carotid artery model. Circulation 2000; 101:2342–4.

55. Mori T, Durand J, Chen Y, et al. Effects of short-term estrogen treatment on the neointimal response to balloon injury of rat carotid artery. Am J Cardiol 2000; 85:1276–9.

56. Spyridopoulos I, Sullivan AB, Kearney M, et al. Estrogen-receptor-mediated inhibition of human endothelial cell apoptosis. Estradiol as a survival factor. Circulation 1997; 95:1505–14.

57. Chandrasekar B, Tanguay JF. Local delivery of 17-beta-estradiol decreases neointimal hyperplasia after coronary angioplasty in a porcine model. J Am Coll Cardiol 2000; 36:1972–8.

58. Rosano GMC, Caixeta AM, Arie S, et al. Acute anti-ischemic effect of estradiol 17 beta in menopausal women with coronary artery disease. Circulation 1996; 94(suppl):I-19 (abstract).

59. Cid MC, Kleinman HK, Grant DS, et al. Estradiol enhances leukocyte binding to tumor necrosis factor (TNF)-stimulated endothelial cells via an increase in TNF-induced adhesion molecules E-selectin, intercellular adhesion molecule type 1, and vascular cell adhesion molecule type 1. J Clin Invest 1994; 93:17–25.

60. Koh KK, Mincemoyer R, Bui MN, et al. Effects of hormone-replacement therapy on fibrinolysis in postmenopausal women. N Engl J Med 1997; 336:683–90.

61. Kim YD, Chen B, Beauregard J, et al. 17beta-Estradiol prevents dysfunction of canine coronary endothelium and myocardium and reperfusion arrhythmias after brief ischemia/reperfusion. Circulation 1996; 94:2901–8.

62. Delyani JA, Murohara T, Nossuli TO, et al. Protection from myocardial reperfusion injury

by acute administration of 17beta-estradiol. J Mol Cell Cardiol 1996; 28:1001–8.

63. Kolodgie FD, Farb A, Litovsky SH, et al. Myocardial protection of contractile function after global ischemia by physiologic estrogen replacement in the ovariectomized rat. J Mol Cell Cardiol 1997; 29:2403–14.

64. Park SJ, Shim WH, Ho DS, et al. The clinical effectiveness of Paclitaxel-coated coronary stents for the reduction of restenosis in the ASPECT Trial. Circulation 2001; 104:II-464.

65. Bailey SR. Local drug delivery: current applications. Prog Cardiovasc Dis 1997; 40:183–204.

66. Camenzind E, Kutryk MJ, Serruys PW. Use of locally delivered conventional drug therapies. Semin Interv Cardiol 1996; 1:67–76.

67. De Scheerder I, Wilczek K, Van Dorpe J, et al. Local angiopeptin delivery using coated stents reduces neointimal proliferation in overstretched porcine coronary arteries. J Invasive Cardiol 1996; 8:215–22.

68. Sousa JE, Costa MA, Abizaid A, et al. Lack of neointimal proliferation after human implantation of Sirolimus-coated stents in human coronary arteries: A quantitative coronary angiography and three-dimensional intravascular ultrasound study. Circulation 2000; 102:r54–r57.

69. Herdeg C, Oberhoff M, Baumbach A, et al. Local paclitaxel delivery for the prevention of restenosis: biological effects and efficacy in vivo. J Am Coll Cardiol 2000; 35:1969–76.

70. Morice MC, Serruys PW, Sousa JE, et al. A randomized comparision of a sirolimus-eluting stent with a standard stent for coronary revascularization. N Engl J Med 2002; 345:1773–80.

71. Moses JW, Leon MB, Popma JJ, et al. Sirolimus-eluting stents versus standard stents in patients with stenosis in a native coronary artery. N Engl J Med 2003; 349:1315–23.

72. Stone GW, Ellis SG, Cox DA, et al. A polymer-based, paclitaxel-eluting stent in patients with coronary artery disease. New Engl J Med 2004; 350:221–31.

73. Sousa JE, Morice MC, Serruys PW, et al. The RAVEL Study: A randomized study with the Sirolimus coated BX velocity balloon-expandable stent in the treatment of patients with de novo native coronary artery lesions. Circulation 2001; 104:II-463 (abstract).

74. Costa MA, Sabate M, Kay IP, et al. Three-dimensional intravascular ultrasonic volumetric quantification of stent recoil and neointimal formation of two new generation tubular stents. Am J Cardiol 2000; 85:135–9.

55

Batimastat: mode of action, preclinical, and clinical studies

Ivan De Scheerder, Xiaoshun Liu, Bernard Chevalier, Guy LeClerc, and Anthony Collias

Cell migration: a target for the control of restenosis • **The matrix metalloproteinases (MMPs)**
• **The role of MMPs in restenosis** • **Batimastat: mode of action** • **Preclinical studies**
• **Clinical studies** • **Results** • **Comparison with the DISTINCT trial** • **Conclusions**
• **Summary**

CELL MIGRATION: A TARGET FOR THE CONTROL OF RESTENOSIS

It has long been considered that restenosis following balloon angioplasty is the result of the formation of excessive neointima. More recently, both animal and human studies have shown that constrictive arterial remodeling is the major determinant of restenosis after balloon angioplasty, and it is responsible for up to 70% of late lumen loss. Arterial remodeling in this context means a structural change of the vessel wall, where reorganization of cells and matrix at sites of injury leads to decreased lumen diameter. At the heart of this remodeling process is the degradation of the extracellular matrix by a group of enzymes known as matrix metalloproteinases (MMPs), secreted predominately by vascular smooth muscle cells (VSMCs) but also macrophages and monocytes.

THE MATRIX METALLOPROTEINASES (MMPs)

The MMPs are a family of zinc-dependent neutral endopeptidases that share structural domains but differ in substrate specificity, cellular sources, and inductivity (see Table 55.1). All the MMPs are important for the remodelling of the extracellular matrix and share the following functional features: (1) they degrade extracellular matrix components, including fibronectin, collagen, elastin, proteoglycans, and laminin; (2) they are secreted in a latent proform and require activation for proteolytic activity; (3) they contain zinc at their active site and they need calcium for stability; (4) they function at neutral pH; and (5) they are inhibited by specific tissue inhibitors of metalloproteinases (TIMPs).

The activity of the MMPs is controlled at the transcriptional level, by activation of the latent proenzymes, and by their endogenous inhibitors, the TIMPs. Whilst the low level expression of most MMPs is generally found in normal adult tissue, it is upregulated during certain physiological and pathological remodeling processes. Induction or stimulation at transcriptional level is mediated by a variety of inflammatory cytokines, hormones, and growth factors, such as (interleukin) IL-1, IL-6,

Table 55.1   Matrix metalloproteinase (MMP) family

Enzyme	MMP classification	Substrate(s)
Collagenases		
Interstitial collagenase	MMP-1	Collagen types I, II, III, VII, and X, gelatin, entactin, aggrecan
Neutrophil collagenase	MMP-8	Collagen types I, II, and III, aggrecan
Collagenase-3	MMP-13	Collagen types I, II, and III, gelatin, fibronectin, laminins, tenascin
Collagenase-4	MMP-18	Not known
Gelatinases		
Gelatinase A	MMP-2	Collagen types I, IV, V, and X, fibronectin, laminins, aggrecan, tenascin-C, vitronectin
Gelatinase B	MMP-9	Collagen types IV, V, and XIV, aggrecan, elastin, entactin, vitronectin
Stromelysins		
Stromelysin 1	MMP-3	Collagen types III, IV, IX, and X, gelatin, fibronectin, laminins, tenascin-C, vitronectin
Stromelysin 2	MMP-10	Collagen IV, fibronectin, aggrecan
Stromelysin 3	MMP-11	Collagen IV, fibronectin, aggrecan, laminins, gelatin
Membrane-type (MT-MMPs)		
MT1-MMP	MMP-14	Collagen types I, II, and III, fibronectin, laminins, vitronectin, proteoglycans; activates proMMP-2 and proMMP-13
MT2-MMP	MMP-15	Activates proMMP-2
MT3-MMP	MMP-16	Activates proMMP-2
MT4-MMP	MMP-17	Not known
MT5-MMP	MMP-24	Activates proMMP-2
MT6-MMP	MMP-25	Not known
Non-classified MMPs		
Matrilysins	MMP-7	Gelatin, fibronectin, laminins, elastin, collagen IV, vitronectin, tenascin-C, aggrecan
Metalloelastase	MMP-12	Elastin
Unnamed	MMP-19	Not known
Enamelysin	MMP-20	Aggrecan
	MMP-23	Not known
Endometase	MMP-26	Not known

Reproduced from Creemers EE, et al. Circ Res 2001; 89(3):201–10.

tumor necrosis factor (TNF)-α, epidermal growth factor (EGF), platelet-derived growth factor (PDGF), basic fibroblast growth factor (bFGF), and CD40. Binding of these stimulatory ligands to their receptors triggers a cascade of intracellular reactions that are mediated through at least three different classes of mitogen-activated protein (MAP) kinases: extracellular signal-regulated kinase, stress activated protein kinase/Jun N-terminal kinases and p38. Activation of these kinases culminates in the activation of a nuclear AP-1 transcription factor, which binds to the AP-1 cis element and activates the transcription of corresponding MMP gene. Other factors, such as corticosteroids, retinoic acid, heparin, and IL-4, have been demonstrated to inhibit MMP gene expression.[1]

THE ROLE OF MMPs IN RESTENOSIS

Although the precise role of MMPs in inducing VSMC migration is not fully understood, there are multiple proposed mechanisms of action, which include the removal of physical restraints by the severing of cell–matrix contacts via integrins or cell–cell contacts via adherins. Additionally, contact with interstitial matrix components may be facilitated and migration may be stimulated through exposure of cryptic extracellular matrix sites, production of extracellular matrix fragments and the release of matrix or cell-bound growth factors.[2] Other recent studies also demonstrate that MMP activity is required for lymphocyte transmigration across endothelial venules into lymph nodes, providing some evidence for the concept that MMPs are important players in transendothelial migration.[3]

Coronary angioplasty inevitably produces a mechanical injury to the vessel. Damage to the endothelia is thought to trigger phenotypic modulation of medial VSMCs, changing them from a normal contractile (differentiated) phenotype to a synthetic (proliferative) state. To enable VSMC migration, remodeling of the basement membrane and the interstitial collagenous matrix that maintains VSMCs in a quiescent state must occur. Intimal thickening

ensues because of the migration of medial VSMCs to the intima, where they proliferate and secrete extracellular matrix proteins. This is supported by studies on aortic explants,[4] in rat carotid arteries,[5] and in human saphenous vein,[2] which have shown that mechanical injury stimulates the production of MMPs. More specifically, remodeling following injury in the rat carotid artery model has been shown to be associated with increased expression of the gelatinases MMP-9 and MMP-2, and subsequently with increased migration and proliferation of VSMCs.[6] Furthermore, the response to arterial balloon injury involves MMP-dependent VSMC migration and can be attenuated by TIMP-I expression. In vivo arterial gene transfer of TIMP-I attenuates neointimal hyperplasia after vascular injury, with a marked reduction in VSMC migration but without altering proliferation.[7] These results confirm that the balance of MMPs/TIMPs is important, and support the supposition that targeting it can be a powerful approach to control the migratory capabilities of the cells and, consequently, control restenosis following balloon angioplasty and stenting.

BATIMASTAT: MODE OF ACTION

Batimastat (4-N-hydroxyamino)-2R-isobutyl-3s-(thiopen-2-ylthiomethyl)-succinyl-l-phenylalanin-n-methylamide, was originally developed by British Biotech Pharmaceuticals as a broad-spectrum metalloproteinase inhibitor (MMPI). It is a low molecular weight (478) peptide mimetic comprised of the peptide residues found on one side of a principal cleavage site in type I collagen, containing a hydroxamate group (Figure 55.1). This group chelates a zinc atom in the active site of the MMP, inhibiting the enzyme reversibly.

The three classes of MMP (collagenases, stromelysins, and gelatinases) are potently inhibited by batimastat, with an IC_{50} in the low nanomolar range. It shows no activity against unrelated metalloproteinases, such as enkephalinase or angiotensin-converting enzyme. These enzymes are critical in matrix degradation and invasion by cancer cells (development of cancer

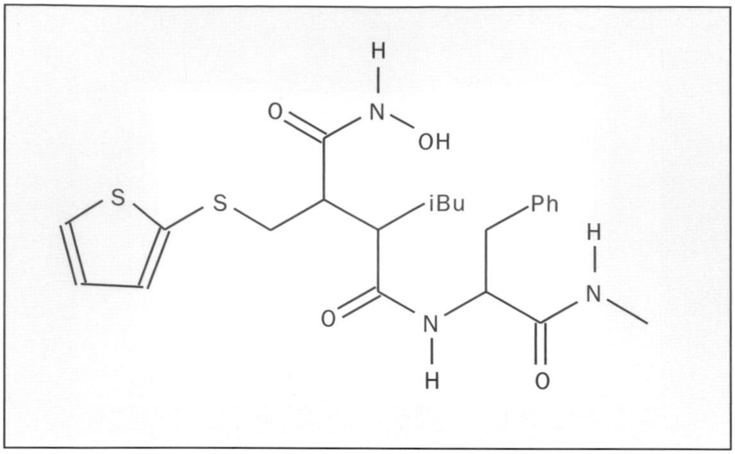

Fig. 55.1   The chemical structure of batimastat.

metastasis), in the process of arterial remodeling after injury, in cytokine receptor shedding, and in the development of restenosis after coronary angioplasty.

Batimastat has been shown to suppress injury-induced phosphorylation of MAP kinase ERK1/ERK2, which is an important signaling pathway of the injury-induced activation of the cells, both restraining the phenotypic modulation and suppressing injury-induced DNA synthesis and migration in VSMC cultures.[8] In an in vitro model of baboon aortic medial explants, batimastat was able to inhibit basal cell migration,[9] and more specifically in a rat carotid model, inhibited intimal thickening after balloon injury by decreasing VSMC migration and proliferation.[10] A study in Yucatán minipigs showed batimastat significantly reduced late lumen loss after balloon angioplasty by inhibition of constrictive arterial remodeling.[11] In studies with other MMPIs, marimastat was also shown to affect the arterial wall following balloon angioplasty in favor of neutral and expansive remodeling,[12] whilst in a double balloon injury model in rabbits, the broad-spectrum MMPI GM6001 was shown to reduce intimal cross-sectional area and collagen content by 40% in stented arteries.[13] These data help support the rationale for the use of a batimastat-loaded stent to help reduce the restenotic response of the artery after stenting.

PRECLINICAL STUDIES

A total of five animal studies, ranging from 5 days to 3 months implantation, have been conducted with the batimastat-loaded Bio*div*Ysio stent. A summary of the preclinical studies is shown in Table 55.2. In all the animal studies, batimastat was loaded on either the Bio*div*Ysio AS or OC stents since these stents are more applicable to the vessel size of the selected animal models.

In all cases stent implantation over-sizing (i.e. balloon/artery ratio >1) was performed to cause an injury to the artery wall that would result in neointimal formation resembling that occurring in stented human coronary arteries. Angiographic data were obtained before and just after implantation of the stent and were compared to that obtained at the end of each study. In some studies, the performance of the batimastat doses was evaluated by histological measurement of neointimal hyperplasia formation and lumen area changes and compared to the performance of the non-drug loaded stents as a control. Appropriate antiplatelet therapy was administered according to the type of study performed.

Short-term studies

The 5 day farm swine study evaluated the subacute safety and re-endothelialization of two

Table 55.2 Preclinical studies: summary

Study	Implantation period	Stent	Total dose/μg batimastat per mm^2 of stent (number of stents implanted)				Animal
			Control	<CTD[b]	CTD[a]	>CTD[c]	
Short term	5 day	Preloaded 15 mm OC stent	0 (6)		0.30 (7)	1.39 (7)	10 farm swine
	1 mth	Non preloaded OC stent	0 (8)		0.30 (8)	1.09 (8)	12 farm swine
	1 mth	Preloaded AS stent	0 (10)		0.30 (10)		10 farm swine
Short & long term	1 & 3 mths	Preloaded AS stent	0 (15)	0.03 (17)	0.30 (30)		26 Yucatán minipigs
Pharmacokinetic	24 h and 1 mth	Preloaded OC stent	0.37 (12) (1 μCi radiolabeled batimastat ^{14}C per stent)				9 New Zealand white rabbits

CTD (clinical trial dose) specification established for larger vessel clinical trials (i.e. BRILLIANT EU) and the actual measured dose for the animal study dose is within this CTD range.

[a] The manufacturing range during the preparation of these stents was 0.30 μg batimastat per mm^2 of stent surface area.

[b] These samples were produced using a less concentrated drug solution to achieve a lower than clinical trial dose.

[c] These samples were prepared as for CTD stents; additional batimastat was added by pipette to increase the dose.

doses of batimastat 0.30 ± 0.13 μg per mm² (CTD) and 1.43 ± 0.20 μg per mm² (>CTD) delivered from the 15 mm Bio*divYsio* batimastat OC stent compared to Bio*divYsio* PC-coated OC stents without batimastat (control). All stents were implanted without problems and there were no deaths during the 5 day follow-up period. All animals were sacrificed at 5 days. The scanning electron micrography (SEM) analysis was performed on all arteries from a total of three animals selected randomly. The rate and extent of endothelialization of the stent struts and the presence of any cellular/biological debris within the stented segment was assessed, and the results showed that batimastat did not interfere with the process of stent endothelialization, the degree of cell coverage being similar to that of the control stent. A continuous and confluent layer of endothelial cells was observed on the inner surface of the stented vessel segments for all stents including control stents. The high degree of endothelial cell coverage over the inner surface of the vessel in each of these cases is consistent with previous observations made by Whelan et al.[14] Some white cells and mural thrombus were also observed (Figure 55.2). It can be

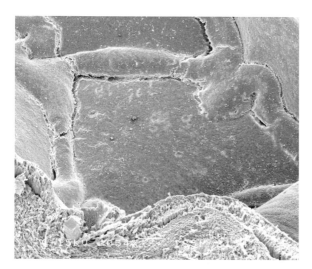

Fig. 55.2 Scanning electron micrograph (SEM) showing continuous endothelial cell coverage of the stent struts after 5-day implantation. Controlled trial dose (CTD) Bio*divYsio* batimastat stent.

concluded that batimastat loaded on to the Bio*divYsio* stent at the CTD or >CTD dose does not affect the in vivo endothelialization process at 5 days in comparison to the control.

Off-line QCA analysis of all stented vessel segments was also performed, and indicated that there were no stent thromboses nor significant differences in percentage stenosis between the control group (3.8%) versus CTD (4.8%) and >CTD (4.4%). The fact that both the controls and the batimastat-loaded stents showed a low stenosis rate demonstrates that the processes of migration, proliferation and remodeling were in their early stages (Figure 55. 3).[15]

The 1 month farm swine studies evaluated safety following implantation of two doses of batimastat loaded on the 18 mm Bio*divYsio* stent in comparison to control stent without batimastat. Two batimastat doses were evaluated as described in Table 55.2. No deaths occurred during the implantation procedure and no subacute death or stent thrombosis was observed during the follow-up period. Histological examination confirmed that all the vessels were patent, without the presence of thrombus in the vessel lumen. All sections showed stent struts to be completely covered, leading to a smooth endoluminal surface. There was no excessive inflammatory response at stent struts in Bio*divYsio* batimastat-treated sections compared to the control sections. Medial and adventitial layers appeared similar in all three groups. The perivascular nerve fibers, the adipose tissue, and adjacent myocardium appeared normal in control and Bio*divYsio* batimastat-treated sections. Therefore, these studies demonstrated that the Bio*divYsio* batimastat stent at CTD and >CTD was well tolerated up to 28 days.

The study of the pharmacokinetics of release of batimastat from the Bio*divYsio* batimastat stent was initiated to investigate the deposition of the drug from the stent in the arterial wall and major organs. These studies used the well established New Zealand white rabbit model where ¹⁴C batimastat-loaded Bio*divYsio* OC stents, at a dose of 0.37 μg per mm², were placed in the left and right iliac arteries and

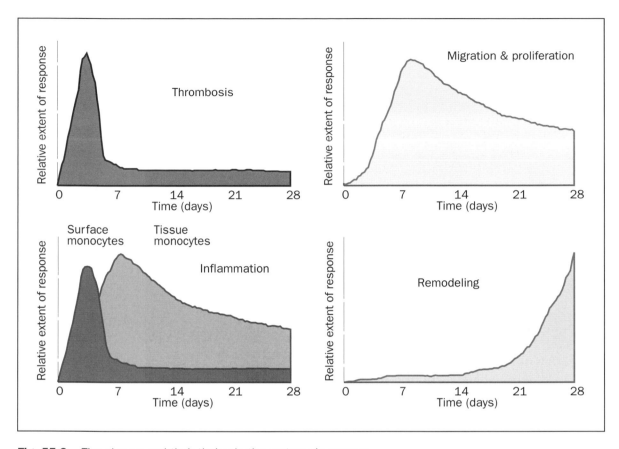

Fig. 55.3 The phases and their timing in the restenosis process.

levels of batimastat deposited in the iliac arteries and solid organs were measured 28 days after stent implantation. A total of 18 Bio*divYsio* batimastat OC stents were implanted in nine rabbits. Three of the nine rabbits were implanted for only 1 day while the remaining six rabbits were implanted for 28 days. The study demonstrated the reproducible release and deposition of drug from the Bio*divYsio* batimastat stent. Release was reproducible at all time points and was first order. Within the first 24 hours, 72.9% ± 4.0% was released and the bulk of loaded drug (94%) was eluted 28 days post implantation. Drug released from each stent is primarily localized to the 15 mm long stented region, and to a lesser degree the adjacent adventitia and regions immediately proximal and distal to the stent. The data follow the expected patterns of release and deposition and indicate that there is unlikely to

be a long-term issue of residual drug within the artery wall after release has terminated. Very little of the drug was found in the distal organs (brain, liver, kidney, spleen, carotid artery, gonad, heart, lung, and intestine), the numbers obtained being so low they could be considered as undetectable.

Long-term studies

The long-term (3-month) safety study was carried out on Yucatán minipigs using two doses of batimastat loaded on the 15 mm Bio*divYsio* stent in comparison to a control stent without batimastat, as outlined in Table 55.2. The evaluation criteria included vessel lumen area, neointimal thickness and area, absence/presence of thrombus, angiographic percentage stenosis, and lumen loss. The quantitative coronary angiography

Table 55.3   Quantitative coronary angiography (QCA) and histology analysis at 3 months

	Control	<CTD	CTD
Injury score	1.6	1.5	1.3
In-stent stenosis (%)	34.10	27.20	22.50
Vessel area (mm^2)	9.4	9.9	9.4
Lumen area (mm^2)	3.2	3.3	3.6
Neointimal area (mm^2)	3.9	3.9	3.3
Intimal/medial ratio	0.74	0.72	0.74
Thrombus present	No	No	No

CTD, clinical trial dose.

(QCA) and histological analysis at 3 months follow-up are presented in Table 55.3.

At 3 months, the stenosis was reduced by 20% and 34% in the <CTD and CTD dose, respectively. These data show a trend in favor of the treatment groups. Histopathology evaluation showed that there were no adverse effects of the drug-loaded stent compared to the controls, and no deleterious phenomenon could be attributed to the drug tested. The intensity of fibrosis, hemorrhages and inflammatory cell infiltration were not significantly different from the control group at 3 months.

CLINICAL STUDIES

One clinical registry has been performed to evaluate the safety of the Bio*divYsio* batimastat stent in countries outside the United States.

The BRILLIANT-EU (Batimastat – BB94 – anti-Restenosis trIaL utiLizIng the Bio*divYsio* locAl drug delivery PC-steNT) was a multicenter, prospective, non-controlled, European-based single pilot trial performed at eight interventional cardiovascular sites in Belgium, 10 sites in France, and two sites in the Netherlands (Table 55.4). The primary purpose of this multicenter, prospective registry was to evaluate the acute safety and effectiveness of the Bio*divYsio* batimastat OC stent (2.0 μg bati-

mastat per mm^2 of stent surface area) in patients with a single, de novo lesion ≤25.0 mm in length, requiring endovascular stenting following percutaneous transluminal coronary angioplasty (PTCA). The primary objective was to evaluate the occurrence of MACE (death, recurrent myocardial infarction or clinically driven target lesion revascularization) 30 days post procedure. The secondary objectives were to evaluate the binary restenosis, incidence of (sub)acute stent thrombosis at 30 day follow-up, MACE at 6 and 12 months, and the QCA endpoints at 6 months. This study was designed to allow a comparison with the patient population and the results of a larger randomized DISTINCT (Bio*divYsio* stent in controlled clinical trial) study previously conducted in the United States.

Study design

A total of 173 (134 male and 39 female) symptomatic patients with stable angina pectoris (Canadian Cardiovascular Society 1, 2, 3 or 4) or unstable angina pectoris with documented ischemia (Braunwald Class IB-C, IIB-C or IIIB-C) or documented ischemia with a single de novo lesion in a coronary artery suitable for treatment with a single Bio*divYsio* DD OC coated coronary stent preloaded with batimastat

Table 55.4 Structure of the BRILLIANT-EU study	
Purpose	To evaluate the acute safety and effectiveness of the Bio*divYsio* batimastat stent
Structure	Multicenter, prospective, non-controlled study
Study devices	11 mm, 15 mm, 18 mm, 22 mm, and 28 mm Bio*divYsio* batimastat stents in diameters 3.0 mm, 3.5 mm, and 4.0 mm
Batimastat dose	0.30 µg batimastat per mm^2
Enrollment	European study 150 patients
Clinical sites	22 sites in France, Belgium, and The Netherlands
Clinical follow-up	All patients will undergo clinical follow-up at 30 days, 6, and 12 months post procedure
Angiographic follow-up	Patients will undergo angiographic follow-up at 6 months post procedure
Primary endpoint	MACE (death, recurrent myocardial infarction or clinically driven target lesion revascularization) at 30 days
Secondary endpoints	Binary restenosis at 6 months follow-up (defined as ≥50% diameter stenosis by QCA). Quantitative coronary angiography endpoints including late loss, loss index, late absolute MLD at 6 month incidence of (sub)acute stent thrombosis (SAT) to 30 day follow-up MACE at 6 months and 12 months
Principal investigators	Dr de Scheerder, UH Gasthuisberg, Leuven Dr Chevalier, Centre Cardiologique du Nord, Paris

of 11 mm, 15 mm, 18 mm, 22 mm or 28 mm length by 3.0 mm, 3.5 mm or 4.0 mm diameter were included in the study, providing they met the selection criteria.

All patients were required to agree to a 6 month clinical and angiographic follow-up and had to be over 18 years old. The reference vessel diameter of the treated lesion was visually estimated >2.75 mm and <3.5 mm in diameter, target lesion stenosis >50% and <100%. Non-calcified lesions, de novo lesions within a native coronary artery, ≤25 mm long, requiring one appropriately sized Bio*divYsio* batimastat OC stent were included. The following patient categories were excluded from the study: patients with ostial and bifurcation lesions, left ventricular ejection fraction <30%, known hypersensitivity or contraindication to aspirin or stainless steel, or a sensitivity to contrast dye, allergy to heparin or ticlopidine.

The ethics committee at each center approved the protocol. The consent form or modification based on local independent ethics committee recommendations was completed by all enrolled subjects and signed by the operating physician.

Medication

All patients were premedicated with acetyl salicylic acid (aspirin) (160 mg/d) orally. Oral clopidogrel 300 mg or ticlopidine 500 mg was given before PTCA. Heparin (100 U/kg) after insertion of the arterial sheath was weight adjusted and administered as needed to maintain an activated clotting time (ACT) of approximately 250–300 sec (if a glycoprotein IIb/IIIa blocker is used, an ACT of 150–200 sec suffices). Intracoronary nitroglycerin 50–200 µg was administered immediately prior to baseline angiography, post-stent deployment, and after final postdilatation angiography. Aspirin was continued indefinitely and clopidogrel 75 mg or ticlopidine (250 mg/d) was prescribed for 28 days in all cases.

Quantitative coronary angiographic analysis (QCA)

Preprocedural, postprocedural and at 6 month follow-up angiography was performed in at least two orthogonal projections after intracoronary injection of nitrates. Quantitative analyses were performed by an independent core laboratory (Brigham and Women's, Boston, MA). The distal end of the guiding catheter was used for calibration in each analyzed projection. The in-lesion segment was defined as the stent plus 5 mm proximal and 5 mm distal to the edge or the nearest branch. Reference vessel diameter (RVD), minimal luminal diameter (MLD), and degree of stenosis (as percentage of diameter) were measured before dilatation, at the end of the procedure, and at a 6 month follow-up. In-stent and in-lesion restenosis were defined as >50% diameter stenosis at follow-up, located within the stent and target lesion, respectively. Late loss was defined as MLD after the procedure minus MLD at follow-up.

Clinical follow-up

All patients were asked to return to the investigative site for a clinical visit four weeks ± one week post procedure to repeat clinical labs and monitor acute clinical events. All patients were contacted by telephone by the investigative site at three months ± 1 week for a safety evaluation. At 6 months post procedure, all subjects were required to return to the investigative site for a repeat coronary angiography whether they were experiencing symptoms or not. If a patient had a positive exercise stress test at any time up to and including the required follow-up, a repeat angiogram was performed.

Definitions and statistics

Safety Analysis patient set was defined as all patients who received the Bio*divYsio* batimas-

tat OC stent. Per Protocol Analysis patient set was defined as all patients in the Safety Analysis set who did not deviate from the protocol. The main analyses were performed on the basis of intention-to-treat principle. Categorical variables were summarized using counts and percentages. Categorical variables were compared by using the Fisher exact t-test. Continuous variables were summarized using means, standard deviations, minimum and maximum and median for variables not showing a normal distribution. For comparison of subgroups, the unpaired two-tailed Student's t-test was used. Results were considered statistically significant at $p<0.05$.

RESULTS

Demographic characteristics, procedural and in-hospital outcomes

The baseline clinical and angiographic characteristics are summarized in Table 55.5. In total, 173 patients were enrolled in the study and had at least one study stent implanted. Nine patients (5%) were excluded from the Per Protocol Analysis, among which six violated the inclusion/exclusion criteria for the study and four (one violated the inclusion/exclusion) had a second stent placed in the study vessel. The mean age was 61 with a range from 34 to 83 years old. Hypercholesterolemia (62%), hypertension (46%), and family coronary history (43%) were the most frequently reported risk factors. The majority of patients (69%) had one diseased vessel and the mean left ventricular ejection fraction was 67%. Fifty-nine patients (34%) had experienced a previous MI, 22 patients (13%) had undergone previous PTCA and four patients (2%) had undergone previous CABG. At preprocedural evaluation, 100 patients (58%) had unstable angina pectoris (including class 4), 56 patients (32%) patients had stable angina (Class 1,2,3), and 17 patients (10%) had silent ischemia.

The most frequent location of the target lesion was the mid left anterior descending vessel (39 patients, 23%), proximal left descending vessel (37 patients, 21%), and mid right coronary artery (35 patients, 20%). Mean

Table 55.4 Baseline clinical and lesion characteristics

	BRILLIANT-EU (n = 173) (%)	DISTINCT (n = 313) (%)
Male	77	71
Mean age (years)	60.6 ± 10.6 (34–83)	60.2 ± 10.3
Risk factors		
Family history of coronary heart disease (CHD)	43	60
Hypercholesterolemia	62	61
Hypertension	46	53
Peripheral vascular disease	11	6
Previous stroke	6	4
Diabetes	13	21
Current smokers	32	25
History of:		
Previous myocardial infarction (MI)	34	37
Previous percutaneous transluminal coronary angioplasty (PTCA)	13	18
Previous coronary artery bypass graft (CABG)	2	4
Angina status		
Stable angina	36	55
Unstable angina	54	44
Silent ischemia	10	7
Number of diseased vessels		
1 vessel	69	60
2 vessels	21	22
3 vessels or more	10	18
Target vessels		
LAD	45	46
RCA	35	32
LCX	18	22
Ramus	2	0
Lesion length (mm)	11.5 ± 5.0 (4–25)	14.44 ± 6.12*

Values are mean ± SD or n (%); LAD, left anterior descending artery; RCA, right coronary artery; LCX, left circumflex artery.
[a]According to (American College of Cardiology/American Heart Association ACC/AHA) classification. *$p<0.001$.

lesion length was 11.5 ± 5.0 mm (range: 4–25 mm). The most commonly recorded target lesion classification was type B1 (86 patients, 50%).

The majority of patients received either a 15 mm stent (71 patients, 41%), an 18 mm stent (38 patients, 22%) or an 11 mm stent (32 patients, 18%). Mean balloon diameter and length were 3.3 mm and 16.6 mm, respectively. Mean maximum balloon inflation pressure was 13.3 atm. Delivery balloon rupture occurred in four patients (2%) during the stent placement. The stent was adequately positioned in 170 patients (98%). Three patients (2%) experienced a residual dissection after stent placement. Two patients (1%) experienced three postprocedural complications in-hospital. One experienced a pseudoaneurysm or arteriovenous fistula at arterial access site requiring surgery and blood loss requiring transfusion. One patient experienced hypotension.

There were no MACE resulting from the angioplasty or stenting procedure. Two non Q-wave MI occurred postprocedural during hospitalization. Technical device success, defined as intended stent successfully implanted as the first stent, was achieved in 162 patients (99%). Clinical device success, defined as technical device success in the absence of MACE was achieved in 160 patients (98%). Procedural success, defined as ≥20% reduction in percentage stenosis of the target lesion from immediately prior to intervention to immediately after stent deployment and ≤50% diameter stenosis immediately after stent deployment, using the assigned treatment alone was achieved in 158 patients (97%) of the patients.

Clinical results

Short-term (up to 30 days) results

At the 30 day (± 7 days) follow up, one cardiac death was reported. There were no significant changes in blood parameters either immediately post procedure or at 30 day follow-up. There were no reports of Q-wave MI, CABG or repeated angioplasty up to 30 days post procedure. In addition, there were no reported cases of (sub)acute thrombosis. The MACE-free rate at 30 days was 98%.

The 6 month follow-up

Between 30 days and 6 months post procedure, 32 MACE were reported (18%), one patient experienced cardiac death (ventricular fibrillation), two patients had non-Q wave MI and one experienced CABG and 28 patients underwent TLR (Table 55.6).

The 12 month follow-up

Three events were reported between 6 months and 12 months post procedure (one CABG and two TLR). No patient experienced late stent thrombosis during the study (Table 55.6).

Angiographic outcome

Angiographic data were available from 146 patients (Table 55.7). Mean reference vessel diameter (defined as the average of normal segments within 10 mm proximal and distal to the target lesion from two views using QCA) was similar at pre-PTCA, post-stent implantation and at 6 months post procedure (2.93 ± 0.41, 2.99 ± 0.41 and 2.90 ± 0.40 mm respectively). Pre-PTCA, mean MLD in the target lesion was 1.01 ± 0.34 and mean DS of the lesion was $65.35 \pm 10.82\%$. After the procedure, the MLD have increased to 2.50 ± 0.45 in-lesion and 2.81 ± 0.36 in-stent respectively. And mean diameter stenosis has decreased to 16% in-lesion and 5.75% in-stent, respectively. At 6 months post procedure, mean MLD were 1.81 ± 0.63 mm in-lesion, and 1.93 ± 0.67 in-stent, mean DS were $37.65 \pm 20.20\%$ in-lesion and 33.33 ± 21.83 in-stent, respectively. Mean acute gain were 1.48 ± 0.46 in-lesion and 1.81 ± 0.38 mm in-stent, mean late loss were 0.68 ± 0.59 in-lesion and 0.88 ± 0.63 in-stent and mean loss index were 0.50 ± 0.39 in-lesion and 0.48 ± 0.48 in-stent, respectively. At 6 month follow-up angiographic assessment, 35 patients (21%) had a binary in-lesion restenosis and 33 (20%) patients reported binary in-stent restenosis.

Table 55.6   Ranked major cardiac events (MACE) by descending severity and number of events during 6 month follow-up

MACE	BRILLIANT-EU (n = 173)(%)				
	In hospital n (%) patients	Up to 30 dy follow-up n (%) patients	Up to 6 month follow-up n (%) patients	Up to 12 mth follow-up n (%) patients	No. of events
Cardiac death	0 (0)	1 (1)	2 (1)	2 (1)	2
Q-Wave MI	0 (0)	0 (0)	0 (0)	0 (0)	0
Non-Q Wave	2 (1)	2 (1)	5 (3)	5 (2)	5
CABG	0 (0)	0 (0)	1 (1)	2 (1)	2
TLR	0 (0)	0 (0)	27 (16)	29 (17)	32
Total MACE	2 (1)	3 (2)	32 (18)	35 (20)	41

MI, myocardial infarction; MACE, major adverse cardiac events; CABG, coronary artery bypass graft; TLR, target lesion revascularization.

COMPARISON WITH THE DISTINCT TRIAL

This study was set up to allow a comparison of the patient population and the results with the larger randomized DISTINCT study previously conducted in the United States. Demographic and clinical data were comparable between the two studies (see Table 55.5). Angiographic characteristics were also similar. The lesion length was longer in the DISTINCT study (14.4 vs 11.5, $p<0.001$). Before treatment, the stenosis in the targeted artery was severe in the DISTINCT study (MLD: 0.81 vs 1.01, $p<0.001$; %DS 72% vs 65%, $p<0.001$) resulted in a greater acute gain (2.03 vs 1.81, $p<0.001$). However, the in-stent late loss was higher in the DISTINCT study (0.94 vs 0.88, $p = 0.41$) at 6 months follow-up (Table 55.7). Nevertheless, the Bio*divYsio* batimastat OC stent showed no improvement in the restenosis rate (21%) and overall MACE (20%) at 6 and 12 months when compared to the non-drug coated Bio*divYsio* stent used in the DISTINCT study where the reported adjudicated restenosis rate and MACE were 19.7% and 17%, respectively (Table 55.8).

CONCLUSIONS

The 5 day, 1 month, and 3 month preclinical data are available for PC stents loaded with the clinical trial dose (CTD) of batimastat. Histological analysis showed that the degree of fibrosis, hemorrhage, and inflammatory cell infiltration was not significantly different between the control and CTD stents at all three time points. Data for 5 day and 1 month are available for stents containing greater than three times the clinical trial dose (CTD). Taken together, these studies demonstrate that the Bio*divYsio* batimastat stent is well tolerated in appropriate animal models for the evaluation of restenosis after stent implantation in coronary arteries. The pharmacokinetics release data for the Bio*divYsio* batimastat stent follow the expected patterns of release and deposition

Table 55.7 QCA data: comparison between BRILLIANT-EU and DISTINCT studies

	BRILLIANT-EU	DISTINCT	p-value
Pre procedure:	n = 163	n = 313	
RVD (mm)	2.93 ± 0.41	2.95 ± 0.48	0.65
MLD (mm)	1.01 ± 0.34	0.81 ± 0.37	<0.001
%DS	65.20 ± 10.70	72.27 ± 11.92	<0.001
Post Procedure:	n = 163	n = 146	
RVD (mm) in lesion	2.99 ± 0.41	2.92 ± 0.47	0.16
MLD (mm) in lesion	2.50 ± 0.45	–	–
%DS in lesion	16.54 ± 8.39	–	–
Acute gain (mm) in lesion	1.48 ± 0.46	–	–
MLD (mm) in stent	2.81 ± 0.36	2.87 ± 0.43	0.18
%DS in stent	5.75 ± 8.37	2.87 ± 12.08	0.02
Acute gain (mm)	1.81 ± 0.38	2.03 ± 0.49	<0.001
Follow-up	n = 146	n = 143	
RVD (mm) in lesion	2.90 ± 0.40	2.90 ± 0.45	1.00
MLD (mm) in lesion	1.81 ± 0.63	–	–
%DS in lesion	37.99 ± 19.61	–	–
Late loss (mm) in lesion	0.68 ± 0.59	–	–
Loss index in lesion	0.50 ± 0.39	–	–
Binary RR (%) in lesion	21	–	–
MLD (mm) in stent	1.93 ± 0.67	1.94 ± 0.67	0.90
%DS in stent	33.33 ± 21.83	33.27 ± 20.67	0.98
Late loss (mm) in stent	0.88 ± 0.63	0.94 ± 0.61	0.41
Loss index in stent	0.48 ± 0.48	0.48 ± 0.33	1.00
Binary RR (%) in stent	20	19.7	nsd

RVD, reference vessel diameter; MLD, minimal luminal diameter; DS, diameter stenosis; nsd, no significant difference.

and indicate that there is unlikely to be a long-term issue of residual drug within the artery wall after release has terminated. The preclinical data at 3 months with the Bio*divYsio* batimastat stent showed a change in the rate of stenosis, where a reduction of 20% and 34% in the <CTD and CTD dose, respectively, as measured by QCA was observed. These data showed a trend in favor of the treatment groups.

In addition to the preclinical studies the clinical studies demonstrate that stent-based

Table 55.8   12 months follow-up clinical outcomes: comparison between BRILLIANT-EU and DISTINCT

	BRILLIANT-EU n = 173 (%)	DISTINCT n = 313 (%)	p value
Cardiac death	1	1	NS
Q Wave MI	0	1	NS
Non-Q Wave	3	1	NS
CABG	1	3	NS
TLR	15	11	NS
Total MACE	20	17	NS

MI: myocardial infarction; MACE: major adverse cardiac events; TLR: target lesion revascularization; CABG: coronary artery bypass graft surgery; NS: no significant difference.

delivery of batimastat in coronary artery using the Bio*divYsio* DD stents is a feasible and safe procedure. Results from the BRILLIANT study, however, did not show a positive effect of the Bio*divYsio* batimastat OC stent on total lesion revascularization and binary restenosis.

SUMMARY

The data suggest that the Bio*divYsio* batimastat OC stent is safe during the period of drug elution from the stent (pharmacokinetic studies have shown that 94% of the batimastat will have eluted from the PC coating after 1 month). The final 12 month results, particularly with no observed acute, sub(acute) and late thrombotic events suggest that the presence of batimastat in the coating is neither associated with an increased occurrence of MACE or serious adverse events, nor a delayed re-endothelialization, therefore the Bio*divYsio* batimastat OC stent is safe for use in patients. However, the comparable angiographic and clinical outcomes to the non-drug eluted PC coated Bio*divYsio* stents demonstrate that the Bio*divYsio* batimastat OC stent has no additional beneficial effect on restenosis.

REFERENCES

1. Hidalgo M, Eckhardt SG. Development of matrix metalloproteinase inhibitors in cancer therapy. J Natl Cancer Inst 2001; 93(3):178–93.
2. Jason LJ, Guillaume JJM, Van Eyes GD, et al. Injury induces dedifferentiation of smooth muscle cells and increased matrix-degrading metalloproteinase activity in human saphenous vein. Arterioscler Thromb Vasc Biol 2001; 21(7):1146–51.
3. Faveeuw C, Preece G, Ager A. Transendothelial migration of lymphocytes across high endothelial venules into lymph nodes is affected by metalloproteinases. Immunobiology 2001; 98(3):688–95.
4. James TW, Wagner R, White LA, et al. Induction of collagenase and stromyelysin gene expression by mechanical injury in a vascular smooth muscle-derived cell line. J Cell Physiol 1993; 157(2):426–37.
5. Jenkins GM, Crow MT, Bilato C, et al. Increased expression of membrane-type matrix metalloproteinase and preferential localization of matrix metalloproteinase-2 to the neointima of balloon-injured rat carotid arteries. Circulation 1998; 97:82–90.

6. Bendeck MP, Zempo N, Clowes AW, et al. Smooth muscle cell migration and matrix metalloproteinase expression after arterial injury in the rat. Circ Res 1994; 75:539–45.

7. Dollery CM, Humphries SE, McClelland A, et al. Expression of tissue inhibitor of matrix metalloproteinases 1 by use of an adenoviral vector inhibits smooth muscle cell migration and reduces neointimal hyperplasia in the rat model of vascular balloon injury. Circulation 1999; 99:3199–205.

8. Lovdahl D, Thyberg J, Hultgardh-Nilsson A. The synthetic metalloproteinase inhibitor batimastat suppresses injury-induced phosphorylation of MAP kinase ERK1/ERK2 and phenotypic modification of arterial smooth muscle cells in vitro. J Vasc Res 2000; 37(5):345–54.

9. Kenagy RD, Vergel S, Mattsson E, et al. The role of plasminogen, plasminogen activators, and matrix metalloproteinases in primate arterial smooth muscle cell migration. Arterioscler Thromb Vasc Biol 1996; 16(11): 1373–82.

10. Zempo N, Koyama N, Kenagy RD, et al. Regulation of vascular smooth muscle cell migration and proliferation in vitro and in injured rat arteries by a synthetic matrix metalloproteinase inhibitor. J Vasc Biol 1996; 16(1):28–33.

11. De Smet BJG, De Kleijn D, Hanemaaijer R, et al. Metalloproteinase inhibition reduces constrictive arterial remodeling after balloon angioplasty: a study in the atherosclerotic yucatán micropig. Circulation 2000; 101:2962–7.

12. Sierevogel MJ, Pasterkamp G, Velema E, et al. Oral matrix metalloproteinase inhibition and arterial remodeling after balloon dilation—an intravascular ultrasound study in the pig. Circulation 2001; 103:302–7.

13. Li CW, Cantor WJ, Robinson R, et al. Matrix metalloproteinase inhibitor GM6001 selectively reduces intimal hyperplasia and intima collagen in stented but not balloon treated arteries. Can J Cardiol 2000; 16(suppl F): 143F.

14. Whelan DM, van der Giessen WJ, Krabbendam SC, et al. Biocompatibility of phosphorylcholine coated stents in normal porcine coronary arteries. Heart 2000; 83(3):338–45.

15. Edelman ER, Rogers C. Pathobiologic responses to stenting. Am J Cardiol 1998; 81(7A):4E–6E.

56

The FIM trial: sirolimus eluting stents

Alexandre Abizaid, Mariano Albertal, and J Eduardo Sousa

Introduction • **The pilot clinical trial** • **Follow-up** • **Conclusion**

INTRODUCTION

Sirolimus, or rapamycin, was first isolated 30 years ago from *Streptomyces hygroscopicus*, a soil microorganism. This macrolide antibiotic was found to have potent immunosuppressant and antimitotic properties. The drug binds to a high affinity cytosolic receptor protein FK506 binding protein-12 (FKBP-12),[1] leading to an inhibition of TOR (target of rapamycin). The latter prevents downregulation of the tumor suppressor gene p^{27}, which is a powerful inhibitor of cyclin-dependent kinase (CDK) activity and block progression of the cell cycle at the G_1–S transition (Figure 56.1).

The drug is lipophilic and thus is readily taken up across the cell membrane. In vitro data have shown that the drug inhibits vascular smooth muscle and endothelial cell proliferation. Furthermore, in a pig model, sirolimus eluting stents containing 185 µg of sirolimus showed a 50% reduction in neointimal proliferation.[2]

THE PILOT CLINICAL TRIAL

The pilot clinical trial of sirolimus-eluting Bx Velocity stent (FIM) enrolled patients with de novo (non-complex) native coronary artery

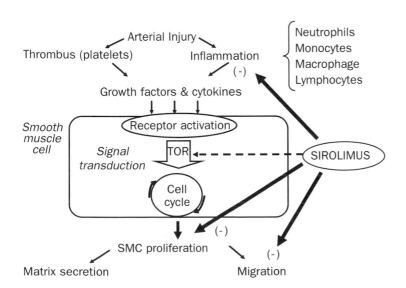

Fig. 56.1 Mechanism of action of sirolimus. Sirolimus binds to FK506 binding protein-12 in the cell cytoplasm, leading to inhibition of target of rapamycin (TOR). Inhibition of TOR prevents progression from the G_1 to the S phase.

lesions from São Paulo, Brazil ($n = 30$) and Rotterdam, The Netherlands ($n = 15$).[3–5] Two different formulations of sirolimus eluting stents were used [slow release (SR), $n = 30$; fast release (FR), $n = 15$]. The polymer coating of the stents contains 185 μg sirolimus at a 30% drug-to-polymer ratio.

A total of 39 patients presented with stable angina symptoms and six had unstable angina. The mean age group was 56 ± 10 years, 64% were male. The incidence of a prior myocardial infarction was 42%, prior percutaneous intervention 4%, smoking 57%, and 14% of the patients had diabetes mellitus. Stent deployment was performed with predilatation in all patients (balloon size 2.5 mm, length 17 ± 3.07 mm and maximum pressure 9.15 ± 2.3), achieving 100% success rate. Postdilatation was required in 14 patients (31%). The number of stents utilized was 1.1 ± 0.3, five patients (11%) requiring two stents.

FOLLOW-UP

In the São Paulo cohort, angiographic and intravascular ultrasound (IVUS) follow-up was performed at 4 and 12 months, revealing a striking binary restenosis rate of 0% at 4 and 12 month follow-up. Moreover, changes in in-stent and in-lesion minimal luminal diameter (MLD) were very small at 4 and 12 month follow-up (see Figure 56.2 and Table 56.1). Neointimal hyperplasia, assessed by IVUS, was virtually absent in both formulations at 4 and 12 months (neointimal volume <11 mm³, <4% volume obstruction, see Figure 56.3). Meanwhile, the Rotterdam cohort underwent angiographic and IVUS assessment at 6 and

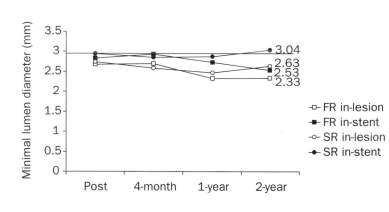

$p = 0.053$, in-lesion MLD FR vs. SR
$p = 0.003$, in-stent MLD FR vs. SR

Fig. 56.2 Post-procedural, 4, 12, and 24 month follow-up minimal luminal diameter (MLD) of fast-release (FR) and slow-release (SR) sirolimus eluting stents (São Paulo cohort).

Table 56.1 Angiographic assessment at 4 and 12 month follow-up (data from the São Paulo Cohort)

Follow-up:	In-stent late loss		In-lesion late loss	
	4 months	*12 months*	*4 months*	*12 months*
Fast release	−0.02 ± 0.3	0.10 ± 0.03	−0.1 ± 0.3	0.24 ± 0.3
Slow release	0.09 ± 0.3	0.09 ± 0.4	0.16 ± 0.3	0.18 ± 0.3

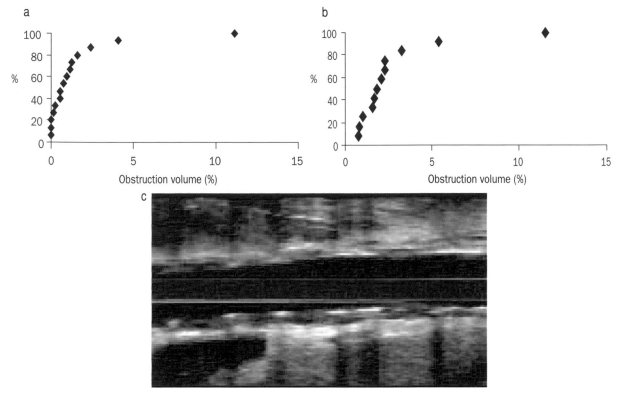

Fig. 56.3 Cumulative distribution curves of percentage obstruction volumes in fast (a) and slow-release (b) sirolimus eluting stents at 12 month follow-up. (c) Longitudinal IVUS reconstruction illustrates the virtual absence of in-stent intimal hyperplasia at 12 months.

18 months, reproducing these remarkable results.

There were no adverse events at 12 month follow-up in the São Paulo cohort, however, one patient experienced late occlusion of the stented artery at 14 months after stenting. The latter appeared to be due to progression of a non-critical proximal lesion (Figure 56.4). Another patient developed a left circumflex ostial lesion and underwent coronary bypass surgery 24.5 months after the index procedure, however, the left circumflex stent presented minimal in-stent neointimal proliferation. Only one patient (fast-release group) had a 52% diameter stenosis within the lesion segment, which required repeat revascularization. Thus, the overall target-vessel revascularization rate was 10% (3/30) at 2 years. No patient developed in-stent restenosis. A total of 28/30 patients from the São Paulo cohort underwent IVUS evaluation at 2 year follow-up, showing a sustained suppression of neointimal proliferation (Figure 56.5).

CONCLUSION

Although the present study included a small number of patients with non-complex lesions, the seminal observation of a long lasting suppression in neointimal growth by sirolimus eluting stents in addition to their excellent safety profile have dramatically changed the world of interventional cardiology.

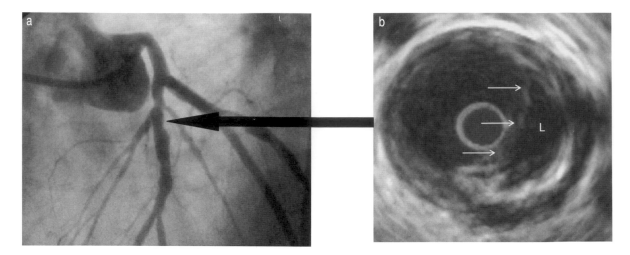

Fig. 56.4 (a) Angiography of the left anterior descending artery showing a non-significant stenosis at the proximal edge of the stent (arrow) at 12 month follow-up. (b) IVUS cross-sectional image at the site of the lesion shows an eccentric plaque with a large lipid pool (L) delimited by a fibrous cap (arrows). This vessel was occluded 2 months later.

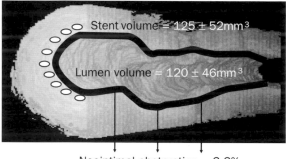

Fig. 56.5 A three-dimensional IVUS reconstruction revealing minimal neointimal growth at 2 year follow-up sirolimus eluting stent implantation (slow-release group, São Paulo cohort).

REFERENCES

1. Sun J, Marx SO, Chen HJ, et al. Role for p27(Kip1) in vascular smooth muscle cell migration. Circulation 2001; 103:2967–72.

2. Suzuki T, Kopia G, Hayashi S, et al. Stent-based delivery of sirolimus reduces neointimal formation in a porcine coronary model. Circulation 2001; 104:1188–93.

3. Sousa JE, Costa MA, Sousa AG, et al. Two-year angiographic and intravascular ultrasound follow-up after implantation of sirolimus-eluting stents in human coronary arteries. Circulation 2003; 107:381–3.

4. Sousa JE, Costa MA, Abizaid AC, et al. Sustained suppression of neointimal proliferation by sirolimus-eluting stents: one-year angiographic and intravascular ultrasound follow-up. Circulation 2001; 104:2007–11.

5. Sousa JE, Costa MA, Abizaid A, et al. Lack of neointimal proliferation after implantation of sirolimus-coated stents in human coronary arteries: A quantitative coronary angiography and three-dimensional intravascular ultrasound study. Circulation 2001; 103:192–5.

57

Tacrolimus eluting stents

Eberhard Grube

Introduction • **Preclinical studies** • **Clinical studies** • **Discussion**

INTRODUCTION

Inflammation is one of the major determinants of neointimal formation after stent implantation. Recently published studies have demonstrated the benefit of drug eluting stents carrying the antiproliferative and antiinflammatory agents, sirolimus (rapamycin) or paclitaxel, for inhibition of reactive neointimal proliferation. Given these initial experiences, additional antiproliferative agents might also have the potential to improve the long-term outcome after percutaneous stent placement due to an effective suppression of the reactive neointimal in-stent cell proliferation.

Tacrolimus (FK506) is a well known potent antiproliferative and immunosuppressive agent with proven inhibitory activity on human vascular smooth muscle cells.[1,2] The compound has the structure of a macrolide antibiotic. Although, structurally, the binding domain of the tacrolimus molecule appears similar to rapamycin, both compounds have distinct mechanisms of action. Cell culture experiments indicate that tacrolimus could allow earlier endothelial regeneration than sirolimus,[1] which facilitates re-endothelialization of the damaged vessel wall. On the other hand, the inhibitory activity on human vascular smooth muscle cells with tacrolimus is about 100 times lower than with sirolimus.[1,2]

In order to evaluate both the safety and efficacy of tacrolimus in the treatment of coronary artery disease via a drug eluting stent system, two product development lines of tacrolimus eluting stents were created in the past. One development line focused on a tacrolimus eluting version of a coronary stent graft, where tacrolimus elutes from the expanded polytetrafluoroethylene (ePTFE) foil of the stent graft. The other development line was based on tacrolimus release from a new coronary stent design that utilized a nanoporous aluminum oxide ceramic layer on to the stent surface as drug carrier, without using additional polymeric formulations for stent coating and drug elution.

PRECLINICAL STUDIES

As shown in early animal models done by Wieneke et al.,[3] tacrolimus eluting stents coated with a biocompatible ceramic layer had the potential to reduce neointimal formation following stent implantation. Histological examination revealed that tacrolimus led to a marked reduction of inflammatory cells close to the stent struts. This reduced infiltration of macrophages and lymphocytes could be attributed to tacrolimus' inhibitory effect on the release of interleukin (IL)-2 and other cytokines.[4] Since macrophages,[5] and lymphocytes,[6] are claimed to play a key role in the inflammation cascade after stent implantation, thus promoting the formation of neointima, tacrolimus appears to have the potential to effectively interrupt the in-stent restenosis cascade. Moreover, histological data showed a good re-endothelialization within tacrolimus eluting stents that might suggest the beneficial effect of a higher activity of tacrolimus against smooth muscle cells compared to endothelial cells. In addition, tacrolimus-mediated inhibition of FasL expression might contribute to the complete re-endothelialization seen in this preclinical study by inhibition of apoptosis of endothelial cells. Based on these findings, clinical studies had been started (PRESENT I, EVIDENT).

However, a following animal study reported by Scheller et al. revealed new controversial results.[6] In this study, it could be confirmed that the tacrolimus stent coating is safe and effective in restenosis prevention. However, only stents coated with high dose tacrolimus could produce an antiproliferative effect comparable to that seen with paclitaxel and sirolimus stents. Tacrolimus stent coating based on the nanoporous ceramic (AlOx) technology was less effective than coating on a polymer basis or direct coating of e-polished bare metal stents. These data finally led to a change of the stent design tested in clinical practice (PRESENT II, PRESET).

CLINICAL STUDIES

Tacrolimus eluting stent for the treatment of vein graft lesions

The EVIDENT study
The EVIDENT study investigates the safety of the 16 mm coronary stent graft (CSG) loaded with 352 μg FK506 (tacrolimus) in treatment of saphenous vein graft stenoses. The primary endpoint was major adverse cardiac event (MACE) at 30 days. The enrollment was completed in January 2003 with 32 patients included. No adverse events were observed up to 30 days post-stent implantation. The com-

plete 6 month follow-up data are not yet available. However, based on the current 6 month follow-up data on 11 patients, the preliminary restenosis rate is 27%, which is similar to the restenosis rate observed with the standard CSG under similar conditions.

Tacrolimus eluting stent for the treatment of native coronary lesions

The PRESENT I, PRESENT II, and PRESET studies
The PRESENT studies investigated the safety of the Flex ceramic stent (ceramic-coated stainless steel) in a non-drug-loaded and a tacrolimus-loaded version. Based on the early preclinical strudies, the stent design consisted of a ceramic stent coating as drug carrier matrix, without using polymeric formulations for stent coating and drug elution.

In PRESENT I, it was planned to treat 30 patients with a Flex ceramic stent of 16 mm length loaded with 60 μg tacrolimus and compare the results from 30 patients with a Flex ceramic stent without drug. However, because there were two cases of target vessel revascularization out of 22 patients treated with the Flex ceramic stent with a low dose of tacrolimus (60 μg) in April 2002, it was recommended by the data safety monitoring board to stop further inclusion in both arms of the study and to increase the dose of the antiproliferative agent to 230 μg.

A further 30 patients were then enrolled in a separate high dose arm of the study (PRESENT II). However, the preliminary MACE rate of PRESENT II at 6 month follow-up was 32% (8/25 pts), with a need for target lesion revascularization in 7 out of 25 patients due to recurrent neointimal lumen renarrowing. Given these results as well as further experiences from animal models reported by Scheller et al.,[7] it was decided to discontinue the use of the ceramic stent coating for drug delivery, because it was believed to abolish the beneficial antiproliferative properties of tacrolimus.

Therefore, a third arm of this study series was conducted, applying the drug directly on to the e-polished stent surface without using any additional stent coatings. The randomized

PRESET study is now evaluating safety and efficacy of the e-polished tacrolimus-eluting Flex stent (JOSTENT® Flex Progress), loaded with the high dose of tacrolimus, similar to PRESENT II ($1.7 \mu g/mm^2$ tacrolimus), compared with the bare metal Flex stent with a total of 120 patients in each arm. The complete 6 month follow-up data are supposed to be available in 2004.

DISCUSSION

The experience of both the PRESENT and EVIDENT studies demonstrates the impact of specific stent designs, especially the drug carrier characteristics, on patient outcome. Tacrolimus is known and used in other therapeutic areas due to its antiproliferative and antiinflammatory properties, and there is evidence of efficacy in treatment of coronary lesions in preclinical studies. However, clinical experience using a stent graft as well as a ceramic-coated stent for drug delivery did not demonstrate a striking benefit of this treatment concept for inhibiting the proliferative vessel response sufficiently. This has been confirmed in the most recent animal study, in which the use of ceramic coating as carrier for tacrolimus (as used in PRESENT I and II) creates increased neointimal formation. Whereas a direct comparison of e-polished stents with and without tacrolimus (as used in PRESET) demonstrated a significant reduction of neointimal formation using direct-coated tacrolimus eluting stents.[6] Therefore, the ongoing PRESET study should provide important additional insights, which may clarify the still unknown potential of tacrolimus for the prevention of neointimal proliferation in clinical practice without being affected by any additional artificial stent surface compounds.

REFERENCES

1. Mohacsi PJ, Tüller D, Hulliger B, Wijngaard PLJ. Different inhibitory effects of immunosuppressive drugs on human and rat aortic smooth muscle and endothelial cell proliferation stimulated by platelet-derived growth factor or endothelial cell growth factor. J Heart Lung Transplant 1997; 16:484–92.

2. Matter MC, Wnendt S, Kurz DJ, et al. Tacrolimus, but not sirolimus targets human vascular smooth muscle cells, but spares endothelial cells – Implications for drug-eluting stents. Eur Heart J 2002; 4(suppl):143 (abstract).

3. Wieneke H, Dirscho, Sawitowski T, et al. Synergistic effects of a novel nanoporous stent coating and tacrolimus on intima proliferation in rabbits. Catheter Cardiovasc Interv 2003; 60:399–407.

4. Sakuma S, Higashi Y, Sato N, et al. Tacrolimus suppressed the production of cytokines involved in atopic dermatitis by direct stimulation of human PBMC system (comparison with steroids). Int Immunopharmacol 2001; 1:1219–26.

5. Rogers C, Welt FG, Karnovsky MJ, Edelman ER. Monocyte recruitment and neointimal hyperplasia in rabbits: coupled inhibitory effects of heparin. Arterioscler Thromb Vasc Biol 1996; 16:1312–18.

6. Meuwissen M, Piek JJ, van der Wal AC, et al. Recurrent unstable angina after directional coronary atherectomy is related to the extent of initial coronary plaque inflammation. J Am Coll Cardiol 2001; 37:1271–6.

7. Scheller B. Preclinical evaluation of tacrolimus stent coating. (Unpublished data, 2003.)

58

Everolimus eluting stents

Eberhard Grube and Lutz Buellesfeld

Introduction • Everolimus • PLA polymer: history, pharmacology, toxicology of polymer • Stent design • Preclinical studies and results • Clinical studies • Results • Conclusion

INTRODUCTION

Long-term clinical efficacy of intracoronary stenting is limited by restenosis, which occurs in 15–30% of patients. In-stent restenosis is solely due to neointimal hyperplasia, which is a response to stent-induced mechanical injury and a foreign body response. The vessel wall becomes acutely and chronically inflamed, with elaboration of cytokines and growth factors that activate smooth muscle cell migration and proliferation. Early experimental data suggested that inhibition of cell cycle progression with rapamycin (or sirolimus) might be an effective strategy to prevent restenosis. These observations established the potential benefit of local application of antiproliferative or antiinflammatory agents via drug eluting stents for the treatment of coronary lesions. However, the treatment effect depends on the drug as well as stent design and coating. In order to evaluate both safety and efficacy of everolimus in the treatment of coronary artery disease via a drug eluting stent, a new stent system has been designed using a new bioabsorbable polymer (PLA) carrying the agent everolimus.

EVEROLIMUS

Everolimus is an orally active derivative of the immunosuppressant sirolimus (rapamycin).

The parent drug, rapamycin, is a macrolide synthesized by *Streptomyces hygroscopicus*. Everolimus, like rapamycin, blocks growth-factor derived cell proliferation, arresting the cell cycle at the G_1 to S phase.[1] This mechanism of action differs from that of CysA and tacrolimus, which inhibit proliferation earlier in the cell cycle (G_0 to G_1 phase). Everolimus does not inhibit the synthesis of growth factors, but blocks growth factor-driven signal transduction in the cellular responses to alloantigens. In particular, interleukin (IL-)2 and IL-15 driven proliferation are inhibited, which is explained by the block of p70S6 kinase.[2]

The everolimus effect is not restricted to T-lymphocytes, but potentially affects other hematopoietic and non-hematopoietic cells, including smooth muscle cells.[3] Thus, the inhibitory action of everolimus on smooth muscle cell proliferation, evidenced in animal models of vessel obliteration has triggered an interest in everolimus as stent coating for local inhibition of in-stent restenosis.

PLA POLYMER: HISTORY, PHARMACOLOGY, TOXICOLOGY OF POLYMER

In humans poly(D, L-lactide), or poly(lactic acid) (PLA) was first used in maxillofacial surgery.[3] Since then, PLA has become one of the most commonly used biodegradable polymers for more than three decades in a variety of medical applications. Biodegradable PLA and its copolymers have been successful in the areas of controlled drug delivery systems,[3-6] plastic reconstructive surgery,[7] bone fracture repairs, etc.[4] Extensive research has also been conducted on the use of these polymers as controlled-release polymer matrix for bioactive agents for animals and man, such as anticancer agents,[8] antitubercular drug carriers (for isoniazid and rifampicin),[9] peptides and proteins,[10] and antibiotics.[11]

PLA devices are known to degrade by chemical, thermal, mechanical, and physical mechanisms, whereas chemical degradation is predominant. The biocompatibility of lactide/glycolide polymers as controlled-release matrix of the bioactive agents is well documented: today, these are the most comprehensively investigated biodegradable polymers for drug delivery.

STENT DESIGN

For preclinical and clinical evaluation of the safety and efficacy of both everolimus and the PLA stent coating, a new stent was introduced based on the bare metal S-Stent scaffold (Biosensors International). The ultra-thin 'composite' coating, which contains the immunosuppressive drug within a polyhydroxyacid biodegradable polymer matrix, provides high adhesion to the metal substrate, controlled resorption characteristics, high surface availability of the active agent, high mechanical flexibility, abrasion resistance, and strength. The drug release is based on a rapid resorption of an amorphous glassine solid without any topcoat. Both the polymer and the immunosuppressive drug are resorbed into the surrounding tissue at roughly equal rates, leaving only the bare metal stent implant (Figure 58.1).

PRECLINICAL STUDIES AND RESULTS

The everolimus eluting stent with a PLA polymer coating was implanted in juvenile farm swine, using different dosings of the drug everolimus.[12,13] The animals were divided into six groups: bare metal S-Stents; polymer only-

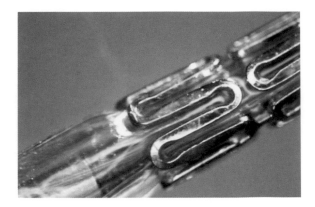

Fig. 58.1 Biosensor everolimus eluting stent with bioerodable polymer coating.

coated S-stents; low dose everolimus eluting S-Stents; high dose everolimus eluting S-Stents; low-dose Sirolimus eluting S-Stents; and high dose Sirolimus eluting S-Stents. At the time of implant, quantitative coronary angiography (QCA) was performed to measure the diameter of the vessels both before and after stent implantation. At 28 days, the animals were again subjected to QCA in the area of the stent, prior to sacrifice. Follow-up QCA at 30 days revealed a statistically significant reduction in late loss index in high dose everolimus eluting S-Stents $(0.23, p<0.05)$, compared to other groups (bare metal S-Stents: 0.44, polymer-coated S-Stents: 0.56, low dose everolimus-eluting S-Stents: 0.27, low dose sirolimus-eluting S-Stents: 0.32, high dose sirolimus-eluting S-Stents: 0.29) (Figure 58.2). Pathology examination revealed no thromboses or inflammatory changes related to the drug eluting stents. In general, the vessels appeared to be well healed with a well established endothelial layer, and evidence of complete healing and vessel homeostasis at 28 days.

These data suggest the biocompatibility and efficacy of everolimus eluting stents compared to bare metal stents at 30 days. This demonstrates that everolimus eluting stents significantly inhibit smooth muscle cell proliferation, and permit complete re-endothelialization without delayed vessel wall healing in a porcine coronary artery model. These data formed the basis for initial clinical studies of the everolimus-eluting stent. Figures 58.3–58.6 show typical examples of stent cross-sections taken from pig coronary arteries.

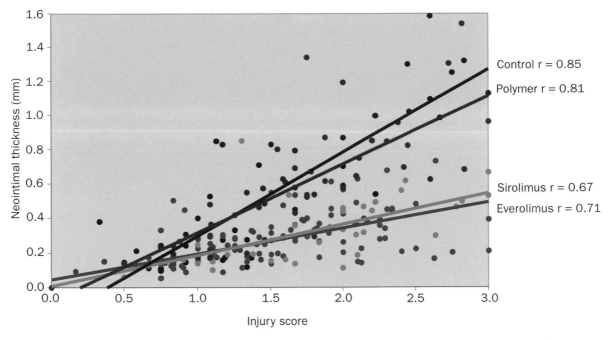

Fig. 58.2 Demonstration of the significant effect that everolimus and sirolimus exert on neointimal response in the 28 day swine over-stretch model vs bare metal and PLA polymer-coated controls. (Reproduced courtesy of Saibal Kar, MD, Cedar Sinai Medical Center, Los Angeles, CA.)

CLINICAL STUDIES

The FUTURE I feasibility study

The FUTURE I trial evaluated both safety and feasibility of an everolimus eluting stent system for the treatment of de novo coronary lesions. FUTURE I was a prospective, single center, single blinded, randomized trial including 27 and 15 patients with native de novo coronary lesions allocated for drug and control groups respectively.

Study endpoints
The primary endpoint was 30 day major adverse cardiac event (MACE)-free survival. MACE was defined as death from any cause, Q-wave myocardial infarction (MI), target vessel revascularization, and stent thrombosis. Q-wave MI was defined as development of Q-waves in two or more contiguous leads with postimplantation elevated creatine kinase-myocardial band (CK-MB) isoenzyme levels. Target vessel revascularization included coronary artery bypass graft (CABG) surgery as well as repeat percutaneous intervention on the

stented vessel. Secondary endpoints were device success, MACE, and restenosis rate at 6 month follow-up.

Device description
The control stent was the commercially available S-Stent. The drug eluting stent was the same stent coated with a bioabsorbable hydroxyacid on-strut polymer which carries and releases the antiproliferative agent everolimus.

Study population
Patients were randomly assigned to receive either the bare S-Stent ($n = 15$) or the Everolimus eluting stent ($n = 27$). Patients were included in FUTURE I if angiography showed lesion lengths ≤18 mm, diameter stenosis between 50% and 99%, and vessel diameter between 2.75 and 4.0 mm. Patients were excluded if they had diabetes mellitus, an acute myocardial infarction within the past 4 weeks prior to intervention; in-stent restenosis or a left ventricular ejection fraction <30%.

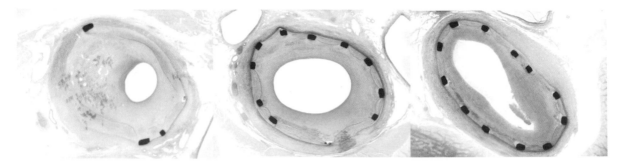

Fig. 58.3   Bare stent histology 1.3 balloon to artery (B/A) ratio.

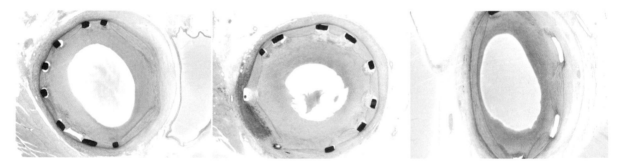

Fig. 58.4   Polymer-only stent histology, 1.3 B/A ratio.

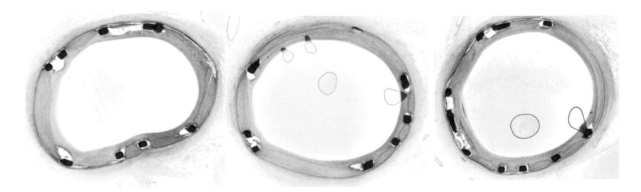

Fig. 58.5   High dose everolimus-coated stent histology, 1.33 B/A ratio.

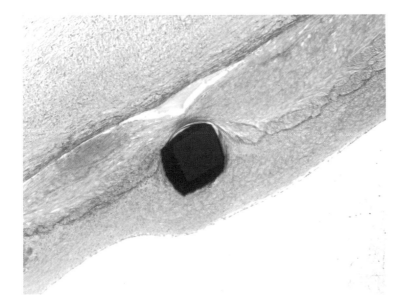

Fig. 58.6 Example of endothelial healing over everolimus-coated stent in swine at ×91 magnification (Biosensors S-Stent).

Follow-up

Clinical evaluation was conducted 1, 6, and 12 months after stent implantation. Coronary angiographic and intravascular ultrasound (IVUS) imaging were performed before and after stent implantation and at the 6 month follow-up visit.

RESULTS

Baseline demographics and lesion characteristics were similar between both study groups, as shown in Table 58.1.

Major adverse cardiac event at 30 days and 6 months (MACE)

At 30 days after stent implantation, there were no (0%) incidents of MACE or stent thrombosis in either cohort, indicating a comparable safety profile for the everolimus eluting stent relative to the uncoated control stent. At 6 months, the non-adjudicated MACE rate was 7.7% (2 events/26 patients) for the everolimus group compared with 8.3% (1 events/12 patients) in the control group. The two MACE in the everolimus group were one chronic obstructive pulmonary disease (COPD)-related non-cardiac death and one target lesion revascularization (TLR) due to an in-segment restenosis distal to the study stent (Table 58.2).

Quantitative coronary angiography (QCA) at 6 months

All 6 month quantitative angiographic indices (minimum lumen diameter, percentage diameter stenosis, lumen loss) were significantly ($p < 0.001$) improved in the everolimus stent group compared with the control. The binary in-stent restenosis rate was 0.0% in the everolimus eluting stent group versus 9.1% in the control. The in-segment restenosis rate was 4.0% (1/25) versus 9.1% (1/11), respectively. The in-stent late loss decreased from 0.83 mm (control) to 0.10 mm (everolimus stent) (Table 58.3).

Intravascular ultrasound (IVUS) at 6 months

At 6 months, the percentage neointimal volume was significantly ($p = 0.001$) lower in the everolimus group (2.9 ± 1.9) compared with the control group (22.4 ± 9.4) (Table 58.4). In addition, there were no late acquired incomplete stent appositions in either group.

Table 58.1   Patient demographics and lesion characteristics

	Everolimus group (%) (n = 27)	Control group (%) (n = 15)	p
Age (years)	64.2	65.6	ns
Male	85.2	86.7	ns
Current smoker	29.6	28.6	ns
Hypertension	85.2	66.7	ns
Hyperlipidemia	70.4	86.7	ns
Prior MI	7.4	20.0	ns
Prior PCI	29.6	20.0	ns
CCS III or IV	11.5	0.0	ns
Target vessel			
RCA	40.7	26.7	ns
LAD	40.7	60.0	ns
Cx	18.5	13.3	ns
ACC/AHA lesion grade			
A	33.3	26.7	ns
B1	40.7	60.0	ns
B2	22.2	13.3	ns
C	3.7	0.0	ns
Lesion length (mm)	9.17	8.32	ns

MI, myocardial infarction; PCI, percutaneous coronary intervention; CCS, Canadian Cardiovascular Society Classification; RCA, right coronary artery; LAD, left anterior descending artery; ACC/AHA, American College of Cardiology/American Heart Association; ns, not significant.

Table 58.2   30 day and 6 month major adverse cardiac event (MACE)

	Everolimus group	Control group	p
MACE at 30 day follow-up	0 (0%)	0 (0%)	ns
MACE at 6 month follow-up	2/26 (7.7%)	1/12 (8.3%)	ns
Death	1/26 (3.8%)[a]	0 (0%)	ns
Q-wave MI	0 (0%)	0 (0%)	ns
Non-Q-wave MI	0 (0%)	0 (0%)	ns
TLR	1/26 (3.8%)	1/12 (8.3%)	ns

[a] COPD-related death. TLR, target lesion revascularization; ns, not significant.

Table 58.3 **Quantitative coronary angiography (QCA) results (in-stent) at 6 months**

	Everolimus group (n = 27)	Control group (n = 15)	p
MLD (mm)			
Pre	1.12	1.11	ns
Post	3.07	2.94	ns
F/U	2.98	2.11	<0.0001
%DS			
Pre	64.09	62.12	ns
Post	1.79	1.73	ns
F/U	2.73	27.2	0.0009
Late loss (mm)	0.10	0.83	<0.0001
Restenosis (%)	0.0% (0/25)	9.1% (1/11)	ns

MLD, minimal luminal diameter; DS, diameter stenosis; F/U, follow-up; ns, not significant.

Table 58.4 **Quantitative computerized ultrasound analysis (QCU) results**

	Everolimus group (n = 24)	Control group (n = 11)	p
Neointimal area (mm^2)	0.5 ± 0.4	2.2 ± 1.3	<0.001
Neointimal volume index (mm^3/mm)	0.2 ± 0.2	1.7 ± 0.7	<0.001
Minimum lumen area (mm^3)			
Post	7.0 ± 2.2	6.4 ± 1.2	
F/U	6.9 ± 2.6	4.6 ± 1.5	
Cross-sectional narrowing (%)	6.9 ± 5.3	31.8 ± 14.2	<0.001

CONCLUSION

This randomized, single blinded feasibility study established an acceptable safety profile for the everolimus eluting stent with a biodegradable coating system, with a very low MACE rate up to 6 months post-stent implantation. The primary endpoint, incidence of 30 day MACE, was 0% in both groups, and with all patients treated for 3 months with clopidogrel, no stent thromboses were reported in either group. The everolimus stent group demonstrated significant and concordant improvements in the more sensitive IVUS and QCA parameters with an 88% reduction of in-stent late loss from 0.83 mm in control to 0.10 mm in the everolimus eluting stent group and an 87% reduction of the percentage neointimal volume from 22.4% to 2.9%, respectively.

Moreover, the in-stent late loss of 0.10 mm suggests that the dosage as well as the release pattern of everolimus disrupts the restenotic cascade, while allowing sufficient neointimal growth to promote healing and avoid late stent thrombosis. FUTURE II will provide further insight into the clinical effects of this promising stent technology in a larger patient cohort.

REFERENCES

1. Nashan B. The role of everolimus (everolimus, RAD) in the many pathways of chronic rejection. Transplant Proc 2001; 33:3215–20.
2. Neuhaus P, Klupp J, Langrehr JM. mTOR inhibitors: an overview. Liver Transplant 2001; 7(6):473–84.
3. Getter I, Cutright DE, Bhaskar SN, Augsburg JK. A biodegradable intraosseous appliance in the treatment of mandibular fractures. J Oral Surg 1969; 30:344–8.
4. Rokkanen P, Bostman O, Vainionpaa S, et al. Biodegradable implants in fracture fixation: early results of treatment of fractures of the ankle. Lancet 1985; 1:1442–4.
5. Bercovy M, et al. Carbon-PGLA prostheses for ligament reconstruction – experimental basis and short results in man. Clin Orthop 1985; 196:159–68.
6. Hashizoe M, Ogura Y, Takanashi T, et al. Biodegradable polymeric device for sustained intravitreal release of ganciclovir in rabbits. Curr Eye Res 1997; 16:633–9.
7. Moe KS, Weisman RA. Resorbable fixation in facial plastic and head and neck reconstructive surgery: an initial report on polyactic acid implants. Laryngoscope 2001; 111(10):1697–701.
8. Strobel JD, et al. Controlled release systems for anticancer agents. Proc Int Symp Control Rel Bioact Mat 1987; 14:261.
9. Dutt M, Kuller GK. Liposomes and PLG microparticles as sustained release antitubercular drug carriers – an in vitro-in vivo study. Int J Antimicr Agents 2001; 18:245–52.
10. Maulding HV. Prolonged delivery of polypeptides by microcapsules. J Controlled Release 1987; 6:167.
11. Tice TR, Rowe CE, Gilley RM, Setterstrom JA, Mirth DD. Development of microencapsulated antibiotics for topical administration. Proc Int Symp Control Rel Bioact Mat 1986; 13:169.
12. Honda H, Kar S, Honda T, et al. Everolimus-eluting stents significantly inhibit neointimal hyperplasia in an experimental pig coronary model. Am J Cardiol 2002; 90(suppl 6A):73H.
13. Honda T, Kar S, Honda H, et al. Stent-based delivery of everolimus leads to complete vessel wall healing without toxicity in a 90-day porcine model. Am J Cardiol 2002; 90(suppl 6A):80H.

59

The Quanam drug eluting stent and the SCORE trial

Eberhard Grube

Introduction • The QuaDDS QP2 eluting stent system • Preclinical studies • Clinical studies • Preclinical studies: after SCORE • Conclusions

INTRODUCTION

In-stent restenosis is a result of neointimal hyperplasia, which is a response to stent-induced mechanical injury as well as a type of 'foreign body response'. The vessel wall becomes acutely and chronically inflamed, with elaboration of cytokines and growth factors that activate smooth muscle cell migration and proliferation. Therefore, inhibition of cell cycle progression with antiproliferative or antiinflammatory agents was believed to be, in the late 1990s, an effective strategy to prevent restenosis. The first clinical program, the Quanam's drug-eluting stent program, was designed to control neointimal proliferation by delivering high doses of an antineoplastic agent to vessel endothelium, treating restenosis as a 'cancer of the blood vessels'. Quanam developed the QuaDDS stent (Figure 59.1) to inhibit neointimal proliferation by providing chemotherapeutic doses of the paclitaxel-derivative 7-hexanoylpaclitaxel (QP2) to vessel walls for up to 6 months.

THE QuaDDS QP2 ELUTING STENT SYSTEM

The drug: QP2

QP2, as shown in Figure 59.2, is structurally similar to paclitaxel, but it has greater lipophilicity and cellular retention.[1] These properties allow QP2 to pass easily through the cell membrane and sustain its activity in and around treated cells. In the cell, QP2 works by inhibiting microtubule formation,[2] and blocking cell division.[3]

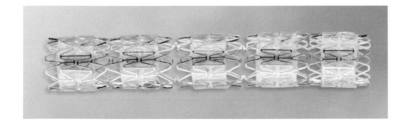

Fig. 59.1 The QuaDDs stent.

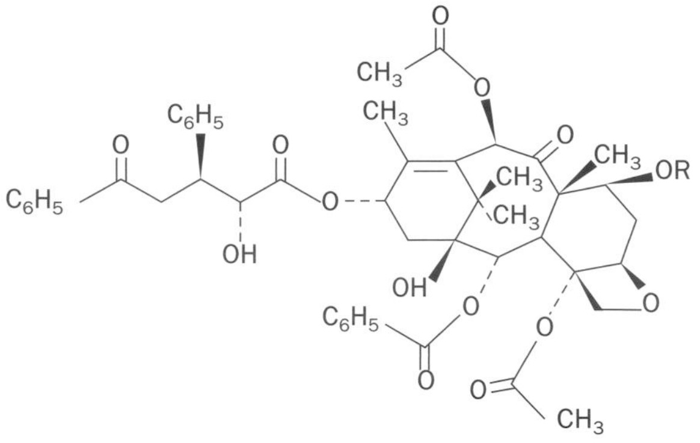

Fig. 59.2 The structure of QP2 (7-hexanoylpaclitaxel).

The drug delivery system: acrylate polymer sleeves

Drug elution from the QuaDDs stent was based on polymer sleeves because of their high drug loading capabilities. The acrylate polymer sleeve was a seamless tube cut into 2 mm lengths that were mounted on to the stent. Each sleeve measured 0.0020 inches in thickness leading to a total stent thickness (metal stent plus polymer sleeve) of 0.0075 inches. Given these sleeves, drug dosages up to 4000 μg QP2 on a 17 mm stent could be delivered. For example, a 16 mm Boston Scientific TAXUS stent contains 108 μg paclitaxel (Boston Scientific Corporation).

QP2 was dissolved in a solvent that was then absorbed into the polymer at a specified volume of solution. The solvent was removed by vacuum-drying. When dry, the 2 mm polymer sleeves, each containing 800 μg of QP2, were mounted on to a QueST stent (Figure 59.1). The number of sleeves per stent varied with the length of the stent, with a 17 mm stent containing five sleeves for a total loaded dose of 4000 μg of QP2.

Drug release studies performed in a rabbit iliac artery model indicated that QP2 was released from the QuaDDS stent for 6 months and was confined to the area under the stent and immediately adjacent tissues.[5] Specifically, 80% of QP2 was released within the first 90 days after implantation, and drug release continued for 180 days. The amount of drug 1 cm proximal and distal from the stent edges was 1/100 to 1/10 of the amount under the stent, and no drug was detectable in organ tissues tested.

The bare stent platform: QueST

Because commercially available stents could not maintain radial integrity under the compressive force of the thick polymer sleeves, Quanam developed a novel stent platform. In fact, mounting the QP2-polymer sleeves on commercially available stents was found to cause stent recoil and sagging and draping of the polymer membrane into the lumen.

The QueST bare metal coronary stent was designed to maintain its radial integrity under the compressive force applied by 4 to 6 acrylate polymer sleeves. The QueST stent was laser cut from 316 L surgical-grade stainless steel into 3.8 mm long individual segments that were connected by intersegmental connecting links.

PRECLINICAL STUDIES

Quanam conducted preclinical studies to determine the biocompatibility of the components of the QuaDDS stent system. The acrylate polymer was tested in vitro and in vivo (rats, rabbits, pigs) and was found to be biocompatible. Studies to determine the effect of QP2 on neointima indicated that QP2 reduced neointimal proliferation at 4 weeks, but no later evaluations were available.

The QuaDDS stent was studied in rabbit iliac and porcine coronary artery models. Total doses of 1500 μg and 3200 μg were evaluated 4 and 8 weeks after implantation. The results indicated a significant reduction in neointimal thickening with no thrombus, acute inflammation, fibrosis, foreign body reactions or medial thinning. Chronic inflammation and the presence of granulation tissue was minimal; cellular necrosis was mild to moderate.[2]

CLINICAL STUDIES

Early, single-arm studies

The BARDDS registry was an open-label study conducted at two sites in South America. At

11 months post implant, the only major adverse cardiac events (MACE) reported were two target vessel revascularizations (6%; 2/32) for stenosis occurring outside of the QuaDDS study stent. Of 32 patients who received a QuaDDS stent and were followed up for at least one year, a subgroup of 13 underwent angiographic and intravascular ultrasound (IVUS) re-evaluation at 11 months, which revealed no evidence of significant neointimal proliferation in the QuaDDS stents. At follow-up, the mean percentage diameter stenosis had been reduced from 84% to 6.3% and minimum lumen diameter had increased from 0.6 mm to 2.9 mm.[6]

The SCORE trial

The Study to Compare Restenosis Rates Between QueST and QuaDDS-QP2 (SCORE) was a randomized, open label, controlled trial comparing the safety and performance of the QuaDDS stent with the bare QueST stent or other bare metal stent for the treatment of de novo coronary artery lesions. The purpose of the study was to establish the superiority of the QuaDDS stent over bare metal stents for reducing restenosis after stent implantation.

The primary endpoint of the study was target vessel revascularization rate at 6 months post implantation. Additional endpoints included restenosis at 6 months as measured by quantitative coronary angiography (QCA) and intravascular ultrasound (IVUS).

Enrollment began in February 2000 at a total of 19 sites in Germany, France, Italy, the Czech Republic, Australia, and New Zealand. Planned enrollment for SCORE was 400 patients based on 80% power to detect a 10% reduction of restenosis in the treatment group with a one-sided level of significance of 0.05. In 19 April 2001, enrollment in SCORE was terminated with 266 patients enrolled due to an unexpectedly high rate of adverse cardiac events.

Study population

Patients were randomly assigned to receive either the QuaDDS stent ($n = 128$) or a bare control stent (QueST $n = 112$; other bare metal stent $n = 26$; total control group $n = 138$).

Aspirin (100 mg daily) and clopidogrel or ticlopidine (500 mg daily) were prescribed for 6 months post procedure.

Eligible patients had angiographically confirmed de novo lesions of ≤30 mm in length in native coronary arteries, lumen narrowing >50%, and vessel diameters between 3.0 mm and 4.0 mm. Patients with lesions requiring more than one stent for full lesion coverage were excluded from the study. Clinical exclusion criteria included history of acute myocardial infarction; left ventricular ejection fraction <30%; stroke within the past 6 months; renal dysfunction as defined by serum creatinine >1.7 µg/100 ml; or contraindication to aspirin, heparin, ticlopidine or stainless steel. Baseline patient characteristics are shown in Table 59.1.

Follow-up

Clinical evaluation was conducted 1, 6, and 12 months after stent implantation. Coronary angiography was performed before the procedure, immediately post procedure, and 6 months post procedure. A subset of patients was examined by IVUS immediately post procedure and at the 6 month follow-up visit.

Early safety analysis

According to an early safety analysis performed in April 2001, the MACE rate was 18% in the QuaDDS group compared with only 2% in the control group. Among QuaDDS patients, 12 stent thromboses, 5 cardiac-related deaths (3 associated with thrombosis), and 20 myocardial infarctions (10 associated with thrombosis) were reported. Among control patients there were no stent thromboses or cardiac-related deaths and 3 myocardial infarctions. These unacceptable safety findings led to the decision to stop trial enrollment.

Final safety analysis

For a qualified detail analysis, a new trial database was created and an independent clinical events committee (CEC) adjudicated all major adverse cardiac events. These new processes focused on safety and antiplatelet medication

Table 59.1   Baseline demographics and clinical characteristics in the SCORE trial

Characteristic	QuaDDS (n = 128)	Control (n = 138)
Gender (male)	81% (104)	78% (107)
Age (years, min, max)	61 (33, 79)	63 (34, 80)
Diabetes	20% (25)	21% (29)
Hypertension	68% (87)	64% (88)
Previous myocardial infarction	39% (50)	41% (56)
Mean reference vessel diameter (mm)	3.24	3.27
Lesion length (mm)	11.1	11.2
Diameter stenosis (%)	85.1%	84.7%

compliance. With the data collected from this more intensive trial monitoring, the SCORE data were again analyzed in May 2002. Under the new system, the number of patients followed up increased markedly from 114/266 to 261/266, as did the number of MACE events identified.

MACE rates as adjudicated by the CEC in September 2002 are shown in Table 59.2. The higher MACE rate in the QuaDDS group (49.2%) versus the control group (30.4%) was primarily due to more stent thromboses in the QuaDDS group (11.7%) than in the control group (2.2%). In addition, more myocardial intarctions occurred in the QuaDDS group (21%) compared with the control group (3%).[7]

Quantitative coronary angiography (QCA) at 6 months

Six month angiography was performed in 81% of QueST-treated patients and 80% of QuaDDS-treated patients. Quantitative coronary angiography results are shown in Table 59.3.

Table 59.2   Major adverse cardiac events reported in the SCORE trial between February 2000 and June 2002

Event	QuaDDS (n = 128)	Control (n = 138)
Total MACE (non-hierarchical)	49.2%	30.4%
Cardiac death	5 (4%)	0 (0%)
Myocardial infarction (MI)	27 (21%)	4 (3%)
Target vessel revascularization (TVR)	42 (33%)	7 (5%)
Target lesion revascularization (TLR)	27 (21%)	35 (25%)
Stent thrombosis	16 (11.7%)	5 (2.2%)

Table 59.3   Quantitative analysis of stented vessels in the SCORE trial 6 months after stent implantation

	QuaDDS	Control	p
Diameter stenosis (%)	20.4 ± 23.9 (n = 99)	41.3 ± 25.4 (n = 103)	0.0001
Binary (>50%) restenosis (%)	6.4% (6/94)	36.9% (38/103)	0.001
Late lumen loss (mm)	0.35 ± 0.73 (n = 98)	0.65 ± 0.71 (n = 102)	0.0039
Acute gain (mm)	1.37 ± 0.50 (n = 125)	1.36 ± 0.55 (n = 133)	0.88
Loss index[a]	0.27 ± 0.63 (n = 99)	0.58 ± 0.41 (n = 103)	0.0001

[a] Loss index = Late loss/acute gain.

Percentage diameter stenosis was significantly (p = 0.0001) lower in the QuaDDS group (17.1%) than in the QueST group (41.3%). Similarly, late loss was significantly (p = 0.0039) lower in the QuaDDS group (0.35 mm) compared with the QueST group (0.65 mm). However, percentage diameter stenosis in the QueST group was higher than is usual with commercially available uncoated stents.

Accordingly, there was significantly (p = 0.0001) less binary restenosis in the QuaDDS group compared with the control group.

Intravascular ultrasound (IVUS) at 6 months

Core lab IVUS analysis in a selected subset of patients showed significantly (p<0.001) reduced neointimal volume in the QuaDDS group (11.3 mm³) compared with the control group (127 mm³).[8] In the QuaDDS group, neointima was either undetectable or appeared as a thin layer on part of the stent struts. In the control group, almost all stent struts were covered with neointima throughout the stented segment. This was accompanied by a significantly (p = 0.001) larger minimum lumen area in the QuaDDS (6.40 mm²) group compared with the control (4.97 mm²) group.

Summary of SCORE findings

Although the QuaDDS stent reduced neointimal proliferation by 56–70% compared with the control stents in the SCORE trial, the rate of major adverse cardiac events was unacceptably high in both groups, with the QuaDDS group significantly higher than the control group. Specifically, stent thrombosis was responsible for 50% of the myocardial infarctions among QuaDDS-treated patients, with side branch occlusion being a major contributor. This unfavorable safety outcome led the investigators to question the possible underlying causes, such as polymer, drug dose, duration of drug release, and stent platform, and revisit the QuaDDS preclinical data. In order to find explanations, further porcine studies were then conducted, particularly to assess local vascular responses to QP2 and the polymer sleeves.

PRECLINICIAL STUDIES: AFTER SCORE

A new animal study was initiated in April 2000 to assess the local vessel response of nondiseased, non-injured porcine coronary arteries to the QuaDDS stent loaded with polymer sleeves containing QP2. One bare control stent (n = 8) and one QuaDDS stent (n = 16) were placed in a coronary artery of 12 female pigs, with the exception of one pig that did not receive a control stent. Half of the control stents were QueST stents (n = 4) and half were commercially available coronary stents (n = 4).

Hematology and blood chemistry, as tested pre-implantation and at harvest (6, 9, or 12 months), yielded equivalent results for all animals, indicating that the QuaDDS stent did not produce toxic effects. However, histopathologic assessments uncovered differences in vessel response to the three types of stents. In the four commercial control stents, in-stent restenosis was minimal (n = 2) and mild (n = 2). In the four QueST control stents, in-stent restenosis was mild (n = 2) and moderate (n = 2), and in the 16 QuaDDS stents, in-stent restenosis was mild (n = 2), moderate (n = 4), and extensive (n = 10).

In vessels examined at 6 months post implantation, polymer sleeves were surrounded by thrombus that did not organize. In addition, negative vessel remodeling was partly present proximal and distal to the stent in QuaDDS-treated vessels. In contrast, control stents did not stimulate positive or negative remodeling. At 12 months post implantation, the QuaDDS stent was associated with total occlusions and neointimal variations including organizing thrombus and fibrocellular tissue. QuaDDS-treated vessels had become severely stenotic with lumen loss reaching >90% and the neointima on these stents appeared to be hyperproliferative. In addition, negative remodeling proximal and distal to the stent increased between 6 and 12 months.

An additional animal study was conducted to evaluate the potential contribution of the polymer sleeves to the safety events seen in the SCORE study. QuaDDS stents with polymer sleeve only but no drug (n = 15) or QueST bare metal stent (n = 6) were implanted in nondiseased, non-injured porcine coronary arteries. At 1-month follow-up, the mortality in the QuaDDS polymer-only stent group was 29% (2/7) compared with 0% (0/3) in the control group. Mortality among pigs evaluated at 3 months post implantation was 63% (5/8) in QuaDDS polymer-only group compared with 0% (0/3) for the control group. Of the total seven deaths in the QuaDDS-treated pigs, six were determined to be of cardiac origin. At 1-month follow-up, angiographic restenosis was present in both groups, but significantly ($p<0.05$) higher in the QuaDDS polymer-only group (56% ± 19) compared with the control group (33% ± 23) (Figure 59.3). Histopathological examination of vessels from the QuaDDS polymer-only group revealed an

a

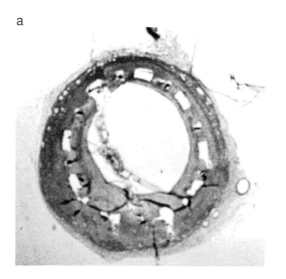

b

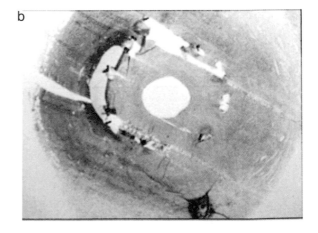

Fig. 59.3 Porcine coronary artery 90 days after stent implantation. (a) Control (b) QuaDDS polymer only.

intense inflammatory reaction with frequent granulomas and fibrosis often associated with severe narrowing or occlusion.

CONCLUSIONS

Based on these results, it was concluded that the QuaDDS polymer sleeves are not an acceptable platform for local drug delivery to coronary vessels due to excessive thrombotic and inflammatory response. The histopathologic findings in these two preclinical studies argue that the polymer is the likely cause of the unacceptably high adverse event rate among QuaDDS-treated patients in the SCORE trial. However, SCORE demonstrated efficacy of a drug eluting stent system in clinical practice in reducing neointimal proliferation in treatment of coronary artery disease and therefore, this study provided the first 'proof' of the drug eluting stent concept.

REFERENCES

1. Kingston DGI. The chemistry of TAXOL. Pharmacol Ther 1991; 52:1–34.
2. Silber S, Grube G, Fitzgerald P. The Quanam QuaDDS-QP2 Stent. In: Serruys PW, Rensing BJ, (eds), Handbook of Coronary Stents, 4th edn. Martin Dunitz: London 2002:343–7.
3. Landzberg BR, et al. Pathophysiology and pharmacological approaches for prevention of coronary artery restenosis following coronary artery balloon angioplasty and related procedures. Prog Cardiovasc Dis 1997; 39(4):361.
4. Morice MC, Serruys PW, Sousa JE, et al. for the RAVEL Study group. A randomized comparison of a sirolimus-eluting stent with a standard stent for coronary revascularization. New Engl J Med 2002; 346:1773–80.
5. Stertzer SH. Evaluation of in-vitro release of 3H-labeled QP-2 in rabbit iliac arteries. 6th International Local Drug Delivery Meeting and Cardiovascular and Molecular Strategies, Geneva, Switzerland, January 2000.
6. de la Fuente LM, Miano J, Mrad J et al. Initial results of the Quanam drug eluting stent (QuaDS-QP-2) Registry (BARDDS) in human subjects. Catheter Cardiovasc Interv 2001; 53(4):480–8.
7. Grube E. The SCORE randomized trial: QuaDDS-QP2 stent with a polymer sleeve delivery system. Lessons learned from a pioneering study. Transcatheter Cardiovascular Therapeutics, Washington, DC September 2002.
8. Kataoka T, Grube E, Honda Y, et al. 7-Hexanoyltaxol-eluting stent for prevention of neointimal growth. An intravascular ultrasound analysis from the Study to COmpare REstenosis rate between QueST and QuaDS-QP2 (SCORE). Circulation 2002; 106:1788–93.

60

The Boston Scientific paclitaxel eluting stent: TAXUS I and II

Eberhard Grube

Introduction • The TAXUS drug delivery system • The TAXUS I feasibility study • Results
• TAXUS II two-dose formulation study • Results
• TAXUS program: current status and perspective

INTRODUCTION

The TAXUS program at Boston Scientific Corporation is exploring both safety and performance of the TAXUS polymer-based, paclitaxel eluting stent, which delivers low dose paclitaxel to the vessel wall during the initial phase of the restenotic process following stent implantation. The microtubule inhibitor, paclitaxel, has been shown to interrupt key cellular and molecular processes associated with the restenotic cascade.[1,2]

The objective of the TAXUS polymer-based, paclitaxel eluting stent system is to deliver the minimum effective dose of paclitaxel for the shortest duration using controlled biphasic drug delivery targeted to the initial phase of the restenotic cascade. The TAXUS stent is designed to blunt the vessel's initial response to injury, thus preventing restenosis due to neointimal proliferation, while still allowing vascular healing through endothelialization.

THE TAXUS DRUG DELIVERY SYSTEM

Paclitaxel eluting stents in the TAXUS I and II trials were NIR™ Conformer stents coated with paclitaxel loaded into a proprietary polymer coating.

Polymer-based drug delivery was chosen for the TAXUS stent system to physically retain the drug, provide homogeneous coverage of the stent surface, prevent mechanical disruption of the drug during implantation, and control release of paclitaxel from the stent. The key advantage of polymer-based drug delivery is controlled release of paclitaxel into the vessel environment so that the lowest effective dose can be delivered within the critical time period following stent implantation.

The polymer is of the class known as 'polyolefins'. It was developed to combine coating integrity, biovascular compatibility, long-term biostability, heat stability, and stability under various sterilization techniques. In addition, the polymer's elastomeric quality makes it ideal for coating directly on to stent struts in that the elastic properties maintain uniform coverage even after crimping, expansion, and manipulation.

The TAXUS paclitaxel eluting stents have a dose density of 1 μg/mm^2 paclitaxel (loaded drug per stent surface area). For example, in the current TAXUS stents on the Express™

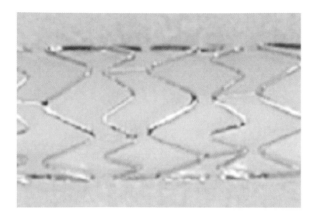

Fig. 60.1 The TAXUS NIRx stent.

platform 108 μg paclitaxel is loaded on to the 16 mm stent and 209 μg on the 32 mm stent. Actual dose released from the stent is a function of the drug-to-polymer ratio, which is termed the 'release formulation.' Higher drug-to-polymer ratios result in faster and higher levels of drug release. For this reason, the slow release TAXUS stent has a lower drug-to-polymer ratio than the moderate release TAXUS stent. In both the slow and moderate release formulations, release of paclitaxel from the polymer matrix is 'biphasic', with an early burst phase of active drug release in the first 48 hours followed by a slower release of smaller amounts of the active drug over the subsequent 8 days.

The TAXUS™ NIRx stent used in the TAXUS I and II trials was a stainless steel NIR™ Conformer stent coated with 1 μg/mm² paclitaxel loaded into the polymer drug delivery system (Figure 60.1, Table 60.1). The NIR stent is made from sheets of 316 LS surgical grade stainless steel, photochemically etched into a prespecified geometric pattern, which is then folded and welded to make cylindrical stents. The geometry is a continuous, uniform multicellular design, with adaptive cells capable of differential lengthening. This enables the stent to be flexible in the unexpanded configuration. The NIRx stent was premounted on an Advance™ monorail-style balloon delivery catheter for implantation. All stents in the

Table 60.1 TAXUS I and II trial comparison		
	TAXUS I *Germany*	*TAXUS II* *International*
Purpose	Feasibility	Two-dose efficacy
Lesion	De novo	De novo
Control	Uncoated control	Uncoated control
Design	Randomized (1:1)	Randomized (1:1)
Total loaded dose	1 μg/mm²	1 μg/mm²
Release formulation	Slow release	Cohort I: Slow release Cohort II: Moderate release
Patient enrollment	61	536
Primary endpoint	30 day major adverse cardiac events (MACE)	6 month % in-stent net volume obstruction (IVUS)

IVUS, intravascular ultrasound.

TAXUS I and II trials were 15 mm in length and either 3.0 mm or 3.5 mm in diameter.

THE TAXUS I FEASIBILITY STUDY

The TAXUS I trial evaluated both the safety and feasibility of the slow release formulation TAXUS stent (TAXUS-SR) in the treatment of de novo coronary lesions.[3] TAXUS I was a randomized, double blinded, controlled trial comparing the slow release TAXUS-SR NIRx stent with the uncoated NIR™ Conformer stent. This study enrolled a total of 61 subjects at three sites in Germany (Siegburg, Munich, and Trier).

Hypothesis

The initial hypothesis was that the TAXUS stent would have a safety profile comparable to the bare NIR stent with respect to major adverse cardiac events (MACE) 30 days after implantation. MACE was defined as death from any cause, Q-wave myocardial infarction (MI), target vessel revascularization, and stent thrombosis. Q-wave MI was defined as development of Q-waves in 2 or more contiguous leads with postimplantation elevated creatine kinase-myocardial band (CK-MB) isoenzyme levels. Target vessel revascularization included coronary artery bypass graft (CABG) surgery as well as repeat percutaneous intervention on the stented vessel.

Study population

Patients were randomly assigned to receive either the bare NIR stent ($n = 30$) or the TAXUS NIRx stent ($n = 31$). Patients were included in TAXUS I if angiography showed lesion lengths ≤12 mm, diameter stenosis between 50% and 99%, and vessel diameter between 3.0 mm and 3.5 mm. Patients were excluded if they had a history of acute MI; in-stent restenosis; a left ventricular ejection fraction <30%; a stroke within the past 6 months; renal dysfunction as defined by serum creatinine above 1.7 µg/ 100 mL; or contraindication to aspirin, clopidogrel, or ticlopidine. Lesions requiring more

than one stent for full lesion coverage were also excluded.

Follow-up

Clinical evaluation was conducted 1, 6, and 12 months after stent implantation, and annual follow-up will be continued until 5 years post implantation. Coronary angiographic and intravascular ultrasound imaging were performed before and after stent implantation and at the 6 month follow-up visit.

RESULTS

Baseline demographics and lesion characteristics were similar between the TAXUS and control groups, as shown in Table 60.2. The majority of patients (59) had de novo lesions; two patients had restenotic lesions.

Major adverse cardiac event (MACE)

At 30 days after stent implantation, there were no (0%) incidents of MACE or stent thrombosis in either cohort, indicating a comparable safety profile for the TAXUS stent relative to the uncoated control stent.

At 6 months, the MACE rate was 0% (0 events/31 patients) for the TAXUS group compared with 7% (2 events/30 patients) in the control group, although this difference was not statistically significant. The two MACE in the control group were target lesion revascularizations (TLR) due to diffuse in-stent restenosis.

One year after stent implantation MACE rates were 3% (1/31) in the TAXUS group and 10% (3/30) in the control group (Table 60.3). The single MACE in the TAXUS group was due to TLR in a lesion remote from the target lesion. MACE in the control group was attributed to four TLRs in three patients – three percutaneous coronary target lesion reinterventions and one coronary artery bypass grafting which included the target lesion. No stent thromboses were reported at any time during the first year after implantation in either treatment group.

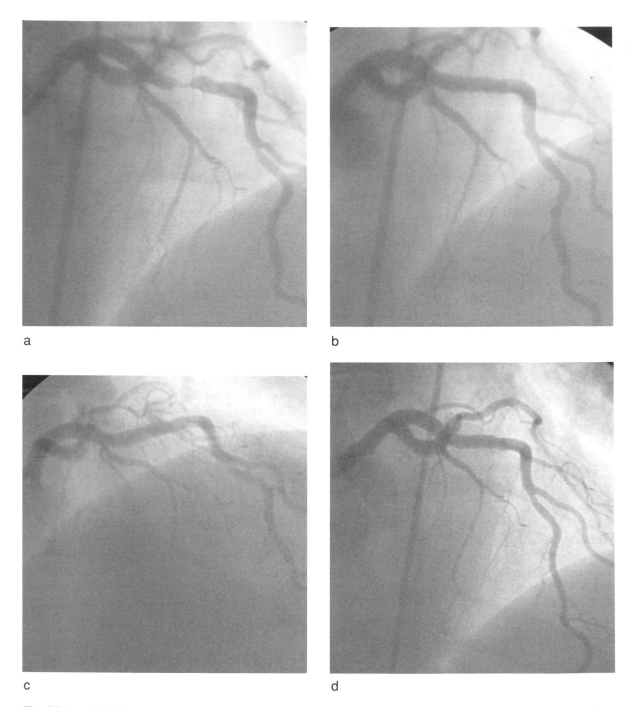

Fig. 60.2 TAXUS I angiographic images. (a) Baseline, (b) post procedure, (c) at 6 months, (d) at 18 months.

The goals of the TAXUS II trial were 2-fold: (1) to evaluate the safety and efficacy of the TAXUS stent for treatment of standard risk, de novo lesions, and (2) to compare the effect of two-dose formulations (slow and moderate) of the TAXUS stent.

The primary endpoint was percentage in-stent net volume obstruction measured by

Table 60.5   TAXUS I intravascular ultrasound analysis at 6 month follow-up

Lesion characteristic	TAXUS	Control	p
Minimal lumen area (mm^3)	5.57 ± 1.21 ($n = 26$)	4.77 ± 1.31 ($n = 26$)	0.0268
Normalized neointimal hyperplasia (mm^3)	14.82 ± 10.83 ($n = 26$)	21.57 ± 10.71 ($n = 26$)	0.0283

IVUS. This endpoint was selected because it provides a precise, three-dimensional measure of neointimal formation that serves as the basis for restenosis assessment.

Hypothesis

The hypothesis for the TAXUS II trial was that TAXUS stents would have reduced neointimal hyperplasia as measured by percentage in-stent net volume obstruction.

Study population

The TAXUS II trial enrolled 536 patients into two consecutive but independent cohorts. Cohort 1 consisted of patients randomized to the TAXUS slow release (SR) stent ($n = 131$) or control stent ($n = 136$). Cohort 1 was enrolled from patients at 28 centers in 12 countries including Europe, Canada, and Australia. After review of Cohort 1 30 day safety data by a safety data monitoring board, enrollment of Cohort 2 began. Cohort 2 randomized patients to the TAXUS moderate release (MR) stent ($n = 135$) or uncoated control stent ($n = 134$).

Patients were eligible for this study if they were diagnosed with stable or unstable angina or silent ischemia, were candidates for coronary artery bypass graft, and not pregnant, lactating or intending to become pregnant. Angiographic inclusion criteria specified a de novo target lesion with diameter stenosis between 50% and 99%, length ≤12 mm, located in a vessel between 3.0 mm and 3.5 mm in diameter. Patients were excluded if they had a coronary

intervention within the past month, left ventricular ejection fraction <30%, evolving myocardial infarction, unprotected left main coronary disease, or diffuse disease requiring more than one 15 mm stent for full lesion coverage.

Follow-up

Coronary angiographic and intravascular ultrasound imaging were performed before and after stent implantation and at the 6 month follow-up visit. Clinical evaluation was conducted at 1, 6, and 12 months after stent implantation and annually for 5 years thereafter.

RESULTS

The baseline demographics and lesion characteristics were similar between the TAXUS-SR, TAXUS-MR and both control groups (Table 60.6). Because no significant clinical differences were found between the control groups, the data for these groups were combined to create a combined control group for comparison with the TAXUS stents.

Major adverse cardiac event (MACE)

At 30 days post procedure, MACE rates were not significantly different among the three groups: TAXUS-SR 2.3%, TAXUS-MR 2.2%, and control 4.4% ($p = 0.40$ for comparison of each TAXUS group with the control group). One month after stent implantation, there were no (0%) stent thromboses in either of the TAXUS groups or the control group.

Table 60.6 TAXUS II baseline demographics and clinical characteristics			
Characteristic	TAXUS-SR (n = 131)	TAXUS-MR (n = 135)	Control (n = 270)
Gender (male)	70	76	78
Age (years, min, max)	61.5 ± 10.5	59.3 ± 10.5	59.8 ± 9.7
Minimal luminal diameter (MLD) (mm)	1.0 ± 0.3	1.0 ± 0.3	1.0 ± 0.4
Lesion length (mm)	10.6 ± 3.9	10.2 ± 4.8	10.6 ± 4.1
Diameter stenosis (DM) (%)	63 ± 10	65 ± 10	65 ± 11
Mean reference vessel diameter (mm)	2.8 ± 0.4	2.7 ± 0.5	2.8 ± 0.5

At 6 months post procedure, MACE rates in the TAXUS-SR group (8.5%; $p = 0.0035$) and TAXUS-MR (7.8%; $p = 0.0019$) group were significantly lower than in the control group (19.8%). This reduction was predominantly due to reductions in target vessel revascularizations (Table 60.7). Only one of the 10 target lesion revascularizations in the TAXUS-treated patients was performed for restenosis occurring within the study stent segment.

At 12 months post procedure, the MACE rates in the TAXUS groups (SR: 10.9% and MR: 9.9%) continued to be significantly lower than in the control group (21.7%).

Quanitative coronary angiography (QCA)

At 6 months, all quantitative angiographic indices (minimum lumen diameter, percentage diameter stenosis, late lumen loss) were significantly ($p<0.0001$) improved in the TAXUS-SR and TAXUS-MR groups compared with the control group (Table 60.8).

The 6 month binary in-segment restenosis rate was significantly lower in the TAXUS-SR (5.5%; $p = 0.0001$) and TAXUS-MR (8.6%; $p = 0.001$) groups compared with the control group (22%). Similarly, binary restenosis in the in-stent analysis was significantly lower for TAXUS-SR (2.3%; $p = 0.0001$) and TAXUS-MR

(4.7%; $p = 0.0001$) groups as compared with the control group (19%).

Incidence of aneurysm was slightly, but not significantly, higher in the TAXUS-SR group (2.3%; 4/128) than the TAXUS-MR (0.8%; 1/128) and control (1.6%; 4/256) groups.

Intravascular ultrasound (IVUS)

The primary endpoint of percentage in-stent net volume obstruction was significantly reduced in the TAXUS-SR (7.8 ± 9.7%) and TAXUS-MR (7.9 ± 9.9%) groups compared with the control group (21.9 ± 17.5%, $p<0.0001$) (Table 60.9). Vessel volume was comparable in all groups without significant change from baseline to follow-up, indicating that the improvement was not due to vessel enlargement. The IVUS assessment showed no significant difference in late-acquired incomplete stent apposition between the two groups.

Summary of TAXUS II findings

These findings demonstrate the safety and superior performance of the TAXUS-SR and TAXUS-MR stents over uncoated control stents for the reduction of restenosis up to 12 months after treatment of de novo coronary artery lesions. Patients receiving TAXUS-SR and

Table 60.7   Major adverse cardiac events (MACE) in TAXUS II at 6 and 12 months

	Control (n = 270)	TAXUS-SR (n = 131)	p[a]	TAXUS-MR (n = 135)	p[b]
6 month MACE					
Overall	19.8%	8.5%	0.003	7.8%	0.002
Death	0.4%	0%		0%	
Myocardial infarction					
• Q-wave	0.8%	0%	1.00	0%	1.00
• non-Q wave	4.6%	1.5%	0.16	2.3%	0.40
Target vessel revascularization (TVR)					
• Overall	16.0%	7.7%	0.026	6.2%	0.006
– Target lesion	13.3%	4.6%	0.008	3.1%	0.001
– Non-target lesion	2.7%	3.1%	0.76	2.3%	1.00
– CABG	0.8%	0.8%	1.00	0.8%	1.00
12 month MACE					
Overall	21.7%	10.9%	0.0082	9.9%	0.0048
Death	0.8%	0.0%	1.0000	0.0%	1.0000
Myocardial infarction					
• Q-wave	1.1%	0.8%	1.0000	1.5%	1.0000
• Non-Q wave	4.2%	1.6%	0.2354	2.3%	0.4026
Target vessel revascularization (TVR)					
• Overall	17.5%	10.1%	0.0704	6.9%	0.0034
– Target lesion	14.4%	4.7%	0.0035	3.8%	0.0010
– Non-target lesion	3.0%	3.1%	1.0000	1.5%	0.5069
– CABG	1.1%	3.1%	0.2244	1.5 %	1.000

[a] Comparison of TAXUS-SR vs control. [b]comparison of TAXUS-MR vs control.
Numbers are percentages (event rates). Event rates are number of patients who experienced the outcome divided by number of patients eligible for the outcome.
One month MACE are included in the cumulative 6 month MACE. Overall TVR numbers do not add up to 100% as some patients had more than one TVR event.

TAXUS-MR stents displayed significant improvements in all key angiographic, intravascular ultrasound, and clinical endpoints compared with control patients. No significant differences in these parameters were reported between the two TAXUS groups.

These data provide proof of principle that 1 μg/mm^2 of paclitaxel delivered via a TAXUS

Table 60.8   TAXUS II angiographic analysis at 6 month follow-up

Lesion characteristic	TAXUS-MR (n = 135)	TAXUS-SR (n = 131)	Control (n = 270)	p
Minimal lumen diameter (MLD) (mm)	2.2 ± 0.5	2.2 ± 0.5	1.8 ± 0.6	0.0001
Diameter stenosis (DS) (%)	18 ± 12	20 ± 12	33 ± 18	0.0001
Binary restenosis (> 50%)	4.7%	2.3%	19%	0.0001
Late lumen loss (mm)	0.30 ± 0.39	0.31 ± 0.38	0.78 ± 0.47	0.0001
Reference vessel diameter (mm)	2.7 ± 0.4	2.8 ± 0.4	2.6 ± 0.5	0.040

Table 60.9   TAXUS II intravascular ultrasound analysis at 6 month follow-up

Lesion characteristic	TAXUS-SR (n = 131)	TAXUS-MR (n = 135)	Control (n = 270)	p
Vessel volume (mm^3)	255 ± 68	234 ± 71	248 ± 63	ns
Volume obstruction (%)	7.9 ± 9.9	7.8 ± 9.7	21.9 ± 17.5	0.0001

ns, not significant.

drug eluting stent reduces the neointimal processes that lead to restenosis.

TAXUS PROGRAM: CURRENT STATUS AND PERSPECTIVE

The TAXUS I and II trials provide proof of principle that polymer-based delivery of paclitaxel to the vessel endothelium immediately after stent implantation can blunt the initial vessel response to injury and prevent restenosis, while still allowing vascular healing with endothelialization. Together, these trials form a foundation of safety and superior performance of the paclitaxel eluting TAXUS stents in treating de novo coronary lesions.

There is consistency in degree of improvement across the TAXUS studies, as well as low MACE rates that are comparable to rates with bare metal stents. Reductions in late lumen loss in TAXUS-treated vessels compared with controls were remarkably similar in TAXUS I (0.36 mm) and TAXUS II (SR = 0.31 mm; MR = 0.30 mm). The consistency in the more sensitive angiographic and IVUS measures argues that the TAXUS system produces a reproducible biologic effect independent of trial and batch of coated stents, and across the indications studied to date. Taken together, the TAXUS I and II trials have established an acceptable safety and efficacy profile for reduction of restenosis in de novo coronary artery lesions.

The continuing goal of the TAXUS program is to identify the TAXUS stent formulation that is effective in reducing restenosis in progressively more complex coronary lesions and other diseased vessel beds. The TAXUS I and II trials indicate that TAXUS stents safely reduce restenosis after stent implantation in standard risk, de novo coronary lesions.

In order to evaluate safety and efficacy of this stent concept in larger patient populations as well as more complex lesion subsets, the TAXUS IV, V, and VI trials are now ongoing, providing further insight into this new and promising technology.

REFERENCES

1. Sollott SJ, Cheng L, Pauly RR, et al. Taxol inhibits neointimal smooth muscle cell accumulation after angioplasty in the rat. J Clin Invest 1995; 95(4):1869–76.

2. Axel DI, Kunert W, Goggelmann C, et al. Paclitaxel inhibits arterial smooth muscle cell proliferation and migration in vitro and in vivo using local drug delivery. Circulation 1997; 96(2):636–45.

3. Grube E, Silber S, Haupmann KE, et al. TAXUS I: Six- and twelve-month results from a randomized double blind trial on a slow-release paclitaxel-eluting stent for de novo coronary lesions. Circulation 2003; 106:38–42.

61

Clinical results with non-polymer based taxol eluting stents. The European evaLUation of pacliTaxel Eluting Stent (ELUTES) trial

Ivan De Scheerder, Bernard Chevalier, Edoardo Camenzind, and Anthony Gershlick, on behalf of the ELUTES investigators

Introduction • Methods • Results • Discussion • Conclusions

INTRODUCTION

Percutaneous coronary intervention (PCI) is an accepted method for treating atheromatous coronary disease. The value of stents over angioplasty alone has been demonstrated,[1,2] reducing the incidence of recurrence to between 15% and 20%. Restenosis in stented patients is almost totally due to the presence of in-stent tissue, caused by the migration of smooth muscle cells (SMCs) from the media of the vessel wall into the intima, where further proliferation and production of extracellular matrix (ECM) takes place. Approximately 1.5 million interventional procedures are undertaken worldwide annually and at 15% recurrence this equates to a potential need for 200 000 repeat procedures. Certain patients, such as diabetics, have an increased risk of recurrence, approaching 40%.[3] Restenosis almost wholly accounted for the difference between surgically treated patients and those undergoing PCI with stents in the ARTS trial.[4]

Preventing recurrence may be possible by delivering a drug, such as paclitaxel, which enhances polymerization of cellular microtubules and thus prevents mitosis, via the stent, locally inhibiting the proliferative process without producing systemic side effects. Studies in vitro,[5,6] and in animal models have shown that paclitaxel delivered locally reduces restenosis by such mechanisms,[7–9] with a dose-dependent benefit in a one month porcine artery model and no late thrombotic deaths.[10] The European evaLUation of pacliTaxel Eluting Stent (ELUTES) trial was a multicenter, randomized, controlled, triple blinded clinical study designed to evaluate the safety and efficacy of a paclitaxel eluting stent.

METHODS

A proprietary process (Cook Corp.) was used to coat paclitaxel to the abluminal bare metal surface of V-Flex Plus™ stents at four dose

Table 61.1   The ELUTES trial: inclusion and exclusion criteria

Inclusion	Exclusion
Age: 18 years +	LVEF <35%
Acceptable candidate for CABG	Enrollment in another trial
Agreed to return for clinical and angiographic follow-up	Women of child bearing potential Comorbidity
Lesion in native vessel	
Lesion type A, B1	Life expectancy <1 year
	Refusal blood transfusion, history coagulopathy
	Hypersensitivity stainless steel, contrast aspirin,
	clopidogrel, ticlopidine
	Multiple lesions requiring staged procedure
	Myocardial infarction <72 h prior
	Total occlusions
	Lesion length >15 mm
	Target reference diameter <2.75 or >3.5 mm
	Angiographic evidence of thrombus

CABG, coronary artery bypass graft; LVEF, left ventricular ejection fraction.

densities ($0.2 \,\mu g/mm^2$, $0.7 \,\mu g/mm^2$, $1.4 \,\mu g/mm^2$, and $2.7 \,\mu g/mm^2$ stent surface area), which were compared with uncoated stents. Consenting patients fulfilling the inclusion criteria (Table 61.1) and with single de novo, type A or B1 lesions, <15 mm long in a native coronary artery were entered into the study and data captured on standardized case report forms. The study was conducted with ethical committee approval in accordance with the Declaration of Helsinki at 10 investigative sites. Stents of either 3.0 mm or 3.5 mm diameter and 16 mm long were used in a predefined random computer-generated tabulated order. Randomization ensured near equal numbers in each of the five arms.

Angioplasty and stent procedure

Angioplasty and stent placement were performed using a radial or femoral approach and a monorail technique. Following predilation, the premounted stent was delivered by low pressure inflation and post dilated, if necessary, to achieve a minimal residual stenosis (<10%). If a second stent was required (e.g. for an edge tear) an open-label uncoated V-Flex Plus™ stent was used.

Antiplatelet therapy

Adjunct medications included aspirin and procedural heparin. Experience with vascular brachytherapy and preclinical data meant that clopidogrel or ticlopidine was mandated for 3 months due to potential delayed re-endothelialization.

Study endpoints

Primary *efficacy* endpoints were 'percentage diameter stenosis' and 'late loss' at 6 months

<table>
<tr><td colspan="1">

Table 61.2 The ELUTES trial: data acquisition, endpoints, and definitions

</td></tr>
</table>

Data collected

- Patient eligibility and history

- Lesion characteristics pre and post procedure

- Balloon and stent inflation data

- Cardiac enzymes pre and post procedure

- In-hospital complications

- 1 month clinical outcome

Primary efficacy endpoints

- Late loss, diameter stenosis, and binary restenosis at 6 months

Primary safety endpoints

- At 1 and 6 months, including Q- and non-Q wave infarction

- Need for CABG, PCI

- Total and subtotal occlusions

- Death

Q-wave myocardial infarctions were defined by the postprocedure presence of new Q-waves greater than 0.04 sec in two contiguous leads. Non-Q wave myocardial infarctions were defined as having peak CK or CK-MB values greater than twice the upper limit of normal. CABG, coronary artery bypass graft; PCI, percutaneous coronary intervention.

measured by angiographic analysis. Primary *safety* endpoints were MACE (as defined in Table 61.2) at 1 and 6 months adjudicated by an independent clinical events committee. Secondary endpoints and definitions are also shown in Table 61.2.

Angiographic analysis

Intracoronary nitrate was administered prior to image acquisition. A blinded independent angiographic core laboratory (The Cardiovascular Angiography Analysis Lab, Baylor College of Medicine) utilized the CAAS II system for standard quantitative coronary angiography (QCA) analysis of periprocedural

and follow-up angiograms. To account for edge effect within stent analysis included 5 mm beyond the stent edges. Investigators reported lesion morphology, side-branch involvement, dissections and TIMI flow.

Study power and statistical analysis

To show improvement in angiographic percentage diameter stenosis from 35% to 20% ($p < 0.05$), the study required a minimum of 32 evaluable patients per group when comparing any one dose versus control. Statistical analysis was performed using Systat v.10 (SPSS, Chicago, IL). Continuous variables are reported as mean and standard deviation and effects across five groups were analyzed by analysis of variance (ANOVA). Post-hoc multiple pair-wise comparisons employed the Bonferroni adjustment. Dichotomous variables were reported in percentages. Group-wise comparisons were performed with a Pearson's chi-square test or Fisher's exact test. All comparisons were performed on an intention-to-treat basis using all patients available with follow-up analysis.

RESULTS

Patient demographics and characteristics

Between January 2000 and April 2001, 192 patients were enrolled. Stent implantation was successful in 99% of patients. Of the 190 stented patients, 39 were randomized to control and 37, 39, 39, and 37 patients to the paclitaxel eluting stent groups (lowest to highest dose density group respectively). There were no significant baseline differences between groups (Table 61.3). The mean age was 60 years; 50% were hypercholesterolemic, and 16% diabetic. Lesion characteristics are described in Table 61.4.

Compliance

One patient suffered two protocol violations due to inter-hospital communication breakdown, receiving a trial thrombolytic *and* a nontrial stent prior to enrollment in ELUTES. The patient died suddenly 10 days post infarct due to an unknown cause.

Table 61.3 The ELUTES trial: patient demographics

	Paclitaxel dose density (µg/mm²)				Control	p-value
	2.7	1.4	0.7	0.2		
Number:	37	39	39	37	39	
Age (yrs)	56 ± 11	61 ± 10	58 ± 9	64 ± 10	61 ± 11	ns
Male gender	30 (81%)	31 (79%)	38 (95%)	27 (73%)	32 (82%)	ns
Diabetics	4 (11%)	8 (21%)	6 (15%)	8 (22%)	4 (10%)	ns
Hypercholesterolemia	22 (59%)	18 (46%)	20 (50%)	18 (49%)	17 (44%)	ns
Hypertension	18 (49%)	14 (36%)	16 (40%)	19 (51%)	21 (54%)	ns
Smoking						ns
Never	5 (14%)	10 (26%)	14 (35%)	15 (41%)	14 (36%)	
Past	15 (41%)	7 (18%)	10 (25%)	10 (27%)	12 (31%)	
Current	16 (43%)	18 (46%)	13 (33%)	8 (22%)	13 (33%)	
Obesity	7 (19%)	6 (15%)	9 (23%)	10 (27%)	4 (10%)	ns
Prior MI	11 (30%)	9 (23%)	18 (45%)	12 (32%)	16 (41%)	ns
Prior CABG	0 (0%)	1 (3%)	0 (0%)	0 (0%)	3 (8%)	ns
No. diseased vessels						ns
1	23 (61%)	20 (51%)	22 (55%)	24 (65%)	20 (51%)	
2	9 (24%)	11 (28%)	12 (30%)	10 (27%)	10 (26%)	
3	2 (5%)	6 (15%)	5 (13%)	1 (3%)	8 (21%)	
4	3 (8%)	2 (5%)	0 (0%)	1 (3%)	1 (3%)	
5	0 (0%)	0 (0%)	1 (3%)	1 (3%)	0 (0%)	

MI, myocardial infarction; CABG, coronary artery bypass graft; ns, not significant.

Clinical and late angiographic follow-up

Mean time for '6 month' angiographic follow-up was 187 ± 18 (range: 113–259) days.

At 6 months one patient had died (see above) and one patient was unavailable for clinical follow-up. Eleven patients refused angiographic follow up:

– Control: $n = 3$
– 0.2 µg/mm²: $n = 3$
– 0.7 µg/mm²: $n = 2$
– 1.4 µg/mm²: $n = 2$
– 2.7 µg/mm²: $n = 1$

Efficacy

Pre procedure there were no significant differences between groups in reference vessel size (2.95 mm–3.03 mm). Vessels were significantly narrowed [mean diameter stenosis (DS)

Table 61.4 The ELUTES trial: lesion characteristics						
	Paclitaxel dose density (μg/mm²)				Control	p-value
	2.7	1.4	0.7	0.2		
Number:	37	39	40	37	39	
Vessel						0.030
LAD	15 (41%)	20 (51%)	9 (23%)	14 (38%)	15 (38%)	
RCA	15 (41%)	9 (23%)	17 (43%)	16 (43%)	11 (28%)	
LCX	7 (19%)	7 (18%)	12 (30%)	6 (16%)	9 (23%)	
Ramus	0 (0%)	3 (8%)	2 (5%)	1 (3%)	4 (10%)	
Vessel type						ns
A	9 (24%)	12 (31%)	7 (18%)	12 (32%)	12 (31%)	
B1	23 (61%)	25 (64%)	29 (73%)	23 (61%)	23 (59%)	
B2	5 (14%)	2 (5%)	3 (8%)	2 (5%)	4 (10%)	
Unknown	0 (0%)	0 (0%)	1 (3%)	0 (0%)	0 (0%)	
Proximal tortuosity						ns
None	14 (38%)	22 (56%)	17 (43%)	17 (46%)	24 (61%)	
Mild	21 (57%)	17 (44%)	19 (48%)	18 (49%)	11 (28%)	
Moderate	2 (5%)	0 (0%)	4 (10%)	2 (5%)	3 (8%)	
Severe	0 (0%)	0 (0%)	0 (0%)	0 (0%)	1 (3%)	
Calcification						ns
None	21 (57%)	19 (49%)	22 (55%)	22 (59%)	26 (67%)	
Mild	13 (35%)	19 (49%)	14 (35%)	14 (38%)	12 (31%)	
Moderate	3 (8%)	1 (3%)	4 (10%)	1 (3%)	0 (0%)	
Unknown	0 (0%)	0 (0%)	0 (0%)	0 (0%)	1 (3%)	
Shape						ns
Concentric	15 (41%)	24 (61%)	18 (45%)	19 (51%)	19 (49%)	
Eccentric	22 (59%)	15 (38%)	22 (55%)	18 (49%)	20 (51%)	
Angulation >45°	4 (11%)	1 (3%)	2 (5%)	4 (11%)	1 (3%)	ns
Other stenosis	2 (5%)	2 (5%)	2 (5%)	2 (5%)	1 (3%)	ns
Ostial	0 (0%)	3 (8%)	0 (0%)	1 (3%)	0 (0%)	ns
Branch	5 (14%)	7 (18%)	3 (8%)	4 (11%)	1 (3%)	ns
Thrombus	0 (0%)	1 (3%)	2 (5%)	0 (0%)	1 (3%)	ns

LAD, left anterior descending artery; RCA, right coronary artery; LCX, left circumflex artery; ns, not significant.

Table 61.5   The ELUTES study: angiographic effectiveness measures

	Paclitaxel dose density (μg/mm²)				Control	p-value*
	2.7	1.4	0.7	0.2		
Procedural results:						
Number:	37	39	38	37	39	–
Lesion length (mm)	11.1 ± 3.1	10.2 ± 3.7	10.6 ± 3.1	11.3 ± 4.4	10.9 ± 3.8	ns
RVD pre (mm)	2.95 ± 0.44	2.93 ± 0.37	2.90 ± 0.39	3.03 ± 0.41	2.99 ± 0.51	ns
RVD post (mm)	2.96 ± 0.38	2.96 ± 0.34	2.95 ± 0.34	3.07 ± 0.38	3.02 ± 0.48	ns
MLD pre (mm)	0.56 ± 0.28	0.56 ± 0.23	0.56 ± 0.25	0.57 ± 0.35	0.53 ± 0.28	ns
MLD post (mm)	2.66 ± 0.41	2.72 ± 0.35	2.63 ± 0.36	2.78 ± 0.46	2.68 ± 0.39	ns
DS pre (%)	81.4 ± 7.44	80.8 ± 7.82	80.6 ± 8.47	81.5 ± 9.72	82.3 ± 7.85	ns
DS post (%)	10.0 ± 9.32	8.08 ± 6.84	10.6 ± 8.30	9.57 ± 9.82	10.5 ± 8.42	ns
	Paclitaxel dose density (μg/mm²)				Control	p-value*
	2.7	1.4	0.7	0.2		
6-month follow-up results						
Number:	32	37	35	34	34	–
MLD (mm)	2.56 ± 0.13	2.26 ± 0.12	2.10 ± 0.13	2.02 ± 0.13	1.98 ± 0.13	0.019
DS (%)	14.1 ± 4.1	23.3 ± 3.8	27.5 ± 3.9	32.8 ± 4.0	33.9 ± 4.0	0.007
Late loss (mm)	0.10 ± 0.12	0.47 ± 0.11	0.47 ± 0.11	0.71 ± 0.11	0.73 ± 0.11	0.002
Binary in-stent restenosis rate	3.1% (1/32)	13.5% (5/37)	14.3% (5/35)	20.6% (7/34)	20.6% (7/34)	0.055

RVD, reference vessel diameter; MLD, minimal luminal diameter, DS, diameter stenosis; ns, not significant.
* High dose vs control.

80%, minimal luminal diameter (MLD) 0.53–0.57 mm] (Table 61.5). Residual stenosis was 8–10%.

Six-month QCA demonstrated benefit in the highest dose density group (2.7 μg/mm²). The percentage DS was reduced from 33.9 ± 26.7% in the control group to 14.1 ± 16.4% ($p<0.0007$) and late loss from 0.73 ± 0.73 mm to 0.10 ± 0.49 mm ($p<0.0002$) (Table 61.5). Binary in-stent restenosis defined as DS≥50% at follow-up was reduced from 20.6% to 3.1% ($p<0.055$) with a

corresponding dose-dependent improvement in MLD from 1.98 ± 0.86 mm in the control group to 2.56 ± 0.61 mm ($p<0.05$). There were no significant benefits seen with intermediate doses.

MLD cumulative distribution curves for control and 2.7 μg/mm² dose density groups are similar at baseline and immediately after stent placement (Figure 61.1). However, at 6 months the distribution in the 2.7 μg/mm² group is similar to immediately after stenting

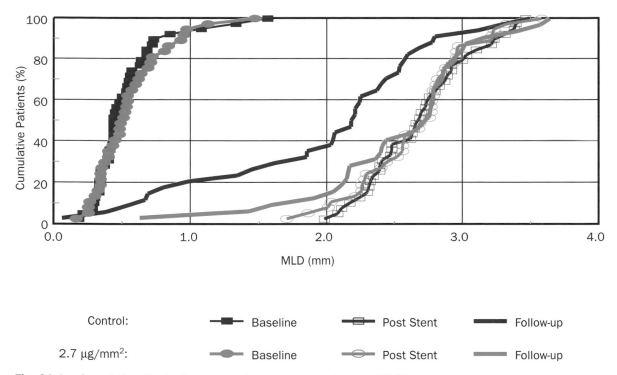

Fig. 61.1 Cumulative distribution graph of mean luminal diameter (MLD).

minimal intimal hyperplasia formation. This result is also clearly demonstrated by the cumulative distribution curves for percentage DS (Figure 61.2).

Safety

One month MACEs are shown in the hierarchical analysis in Table 61.6. There were no 30 day MACE events in the intermediate dose groups. In the 2.7 μg/mm² treatment group, three events were reported. One death occurred in the patient with the two protocol violations as previously described. One subacute thrombosis occurred in a patient with a proximal edge tear following trial stent implantation, necessitating placement of an additional non-trial stent. The patient received redilatation of the trial and non-trial stent at day 8 having presented with chest pain and electrocardiogram (ECG) changes. The third early event was a non-Q wave infarct at the time of stenting due to a spiral distal dissection, fixed using a non-trial stent with resultant TIMI 3 flow. In the control group, there was one subacute thrombosis.

Between 1 and 6 months there were no additional deaths, bypass surgeries, or Q-wave myocardial infarctions (Table 61.7). One non-Q wave MI occurred in the control group and one in the 0.7 μg/mm² dose group. There were three target lesion revascularizations (TLRs) in the control group, two in the 0.2 μg/mm² dose treatment group, and one each in the 0.7, 1.4, and 2.7 μg/mm² dose-treatment groups. This last patient was not the one recorded in the text as suffering restenosis (who, despite in-stent restenosis, did not require TLR) but another patient with worsening of a residual stenosis proximal to the stent left unstented at the time of the original procedure. It is classified as a TLR (rather than target vessel revascularization – TVR) since it was within 5 mm of the proximal edge of the stent. Importantly, there were no further stent thromboses in the highest dose group at 6 months.

DISCUSSION

The true potential of vascular stents is limited by the formation of new tissue within the stent,

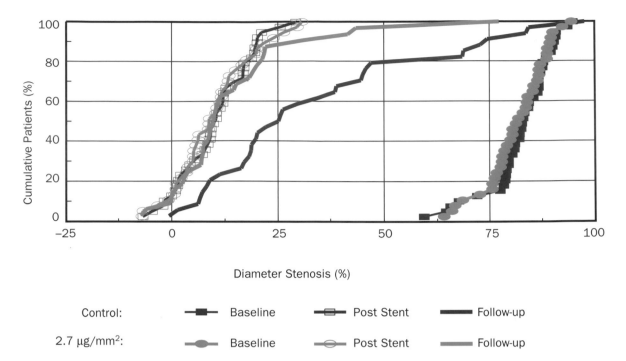

Fig. 61.2 Cumulative distribution graph of percentage diameter stenosis (DS).

Table 61.6 The ELUTES trial: safety data at 30 days

	Paclitaxel dose density ($\mu g/mm^2$)				Control	p-value*
	2.7	1.4	0.7	0.2		
Number	37	39	39	37	38	–
Death	1	0	0	0	0	ns
Q-wave MI	0	0	0	0	0	ns
CABG	0	0	0	0	0	ns
SAT	1	0	0	0	1	ns
Non-Q MI	1	0	0	0	0	ns
Event-free	92%	100%	100%	100%	97%	0.55

SAT, subacute thrombosis. (Other abbreviations as in previous tables).
* p-value for high dose vs control.

which can renarrow the stented lumen potentially necessitating a repeat procedure. Vessel wall injury at the time of stent deployment initiates a well-understood sequence of steps involving stimulation of SMCs, which leave the quiescent G_0 phase of the cell cycle and enter the G_1 and S phases.[11] Coordination of cell cycle events is effected by a series of

Table 61.7   The ELUTES trial: safety data at 6 months

	Paclitaxel dose density ($\mu g/mm^2$)				Control	p-value
	2.7	1.4	0.7	0.2		
Number	37	39	39	37	38	–
Death	1	0	0	0	0	ns
Q-wave MI	0	0	0	0	0	ns
CABG	0	0	0	0	0	ns
SAT	1	0	0	0	1	ns
Non-Q MI	1	0	1	0	1	ns
TLR	1	1	1	2	3	ns
Event-free	89%*	97%	95%	95%	89%*	ns

TLR, target lesion revascularization. (Other abbreviations as in previous tables.)
* p-value for high dose vs control.

cyclin-dependent kinases and requires inactivation of several 'tumor suppressor genes', including p53, p21, p16, p15, p27, and prevention of phosphorylation of the retinoblastoma gene Rb, which is normally promoted by activity of the cyclin/Cdk complexes.[12] Consequently, cells progress toward division, migrate through the internal elastic lamina and undergo further proliferation in the new intima. SMCs make up the majority of the tissue in the first few days only following PCI, with collagen and other ECM proteins increasingly making up the bulk of the new lesion over the following 1–2 months.

While this excess tissue formation affects up to 20% of stented patients, only 10–15% require further intervention. Certain subgroups are, however, at much higher risk of restenosis including diabetics,[3] those with prior in-stent restenosis, long diffuse,[13] or bifurcating lesions,[14] chronic total occlusions,[15] and multivessel disease.[16] In such patients, restenosis rates may reach 45% especially if risks are combined.[3,17]

Paclitaxel and drug eluting stents

Paclitaxel, discovered in the early 1970s,[18] is used primarily as systemic chemotherapy for ovarian and breast carcinoma as well as Kaposi's sarcoma. It promotes the assembly of microtubules from tubulin dimers and stabilizes them by preventing depolymerization resulting in the inhibition of the normal dynamic reorganization of the microtubule network essential for vital interphase and mitotic cellular functions. In addition, paclitaxel induces abnormal arrays or 'bundles' of microtubules throughout the cell cycle and multiple asters of microtubules during mitosis. Cell replication is inhibited in the G_0/G_1 and G_2/M phases. Cell motility, shape, and transport between organelles may also be affected. It has been suggested that paclitaxel has antiinflammatory properties. Paclitaxel is catalyzed by cytochrome P_{450} isoenzymes CYP2C8 and CYP3A4.

The effect of paclitaxel has been tested in vivo, in the rat, rabbit, and pig models, with either local balloon or stents as delivery devices. Hahnel et al.,[5] for example, assessed the effect of paclitaxel released by a biodegradable stent on vascular SMCs and showed a dose-dependent reduction in cell numbers. Exposure to 3.2 nmol or greater over one week resulted in a significant effect. Importantly, this

Table 61.8	The ELUTES trial: preclinical data for paclitaxel			
Species	Stent (S) or other device (e.g. balloon) (D)	Dose	Outcome	Source
Rat			Intima/medial ratio: Control 0.66(0.08) vs Treated 0.18(0.04) (*p<0.0001*)	Sollott et al.[19]
Rat	S	42 μg	Intimal thickness: Control 0.06 mm vs Treated 0.35 mm (*p<0.0001*)	Farb et al.[8]
Rabbit	S		Intima area: Control 1.13 (0.13) mm vs Treated 0.29 (0.07) (*p<0.03*)	Drachman et al.[20]
Rabbit	D: Microporous balloon		8 Wks–Intimal area: Control 0.31 mm² vs Treated 0.193 mm² Evidence positive remodeling– Control: 0.417 mm² vs Treated 0.75 mm²	Herdeg et al.[21]
Rabbit	D: Microporous balloon	10 μmol/L	28 d–Intimal area: Control 0.36(0.29) vs Treated 0.21 (0.11) (*p = 0.01*) Endothelial regeneration by 28 days	Axel et al.[22]
Rabbit	S	Control: 15 μg 90 μg	28 d: Late loss & Intimal area 0.46 (0.04) & 1.86 (0.25) 0.34 (0.07) & 1.75 (0.21) 0.16 ((0.06) & 1.20 (0.13) (*p<0.003 & p<0.05 vs Control*)	Heldman et al.[9]
Porcine	S	175–200 μg	30 d: Intimal thickness Control 669 (357) μm vs Treated 403 (197) (*p<0.05*)	Hong et al.[23]
Porcine	S	Control: 0.2, 15, 187 μg/ stent	4 ws: Late loss & Intimal area	Heldman et al.[10]

was at local doses at least 10^5 below systemic dosage. A summary of the preclinical data is presented in Table 61.8.

From such evidence it is clear that paclitaxel has beneficial effects on inhibiting SMC prolif- eration. However, there is a dose-dependant unwanted inhibition of proliferating endothe- lial cells at doses close to those needed to inhibit SMCs.[24] Others have clearly shown adverse effects on the vessel wall at certain doses.[25] Stents coated with a cross-linked biodegradable polymer (chondroitin and gelatin) loaded with different doses of paclitaxel to the iliac arteries of rabbits reduced mean intimal thickness by 49% and 36% at high doses of 42.0 and 20.2 μg per stent at 28 days. However, incomplete healing was noted with persistent intimal fibrin deposition, intraintimal hemorrhage and increased intimal and adventitial inflammation. The concentration at vessel level is not indicated but based on this and other preclinical data,[10] data suggesting a narrow therapeutic window, we believed a dose finding and safety pilot study was warranted.

ELUTES aimed to determine if there was a trend towards an effective but safe dose of paclitaxel that could be locally delivered in man, on a stent with *no polymer*. The results suggest that even without a polymer, effective doses of paclitaxel can be delivered to the atheromatous arterial wall, inhibiting intimal hyperplasia, and the presence of a dose–response curve indicates a firm link between proprietary process, dose, and biologic effect.

The study was planned as a pilot dosing study, but was powered to show a significant effect if the diameter stenosis (DS) could be reduced from 35% to 20%. The first (efficacy) endpoint was reached with a difference in DS from 33.9% in controls to 14.1% in the highest dose and late loss from 0.73 mm to 0.10 mm. Doses less than the highest (2.7 μg/mm^2 of stent) dose were ineffective, but trends for diameter stenosis and late loss were seen. These data tell us that the minimum effective dose is in the order of 3 μg/mm^2 stent. That dose density is a more important concept than 'total dose',[25] or 'concentration' is illustrated when ELUTES is considered with the ASPECT trial (presented in abstract at TCT (Transcatheter Cardiovascular Therapeutics), Washington 2001) in which paclitaxel was again applied in different dose densities directly to the SUPRA G (rather than the V-Flex, ELUTES) stent. Again, a dose–response

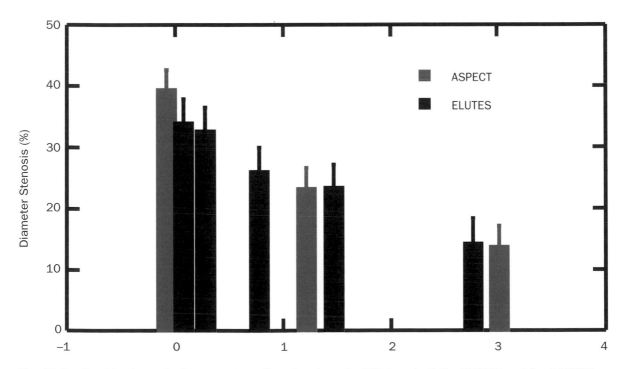

Fig. 61.3 Combined results for percentage diameter stenosis (DS) from both the ELUTES and the ASPECT studies as a function of dose density.

curve was obtained (Figure 61.3). The interesting comparison is the *overall dose* delivered in each study. In ASPECT, with a SUPRA G stent surface of 42 mm^2 the total dose delivered was 130 μg at their 3.1 μg/mm^2 dose density, whereas the V-Flex has only 22 mm^2 surface area resulting in a total dose of 60 μg at the 2.7 μg/mm^2 dose density. The control and highest dose diameter stenosis at follow-up were 33.9% and 14.1% (ELUTES) and 39% and 14% (ASPECT) showing identical biological responses despite different overall amount of drug delivered. Dose density is what matters. The similarity of results confirms the reliability of the application process and emphasizes the effect of paclitaxel on proliferative responses close to the stent strut, where most injury occurs. A useful property of paclitaxel appears to be that it is very lipophilic, being rapidly taken up by cells close to areas of delivery.

The absence of polymer is clearly a potential advantage, overcoming concerns regarding inflammatory effects of polymers,[26] particularly important once the drug has eluted. The proprietary loading process in this study was sufficiently precise to produce a dose–response curve, with no disadvantage in relation to applying the drug without the polymer.

While the ELUTES study illustrates virtual elimination of restenosis in the 6 months following intervention, a major concern is always safety. One important potential negative aspect is on re-endothelialization and therefore thrombotic risk. Partly empirically and partly based on preclinical data, 3 months of antiplatelets was mandated. One month MACE suggests that the paclitaxel-eluting stent is safe at each treatment dose studied. The three early events could not have been due to the presence of the drug on the stent. Importantly, despite no antiplatelet therapy between 3 and 6 months, no stent thromboses occurred, unlike other trials where exceedingly high doses of paclitaxel were used.[27] The SCORE trial, stopped due to excess stent thromboses in the treated arm of the study, used a very high dose of paclitaxel derivative (4000 μg) loaded on to an unusual stent with 2 mm polymer sleeves along its length.[28]

In the current (ELUTES) study the percentage of patients in the highest dose treatment group who were adverse event-free at 6 months was equal to that of the control group (89%).

CONCLUSIONS

Available data suggest that local treatment of the target site with an antiproliferative drug may inhibit or reduce restenosis reducing repeat percutaneous transluminal coronary intervention (PTCA) or coronary artery bypass graft (CABG) rates (and therefore costs). The ELUTES trial demonstrates that paclitaxel can be directly applied to a stent and on eluting from it significantly improves 6 month angiographic outcome following PTCA. Reduction of neointimal hyperplasia following stent placement results in increased vessel lumen, reduced percentage diameter stents, and reduced binary restenosis. Paclitaxel in effective doses (2.7 μg/mm^2 stent) has a safety profile similar to control. The results of the ELUTES trial corroborate the findings of a contemporaneously run trial of a different stent coating agent. The RAVEL trial has shown similar efficacy in the inhibition of restenosis after stenting.[29] While the trials differed in several details, preventing a valid trial-to-trial comparison, both had similar results in virtually eliminating angiographic restenosis at 6 months without apparent safety concerns.

Future study is warranted to address longer-term aspects of coated stent technology for the elimination of restenosis. Long-term follow-up of these patients out to 5 years is ongoing. The results at 6 months alone suggest that new therapeutic options for percutaneous coronary intervention using drug eluting stents will be become standard treatment, and that paclitaxel is an important player.

REFERENCES

1. Serruys PW, de Jaegere P, Kiemeneij F, et al. A comparison of balloon-expandable-stent implantation with balloon angioplasty in patients with coronary artery disease. Benestent Study Group. N Engl J Med 1994; 331(8):489–95.

2. Fischman DL, Leon MB, Baim DS, et al. A randomised comparison of coronary stent placement and balloon angioplasty in the treatment of coronary artery disease. Stent restenosis study investigators. N Engl J Med 1994; 331(8):496–501.

3. Van Belle E, Bauters C, Hubert E, et al. Restenosis rates in diabetics: a comparison of stenting and balloon angioplasty in native coronary vessels. Circulation 1997; 96(5):1454–60.

4. Serruys PW, Unger F, van Hout BA, et al. The ARTS study (Arterial Revascularization Therapies Study). Semin Interv Cardiol 1999; 4:209–19.

5. Hahnel I, Alt E, Resch B et al. Local growth inhibitory effect of paclitaxel released by a biodegradable stent coating on vascular smooth muscle cells. J Am Coll Cardiol 1998; 31(4):278A (abstract).

6. Voisard R, Alt E, Baur R, et al. Paclitaxel-coated biodegradeable stents inhibit proliferative activity and severely damage cytoskeletal components of smooth muscle cells from human coronary plaque material in vitro. Eur Heart J 1998; 376(suppl):P2109 (abstract).

7. Herdeg C, Blattner A, Oberhoff M. Local delivery of paclitaxel in the rabbit carotid artery results in reduced neointima formation and vessel enlargement. Eur Heart J 1997; 18(suppl):460 (abstract 2695).

8. Farb A, Heller PF, Carter AJ. Paclitaxel polymer-coated stents reduce neointima. Circulation 1997; 96(8)(suppl):1-609 (abstract 3394).

9. Heldman IW, Hopkins J, Cheng L. Paclitaxel applied directly to stents inhibits neointimal growth without thrombotic complications in a porcine coronary artery model of restenosis. Circulation 1997; 96(8)(suppl 1):1-288 (abstract 1602).

10. Heldman AW, Cheng L, Jenkins GM, Heller PF, et al. Paclitaxel stent coating inhibits neointimal hyperplasia at 4 weeks in a porcine model of coronary restenosis. Circulation 2001; 103(18):2289–95.

11. Sriram V, Patterson C. Cell cycle in vasculoproliferative diseases: Potential interventions and routes of delivery. Circulation 2001; 103:2414–19.

12. Boehm M, Nabel E. Cell cycle and cell migration: New pieces to the puzzle. Circulation 2001; 103:2879–81.

13. Rozenman Y, Mereuta A, Schechter D, et al. Long-term outcome of patients with very long stents for treatment of diffuse coronary disease. Am Heart J 1999; 138(3):441–5.

14. Melikian N, Di Mario C. Treatment of bifurcation coronary lesions: a review of current techniques and outcome. J Interv Cardiol 2003; 16:507–13.

15. Serruys PW, Hamburger JN, Koolen JJ, et al. Total occlusion trial with angioplasty by using laser guidewire. The TOTAL trial. Eur Heart J 2000; 21:1797–805.

16. Serruys PW, Emanuelsson H, van der Giessen W, et al. Heparin-coated Palmaz-Schatz stents in human coronary arteries. Early outcome of the Benestent-II Pilot study. Circulation 1996; 93:412–22.

17. Elezi S, Kastrati A, Neumann FJ, et al. Vessel size and long-term outcome after coronary stent placement. Circulation 1998; 98(18):1875–80.

18. Riondel J, Jacrot M, Picot F. Therapeutic response to taxol of six human tumors xenografted into nude mice. Cancer Chemother Pharmacol 1986; 17(2):137–42.

19. Sollott SJ, Cheng L, Pauly RR. Taxol inhibits neointimal smooth muscle cell accumulation after angioplasty in the rat. J Clin Invest 1995; 95(4):1869–76.

20. Drachman DE, Edelman ER, Kamath KR. Sustained stent-based delivery of paclitaxel arrests neointimal thickening and cell proliferation. Circulation 1998; 98(17S)(suppl):P7401.

21. Herdeg C, Blattner A, Oberhoff M. Local delivery of paclitaxel in the rabbit carotid artery results in reduced neointima formation and vessel enlargement. Eur Heart J 1997; 18(suppl):460 (abstract 2695).

22. Axel DI, Kunert W, Goggelmann C. Paclitaxel inhibits arterial smooth muscle cell proliferation and migration in vitro and in vivo using local drug delivery. Circulation 1997; 96(2):636–45.

23. Hong MK, Kornowski R, Bramwell O, et al. Paclitaxel-coated Gianturco-Roubin II (GR II) stents reduces neointimal hyperplasia in a porcine coronary instent restenosis model. Coron Artery Dis 2001; 12:513–15.

24. Axel DI, Kunert W, Goggelmann C. Paclitaxel inhibits arterial smooth muscle cell proliferation

and migration in vitro and in vivo using local drug delivery. Circulation 1997; 96(2):636–45.

25. Farb A, Heller PF, Shroff S, Cheng L. Pathological analysis of local delivery of paclitaxel via a polymer-coated stent. Circulation 2001; 104(4):473–9.

26. van der Giessen WJ, Lincoff AM. Marked inflammatory sequelae to implantation of biodegradable and nonbiodegradable polymers in porcine coronary arteries. Circulation 1996; 94(7):1690–7.

27. Liistro F, Colombo A. Late acute thrombosis after paclitaxel eluting stent implantation. Heart 2001; 86:262–5.

28. de la Fuente LM, Miano J, Mrad J, et al. Initial results of the Quanum drug eluting stent (QuaDS-QP-2) registry (BARDS) in human subjects. Catheter & Cardiovasc Interv 2001; 53:480–8.

29. Serruys PW, Morice M-C, Sousa JE, et al. The RAVEL study: a randomised study with the sirolimus coated Bx velocity balloon-expandable stent in the treatment of patients with de novo native coronary artery lesions. Eur Heart J 2001; 22(Suppl):2624 (abstract 484).

62

Intrapericardial drug delivery for the prevention of restenosis

Dongming Hou and Keith L March

Introduction • Current methods for intrapericardial delivery
• Efficacy of experimental intrapericardial delivery of anti-restenosis agents • Conclusions
• Acknowledgments

INTRODUCTION

The major limitation to the long-term efficacy of coronary balloon angioplasty is restenosis at the site of arterial injury. Over the past 20 years, a number of devices have been developed as alternatives to balloon dilation.

Local delivery of a therapeutic agent is a reasonable strategy for administration of highly potent agents to a target vessel wall while minimizing systemic toxicity. More than a decade ago, it was hoped that local intramural delivery would allow for the achievement of high concentrations of pharmacological drugs or therapeutic bioactive agents within the coronary artery wall. Although a variety of endovascular delivery devices was designed for this purpose, the limitations of such delivery were found to include the possibility of increased vascular trauma, low efficiency of localization, inconsistency of delivery, and rapid washout of the agent from the vascular wall following delivery.[1–3] Several studies have shown that a maximum of 0.1–0.6% of agent remains in the artery wall after endovascular local delivery in porcine coronary vessels.[4]

Catheter-based methods for access to the normal pericardial space have been described over the last ten years. Several benefits of agent delivery to the pericardial space have become apparent, including: enhanced consistency of local agent levels; reduced acute systemic delivery of agent; and prolonged exposure of coronary arteries to the therapeutic material.[1] Favorable local pharmacokinetics and consistency of tissue loading following pericardial delivery, in comparison with endoluminal delivery, have been demonstrated with agents instilled into the pericardial fluid achieving intramural coronary concentrations that vary at most by 10–15-fold. Endoluminal delivery results in a remarkably wider intramural concentration range of up to 33 000-fold variability.[2] Figure 62.1, which shows the fractional intramural delivery (FID) after endoluminal and pericardial deliveries, indicates that the intrapericardial approach exhibits a substantially greater reproducibility of localization. Intrapericardial space delivery of nitric oxide donors reduces neointimal proliferation in a porcine coronary overstretch model after two

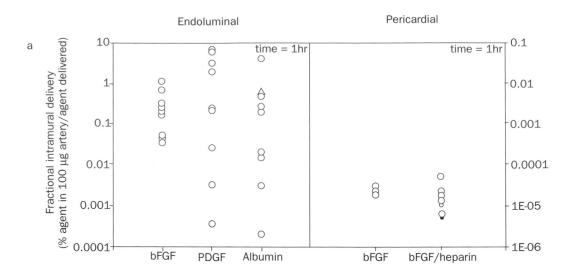

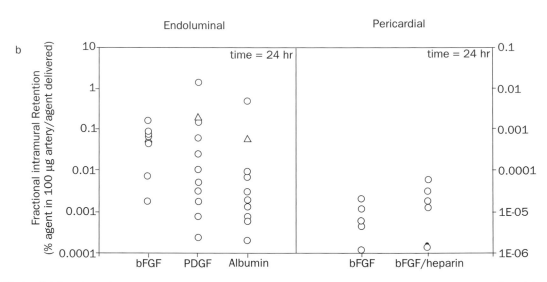

Fig. 62.1 (a) Fractional intramural delivery (FID) expressed as a percentage of each infused agent found in arterial tissue 1 h after delivery. The left panel shows one value for each coronary artery harvested after endoluminal delivery of the agents listed on the x-axis. The right panel shows one value for each coronary artery harvested following intrapericardial delivery of the indicated agents. It is apparent that endoluminal delivery results in a greater degree of variation in FID by several orders of magnitude. (b) Fractional intramural retention (FIR) expressed as a percentage of each infused agent found in arterial tissue 24 h after delivery. As for (a), the left panel shows one value for each coronary artery harvested after endoluminal delivery of the agents listed on the x-axis. The right panel shows one value for each coronary artery harvested following intrapericardial delivery of the indicated agents. It is apparent that endoluminal delivery results in substantially greater degree of variation in FIR. (bFGF, basic fibroblast growth factor; PDGF, platelet-derived growth factor.) (From Stoll HP et al. Pharmacokinetics and consistency of pericardial delivery directed to coronary arteries: direct comparsion with endoluminal delivery. Clin Cardiol 1999; 22(suppl): I-10–I-16, with permission.)

weeks,[5] and in a porcine stent-restenosis model after four weeks.[6] Recently, our experiments have further shown that intrapericardial paclitaxel delivery not only inhibits neointimal proliferation, but also promotes arterial enlargement four weeks after porcine coronary over-stretch.[7] Therefore, we hypothesized that the intrapericardial space may be of potential significance as a therapeutic site for local drug delivery to prevent epicardial coronary artery restenosis.[8]

CURRENT METHODS FOR INTRAPERICARDIAL DELIVERY

The existing delivery strategies for intrapericardial space delivery have recently been widely reviewed.[3] Several methods have been described, which may be broadly divided into techniques which access the pericardial space from outside the pericardial sac ('outside-in') and transvascular approaches that traverse a cardiac chamber and myocardial muscle to enter the pericardial space from the epicardial surface ('inside-out'). The former category utilizes thoracotomy exposure followed by pericardial puncture, or closed percutaneous, transthoracic approaches; while the latter includes transatrial or transventricular access.

Pericardial space administration of therapeutic agents through direct pericardium puncture after thoracotomy is relatively safe. However, it is clearly limited by the surgical procedure. Lazarous et al. reported use of a 6.6 Fr silastic catheter with end port positioned into the pericardial space in dogs following a left thoracotomy.[9] Differential regional uptake of ^{125}I-labeled basic fibroblast growth factor (bFGF) was evaluated by this study.[9]

More recently, practical percutaneous approaches have been described for accessing the pericardial space. The use of a transatrial approach for accessing the pericardial space was reported by Uchida et al. and Verrier et al.[10,11] This method has been shown to provide a safe and rapid delivery of therapeutic agents into the pericardium. Using femoral vein access to position a 6 Fr or 8 Fr-guide catheter in the right atrial appendage under

fluoroscopic guidance, a small perforation is made with a 21 gauge, hollow, radiopaque needle catheter. This catheter may subsequently be exchanged over a guidewire for a tapered-tip 4 Fr aspiration catheter with side ports, permitting pericardial delivery and withdrawal of fluid. We have successfully utilized this procedure in our laboratory and found it may be readily accomplished in less than 5 minutes of operator time. Figure 62.2 shows fluoroscopic images demonstrating transatrial access of the pericardial space. Initially, an 8 Fr guide catheter is placed against the wall of the right atrial appendage. A 0.014 inch guidewire placed inside a 0.038 inch infusion catheter with the stiff tip directed forward is used to pierce the right atrium (Figure 62.2a). The infusion catheter was then introduced into the pericardial space, followed by withdrawal of the inner 0.014 inch wire, and infusion of 2–3 cc radiopaque contrast into the pericardial space (Figure 62.2b).

The transventricular method, first described for adenoviral delivery,[12] and more recently used by Stoll et al. for bFGF intrapericardial space instillation,[13] uses a hollow, helical-tipped catheter designed for controlled penetration through the myocardium into the pericardial sac, under fluoroscopic guidance. In this method, a catheter is placed through a right jugular or carotid sheath and advanced, respectively, into either the right or left ventricle to the cardiac free wall. Upon firm contact with the myocardium, the catheter tip is advanced through the myocardium using a gentle turning motion. After initial advancement, hand infusion of a 1:1 meglumine/normal saline mixture is initiated and contrast location is monitored fluoroscopically. Successful intrapericardial tip placement is identified by accumulation of contrast in the pericardium, and may be followed by delivery and device removal by rotation. The helical exit appears to preclude significant local bleeding, and this procedure has been employed successfully in our laboratory in well over 150 animals, again with a typical procedural time of less than 5 minutes to complete instillation. Figure 62.3 shows intrapericardial contrast delivery via a hollow, helical-tipped catheter.

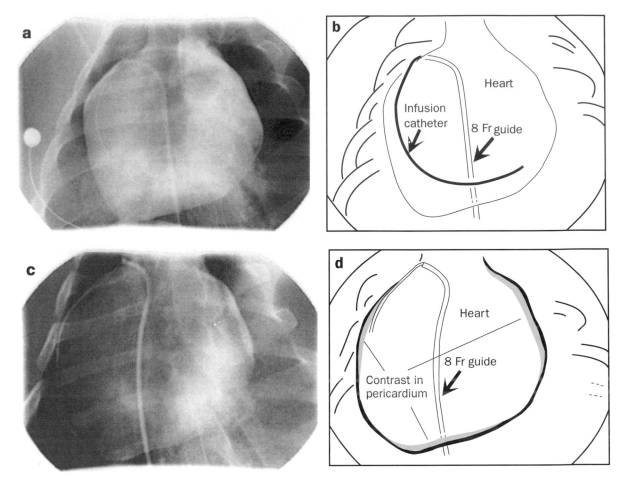

Fig. 62.2 Fluoroscopic images documenting transatrial access of pericardial space. (a) An 8 Fr guide catheter rests against the wall of the right atrial appendage. A 0.014 inch guidewire, premounted inside a 0.038 inch infusion catheter, is then inserted through the guide, and the right atrium atrial pierced with the 0.014 inch wire. This image is represented as a line drawing in (b) for clarity. (c) The infusion catheter is then introduced into the pericardial space and the inner 0.014 inch wire withdrawn, followed by infusion of 2–3 cc of radiopaque contrast into the pericardial space, shown with a line representation in (d).

A percutaneous transthoracic delivery approach has been used by both Landau,[14] and Laham et al.[15] After partial surgical dissection to create a tunnel, a 22-gauge spinal needle assembly was directed at a 15 degree angle to the skin surface of the subxiphoid region and, using fluoroscopy, advanced left of midline, towards the cardiac silhouette and through the diaphragm into the pericardial space. A guidewire and 5 Fr dilator were then serially inserted, and after dilating the puncture tunnel, a 20 cm length of polyethylene tubing was advanced over the wire to the pericardial space.

Recently, a specific transthoracic pericardial access device, PerDUCER®, has been manufactured with a design which is intended to minimize the possibility of myocardial puncture by the access needle in the context of transthoracic access of a non-effused pericardial sac. This device is a needle protectively sheathed with a catheter bearing a hemispherical-shaped side hole at its tip which allows for the suction, capture, and subsequent puncture of the

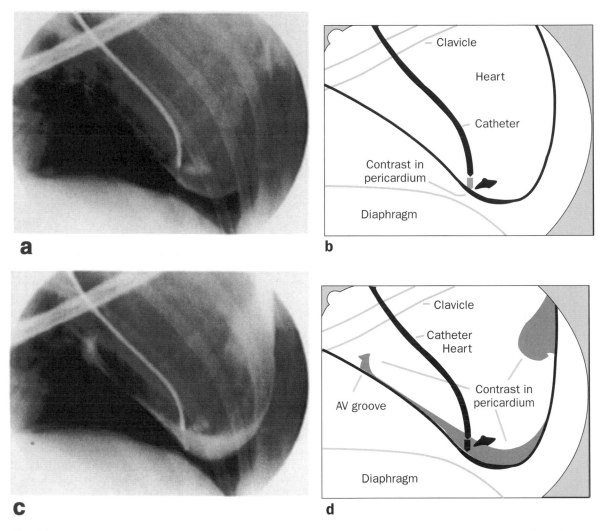

Fig. 62.3 Sequential fluorographic images, obtained during a percutaneous delivery procedure, from the right anterior oblique projection. (a) Cardiac silhouette, with the helix catheter in place transmurally in the right ventricular wall. The instillation of contrast had just begun at the time of angiography; a thin layer of contrast is seen outlining the cardiac edge, confirming pericardial location. This image is represented as a line drawing in (b) for clarity. (c) The same projection after the infusion of approximately 15 cc of a mixture of radiographic contrast and vector suspension, with a line representation in (d). (From March KL et al. Efficient in vivo catheter-based pericardial gene transfer mediated by adenoviral vectors. Clin Cardiol 1999; 22(suppl):I-23–I-29, with permission from Clinical Cardiology Publishing Company, Inc.)

pericardium. Prior to using the access device, a percutaneous tunnel is made below the xiphoid process using a 21 gauge needle introduced nearly parallel to the skin surface, after which a 0.038 inch guidewire and introducer sheath is placed under fluoroscopic guidance into the mediastinum over the anterior pericardium. The PerDUCER® is then positioned through the

sheath onto the anterior (outer) surface of the pericardial sac, which is drawn into the hemispherical-shaped tip by manual suction, and pierced by the needle. Finally, a 0.018 inch guidewire is placed through the needle lumen and advanced several centimeters to confirm its confinement within the pericardial space. The needle is removed and a 4 Fr dilator catheter is

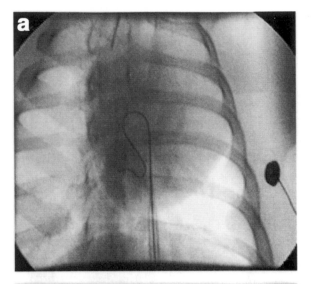

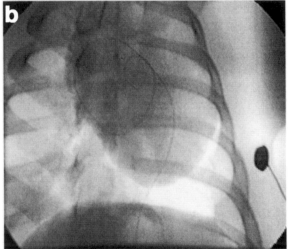

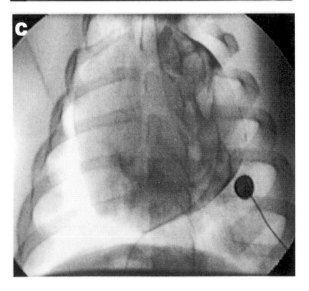

Fig. 62.4 Sequential fluorographic images show anteroposterior (AP) views of a pericardial access procedure. (a) The 0.038 inch guidewire and special introducer sheath are placed into the mediastinum over the anterior pericardium, after a percutaneous tunnel is made below the xiphoid. (b) A 0.018 inch guidewire is placed through the access device. (c) Contrast is injected into pericardial space via a 4 Fr dilator catheter.

inserted over the wire. Successful intrapericardial tip placement is tested by injection of contrast into the pericardial space. Figure 62.4 shows intrapericardial delivery of contrast in this manner. Initial animal and clinical trials indicate that this procedure is a safe and effective method for percutaneous insertion of a guidewire into the normal pericardial space.[7,16] Our experience in more than 75 animals confirms that after an initial learning curve, successful pericardial instillation may typically be accomplished in less than 5 minutes.

EFFICACY OF EXPERIMENTAL INTRAPERICARDIAL DELIVERY OF ANTI-RESTENOSIS AGENTS

Table 62.1 provides a summary of the studies that have investigated intrapericardial placement of anti-restenosis agents. These studies have collectively demonstrated that access to the pericardial space provides for an efficacious, consistent, relatively rapid, minimally invasive administration route for local drug therapy to the coronary vasculature.

Systemic and local endovascular delivery of organic nitric oxide (NO) donor compounds, L-arginine, and adenovirus-mediated transfer of the gene encoding human endothelial constitutive nitric oxide synthase (NOS) have been shown to reduce endothelial dysfunction and neointima formation after balloon injury in several models.[17–20] Recently, a family of diazeniumdiolate-conjugated NO-generating compounds has been described, with the capacity to release NO over a range of release rates, varying significantly among the compounds.[21] Diazeniumdiolated albumin (NONO-Alb) has a particularly prolonged release $T1/2$

Table 62.1   Intrapericardial delivery experience and results

Year	Animal model	Arterial injury	Administered compound	Results	Source
1997	Porcine	Coronary over-stretch	NO donor	Reduces NP	6
1998	Porcine	In-stent restenosis	NO donor	Reduces NP	7
1999	Porcine	Coronary over-stretch	AdeNOS	Reduces NP	8
2000	Porcine	Coronary over-stretch	Paclitaxel	Reduces NP	9

NO, nitric oxide; NP, neointimal proliferation.

of approximately 24 hours. To test the effect of intrapericardial space delivery of NONO-Alb on the coronary injury response after balloon injury,[21] Baek et al. delivered this compound at two dosages (40 mg, low dose and 400 mg, high dose) or unconjugated albumin (40 mg, control) in 18 farm pigs using a helical needle catheter.[5] Animal were sacrificed at 14 days and arterial sections evaluated by histomorphometric analysis. The results revealed that NONO-Alb caused dose-dependent reduction in the neointimal and adventitial area, while also promoting outward vascular remodeling.[5] The reductions in the high dose group were 46% in the neointima ($p<0.05$) and 35% in the adventitial area ($p<0.05$). The reductions in the low dose group were 29% in the neointima and 21% in the adventitial area. Similar results were reported with another diazeniumdiolate compound by Makkar et al. administered in a porcine coronary artery in-stent stenosis model.[6] Pompili et al. reported adenoviral expression of endothelial nitric oxide synthase (AdeNOS) gene in porcine pericardium yields in vivo functional enzymatic activity and inhibits neointimal hyperplasia in coronary arteries after balloon injury.[8] Pigs received catheter-based intrapericardial delivery of AdeNOS (1×10^9 pfu) or control Adnull (1×10^9 pfu) after balloon injury of two epicardial arteries ($n = 8$, per group) and were sacrificed

at day 14. The AdeNOS animals demonstrated higher levels of NO than the Adnull animals (pericardium: 652.3 ± 47.2 vs 275 ± 15.9 nmol, epicardium: 596.1 ± 48.9 vs 330.8 ± 32.6 nmol, respectively $p<0.05$). Histomorphometry indicated that the local increase of NO activity was associated with inhibition of lumen occlusion after coronary balloon injury.

More recently, Hou et al. demonstrated a positive effect of intrapericardial (IPC) instillation of paclitaxel on neointimal proliferation after balloon over stretch of porcine coronary arteries.[8] Over stretch injury of coronary arteries was followed by transthoracic IPC administration of micellar paclitaxel at low dose (LD, 10 mg, $n = 6$), high dose (HD, 50 mg, $n = 7$), or inactive control micelles (C, 50 mg, $n = 5$). Animals were sacrificed 28 days post-balloon dilation. The results demonstrated that neointimal area, maximal intimal thickness, and adventitial thickness were significantly reduced in both LD (0.47 ± 0.04 mm^2; 0.43 ± 0.03 and 0.35 ± 0.02 mm) and HD (0.51 ± 0.06 mm^2; 0.42 ± 0.03 and 0.38 ± 0.03 mm) paclitaxel groups compared with the control group (0.79 ± 0.07 mm^2; 0.56 ± 0.02 and 0.47 ± 0.02 mm; $p<0.001$). Meanwhile, the vessel circumference measured at the external elastic lamina of paclitaxel-treated vessels was again significantly larger than control, contributing importantly (about 67%) to lumen preservation. The IPC

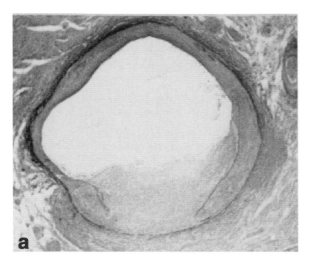

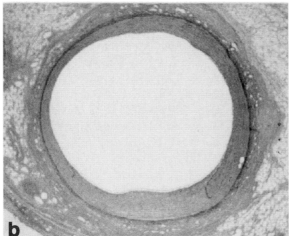

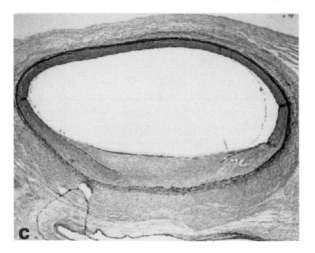

Fig. 62.5 Effect of IPC paclitaxel delivery on coronary arteries 28 days after balloon angioplasty. Verhoff-Van Giesson's staining. (a) Untreated artery segment showing intimal proliferation. (b) and (c), 10 mg and 50 mg paclitaxel-treated segments, respectively. Note reduction in neointima as well as an enlarged vessel lumen vs control. (Magnification ×25.) (From Hou D et al. Intrapericardial paclitaxel delivery inhibits neointimal proliferation and promotes arterial enlargement after porcine coronary overstretch. Circulation 2000; 102:1575–81[9] with permission from Lippincott Williams & Wilkins.)

delivery of a single dose of paclitaxel thus reduced vessel narrowing by reduction of neointimal mass as well as positive vascular remodeling. Figure 62.5 shows the histologic results after IPC paclitaxel delivery.

The data from all these studies collectively indicates that intrapericardial delivery of antiproliferative agents may be a helpful therapeutic strategy for prevention of restenosis.

CONCLUSIONS

Exploration of pericardial administration of anti-restenosis agents has been stimulated by three recent conceptual advances. (1) Recognition of the important role that the pericardial space may play in endogenous modulation of epicardial vessel pathophysiology. (2) Evidence of the pharmacokinetic and localization advantages of intrapericardial space delivery. (3) Development of practical approaches for the non-surgical access to the normal pericardium. Numerous preclinical experimental results have shown inhibition of neointimal proliferation after coronary intervention using intrapericardial strategies. Therefore, it may be concluded that manipulation of the composition of intrapericardial fluid can significantly influence coronary vascular behavior and that administration of antiproliferative agents may indeed provide an efficacious and consistent minimally invasive method for restenosis therapy.

ACKNOWLEDGMENTS

The authors thank Teresa Knight and Kim Irwin for their editorial assistance.

REFERENCES

1. March KL. Method of local gene delivery to vascular tissue. Semin Interv Cardiol 1996; 1:215–23.

2. Stoll HP, Carlson K, Keefer LK, et al. Pharmacokinetics and consistency of pericardial delivery directed to coronary arteries: direct comparison with endoluminal delivery. Clin Cardiol 1999; 22(suppl):I-10–I-16.

3. Hou D, March KL. Intrapericardial approach for therapeutic angiogenesis. In Kornowski R, Leon MB (eds), Handbook of Myocardial Revascularization and Angiogenesis. Martin-Dunitz: London 1999: 189–200.

4. Lincoff AM, Weinberger J. Local drug delivery and endovascular radiation. In Topol EJ (ed), Comprehensive Cardiovascular Medicine, 1st edn. Lippincott-Raven: Philadelphia 1998: 2433–52.

5. Baek SH, Hrabic JA, Keefer LK, et al. Augmentation of intrapericardial nitric oxide level by a prolonged-release nitric oxide donor reduces luminal narrowing after porcine coronary angioplasty. Circulation 2002; 105:2779–84.

6. Makkar RR, Shah PK, Terhakopian A, et al. Intrapericardial delivery of a nitric oxide donor inhibits in-stent stenosis in porcine coronary arteries. Am J Cardiol 1998; 82(suppl 7A):104S.

7. Pompili VJ, D'Souza D, Bohlen G, et al. Adenoviral expression of endothelial nitrc oxide synthase gene in porcine pericardium yields in vivo function enzymatic activity and inhibits neointimal hyperplasia in coronary arteries after balloon injury. Circulation 1999; 100:I-702.

8. Hou D, Rogers PI, Toleikis PM, et al. Intrapericardial paclitaxel delivery inhibits neointimal proliferation and promotes arterial enlargement after porcine coronary overstretch. Circulation 2000; 102:1575–81.

9. Lazarous DF, Shou M, Stiber JA, et al. Pharmacodynamic of basic fibroblast growth factor: route of administration myocardial and systemic distribution. Cardiovasc Res 1997; 36:78–85.

10. Uchida Y, Yanagisawa-Miwa A, Fumitake N, et al. Angiogenic therapy of acute myocardial infarction by intrapericardial injection of basic fibroblast growth factor and heparin sulfate. Am Heart J 1995; 130:1182–8.

11. Verrier RL, Waxman S, Lovett EG, Moreno R. Transatrial access to the normal pericardial space: a novel approach for diagnostic sampling, pericardiocentesis, and therapeutic interventions. Circulation 1998; 98:2331–3.

12. Woody M, Mehdi K, Zipes DP, et al. High efficiency adenovirus-mediated pericardial gene transfer in vivo. JACC 1996; 27:31A.

13. Stoll HP, Szabo A, March KL. Sustained transmyocardial loading with bFGF following single intrapericardial delivery: local kinetics and tissue penetration. Circulation 1998; 98(suppl): I-399.

14. Landau C, Jacobs AK, Haudenschild CC. Intrapericardial basic fibroblast growth factor induces myocardial angiogenesis in a rabbit model of chronic ischemia. Am Heart J 1995; 129:924–31.

15. Laham RJ, Simons M, Tofukuji M, et al. Modulation of myocardial perfusion and vascular reactivity by pericardial basic fibroblast growth factor: insight into ischemia-induced reduction in endothelium-dependent vasodilatation. J Thorac Cardiovasc Surg 1998; 116:1022–8.

16. Seferovic PM, Ristic AD, Marsimovic R, et al. Initial clinical experience with PerDUCER® device: promising new tool in the diagnosis and treatment of pericardial disease. Clin Cardiol 1999; 22(suppl): I-30–I-35.

17. Janssens S, Flaherty D, Nong Z, et al. Human endothelial nitric oxide synthase gene transfer inhibits vascular smooth muscle cell proliferation and neointima formation after balloon injury in rats. Circulation 1998; 97:1274–81.

18. Guo J, Milhoan K, Tuan R, et al. Beneficial effect of SPM-5185, a cysteine-containing nitric oxide

donor, in rat carotid artery intimal injury. Circ Res 1994; 75:77–84.

19. Tarry W, Makhoul R. L-Arginine improves endothelium-dependent vasorelaxation and reduces intimal hyperplasia after balloon angioplasty. Arterioscler Thromb 1994; 14:938–43.

20. Hamon M, Vallet B, Bauters C, et al. Long-term oral administration of L-arginine reduces intimal thickening and enhances neoendothelium-dependent acetylcholine-induced relaxation after arterial injury. Circulation 1994; 90:1357–62.

21. Wink DA, Kasprzak KS, Maragos CM, et al. DNA deaminating ability and genotoxicity of nitric oxide and its progenitors. Science 1991; 254:1001–3.

63

Alternatives to drug eluting stents: safety and efficacy of systemic delivery of antiproliferative therapy to reduce in-stent neointimal hyperplasia

Frank D Kolodgie, Andrew Farb, Herman K Gold, Aloke V Finn, and Renu Virmani

INTRODUCTION

The current approaches for the treatment of coronary atherosclerosis are palliative. Although percutaneous coronary interventions (PCIs) are an attractive alternative to bypass surgery, this therapy is associated with a significant number of treatment failures primarily resulting from in-stent restenosis (ISR). The development of stents together with new antiplatelet strategies has substantially reduced early and late complications of PCIs. Nevertheless, a significant proportion of successfully treated patients continue to experience recurrent ischemic events. These complications for the most part represent ISR along with the risk of coronary disease progression in other lesions left untreated by interven-

tion. Of late, drug eluting stents have emerged as promising therapy for the prevention of ISR. The sustained inhibition of neointimal growth by drug eluting stents, however, may not be achieved since the kinetic properties of a single drug dose may only delay vascular healing with a return of neointimal growth. Long-term suppression of ISR may, therefore, require repeat dosing, perhaps with multiple drugs given at defined intervals. Such complex dosing regimens are not feasible with the current drug eluting stents. As an alternative to local drug delivery, the use of oral agents in combination with improved metal stents may offer a more effective and economical approach to preventing ISR.

MECHANISMS OF RESTENOSIS (Figure 63.1)

Restenosis is defined as a decrease in lumen size resulting from the loss of acute lumen gain achieved at the time of an intravascular interventional procedure. Arterial injury evoked by placement of a stent initiates a complex sequence of cellular and molecular events consisting of smooth muscle cell (SMC) migration and proliferation and matrix secretion culminating in a thickened neointima.[1,2] While the bulk of in-stent restenosis is comprised of extracellular matrix (accumulations of proteoglycans and collagen), the SMC content is typically limited.[3]

Following stenting, there is an initial endothelial denudation and exposure of subintimal components to the bloodstream causing platelet adherence and aggregation, fibrinogen binding, and thrombus formation. Local thrombus deposition confers an essential provisional matrix, in which SMCs can migrate. The migration and proliferation of SMCs is promoted by platelet release of several mitogen and chemotactic factors at the injured site. Moreover, platelet activation also promotes the recruitment of monocytes/macrophages[4] to the injured vessel wall, further contributing to matrix production and cellular proliferation.

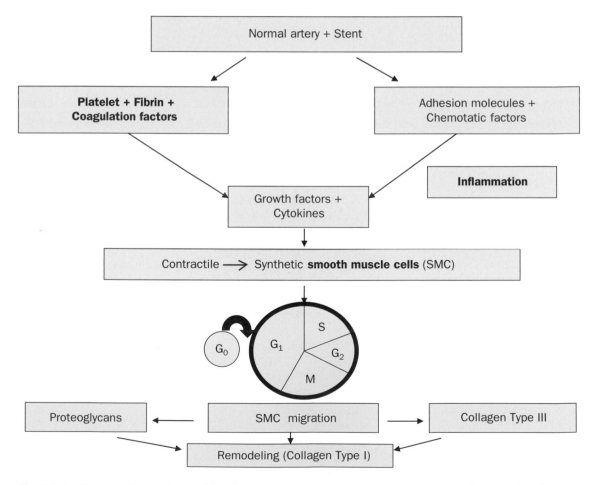

Fig. 63.1 Diagram illustration highlighting general mechanisms of in-stent restenosis; the critical participants are indicated in bold.

Increasing evidence suggests that inflammation is critical to the development of ISR. In animals models, macrophages accumulate to a greater extent with stenting compared with balloon angioplasty alone.[5] Although both types of injury result in early neutrophil responses, stented arteries are associated with prolonged infiltration of macrophages with sustained expression of interleukin-8 (IL-8) and monocyte chemotactic protein (MCP-1).[6] This association, however, becomes more complex in humans with coronary atherosclerosis where the physical relationship of the stent with the various plaque elements augments inflammatory responses. For example, studies from our laboratory demonstrate increased inflammatory density when stent struts are in direct contact with an underlying medial rupture site or when struts penetrate into a lipid core.[7] Further, the extent of inflammatory infiltrate is a predictor of restenosis such that there is a >2-fold higher neointimal inflammatory cell density in stents with restenosis versus non-restenotic stents.[7] Quantitative angiographic studies suggest that late lumen loss independently correlates with expression of the macrophage β_2 integrin Mac-1, which is responsible for leukocyte adhesion to platelets and fibrinogen at injured arterial sites.[8] Moreover, patients with ISR, compared with patients without ISR, have significantly elevated levels of monocyte chemoattractant protein-1 (MCP-1).[9] The contribution of macrophages to the development of restenosis is likely related to their expression of numerous growth factors, cytokines, and enzymes (in particular matrix metalloproteinases).[10]

MOLECULAR TARGETS OF RESTENOSIS

The developing neointimal response to a stent represents a complex interaction among biologically active mediators that regulate cellular proliferation, migration, inflammation, apoptosis, and matrix alterations. Studies of animal models of arterial injury have helped unravel the nature of these relationships since direct data from human disease are limited. Initial studies in the rat model of carotid artery balloon injury demonstrated the role of basic fibroblast growth factor (FGF), released from injured or dying vascular cells, in promoting the proliferation of medial SMCs, whereas platelet-derived growth factor (PDGF) facilitates the migration of SMCs towards the intima.[11,12] Intimal proliferation and matrix accumulation are responsive to PDGF, transforming growth factor-β (TGF-β), angiotensin II, epidermal growth factor, and insulin growth factor 1 (IGF-1).[13] The loss of growth-inhibitory factors such as endothelial derived nitric oxide (NO),[14] or altered heparan sulfate proteoglycan synthesis,[15] may also contribute to the migration and proliferation of SMCs and the inflammatory response associated with restenosis.

With an improved understanding of the molecular mechanism of vascular proliferative diseases, several treatment strategies have emerged that may inhibit or block vascular proliferation. To date, trials with systemic drugs, such as antiplatelet agents, anticoagulants, calcium-channel blockers, angiotensin-converting enzyme inhibitors, cholesterol-lowering agents, and antioxidants to block restenosis have been unsuccessful.[4] These treatment failures may represent species differences in the response to vascular injury, insufficient concentration of drug at the injury site, or lack of chronic dosing. Often, effective doses in animals cannot be achieved in humans because of toxicity. Moreover, animal models of restenosis may be overly simplistic since they generally consist of non-atherosclerotic vessels studied within weeks of injury and may not be representative of the human condition, which takes 6 to 9 months to develop.[16] Finally, the belief that a multifactorial disease can be treated successfully by targeting a single mitogenic factor may be inaccurate.

The poor results of the early clinical trials have shifted the interest in candidate antirestenosis drugs to those with broader pharmacologic activity directed against cell cycle arrest rather than single mitogenic factors.[17] The current generations of antirestenosis agents are targeted to suppress vascular proliferation by cytostatic (sirolimus, everolimus) or cytotoxic (paclitaxel) mechanisms. The cytotoxic approach involves the destruction and death of vascular cells, whereas a cytostatic agent blocks cell cycle progression without inducing cell death. A cytostatic strategy is theoretically more desirable since cytotoxic treatments may result in vessel wall necrosis, potentially leading to increased inflammation, arterial dilatation (positive remodeling), or aneurysms.

THE RATIONALE FOR LOCALIZED DRUG DELIVERY (Table 63.1)

Drug eluting stents comprise a three-component system involving a favorable stent design coupled to a drug carrier and pharmacologic agent. The key advantage of drug eluting stents is that they effectively provide local drug delivery over a defined period limiting the risk of systemic toxicity. Moreover, the agent can be selective to the pathological process for the reduction of thrombosis, restenosis, and/or both. Recent clinical trials with stents loaded with *sirolimus*[18–20] *paclitaxel*[21–24] or *everolimus*[25] demonstrated remarkably low coronary restenosis rates of 0% to 9% from 6 to 12 months. These early impressive results have led some clinicians to conclude that drug eluting stents have solved the problem of ISR. Preclinical studies, however, suggest that the beneficial effects of these devices are attributed to delayed vascular repair and healing is accompanied by a late return of neointimal growth. The recent observation of unexpectedly high wound dehiscence in liver,[26] and lung trans-plant recipients,[27] with prophylactic oral sirolimus offers evidence of delayed healing with these drugs in humans.

LIMITATIONS OF LOCALIZED DRUG DELIVERY (Table 63.1)

There are several potential limitations to using a stent for chronic local drug delivery since the pharmacologic agent cannot be given indefinitely and effective doses may be toxic to the vessel wall. Further, unreliable pharmacokinetics may result in the untimely release of the drug and a loss of efficacy. The potential for long-term adverse effects secondary to polymeric coating poses another concern. The premature breakdown of a polymer coating or its potential to stimulate inflammation may limit any beneficial effect of the drug. In addition, drug eluting stents need to be precisely deployed to avoid geographical miss. In the SIRIUS trial, despite the inhibition of in-stent neointimal growth there remained a persistent problem of restenosis at the peristent margins because these balloon-injured sites remain unprotected by the stent and may not have received significant exposure to the drug (unpublished data 2002, Martin Leon, Lenox Hill Hospital, NY). Furthermore, despite the promising results of drug eluting stents, intravascular ultrasound (IVUS) studies from the RAVEL trial, demonstrate stent malapposition with 'black holes' around stent struts in

---

Table 63.1 Advantages and disadvantages of drug-eluting stents

Advantages	Disadvantages
• Drug delivered directly to the vessel	• Need polymer for prolonged drug delivery
• No systemic toxicity	• Polymers may be toxic
• Can vary dose but cannot control the amount delivered to each patient	• Limited period of drug delivery
• Prolonged delivery of large amount of drug over a fairly long time	• Local toxicity to the vessel wall
	• Release kinetics have to be exactly titrated
	• Cannot vary dose according to the need of the patient
	• Cannot repeat the regimen

21% of sirolimus eluting stents versus 4% in controls.[19] The disappointing performance of stents eluting actinomycin D (ACTION Trial),[28] or QuaDS- (QP2 taxane analog),[29,30] suggests that the choice of drug is a critical element in reducing restenosis. Even if a drug holds promise, potential problems with polymeric coatings, very high concentration of the active drug, extended release kinetics, inhomogeneous strut placement are all undesirable factors.[31] Thus, there are multiple aspects of stent design independent of the drug, which determine its overall clinical success.

RATIONALE FOR ORAL/SYSTEMIC THERAPY
(Table 63.2)

The use of oral/systemic agents in combination with conventional metal stents may potentially lead to an effective approach to prevent ISR, beyond the obvious reduction in cost. The potential toxicity of oral/systemic agents can be reduced or eliminated by giving limited doses timed to critical cellular events. An effective oral/systemic agent would provide more flexibility in the choice of stent allowing for variations in lesion lengths, artery sizes, and anatomic locations. More importantly, repeat dosing schedules could be easily optimized for sustained suppression of neointimal growth. It is also conceivable that an oral/systemic agent might dramatically reduce the need for stent-

ing altogether since in some circumstances, such as in small vessels <2.5 mm in diameter, balloon angioplasty alone is equally successful.[32] Similarly, discrete lesions in large vessels have relatively low restenosis rates with bare metal stents, and the use of an expensive drug eluting stent may be also unnecessary.

LIMITATIONS OF ORAL/SYSTEMIC THERAPY
(Table 63.2)

The principal argument against oral/systemic therapy for preventing ISR is the potential for adverse side effects. Other major reasons for the failure of oral/systemic therapy involve suboptimal dosing intervals, duration of administration, and ineffective retention of the drug at the treatment site. Moreover, required solvents for certain lipophilic drugs (eg. paclitaxel), such as poloxyethylated castor oil (Cremophor EL) or polysorbate 80 (Tween 80), limitis their use as restenosis therapy because of acute hypersensitivity reactions.[33]

THE PRECLINICAL EXPERIENCE WITH SYSTEMIC/ORAL THERAPY

The concept of using cell cycle inhibitors for the prevention of restenosis was initially tested in a coronary swine angioplasty model. Intramuscular administration of rapamycin 3 days before percutaneous transluminal coro-

---

Table 63.2	Advantages and disadvantages of oral/systemic therapy
Advantages	**Disadvantages**
• Flexibility in the choice of stent	• Potential systemic toxicity
• Less toxic to the vessel wall	• Toxic solvents, specifically with lipophilic drugs
• Allows for repeat dosing and combined therapy	• Insufficient amount of drug to the stent-treatment site
• May allow for the treatment of small vessels <2.5 mm where stenting is of little value	• Potential variation in dose at the stent-treatment site
• Can be given in doses timed to critical cellular events	
• Reduced cost over drug eluting stents	

nary angioplasty (PTCA) produced a significant inhibition in coronary stenosis at 14 days.[34] The decrease in SMC proliferation was associated with markedly increased concentrations of p27[kip1] levels and inhibition of pRb phosphorylation within the vessel wall. This study was the first to offer successful proof of the concept of an agent that targets cyclin-dependent kinase activity for the prevention of ISR.

The use of oral inhibitors of cell cycle regulation was further examined in our laboratory in a rabbit model of iliac artery stenting. Rabbits treated with everolimus, an agent of the same macrolide family as sirolimus, demonstrated a marked reduction in neointimal growth at 28 days.[35] In the high dose everolimus group, there was a 49% reduction in mean intimal thickness and a 36% reduction in percentage stent stenosis. Although inhibition of neointimal formation was slightly less pronounced in the low dose everolimus animals, there remained a significant 40% reduction in mean intimal thickness and a 26% reduction in percent stenosis. The results of the low dose regimen showed particular promise since there was efficacy and better toleration of the dose. Moreover, the degree of in-stent neointimal inhibition was similar to that seen with sirolimus eluting stents. Thus, everolimus might potentially provide drug delivery stent-like results without the engineering challenges and potential costs of manufacturing.

The systemic delivery of another promising agent, paclitaxel, was previously avoided because of toxicity of the Cremophor EL solvent. In a recent study from our laboratory, however, we tested a novel albumin stabilized nanoparticle formulation of paclitaxel (nPXL, ABI-007, American Bioscience) developed for systemic use. In a rabbit model of iliac artery stenting, systemic nPXL (2.5–5.0 mg/kg) produced a significant dose-dependent reduction in mean intimal thickness compared with control stents.[36] The neointima of stented arteries treated with nPXL (3.5–5.0 mg/kg) showed incomplete healing at 28 days, with frequent areas of mild to severe focal fibrin deposition and inflammation; these lesions were histologically similar to PXL eluting stent implants in rabbits for 28 days (Figure 63.2). In contrast, control animals and those treated with low dose nPXL showed near complete surface endothelialization while animals treated with ≥3.5 mg/kg demonstrated focal endothelial cell loss in particular, over stent struts. This is the first study of systemic paclitaxel for the reduction of ISR and although in its infancy, the application of nanoparticle technology for the prevention of restenosis is emerging as a promising technique for the selective targeting of vascular lesions.[37]

Long-term results with localized drug delivery in animal models have been disappointing. The primary reason for lack of sustained effect is predicted by delayed vascular healing characterized by persistent intimal fibrin deposition, intraintimal hemorrhage, increased intimal and adventitial inflammation, and incomplete endothelialization. Complete healing is often accompanied by a return of neointimal growth (late lumen loss). For example, the efficacy of a single dose of 5 mg/kg nPXL was gone in our rabbit model by 90 days.[36] In contrast, a second repeat dose of nPXL of 3.5 mg/kg given 28 days after stenting resulted in sustained suppression of neointimal thickness at 90 days with near complete healing. These data emphasized the benefit of repeat dosing for achieving long-term suppression of neointimal growth.

Selective targeted depletion of circulating macrophages with systemic delivery of bisphosphonates (bone-seeking agents that are potent inhibitors of osteoclasts) has also shown promise for the prevention of restenosis. In a rabbit model of balloon angioplasty, liposomal clodronate, a specific macrophage inhibitor belonging to the family of bisphosphonates, produced a transient depletion of circulating blood monocytes and liver and splenic macrophages.[38] The inactivation of macrophages was associated with suppressed neointimal growth in hypercholesterolemic rabbits and rats without adverse side effects. Similar efficacy has been shown in a rabbit model of arterial stenting (unpublished observation, Edelman ER, 2002). Therefore, these studies suggest that selective transient modulation of

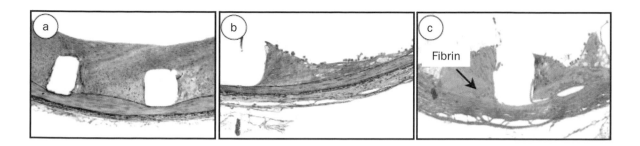

Paclitaxel-eluting stent (42 µg)

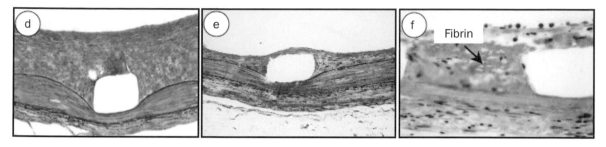

Fig. 63.2 Comparison of the effects of paclitaxel administered as a systemic infusion (a–c) versus local stent delivery (d–f) in an iliac artery stent injury model in the rabbit. (a) A control iliac artery at 28 days (Movat pentachrome, ×200). (b) Iliac artery stent from an animal treated with 5 mg/kg nanoparticle paclitaxel (nPXL, ABI-007, American Bioscience); note the marked reduction in neointimal growth and surface inflammation compared with (a) (Movat pentachrome, ×200). (c) High power view from an animal treated with systemic nPXL. This shows focal fibrin deposition around a stent strut (hematoxylin-eosin, ×400). (d) Control 28 day iliac artery stent from an animal with a paclitaxel eluting stent showing a well healed neointima; note the similarity with (a) (Movat pentachrome, ×20). (e) Paclitaxel eluting stent showing suppression of neointimal growth, similar to that observed with systemic nPXL in (b) (Movat pentachrome, ×200). (f) Focal fibrin accumulation around struts in a paclitaxel eluting stent (hematoxylin-eosin, ×600).

monocytes/macrophages may have important clinical implications in the prevention of in-stent restenosis.

ORAL THERAPY FOR IN-STENT RESTENOSIS: THE CLINICAL EXPERIENCE (Table 63.3)

Therapeutic strategies using an oral approach for the treatment of in-stent restenosis are evolving, and as yet, data from randomized clinical trails are unavailable. There are however, promising results from observational studies of stented patients using immunosuppressive agents for chronic transplant rejection. In a study of 776 renal transplant patients, 13 were treated with stainless steel stent implants for coronary artery stenosis of which

38% were diabetics.[41] All patients were treated with combined immunosuppressive therapy including cyclosporine, prednisone, and aza-thioprine (n = 11); one patient received cyclosporine, prednisone, and mycophenolate mofetil, and one received azathiopine and prednisone only. The cyclosporine whole blood level at the time of coronary intervention was 129 ± 49 ng/dL. Intravascular ultrasound measurements at 14 ± 8 months demonstrated minimal intimal proliferation and angiography showed no ISR. Because various immuno-suppressive agents were used, it is difficult to attribute the anti-restenotic effect to a single or combination of drugs. Early clinical trials with corticosteroids, however, have previously failed to inhibit restenosis.[42,43] In contrast,

Table 63.3 Summary of in-stent restenosis (ISR) prevention studies with oral/systemic therapy

Age/Sex	No. pts	Indication for PCI	Drug	Pre MLD	Post MLD	Follow-up MLD	Follow-up duration	LLL (mm)	ISR (%)	Source
58 ± 6/11 M	13	ACS 9 pts	Cyclo + Pred + AZA[a]	1.02 ± 0.46	3.13 ± 0.43	2.82 ± 0.56	14 ± 8[a]	0.25 ± 0.60	0%	41
–	40	–	Anthra/Antibiotics[b]	–	–	–	3 yrs	–	5%/control 26%	47
57 ± 6/14 M	22	ISR	Sirolimus 6 mg loading 2 mg/d	–	–	9.9 ± 1.8	–	–	86.7%	48
63 ± 12/32 M (ORAR)	34	ACS/23 pts	Sirolimus 6 mg loading 2 mg/30 d (30 d)	De novo 0.6 ± 0.31 / Restenotic 2.76 ± 0.31	2.8 ± 0.26 / 0.4 ± 0.29	2.11 ± 0.31 / 1.6 ± 0.32	6 mths	0.31 ± 0.22 / Rap > 8 ng/ml	18.9% / 50%	50
60 ± 10/26 M (ORBIT)	60	ACS/40 pts	Sirolimus 5 mg loading 2 or 5 mg/d (30 d)	1.11 ± 0.6	2.90 ± 0.57	2.29 ± 0.61	6 mths	0.60 ± 0.61	7%	Waksman et al. 2002 not publ
–	12	ISR	Sirolimus 15 mg loading 2 mg/d (28 d)	–	–	–	4 mths	–	0%	39
–	10	ISR	Sirolimus 6 mg loading 2 mg/d (2 wks)	1.14 ± 0.62	3.32 ± 0.63	–	–	–	0%	40

[a] One patient (pt) received cyclosporine (Cyclo), prednisone (Pred), and mycophenolate mofetil and 1 pt received azathioprine (AZA) and prednisone only.
[b] Patients received polyfunctional alkylating agents (n = 29), anthracycline (Anthra) and antibiotics (n = 20), plant alkaloids (n = 25), antimetabolites (n = 8), and steroid hormones (n = 4).
[c] 3 pt refused follow-up angiography, but had negative stress thallium.
PCI, percutaneous intervention; MLD, maximal luminal diameter; LLL, late lumen loss; ACS, acute coronary syndrome.

recent results from the IMmunosuppressive therapy for the Prevention of REStenosis after Coronary Artery Stent Implantation (IMPRESS study) demonstrate a significant reduction of clinical events and angiographic restenosis rate in patients with persistently high C-reactive protein (CRP) levels treated with prednisone.[44] Animals studies however, suggest that cyclosporine alone inhibits T-lymphocytes and SMC proliferation after vascular injury in experimental models.[45,46] The finding that renal transplant patients treated with coronary stents develop minimal late in-stent intimal proliferation suggests that oral immunosuppressive therapy given to avoid kidney rejection reduces ISR.

The potential for systemic chemotherapy in decreasing coronary ISR in cancer patients has also been recognized. In one preliminary study by Kokolis et al., in 40 patients who received active chemotherapy for cancer and concurrent PCI, there was 0% restenosis at 3 year follow-up.[47]

The success of sirolimus-eluting stents as a platform for local drug delivery has inspired pilot trials of oral sirolimus therapy as an alternative approach for the prevention of ISR. In a recent study, 22 patients with recalcitrant restenosis were given oral sirolimus.[48] In this series, 50% of patients did not fully complete the 30 day prescription because of side effects mainly attributed to leukopenia and elevated triglycerides; the average duration of oral rapamycin therapy prior to discontinuation was 14.5 ± 6.5 days. In this trial, oral sirolimus therapy was associated with target lesion revascularization in 13 (59%) study patients and angiographic restenosis in 86.7% of patients with follow-up angiograms. The lack of efficacy of oral sirolimus in these patients with recurrent restenosis may involve several factors including a previously failed response to radiation therapy or inadequate dosing. Circulating sirolimus blood levels were not obtained so it is difficult to attribute the lack of benefit to insufficient drug concentrations. Experience in renal transplant patients suggests that the monitoring of sirolimus blood concentration is critical. Adverse effects are

markedly reduced when sirolimus target trough levels are lowered to 15 ng/mL.[49] Moreover, there is a large inter- and intra-subject variability in drug clearance, and the time required to reach steady state is typically 5 to 7 days after a dose change.[50] Finally, it is unlikely that these patients would have responded favorably even to a sirolimus eluting stent, since previous radiation failures have been shown to experience a higher rate of thrombosis and restenosis with these devices.[51]

Conversely, other studies of oral sirolimus report the beneficial effects in preventing ISR. In the Oral Rapamycin in Argentina (ORAR) trial, 34 patients with 49 coronary lesions were treated with oral sirolimus for 1 month following stenting.[52] Patients received a loading dose of 6 mg of sirolimus followed by a daily dose of 2 mg for 30 days immediately after successful stent deployment. In contrast to the study by Brara, this dosing regimen was well tolerated with only one patient discontinuing therapy for mild side effects. Diabetes was present in 35% of patients, and 25% of lesions already had ISR. At follow-up, angiographic restenosis and total lesion revascularization (TLR) at 6 months was documented in 26.5% of lesions with 13/49 (18.9%) occurring in de novo lesions and 6/12 (50%) in lesions that previously showed ISR. Neointimal growth was strongly dependent on drug concentration since restenosis in patients with rapamycin levels $\geq$ 8 ng/mL was zero (0/12) compared with 24% (6/25) when blood levels were $\leq$8 ng/mL.

In the Oral Rapamune to inhiBIT restenosis (ORBIT) trial, 60 patients were treated with a loading dose of 5 mg of rapamycin administered immediately before or after percutaneous intervention followed by a maintenance dose of 2 mg or 5 mg/day for 30 days (unpublished data 2002; Ron Waksman, Washington Hospital Center, Washington, DC). Sirolimus blood levels were in the therapeutic range of 4–20 ng/mL. Adverse reactions ranged from mild to severe with two patients discontinuing the drug because of side effects. Quantitative coronary angiography (QCA) at 6 months demonstrated an in-stent restenosis rate of

4.2% with an in-segment restenosis rate of 7.0%; late lumen loss was 0.60 ± 0.61 mm.

ADVERSE SIDE EFFECTS OF SIROLIMUS

The principal side effects of sirolimus are bone marrow suppression and hyperlipidemia.[53] The former usually manifests as a mild thrombocytopenia, and seldom dictates discontinuation of treatment. Severe thrombocytopenia is rare, and there have been no reports to date of bleeding episodes. These side effects are often concentration-related and respond to dosage adjustment. Hyperlipidemia is seldom a cause for discontinuation of therapy and can be treated by conventional lipid-lowering therapy. Other reported side effects include hypocalemia, hyperglycemia, diarrhea, and abnormal liver function tests. For patients at standard risk for transplant rejection, the therapeutic whole blood sirolimus level is 5–15 ng/mL; this dose range also minimizes side effects.[49] In four of five observational studies using sirolimus for the prevention of ISR, reported side effects were noted in approximately 30% of patients with less than 10% resulting in the discontinuation of medication. It is conceivable that the incidence of systemic toxicity can be further minimized by combination therapy with other immunosuppressive or antiproliferative drugs.

OTHER CANDIDATE DRUGS FOR ORAL/ SYSTEMIC PREVENTION OF IN-STENT RESTENOSIS

Other oral/systemic drugs, particularly nanoparticle paclitaxel ABI-007, are currently in early clinical trials for the prevention of ISR. The initial dose-finding study SNAPIST (Systemic NAnoparticle Paclitaxel for In-STent Restenosis) is a four-arm randomized multicenter study evaluating the safety of a single dose of systemically administered ABI-007 at the time of stenting in patients with de novo lesions in a single native coronary artery. After the initial dose finding, this study will be expanded into patients with more complex lesions with multiple vessel disease to elucidate the ability of systemic therapy to simultaneously treat multiple lesions.

ORAL/SYSTEMIC THERAPY FOR RESTENOSIS PREVENTION IN DIABETICS

Another potential therapeutic target for ISR prevention is the peroxisome proliferators-activated receptor (PPARs). PPARs are primarily involved in the regulation of lipid metabolism and homeostasis.[54] Three distinct PPARs (designated PPARα, PPARγ, and PPARβ/δ) have been identified.[55] Recent evidence suggests that PPARS exert antiproliferative and inflammatory effects in vascular cells (endothelial and SMCs), and monocytes/macrophages. PPARγ ligands (thiazolidinediones) are the latest group of drugs for treating Type 2 diabetes and include troglitazone, rosiglitazone, and pioglitazone. Of these, troglitazone is the most potent inhibitor of SMC proliferation.[56] Animal restenosis studies with troglitazone show a reduction in intimal hyperplasia after balloon-induced vascular injury.[57] The efficacy of the PPARγ ligand troglitazone to prevent ISR in patients with Type 2 diabetes mellitus has also been examined. Patients with non-insulin-dependent diabetes mellitus were treated with 400 mg troglitazone for 6 months.[58] The maximal luminal diameter (MLD) in the troglitazone group was significantly greater than in the control group (2.2 ± 0.5 mm vs 1.7 ± 0.5 mm, respectively, $p = 0.0002$). Similar positive results with troglitazone were obtained in small vessels using 2.5 mm diameter stents.[59]

Pioglitazone is another potential candidate drug. In cultured SMC, pioglitazone lowered cell viability by promoting cytokine-induced NO production.[60] When given orally in an in vivo rat model of balloon arterial injury, it decreased maximal neointimal growth by 30% compared with vehicle-treated animals.[57] In a recent clinical study of 44 patients with Type 2 diabetes mellitus, pioglitazone was given to 23 patients following successful coronary stent implantation.[61] After 6 months of treatment, angiographic ISR and target lesion revascularization (TLR) were less frequent in the pioglitazone than control group, although differences were not statistically significant. Neointimal index measured by IVUS, however, was significantly smaller in the pioglitazone group.

Thus far, clinical studies using glitazones for preventing ISR have been limited to a small group of patients and from one investigative group. Although these early results shown promise, larger multicenter clinical trials are necessary to better determine the outcome of PPAR ligands for the treatment of ISR.

CONCLUSIONS

Encouraging early data suggest that oral therapy for in-stent restenosis particularly with sirolimus, may be a viable treatment option compared to drug eluting stents. Multiple stents could be treated simultaneously with repeat doses or combined therapy optimized for individual patients. Importantly, the clinician would have the option to select the most appropriate stent of varying lesion lengths, artery sizes, and anatomic locations. Larger randomized clinical studies are necessary to confirm the safety and efficacy of oral therapy for in-stent restenosis.

REFERENCES

1. Schwartz SM. Smooth muscle migration in atherosclerosis and restenosis. J Clin Invest 1997; 100:S87–9.
2. Schwartz SM. Perspectives series: cell adhesion in vascular biology. Smooth muscle migration in atherosclerosis and restenosis. J Clin Invest 1997; 99:2814–16.
3. Chung IM, Gold HK, Schwartz SM, et al. Enhanced extracellular matrix accumulation in restenosis of coronary arteries after stent deployment. J Am Coll Cardiol 2002; 40:2072–81.
4. Fattori R, Piva T. Drug-eluting stents in vascular intervention. Lancet 2003; 361:247–9.
5. Kollum M, Kaiser S, Kinscherf R, et al. Apoptosis after stent implantation compared with balloon angioplasty in rabbits. Role of macrophages. Arterioscler Thromb Vasc Biol 1997; 17:2383–8.
6. Welt FG, Tso C, Edelman ER, et al. Leukocyte recruitment and expression of chemokines following different forms of vascular injury. Vasc Med 2003; 8:1–7.
7. Farb A, Weber DK, Kolodgie FD, et al. Morphological predictors of restenosis after coronary stenting in humans. Circulation 2002; 105:2974–80.
8. Inoue T, Uchida T, Yaguchi I, et al. Stent-induced expression and activation of the leukocyte integrin Mac-1 is associated with neointimal thickening and restenosis. Circulation 2003; 107:1757–63.
9. Cipollone F, Marini M, Fazia M, et al. Elevated circulating levels of monocyte chemoattractant protein-1 in patients with restenosis after coronary angioplasty. Arterioscler Thromb Vasc Biol 2001; 21:327–34.
10. Inoue S, Koyama H, Miyata T, Shigematsu H. Cell replication induces in-stent lesion growth in rabbit carotid artery with preexisting intimal hyperplasia. Atherosclerosis 2002; 162:345–53.
11. Lindner V, Lappi DA, Baird A, et al. Role of basic fibroblast growth factor in vascular lesion formation. Circ Res 1991; 68:106–13.
12. Majesky MW, Reidy MA, Bowen-Pope DF, et al. PDGF ligand and receptor gene expression during repair of arterial injury. J Cell Biol 1990; 111:2149–58.
13. Dzau VJ, Braun-Dullaeus RC, Sedding DG. Vascular proliferation and atherosclerosis: new perspectives and therapeutic strategies. Nat Med 2002; 8:1249–56.
14. Ignarro LJ, Buga GM, Wei LH, et al. Role of the arginine-nitric oxide pathway in the regulation of vascular smooth muscle cell proliferation. Proc Natl Acad Sci USA 2001; 98:4202–8.
15. Kinsella MG, Wight TN. Modulation of sulfated proteoglycan synthesis by bovine aortic endothelial cells during migration. J Cell Biol 1986; 102:679–87.
16. Virmani R, Kolodgie FD, Farb A, Lafont A. Drug eluting stents: are human and animal studies comparable? Heart 2003; 89:133–8.
17. Gershlick AH. Treating atherosclerosis: local drug delivery from laboratory studies to clinical trials. Atherosclerosis 2002; 160:259–71.
18. Moses JW, Leon MB, Popma JJ, et al. Sirolimus-eluting stents versus standard stents in patients

with stenosis in a native coronary artery. N Engl J Med 2003; 349:1315–23.

19. Serruys PW, Degertekin M, Tanabe K, et al. Intravascular ultrasound findings in the multi-center, randomized, double-blind RAVEL (RAndomized study with the sirolimus-eluting VElocity balloon-expandable stent in the treatment of patients with de novo native coronary artery Lesions) trial. Circulation 2002; 106:798–803.

20. Sousa JE, Costa MA, Sousa AG, et al. Two-year angiographic and intravascular ultrasound follow-up after implantation of sirolimus-eluting stents in human coronary arteries. Circulation 2003; 107:381–3.

21. Colombo A, Drzewiecki J, Banning A, et al. Randomized study to assess the effectiveness of slow- and moderate-release polymer-based paclitaxel-eluting stents for coronary artery lesions. Circulation 2003; 108: 788–94.

22. Grube E, Silber S, Hauptmann KE, et al. TAXUS I: six- and twelve-month results from a randomized, double-blind trial on a slow-release paclitaxel-eluting stent for de novo coronary lesions. Circulation 2003; 107:38–42.

23. Hong MK, Mintz GS, Lee CW, et al. Paclitaxel coating reduces in-stent intimal hyperplasia in human coronary arteries: a serial volumetric intravascular ultrasound analysis from the Asian Paclitaxel-Eluting Stent Clinical Trial (ASPECT). Circulation 2003; 107:517–20.

24. Tanabe K, Serruys PW, Grube E, et al. TAXUS III Trial: in-stent restenosis treated with stent-based delivery of paclitaxel incorporated in a slow-release polymer formulation. Circulation 2003; 107:559–64.

25. Grube E, Sonoda A, Ikeno F, et al. Six- and twelve-month results from first human experience using everolimus-eluting stents with bioabsorbable polymer. Circulation 2004; 109:168–71.

26. Guilbeau JM. Delayed wound healing with sirolimus after liver transplant. Ann Pharmacother 2002; 36:1391–5.

27. King-Biggs MB, Dunitz JM, Park SJ, et al. Airway anastomotic dehiscence associated with use of sirolimus immediately after lung transplantation. Transplantation 2003; 75:1437–43.

28. Serruys PW, Ormiston JA, Degertekin M, et al. Actinomycin eluting stent for coronary revascularization: A randomized feasibility and safety study (The ACTION Trial). J Am Coll Cardiol 2004; 44:1363–7.

29. Liistro F, Stankovic G, Di Mario C, et al. First clinical experience with paclitaxel derivative-eluting polymer stent system implantation for in-stent restenosis. Immediate and long-term clinical and angiographic outcome. Circulation 2002; 105:1883–6.

30. Virmani R, Liistro F, Stankovic G, et al. Mechanism of late in-stent restenosis after implantation of a paclitaxel derivate-eluting polymer stent system in humans. Circulation 2002; 106:2649–51.

31. Hwang CW, Wu D, Edelman ER. Physiological transport forces govern drug distribution for stent-based delivery. Circulation 2001; 104:600–5.

32. Holmes DR, Jr, Hirshfeld J, Jr, Faxon D, et al. ACC Expert Consensus document on coronary artery stents. Document of the American College of Cardiology. J Am Coll Cardiol 1998; 32:1471–82.

33. Loos WJ, Szebeni J, ten Tije AJ, et al. Preclinical evaluation of alternative pharmaceutical delivery vehicles for paclitaxel. Anticancer Drugs 2002; 13:767–75.

34. Gallo R, Padurean A, Jayaraman T, et al. Inhibition of intimal thickening after balloon angioplasty in porcine coronary arteries by targeting regulators of the cell cycle. Circulation 1999; 99:2164–70.

35. Farb A, John M, Acampado E, et al. Oral everolimus inhibits in-stent neointimal growth. Circulation 2002; 106:2379–84.

36. Kolodgie FD, John M, Khurana C, et al. Sustained reduction of in-stent neointimal growth with the use of a novel systemic nanoparticle paclitaxel. Circulation 2002; 106:1195–8.

37. Uwatoku T, Shimokawa H, Abe K, et al. Application of nanoparticle technology for the prevention of restenosis after balloon injury in rats. Circ Res 2003; 92:e62–9.

38. Danenberg HD, Fishbein I, Gao J, et al. Macrophage depletion by clodronate-containing liposomes reduces neointimal formation after balloon injury in rats and rabbits. Circulation 2002; 106:599–605.

39. Arruda JA, Costa MA, Brito FS Jr, et al. Effect of systemic immunosuppression on coronary in-

stent intimal hyperplasia in renal transplant patients. Am J Cardiol 2003; 91:1363–5.

40. Costantini C, Zanultine D, Tarbine S, et al. Oral sirolimus in the treatment of in-stent restenosis. Am J Cardiol.

41. Arruda JA, Costa MA, Brito FS, Jr, et al. Effect of systemic immunosuppression on coronary in-stent intimal hyperplasia in renal transplant patients. Am J Cardiol 2003; 91:1363–5.

42. Lee CW, Chae JK, Lim HY, et al. Prospective randomized trial of corticosteroids for the prevention of restenosis after intracoronary stent implantation. Am Heart J 1999; 138:60–3.

43. Stone GW, Rutherford BD, McConahay DR, et al. A randomized trial of corticosteroids for the prevention of restenosis in 102 patients undergoing repeat coronary angioplasty. Catheter Cardiovasc Diagn 1989; 18:227–31.

44. Versaci F, Gaspardone A, Tomai F, et al. Immunosuppressive therapy for the prevention of restenosis after coronary artery stent implantation (IMPRESS Study). J Am Coll Cardiol 2002; 40:1935–42.

45. Jonasson L, Holm J, Hansson GK. Cyclosporin A inhibits smooth muscle proliferation in the vascular response to injury. Proc Natl Acad Sci USA 1988; 85:2303–6.

46. Voisard R, Seitzer U, Baur R, et al. A prescreening system for potential antiproliferative agents: implications for local treatment strategies of postangioplasty restenosis. Int J Cardiol 1995; 51:15–28.

47. Kokolis S, Dangas G, Mehran R, et al. Use of systemic chemotherapy decreases the rate of in-stent restenosis. Am J Cardiol 2002; 90:(suppl 6A):10H (abstract).

48. Brara PS, Moussavian M, Grise MA, et al. Pilot trial of oral rapamycin for recalcitrant restenosis. Circulation 2003; 107:1722–4.

49. Charpentier B, Groth CG, Backman L, et al. Bicentre hospital experience with sirolimus-based therapy in human renal transplantation: the Sirolimus European Renal Transplant Study. Transplant Proc 2003; 35:58S–61S.

50. MacDonald A. Improving tolerability of immunosuppressive regimens. Transplantation 2001; 72:S105–S112.

51. Degertekin M, Regar E, Tanabe K, et al. Sirolimus-eluting stent for treatment of complex in-stent restenosis: the first clinical experience. J Am Coll Cardiol 2003; 41:184–9.

52. Rodriguez AE, Alemparte MR, Vigo CF, et al. Pilot study of oral rapamycin to prevent restenosis in patients undergoing coronary stent therapy: Argentina single center study (ORAR Trial). J Invasive Cardiol 2003; 15:581–4.

53. Dupont P, Warrens AN. The evolving role of sirolimus in renal transplantation. QJM 2003; 96:401–9.

54. Duval C, Chinetti G, Trottein F, et al. The role of PPARs in atherosclerosis. Trends Mol Med 2002; 8:422–30.

55. Torra IP, Chinetti G, Duval C, et al. Peroxisome proliferator-activated receptors: from transcriptional control to clinical practice. Curr Opin Lipidol 2001; 12:245–54.

56. de Dios ST, Bruemmer D, Dilley RJ, et al. Inhibitory activity of clinical thiazolidinedione peroxisome proliferator activating receptor-gamma ligands toward internal mammary artery, radial artery, and saphenous vein smooth muscle cell proliferation. Circulation 2003; 107:2548–50.

57. Shinohara E, Kihara S, Ouchi N, et al. Troglitazone suppresses intimal formation following balloon injury in insulin-resistant Zucker fatty rats. Atherosclerosis 1998; 136:275–9.

58. Takagi T, Akasaka T, Yamamuro A, et al. Troglitazone reduces neointimal tissue proliferation after coronary stent implantation in patients with non-insulin dependent diabetes mellitus: a serial intravascular ultrasound study. J Am Coll Cardiol 2000; 36:1529–35.

59. Takagi T, Yamamuro A, Tamita K, et al. Impact of troglitazone on coronary stent implantation using small stents in patients with type 2 diabetes mellitus. Am J Cardiol 2002; 89:318–22.

60. Aizawa Y, Kawabe J, Hasebe N, et al. Pioglitazone enhances cytokine-induced apoptosis in vascular smooth muscle cells and reduces intimal hyperplasia. Circulation 2001; 104:455–60.

61. Takagi T, Yamamuro A, Tamita K, et al. Pioglitazone reduces neointimal tissue proliferation after coronary stent implantation in patients with type 2 diabetes mellitus: an intravascular ultrasound scanning study. Am Heart J 2003; 146:E5.

64

Drug eluting stents: a critical perspective*

Renu Virmani, Andrew Farb, and Frank D Kolodgie

Introduction • Mechanism of restenosis • Lessons from preclinical animal studies
• Are polymer coated drug eluting stents risk-free?
• Pathology of balloon expandable stainless steel stents in human arteries
• Temporal differences in arterial healing in humans and animals
• Drug eluting stents vs balloon expandable stents: healing times similar?
• Critical review of clinical studies • Conclusions

INTRODUCTION

Although stenting has significantly reduced restenosis as compared to balloon angioplasty, the unacceptably high incidence of in-stent restenosis has led to the development of drug-eluting stents (DES). There has been a growing expectation among many interventional cardiologists that DES will conquer the problem of in-stent restenosis. Initial results from clinical trials in ideal coronary lesions have shown a significant reduction in the frequency of restenosis at 6 and 12 months. In the largest trials to date, restenosis rates have ranged from 0% to 9% for sirolimus eluting BX Velocity stents compared to 26–34% in uncoated BX Velocity stents (Leon, M. published data).[1] Similarly, paclitaxel eluting stents (TAXUS trials I and II) have also shown promising results at 6 and 12 months with restenosis rates of 2–5% versus 19% in control stents (Colombo, A. Unpublished data).[2] However, these studies have yet to adequately address many complex 'real-world' lesion subsets (e.g. diffuse disease,

bifurcations, ostial lesions, saphenous vein bypass grafts, and stenting of thrombus containing lesions in acute coronary syndromes). Early results of studies conducted of more complicated lesion morphologies suggest that restenosis may be reduced but is certainly not eliminated.[3–5]

MECHANISM OF RESTENOSIS

In balloon angioplasty, the major component of the restenosis process is constrictive negative remodeling (collagen synthesis and cross-linking occurring within the plaque and/or the adventitia) rather than neointimal thickening.[6] Conversely, in-stent restenosis occurs solely as a result of excessive neointimal growth consisting predominantly of extracellular matrix and smooth muscle cells.[7] In-stent neointimal growth is governed by the extent of vessel wall injury, platelet deposition, and the induction of inflammation; these processes are regulated by chemotactic factors, inflammatory cytokines,

---

*The opinions or assertions contained herein are the private views of the authors and are not to be construed as official or as reflecting the views of the Department of the Army or the Department of Defense.

growth factors, and mitotic signals that lead to smooth muscle migration and proliferation.[8] In human stented arteries, neointimal formation is proportional to the circumferential medial injury that is produced during arterial dilatation and stent deployment, contradicting the 'bigger is better' belief that achieving an overly large lumen at the time of stenting results in a superior long-term result.[9,10] Furthermore, stent strut penetration of the necrotic core and persistent chronic inflammation are associated with increased neointimal growth and restenosis.

Most of the early attempts at reducing restenosis by systemic therapy failed probably from an under-appreciation of the mechanical and humoral processes involved and also by the use of single drug therapies with inadequate local tissue concentrations. The current drugs used on DES are significantly more powerful antiproliferative agents, and have been used systemically to treat either malignant neoplasms or as immunosuppressants to prevent organ transplant rejection. These drugs coat the stents by being incorporated in polymers so as to deliver an adequate dosage targeted to the site of arterial injury. Optimally, drugs are eluted slowly for at least the initial 30 days, a time during which proliferation and inflammation are occurring as demonstrated in animal models of stenting.

LESSONS FROM PRECLINICAL ANIMAL STUDIES

Soon after deployment in normal animal arteries, stent struts become covered by a thin layer of platelet/fibrin thrombus accompanied by acute and chronic inflammatory cells. Smooth muscle cell proliferation is observed in the first few days, which peaks in the media at 3 days and in the intima at 7 days. Endothelial coverage of the luminal surface is >80% by 7 days. Proliferation is accompanied by migration of smooth muscle cells from the media into the intima with subsequent synthesis of extracellular matrix in the intima consisting of proteoglycan and collagen.[11,12] These events result in complete coverage of the stent surface by endothelium and a fully healed neointima by 28 days.

Preclinical studies of DES (immunosuppressant and chemotherapeutic agents) in animals have shown that there is a delay in healing characterized by a decrease in neointimal thickness, persistent fibrin deposition, continued proliferation of smooth muscle cells, and impaired endothelialization; a 28 day DES has the morphologic appearance similar to a 7 day balloon expandable non-drug eluting stainless steel stent (Figure 64.1).[13–15] When animal studies have been extended to 3 and 6 months, no differences in neointimal formation had been observed between sirolimus eluting DES and stainless steel balloon expandable stents, and the healing is complete with absence of fibrin (Carter, A. unpublished results). Furthermore, cytotoxic drugs can result in an even *greater* neointimal thickness if there is accompanying necrosis and inflammation, as was seen with actinomycin D eluting stent.[16] These data suggest that DES may only delay rather than prevent long-term healing and neointimal growth.

Polymers used to deliver drugs have shown increased arterial inflammation at 28 days. Granuloma formation with extensive eosinophil infiltration has been observed especially at 3 months with as many as 15–35% of stent implants showing inflammation (Virmani, R. unpublished results). Similar inflammatory reactions have been observed in stainless steel stents but to a far lesser extent. The mechanisms of the granulomatous reaction are poorly understood. However, when an animal has received multiple stents (drug eluting, polymer coating alone, or bare stainless steel), it has been our observation that granulomas are observed in all three stent platforms, reflecting a possible hypersensitivity reaction.

ARE POLYMER COATED DRUG ELUTING STENTS RISK-FREE?

Preclinical and early clinical studies suggested that DES might be the answer to restenosis. However, it is appropriate at this juncture to rethink and critically analyze available data before concluding that the puzzle of restenosis has been solved. Since the release of the sirolimus eluting (CYPHER) stent, a recent

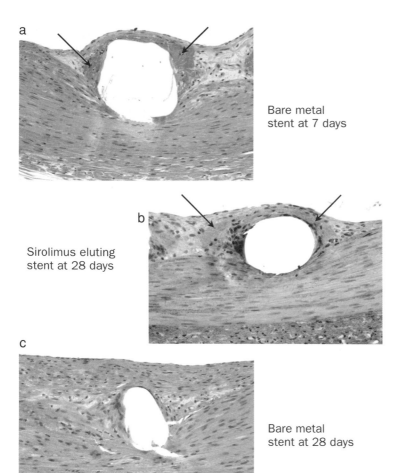

a

Bare metal
stent at 7 days

Sirolimus eluting
stent at 28 days

b

c

Bare metal
stent at 28 days

Fig. 64.1 Delayed healing associated with drug eluting stents. (a) Note the similar degree of fibrin deposition (arrows) in the 28 day sirolimus eluting stent and 7 day bare metal stent, (b) chronic inflammatory cells are more numerous. (c) The 28 day bare metal stent is completely healed; the smooth muscle cell-rich neointima has a rare chronic inflammation around the stent strut and no fibrin deposition.

Food and Drug Administration (FDA) report noted 47 cases of subacute thrombosis in >50 000 CYPHER stents implants; it was recommended that there be greater attention to following specifically labeled deployment guidelines, and greater assurance that the stent is fully deployed and is in contact with the vessel wall.[17] Although the subacute thrombosis rate does not seem high, it should be recognized that these data are derived from voluntary reporting and thus may not represent a true incidence. It is likely that voluntary reporting, at least in the United States, may not reliably reflect the true incidence of adverse clinical outcomes.

Preclinical animal studies reported no excess thrombosis in any study with the exception of inflammation around the stent struts with or without granulomas (or eosinophilic infiltration) associated with non-bioerodable polymers. However, it should be noted that the inflammatory reaction peaks at 90 days post-stenting, while stents are analyzed at only 28 days in most animal studies. Thus, longer periods of DES implant duration may be needed to fully appreciate the local inflammatory responses. Maximum inflammation is observed with polymer combined with drug and is least with a bare metal stent.

In a subset of patients from the RAVEL study that underwent intravascular ultrasound (IVUS), there was a 21% incidence of incomplete stent strut apposition in the sirolimus group compared to a 4% incidence in the control uncoated stent group.[18] The authors were unable to determine if the incomplete apposition occurred at time of stenting or developed over time; however, the higher incidence of malapposition in the CYPHER group strongly suggests strut malapposition is a relatively common finding in arteries with CYPHER stents. Preclinical studies demonstrate that strut malapposition occurs in the setting of an excessive inflammatory response to the polymer and/or drug associated with positive remodeling of the artery.

PATHOLOGY OF BALLOON EXPANDABLE STAINLESS STEEL STENTS IN HUMAN ARTERIES

Immediately after bare metal stent placement, there is platelet and fibrin deposition with acute inflammatory cell infiltration. Platelets and fibrin persist up to 14 and 30 days, respectively, and their presence is further prolonged if the stent struts are embedded in a necrotic core associated with necrotic core prolapse into the lumen. Inflammatory cells (polymorphonuclear leukocytes and macrophages) are present by 1 to 3 days, and macrophages persist for at least 3 months. T-lymphocytes appear at 2–3 weeks and persist beyond 6 months.[8,19] Collections of smooth muscle cells, the main cellular component of the restenotic lesion, are evident by 14 days following stenting. The extracellular matrix, composed initially of proteoglycans and type III collagen, is gradually replaced by type I collagen in stents in place beyond 12 months.

The time course of intimal smooth muscle cell proliferation in relation to in-stent restenosis in humans is not known. Cell proliferation studies in human restenotic coronary atherectomy tissue retrieved from a few days to just beyond one year have generally shown a low proliferation index without the characteristic peak observed at one week in animal models of angioplasty and stenting.[20] Clearly, significantly more rapid proliferative events appear to occur in animals compared to human restenotic coronary arteries. Furthermore, rather than a simple proliferative response, smooth muscle cell migration from within the plaque or media to the expanding neointima

may be a dominant factor contributing to in-stent restenosis in humans.[21]

TEMPORAL DIFFERENCES IN ARTERIAL HEALING IN HUMANS AND ANIMALS

One explanation for the delayed arterial healing responses in humans compared to animals is the presence of an underlying atherosclerotic process, which usually manifests itself in the fifth to sixth decade of life. Arterial interventions in animals are usually performed in young adults, and stents are typically placed in apposition to a normal smooth muscle-rich medial wall without resident inflammatory cells. The absence of an underlying atherosclerotic plaque likely contributes to a more predictable healing response in animals. In contrast, in diseased human coronary arteries, at least 70% of stent struts are in direct contact with the underlying atherosclerotic plaque.[8,19] The morphologic components of the lesion relative to the position of the stent likely affects the local response to healing. For example, stent struts in proximity to a necrotic core are exposed to a paucity of smooth muscle cells and thus heal slower than stents in direct contact with areas of adaptive intimal thickening, which contain an abundance of smooth muscle cells.[19] Similarly, stents overlying calcified, hypocellular, and densely fibrotic plaques also require a longer time to develop a neointima since these plaques must recruit smooth muscle cells from remote areas of the arterial wall to cover the struts.

The differential rate of healing between animals and humans may also be proportional to the longevity of the species. The typical lifespan of a human is >70 years; in contrast, pigs have a lifespan of 16 years, and rabbits 5–6 years. The biological differences in the rate of healing are age-dependent as shown in animal models of cutaneous wounds. This analogy may be appropriate to in-stent restenosis, since the developing neointima is similarly considered a response to traumatic injury. In swine, the extent of cutaneous re-epithelialization declines with age partly because of a decrease in the expression of growth factors.[22]

Furthermore, wound contraction 'remodeling' is accelerated in juvenile as compared with adult pigs. The type of injury is another consideration; wound healing is delayed in traumatic compared to surgically induced injury and in large versus small injury sites.[23,24] Human coronary stenting is often associated with extensive local trauma characterized by plaque splitting and medial disruption. Conversely, most stents in animals are deployed in normal arteries with 1:1.1 stent-to-artery ratio resulting in only mild arterial injury.[21,25]

DRUG ELUTING STENTS VS BALLOON EXPANDABLE STENTS: HEALING TIMES SIMILAR?

Most follow-up clinical studies of coronary artery stents in man utilize angiography or intravascular ultrasound (IVUS). Angiography only looks at the lumen and is unable to determine the quality of the neointimal growth, whereas IVUS can detect tissue growth as long as it is echogenic. From animal studies of stents harvested at 28 days, the neointimal tissue of DES has a greater concentration of fibrin and proteoglycan matrix and fewer smooth muscle cells compared with non-DES. IVUS cannot reliably detect both thrombus and proteoglycans; thus it is not surprising that IVUS studies at 6–12 months following DES placement suggest that either the stent struts are bare or have minimal neointimal growth.[18] Therefore, until better tools for the visualization of the early neointima are available, one is limited to atherectomy specimens or autopsy studies. Only a small number of atherectomy specimens have been examined histologically to date. A recent study of 15 patients treated for in-stent restenosis with QuaDS stents (Quanam Medical Corp) containing the paclitaxel derivative 7-hexanoyltaxol (QP2, a taxane analog) sheds some insight into stent healing in humans.[26] Although at 6 months there was minimal in-stent intimal hyperplasia (late loss = 0.47 ± 1.01 mm), at 12 months there was an aggressive increase in neointimal growth (late loss = 1.36 ± 0.94 mm) resulting in a dramatic 61.5% rate of restenosis.[27] Morphologic exam-ination of atherectomy tissue from a subset of these patients showed persistent fibrin admixed with smooth muscle cells, chronic inflammation, and extensive proteoglycan matrix (Figure 64.2); these findings demonstrate that incomplete neointimal healing was still present even 12 months post stenting.[26]

We have also had the opportunity to examine at autopsy a sirolimus eluting BX Velocity balloon expandable stent from a 71-year-old woman enrolled in the RAVEL trial. The patient received a single sirolimus eluting BX Velocity stent to treat an 80% proximal left anterior descending (LAD) coronary artery stenosis. IVUS and angiography at 6 months showed 0% stenosis with no in-stent neointimal thickening. The patient remained asymptomatic until presentation with unstable angina (16 months after the deployment of the LAD sirolimus eluting stent). Angiography demonstrated a subtotal occlusion of the left obtuse marginal artery. The LAD sirolimus eluting stent showed 0% stenosis. The left obtuse margin (LOM) was successfully stented, but the patient suffered a fatal stroke 24 hours after coronary intervention.[28] At autopsy LAD, the sirolimus eluting stent was widely patent, and there was a minute thrombus at the ostium of a small side branch. Light microscopy showed mild neointimal formation above the stent consisting of smooth muscle cells in a proteoglycan-rich matrix. Fibrin was occasionally identified near the stent strut, especially within the necrotic core and was minimal within the neointima. Inflammatory cells were rarely observed and consisted of giant cells. Scanning electron microscopy showed >80% endothelialization of the stent; there were small foci of poorly formed endothelial cell junctions and rare platelet aggregates close to the side branch ostium associated with pavement shaped endothelial cells.[28] Since *complete* endothelialization of balloon expandable stainless steel stents most likely occurs by 3–4 months in human atherosclerotic arteries, the results of this sirolimus eluting stent supports the hypothesis that endothelialization is delayed in man with DES; complete healing in uncomplicated atherosclerotic stented human arteries

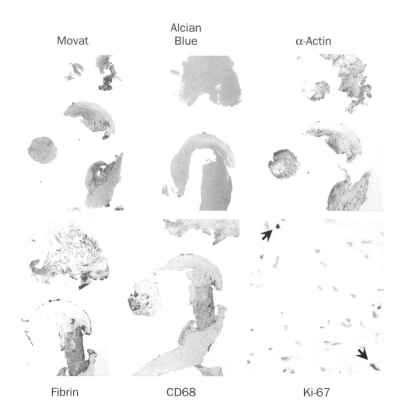

Movat | Alcian Blue | α-Actin

Fibrin | CD68 | Ki-67

Fig. 64.2 A 49-year-old man had a 13 mm long 2400 µg QuaDS-QP2 (7-hexanoyltaxol) coronary stent placed. Angiography at 6 months showed patent stent with only a mild increase in minimal lumen diameter. At 12 months, follow-up angiography demonstrated severe in-stent restenosis, and directional atherectomy was performed. The retrieved tissue consisted of a proteoglycan-rich (green areas in Movat stain and blue areas in alcian blue stain) restenosis lesion containing focal smooth muscle cell collections (α-actin stain). Delayed neointimal healing was present characterized by persistent fibrin deposition (fibrin stain), macrophage aggregates (CD68 stain), and ongoing cell proliferation (Ki-67 stain).

treated with DES may require at least 2 years. Patients who receive DES need to be followed for longer than 24 months in order to fully understand the biological behavior of these novel devices.

CRITICAL REVIEW OF CLINICAL STUDIES

Clinical studies with up to two years follow-up of DES in a limited number of patients show an extremely low rate of restenosis in selected lesions.[29,30] It should be recognized that the selection of the control stent (to which the DES is being compared) can have a major influence on the reported advantage of DES over bare metal stents. Arterial responses differ between stents of varying design.[31,32] Studies of DES sponsored by industry use their own non-DES (already on the market) as the control device. The restenosis rates in the control groups of DES studies have varied greatly (Figure 64.3). A control metal stent that does not produce the

smallest possible neointimal response and has a relatively high restenosis rate can project an exaggerated perceived advantage of the DES. Therefore, greater attention should be paid to the control stent groups to assure that restenosis rates in the non-DES arteries reflect expected real-world outcomes. By this approach, one can avoid overhyping the benefit of DES, which is of great importance secondary to the high cost of DESs. Finally, one should also look beyond angiographic variables and focus on significant clinical outcomes: patient symptoms, quality of life, future presentations with unstable angina or acute myocardial infarction, and overall mortality.

CONCLUSIONS

Careful follow-up beyond two years by improved imaging techniques to better visualize arterial wall are needed along with histologic studies to prove that drug eluting stents

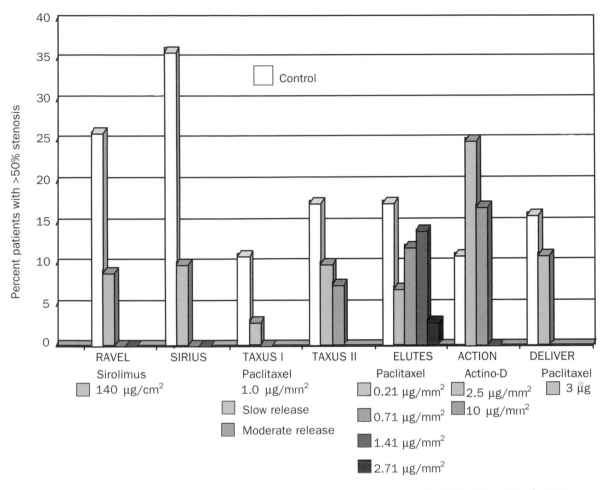

Fig. 64.3 Clinical trials of drug eluting stents. Note varying rates of restenosis among the control groups ranging from <15% in the TAXUS I and ACTION trials to >35% in the SIRIUS trial.

(DES) are the answer to in-stent restenosis. Stent malapposition and aneurysms must be closely followed for the development of hypersensitivity to stent polymers and/or drug. The issue of a possible increased frequency of subacute thrombosis in DES requires further study. We must make sure that stent polymers are safe and do not crack and flake from the stent during deployment. New drugs and polymers along with better understanding of the pharmacokinetics of DES in atherosclerotic arteries in animal models would be valuable to further improve this promising technology. Perhaps the most important aspect of DES is the platform on which the drug is delivered; new designs to improve stent performance must not be abandoned. Finally, while reaching for the magic stent, we must not forget that systemic therapy may also hold promise and may be more economical.

REFERENCES

1. Morice MC, Serruys PW, Sousa JE, et al. A randomized comparison of a sirolimus-eluting stent with a standard stent for coronary revascularization. N Engl J Med 2002; 346:1773–80.
2. Grube E, Silber S, Hauptmann KE, et al. TAXUS I: six- and twelve-month results from a randomized, double-blind trial on a slow-release paclitaxel-eluting stent for de novo coronary lesions. Circulation 2003; 107:38–42.

3. Colombo A, Orlic D, Stankovic G, et al. Preliminary observations regarding angiographic pattern of restenosis after rapamycin-eluting stent implantation. Circulation 2003; 107:2178–80.

4. Lemos PA, Saia F, Ligthart JM, et al. Coronary restenosis after sirolimus-eluting stent implantation: morphological description and mechanistic analysis from a consecutive series of cases. Circulation 2003; 108:257–60.

5. Lemos PA, Lee CH, Degertekin M, et al. Early outcome after sirolimus-eluting stent implantation in patients with acute coronary syndromes: insights from the Rapamycin-Eluting Stent Evaluated At Rotterdam Cardiology Hospital (RESEARCH) registry. J Am Coll Cardiol 2003; 41:2093–9.

6. Mintz GS, Popma JJ, Pichard AD, et al. Arterial remodeling after coronary angioplasty: a serial intravascular ultrasound study. Circulation 1996; 94:35–43.

7. Virmani R, Farb A. Pathology of in-stent restenosis. Curr Opin Lipidol 1999; 10:499–506.

8. Farb A, Weber DK, Kolodgie FD, et al. Morphological predictors of restenosis after coronary stenting in humans. Circulation 2002; 105:2974–80.

9. Farb A, Virmani R, Atkinson JB, et al. Long-term histologic patency after percutaneous transluminal coronary angioplasty is predicted by the creation of a greater lumen area. J Am Coll Cardiol 1994; 24:1229–35.

10. Kuntz RE, Gibson CM, Nobuyoshi M, et al. Generalized model of restenosis after conventional balloon angioplasty, stenting and directional atherectomy. J Am Coll Cardiol 1993; 21:15–25.

11. Carter AJ, Laird JR, Farb A, et al. Morphologic characteristics of lesion formation and time course of smooth muscle cell proliferation in a porcine proliferative restenosis model. J Am Coll Cardiol 1994; 24:1398–405.

12. Kollum M, Kaiser S, Kinscherf R, et al. Apoptosis after stent implantation compared with balloon angioplasty in rabbits. Role of macrophages. Arterioscler Thromb Vasc Biol 1997; 17:2383–8.

13. Farb A, John M, Acampado E, et al. Oral everolimus inhibits in-stent neointimal growth. Circulation 2002; 106:2379–84.

14. Farb A, Heller PF, Shroff S, et al. Pathological analysis of local delivery of paclitaxel via a polymer-coated stent. Circulation 2001; 104:473–9.

15. Kolodgie FD, John M, Kuhurana C, et al. Sustained reduction of in-stent neointimal growth with the use of novel systemic nanoparticle paclitaxel. Circulation 2002; 106:1195–8.

16. Serruys PW, Ormiston JA, Degertekin M, et al. Actinomycin eluting stent for coronary revascularization: A randomized feasibility and safety study (The ACTION Trial). J Am Coll Cardiol 2004; 44:1363–7.

17. FDA News. http://www.fda.gov/bbs/topics/NEWA/2003/NEWOO919.html

18. Serruys PW, Degertekin M, Tanabe K, et al. Intravascular ultrasound findings in the multicenter, randomized, double-blind RAVEL (RAndomized study with the sirolimus-eluting VElocity balloon-expandable stent in the treatment of patients with de novo native coronary artery Lesions) trial. Circulation 2002; 106:798–803.

19. Farb A, Sangiorgi G, Carter AJ, et al. Pathology of acute and chronic coronary stenting in humans. Circulation 1999; 99:44–52.

20. O'Brien ER, Alpers CE, Stewart DK, et al. Proliferation in primary and restenotic coronary atherectomy tissue. Implications for antiproliferative therapy. Circ Res 1993; 73:223–31.

21. Virmani R, Kolodgie FD, Farb A, et al. Drug eluting stents: are human and animal studies comparable? Heart 2003; 89:133–8.

22. Yao F, Visovatti S, Johnson CS, et al. Age and growth factors in porcine full-thickness wound healing. Wound Repair Regen 2001; 9:371–7.

23. Forrester JS, Fishbein M, Helfant R, et al. A paradigm for restenosis based on cell biology: clues for the development of new preventive therapies. J Am Coll Cardiol 1991; 17:758–69.

24. Schwartz RS, Huber KC, Murphy JG, et al. Restenosis and the proportional neointimal response to coronary artery injury: results in a porcine model. J Am Coll Cardiol 1992; 19:267–74.

25. Taylor AJ, Gorman PD, Kenwood B, et al. A comparison of four stent designs on arterial injury, cellular proliferation, neointima formation, and arterial dimensions in an experimental porcine model. Catheter Cardiovasc Interv 2001; 53:420–5.

26. Virmani R, Liistro F, Stankovic G, et al. Mechanism of late in-stent restenosis after implantation of a paclitaxel derivate-eluting polymer stent system in humans. Circulation 2002; 106:2649–51.

27. Liistro F, Stankovic G, Di Mario C, et al. First clinical experience with paclitaxel derivative-eluting polymer stent system implantation for in-stent restenosis. Immediate and long-term clinical and angiographic outcome. Circulation 2002; 105:1883–6.

28. Guagliumi G, Farb A, Musumeci G, et al. Images in cardiovascular medicine. Sirolimus-eluting stent implanted in human coronary artery for 16 months: pathological findings. Circulation 2003; 107:1340–1.

29. Sousa JE, Costa MA, Sousa AG, et al. Two-year angiographic and intravascular ultrasound follow-up after implantation of sirolimus-eluting stents in human coronary arteries. Circulation 2003; 107:381–3.

30. Degertekin M, Serruys PW, Foley DP, et al. Persistent inhibition of neointimal hyperplasia after sirolimus-eluting stent implantation: long-term (up to 2 years) clinical, angiographic, and intravascular ultrasound follow-up. Circulation 2002; 106:1610–13.

31. Rogers C, Edelman ER. Endovascular stent design dictates experimental restenosis and thrombosis. Circulation 1995; 91:2995–3001.

32. Rogers C, Tseng DY, Squire JC, et al. Balloon-artery interactions during stent placement: a finite element analysis approach to pressure, compliance, and stent design as contributors to vascular injury. Circ Res 1999; 84:378–83.

Index